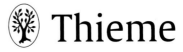

MR Imaging
of the Spine and Spinal Cord

Detlev Uhlenbrock, M.D.
Professor
Department of Radiology
St.-Josefs-Hospital
Dortmund, Germany

With contributions by
D. Brechtelsbauer, J. F. Debatin, A. J. Felber, S. Felber, H. Henkes, P. Hilfiker, P. Kreisler, D. Kühne, V. Kunze, S. E. Mirvis, R. Schultheiß, K.-H. Trümmler, D. Uhlenbrock, W. Weber

Translated by Grahame Larkin, M.D.

1305 illustrations

Thieme
Stuttgart · New York

Library of Congress Cataloging-in-Publication Data is available from the publisher.

This book is an authorized translation of the German edition published and copyrighted 2001 by Georg Thieme Verlag, Stuttgart, Germany. Title of the German edition: MRT der Wirbelsäule und des Spinalkanals

Translator: Grahame Larkin, M.D., Bonn, Germany

Important Note: Medicine is an ever-changing science undergoing continual development. Research and clinical experience are continually expanding our knowledge, in particular our knowledge of proper treatment and drug therapy. Insofar as this book mentions any dosage or application, readers may rest assured that the authors, editors, and publishers have made every effort to ensure that such references are in accordance with **the state of knowledge at the time of production of the book.**

Nevertheless, this does not involve, imply, or express any guarantee or responsibility on the part of the publishers in respect to any dosage instructions and forms of applications stated in the book. **Every user is requested to examine carefully** the manufacturers' leaflets accompanying each drug and to check, if necessary in consultation with a physician or specialist, whether the dosage schedules mentioned therein or the contraindications stated by the manufacturers differ from the statements made in the present book. Such examination is particularly important with drugs that are either rarely used or have been newly released on the market. Every dosage schedule or every form of application used is entirely at the user's own risk and responsibility. The authors and publishers request every user to report to the publishers any discrepancies or inaccuracies noticed.

© 2004 Georg Thieme Verlag, Rüdigerstrasse 14, D-70469 Stuttgart, Germany
http://www.thieme.de
Thieme New York, 333 Seventh Avenue, New York, NY 10001, USA
http://www.thieme.com

Typesetting by primustype R. Hurler GmbH, D-73274 Notzingen,
Typeset on Textline/HerculesPro
Printed in Germany by Druckhaus Götz, Ludwigsburg

ISBN 3-13-130941-5 (GTV)
ISBN 1-58890-264-1 (TNY)   1 2 3 4 5

Preface

In terms of hardware and software development, magnetic resonance imaging is still subject to rapid change. For this reason the procedure is undergoing considerable improvement and refinement. The radiologist must accept this development process and ensure that improvements are quickly incorporated into routine. These include the use of new sequences, verification of examination records, and a refinement of diagnostic interpretation, which is frequently necessary as a result. Owing to an increase in resolution and the use of sequences with enhanced contrast-to-noise ratio, such as the STIR sequence, diagnostic significance is now considerably higher than it was 6 to 7 years ago. Anyone who in the light of such aspects is unable or unwilling to learn will soon lose touch.

The necessity of continuous learning remains, and books are an important aid in this process. Furthermore, constant updating is absolutely essential, which was the reason behind publishing this book. It demonstrates impressively how quickly examination technology and the diagnostic significance of the procedure have changed for the vertebral column and spinal canal over the last few years.

A number of authors have cooperated in writing this book. The aim was to engage particularly well-qualified colleagues for the various sections of the chapters. The editor hopes that this has proven successful.

One or two readers may be surprised to see that a book about the vertebral column and spinal canal region has reached such a length. Admittedly, I did not expect it either. However, if one takes a look at the various sections within the chapters, one will realize that nothing is of undue length.

Apart from those contributors whose are named on the front of the book, there are others who have also made a contribution, in some cases a very important one that was necessary to ensure the success of the book. In this connection I would like to particularly express my gratitude to those who have contributed to rounding off the chapters by providing illustrations. I am particularly indebted to Dr. Carlos Hartung in Rheine who had set aside some interesting illustrative examples for me beforehand, because he knew that I would approach him. I would also like to take the opportunity of expressing my sincere gratitude to Dr. Heinen from the St. Johannes-Hospital in Arnsberg.

Last but not least I would like to say a sincere thank-you to the members of staff at Thieme publisher's. I hope that the book will be well received and that colleagues entrusted with interpreting magnetic resonance images will enjoy using it.

Dortmund, autumn 2003   Detlev Uhlenbrock

Contributors' Addresses

Dirk Brechtelsbauer, M.D.
Department of Neuroradiology
University of Würzburg
Würzburg, Germany

Jörg F. Debatin, M.D.
Professor
Central Institute of
Radiodiagnostics
University Medical Center GHS
Essen
Essen, Germany

Alexandra J. Felber, M.D.
MRI and MR Spectroscopy
University Medical Center
Innsbruck
Innsbruck, Austria

Stephan Felber, M.D.
Professor
Department of Radiology II
University Medical Center for
Radiodiagnostics
Innsbruck, Austria

Hans Henkes, M.D.
Associate Professor
Alfried-Krupp Hospital
Clinic for Radiology and
Neuroradiology
Essen, Germany

Paul René Hilfiker, M.D.
University Hospital Zürich
Institute for
Diagnostic Radiology
Zürich, Switzerland

Peter Kreisler
Medical Technology
MRI application development
Siemens AG
Erlangen, Germany

Dietmar Kühne, M.D.
Professor
Alfried-Krupp Hospital
Clinic for Radiology and
Neuroradiology
Essen, Germany

Volker Kunze, M.D.
Oldenburg Municipal Clinics
Institute for Radiology and
Nuclear Medicine
Oldenburg, Germany

Stuart E. Mirvis, M.D.
Professor
University of Maryland
Department of Radiology
Medical Center
Baltimore, Maryland
USA

Rolf Schultheiß, M.D.
Associate Professor
Dortmund Municipal Clinics
(Clinic Center North)
Neurosurgical Clinic
Dortmund, Germany

Karl-Heinz Trümmler
Medical Technology
Siemens AG
Cologne, Germany

Detlev Uhlenbrock, M.D.
Professor
Department of Radiology
St.-Josefs-Hospital
Dortmund, Germany

Werner Weber, M.D.
Alfried-Krupp Hospital
Clinic for Radiology and
Neuroradiology
Essen, Germany

Contents

1 Physics and its Application

K.-H. Trümmler, P. Kreisler

2 MRI and Spinal Surgery—Indications Based on the Spectrum of Surgical Therapeutic Options

R. Schultheiß

3 Malformations of the Spinal Canal

D. Uhlenbrock, D. Brechtelsbauer

4 Degenerative Disorders of the Spine

159

D. Uhlenbrock

5 Tumors of the Spine and Spinal Canal

269

D. Uhlenbrock, V. Kunze

6 Inflammatory Disorders of the Spine and Spinal Canal

357

D. Uhlenbrock, H. Henkes, W. Weber, S. Felber, D. Kühne

7 Use of MRI in Acute Spinal Trauma

437

S. E. Mirvis

8 Vascular Disorders of the Spinal Canal

467

A.J. Felber, S. Felber, H. Henkes, D. Kühne

9 Functional Analysis and Surgery of the Spine in an Open MR System

491

P. Hilfiker, J.F. Debatin

Index

511

1   Physics and its Application

K.-H. Trümmler and P. Kreisler

Contents

Basic Principles

Protons in a Magnetic Field

The human body is composed of more than 60 % water. Water is, therefore, the most common molecule in our body. Furthermore, hydrogen, as part of the water molecule, has a very high detection rate for measuring *nuclear magnetic resonance*. For these reasons hydrogen is the ideal element for imaging. The atomic nucleus of hydrogen has only one nuclear particle, the proton. The proton spins on its own axis with its positive elementary charge. This intrinsic rotation of the proton is called *nuclear spin.*

The rotation of the electric charge generates a characteristic magnetic field around the proton. This is the *magnetic moment*, μ, of the proton. μ causes the orientation of the protons to be in-

Protons with no magnetic field present

Protons in a magnetic field

External magnetic field B_0 in Z direction

$M_Z =$ ⬤ + ⬤

| Protons aligned antiparallel | Protons aligned parallel |

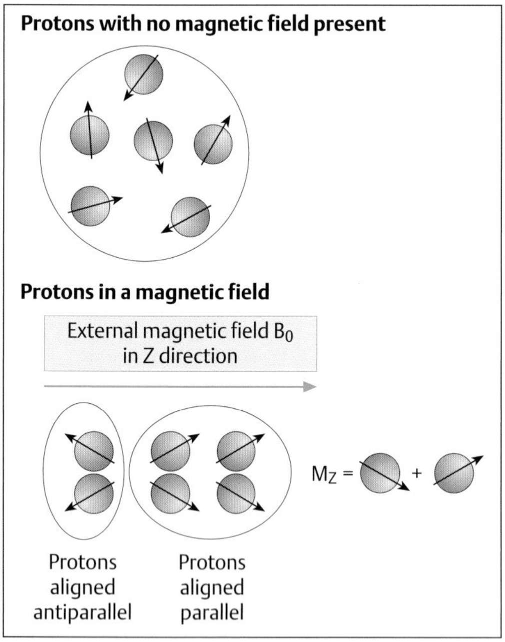

Fig. 1.1 Protons in a magnetic field
Top: In the absence of a magnetic field the magnetic moments of the protons are aligned statistically and their effects neutralize each other.
Bottom: Within the magnetic field B_0 the majority of the protons are aligned parallel to the applied field while the minority are aligned antiparallel. The resulting longitudinal magnetization (M_Z) of the tissue is the prerequisite for producing MR images.

fluenced by an external *magnetic field B_0*. In field B_0, the majority of the protons align themselves parallel to the direction of the field. A minority of protons align themselves in the opposite direction (antiparallel). This is the ground, or equilibrium, state. Since more protons align themselves parallel rather than antiparallel, their magnetic moments μ are summed up to produce a *net magnetization M*. In the equilibrium state, M is always parallel to B_0 in Z direction, which is why it is called the *longitudinal magnetization M_Z.*

Apart from setting up the longitudinal magnetization M_Z, B_0 also forces the protons into a precession movement around the Z-axis of the field, similar to a rotating spinning top precessing around the gravitational field of the earth. This rotation, or precession, frequency of the protons is also called the *Larmor frequency ω_0* and is proportional to the strength of the magnetic field (Fig. 1.1).

$$\omega_0 = \gamma \times B_0$$
γ = gyromagnetic ratio = 42 MHz per tesla for protons

Excitation

MR systems have special receiver coils for picking up the signal sent back by the protons from the human body. These signals represent the raw data for reconstructing the MR image. The receiver coils of MR systems are oriented transversely to B_0 in the XY plane, which explains why the longitudinal magnetization M_Z does not induce a signal.

In order to measure a signal, M_Z must be rotated into the transverse direction (XY plane). A magnetization that points in the transverse direction is referred to as the *transverse magnetization* or M_{XY}. The rotation of M into the transverse plane (M becomes M_{XY}) is called excitation. This is brought about by a radio-frequency pulse (RF pulse) that is sent by the transmitter coil at the appropriate frequency ω_0 (= Larmor frequency).

After excitation the protons are in the excited state. The magnetization has been flipped by 90° out of the Z direction into the XY plane (90° excitation) and rotates at the Larmor frequency ω_0. The longitudinal magnetization M_Z no longer exists ($M_Z = 0$); it has become the transverse magnetization M_{XY}. M_{XY} now induces a voltage, the MR signal, whose strength is proportional to the magnitude of M_{XY}.

Directly after excitation, the process of *relaxation* begins in which the protons leave the excited state and return to their state of equilibrium.

Relaxation

There are two relaxation mechanisms that describe the transition from excitation back to the equilibrium state:

▪ Longitudinal Relaxation Time T1

During longitudinal relaxation, longitudinal magnetization M_Z recovers. Once longitudinal relaxation ends, the total magnetization is once again parallel to the applied field, the protons are in the state of equilibrium and the longitudinal magnetization M_Z has regained its initial value prior to excitation ($M_Z = 100\%$).

T1 time describes the rate at which the protons return from the excited state to the state of equilibrium.

The T1 relaxation times of tissues differ from each other:

- in tissues with a long T1 time relaxation occurs slowly,
- in tissues with a short T1 time relaxation occurs rapidly.

The associated relaxation process is called longitudinal relaxation, or T1, because the protons "relax" from the excited state back into the longitudinal direction of the magnetic field. Another term for T1 relaxation is *spin-lattice relaxation* because the energy absorbed by the protons (spins) during excitation is released to the surrounding tissue (lattice) during relaxation (Fig. 1.2).

▪ Transverse Relaxation Time T2

The signal that the transverse magnetization M_{XY} induces after excitation is referred to as FID (free induction decay). The FID signal is high immediately after excitation and then becomes rapidly smaller as time progresses.

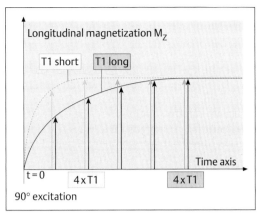

Fig. 1.**2** **Relaxation.** Immediately after excitation $M_Z = 0$ because the 90° excitation pulse has rotated the total longitudinal magnetization from the Z direction into the XY plane. After excitation M_Z recovers with increasing time. Tissues with a short T1 time relax more rapidly than tissues with a long T1 time. The increase in M_Z follows an exponential function. After approximately four times the T1 time of the tissue, T1 relaxation has finished, and M_Z has reached its initial state before excitation (100 % M_Z). During T1 relaxation the energy that the protons have absorbed during excitation is released back to the tissue as heat.

How Does this Signal Decay Occur?

Immediately after excitation all the protons precess in phase and their magnetic moments add up to form a large M_{XY} and thus a large summation signal. Afterwards the protons are disturbed in their precession by their neighbors (i.e., other protons and molecules). Thus dephasing occurs, M_{XY} becomes smaller, and the summation signal declines.

How are the Protons Disturbed?

Each proton as well as each molecule has magnetic properties that locally alter the main external magnetic field B_0 of the magnet in their immediate vicinity. These tissue-specific effects are variable both in their size and over time. They depend:

- on the chemical binding state,
- on the electrical and magnetic properties of the tissue.

If only a single proton is observed, the effects that its neighbors exert are so complex that it is impossible to quantify them. With a whole host of protons as in the human body, however, the effects on one proton obey statistical laws and the net behavior of the protons becomes predictable, appearing in a temporal relationship to the transverse magnetization M_{XY}.

Because the precession frequency of the protons is related to the strength of the local magnetic field, the field variations produced by the adjacent atoms influence the precession frequency in an unpredictable way. The protons precess somewhat faster or more slowly, depending on whether the main external field chances to be intensified or weakened by the tissue-specific effects. This results in divergence, the protons dephase, M_{XY} and the signal become smaller (Fig. 1.**3**).

The dephasing of the protons after excitation is a relaxation process. The rate at which the protons dephase is characterized by the time T2.

The T2 relaxation times of tissues differ from each other:

- in tissues with a long T2 time, relaxation occurs slowly,

- in tissues with a short T2 time, relaxation occurs rapidly.

T2 time and signal decay are directly proportional:

- A long T2 time means that the protons affect each other only slightly, resulting in slow dephasing and hence slow decay of the signal.
- A short T2 time means that the protons affect each other strongly, resulting in rapid dephasing and thus rapid decay of the signal.

The Effects of Inhomogeneities

All the observations made so far with respect to transverse relaxation and the T2 time of the tissues are only valid when the magnet induces an ideal homogeneous magnetic field B_0, so that only tissue-specific effects can produce T2 relaxation and external disturbances are irrelevant.

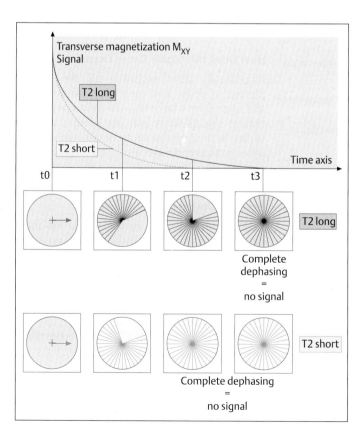

Fig. 1.**3** **Dephasing.** Tissue-specific effects on the precession frequency of the individual protons cause dephasing. Dephasing can be visualized as a fanning out of the proton population. This fanning out causes the protons to "look" in different directions and their magnetic moments no longer sum up. This results in a reduction of M_{XY} and signal loss. Tissues with a short T2 time lose their signal more rapidly because their relaxation is faster than in tissues with a long T2 time.

What is a Homogeneous Magnetic Field?

An ideal homogeneous magnetic field is achieved when there are no fluctuations from the ideal field strength within the measurement range. Modern magnets do indeed reach a very high degree of homogeneity, but full 100 % homogeneity is not achieved. Apart from that, the patient's presence disturbs the homogeneity.

What Effects do Inhomogeneities Have?

Because inhomogeneities are no more than fluctuations of the magnetic field, they result in different precession frequencies of the protons. This difference in precession frequencies causes an additional dephasing of the protons, which is superimposed over the tissue-dependent dephasing (T2 relaxation).

This is why in a real magnetic field with inhomogeneities the FID (free induction decay) decreases more rapidly than in an imaginary, completely homogeneous field.

The time constant T2, which is calculated in the real magnetic field with the aid of the FID, is therefore referred to as *time constant T2**. The * indicates that this is a time constant that does not reflect the true tissue parameter T2, but rather that a second dephasing process is superimposed, which is dependent upon the quality of the field. The inhomogeneities cause the protons to dephase more rapidly. Therefore T2* is usually significantly shorter than T2.

How Can the Effects of Inhomogeneities Be Avoided?

Because the inhomogeneities of the external field are temporally constant, it is possible to compensate for their effect. With the aid of a second RF pulse (after the 90° excitation pulse), the 180° rephasing pulse, a signal is generated whose amplitude is not influenced by the inhomogeneities. This signal is called a *spin echo (SE)*. Acquisition sequences using a 90–180° pulse sequence to generate an image whose signals are independent of inhomogeneities are referred to as SE sequences. Sequences without the 180° rephasing pulse are called gradient echo (GRE) sequences, the analogous signal being the gradient echo (GRE).

The 180° rephasing pulse compensates exclusively for the temporally constant inhomogeneities of the external magnetic field. However, the tissue-specific dephasing processes that result in T2 relaxation are not influenced. The intensity of the echo signal after a 180° rephasing pulse is therefore entirely dependent upon the tissue-specific T2 effects.

Various Image Contrasts

T1 contrast (T1-weighted image). Here image contrasts result primarily from the T1 differences of the tissues. The effects of T2 and proton density (PD influences) are minimized (yet still exist).

T2 contrast (T2-weighted image). In a T2-weighted image, contrasts result primarily from the T2 differences of the tissues. The effects of T1 and PD influences are minimized (yet still exist).

PD contrast (PD-weighted image). In a PD-weighted image, contrasts result primarily from the PD differences of the tissues. The effects of T1 and T2 are minimized (yet still exist).

T1-Weighted Image

■ Repetition Time TR

The acquisition of only one echo is not enough for the entire raw-data set of one MR image because it contains too little spatial information to reconstruct the image. An echo signal forms only one line in the raw-data set.

The size of the raw-data set depends on the acquisition matrix of the MR image. For a matrix size of 256 × 256 pixels, 256 raw-data lines must be read in.

For the acquisition of each raw-data line, the slice usually has to be excited again. The time between two excitations is the repetition time TR.

One slice package containing several slices (multislice scan) can be acquired during the time TR, with the number of slices depending on the time TR.

■ TR Time and T1 Contrast

The T1 contrast of an MR image is regulated with the aid of the TR time.

What Happens When TR Time is Long (TR >2500 ms)?

TR time can be selected so long that the net magnetization returns to its original position parallel to the magnetic field between the excitations. This is the case when TR time is set at four times as long as the T1 time of the tissue. In this case the protons have enough time for more or less complete T1 relaxation, and the state of equilibrium (= 100 % M_Z) is always reached before the next excitation.

Because TR time is so long that T1 relaxation between two excitations is fully concluded in all tissues, there are no T1 contrasts visible on the image. (The image shows PD contrast; see p. 10.)

What Happens When TR Time is Short (TR = 400–800 ms)?

For a more understandable presentation, four time points will be considered (Fig. 1.**4**):

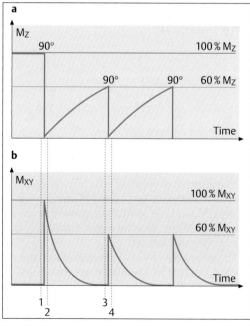

a

M_Z

90°   100 % M_Z

          90°   90°   60 % M_Z

                                       Time

b

M_{XY}

                                 100 % M_{XY}

                                 60 % M_{XY}

                                       Time

1   3
   2   4

Fig. 1.**4 a,b Course of M_Z and its effect on the signal.** The upper part of the illustration shows the Z magnetization and the course of T1 relaxation. The lower part of the illustration shows the transverse magnetization M_{XY} and the signal and course of T2 relaxation. The time points 1–4 are explained in the text.

Time 1. Immediately before the first 90° excitation there is a state of equilibrium.

M_{Z1} = 100 %
M_{XY1}= 0

Time 2. Immediately after the first 90° excitation: the excitation causes the magnetization to flip out of the Z direction into the XY plane.

M_{Z2} = 0
M_{XY2}= 100 %

With increasing time M_Z is set up again as a result of T1 relaxation.

Time 3. Immediately before the next 90° excitation: TR time is so short that M_Z cannot be set up 100 %. At this point of time M_{Z3} is generated only by those protons that have relaxed during the (short) TR interval.

M_{Z3} <100 % (in this example 60 %)
M_{XY3} = 0 (due to the rapid T2 relaxation)

Time 4. Immediately after the next 90° excitation: The 90° excitation pulse flips only the Z magnetization into the XY plane, which was set up in Z direction as M_Z during the previous TR interval.

M_{XY4} = M_{Z3} (= 60 % in this example).

The result is a reduced signal on the MR image.

Saturation. Incomplete T1 relaxation during a short TR interval results in signal reduction on the MR image. This process is referred to as saturation. During a short TR interval the brightness of the tissues is determined largely by their T1 time:

● tissues with a long T1 time appear dark because they are more highly saturated,
● tissues with a short T1 time appear brighter because they are less saturated.

What Happens When TR Time is Very Short (TR = < 300 ms)?

If the TR interval is continually shortened, the saturation of all the tissues increases. Consequently they become hypointense and appear with little contrast.

Which TR Time for a T1-Weighted Image?

A TR time of 400–800 ms has proven itself for the acquisition of T1-weighted images (Fig. 1.**5**).

■ Contrasts of a T1-Weighted Image

The brightness of the tissues depends on their T1 time and thus on their saturation:

- water with the longest T1 time appears very dark,

- brain gray matter has a longer T1 time than white brain substance and is darker than the latter,
- fat has the shortest T1 time and is very bright.

T2-Weighted Image

The T2 contrast of an MR image is regulated with the aid of the echo time TE.

■ Echo Time TE

TE is the time between the excitation pulse and the recording of the echo signal.

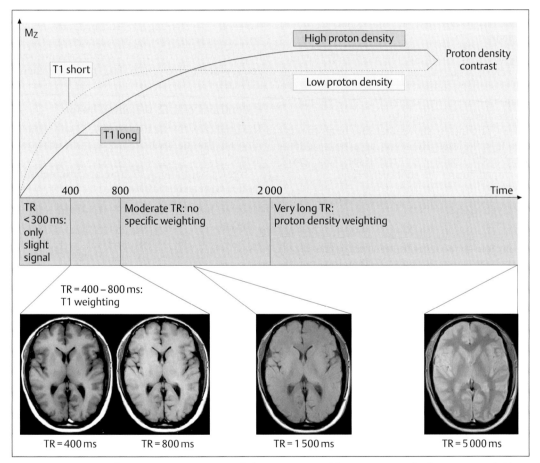

Fig. 1.**5 TR time and T1 contrast.** Because of the different T1 times of the tissues, T1 contrasts can be generated on MR images when the T1 relaxation of the tissues has elapsed to varying degrees within the TR time. With a TR time of 400–800 ms the T1 relaxation in tissues with a short T1 time has elapsed further than in tissues with a long T1 time, and the 90° excitation pulse flips (in tissues with a short T1 time) a larger mag-netization (than in tissues with a longer T1 time). Therefore the signal of tissues with a short T1 time is larger than the signal of tissues with a long T1 time. The images demonstrate a strong T1 contrast. If the TR time is prolonged, contrast becomes less because the longitudinal magnetization M_Z of all the tissues returns to 100 %. With a very long TR time the contrast is PD contrast.

If the signal is recorded at the echo time point then dephasing in the tissues, and thus also the signal, varies in strength (depending on the T2 time).

The signal differences measured are a reflection of the T2 effect:

- If the echo time TE is short, then the protons have little time to dephase and the T2 effect on the image is small.
- With a long TE echo time the protons have enough time to dephase and the T2 effect on the image is large.

■ **TE Time and T2 Contrast**

What Happens When TE Time is Short (TE < 30 ms)?

Dephasing has advanced only slightly by the time the echo is acquired; the protons of all tissues are still precessing almost in phase. Because of the small amount of dephasing, M_{XY} is large and all tissues appear hyperintense.

Low T2 contrast shows that M_{XY} of all the tissues is still almost the same because no differences in the dephasing of the tissues have as yet developed during the short echo time.

What Happens When TE Time is Longer (TE = 70–150 ms)?

The tissue-specific effects are allowed to act on the protons for a longer time so that dephasing of all the tissues has advanced further. In comparison with an image with a short echo time TE, the signal from all the tissues has become smaller due to the increased amount of dephasing. In tissues with a short T2 time, however, dephasing has progressed further than in tissues with a long T2 time.

The tissues on the image appear with varying intensity:

- tissues with a short T2 time appear dark because dephasing has progressed further,
- tissues with a long T2 time appear bright because dephasing has progressed less.

Contrasts are a qualitative reflection of the T2 times of the tissues. Such an image is referred to as T2-weighted.

What Happens When TE Time is Very Long (TE >200 ms)?

Dephasing has progressed even further; all the tissues have lost even more signal.

Tissues with short T2 times are no longer displayed. Because the protons are completely dephased, $M_{XY} = 0$ and can no longer induce any signal.

Tissues with moderate T2 times are hypointense due to the relatively large amount of dephasing of the protons.

Only tissues with very long T2 times, e.g., fluids, still appear bright due to the small amount of dephasing.

A very strong T2 contrast is visible on the image. The echo time however is too long to display tissues with short and moderate T2 times.

Which TE Time for a T2-Weighted Image?

For good T2-weighting a TE time of approximately 70–150 ms is appropriate in the majority of scans because with this TE time T2 contrasts are very good without too much loss of image signal (Fig. 1.**6**).

■ **Contrasts of a T2-Weighted Image**

The brightness of the tissues depends on their T2 time and thus on their dephasing at the echo time point.

Tissues with a long T2 time are brighter than tissues with a short T2 time:

- water has the longest T2 time and appears bright,
- brain gray matter has a longer T2 time than white brain substance and is slightly brighter than the latter.

Further Preconditions for a T1- and T2-Weighted Image

Which Echo Time TE for a T1-Weighted Image?

On a T1-weighted image T2 effects should be minimal.

Conclusion: The shorter the TE time, the less time the protons have to dephase. A short TE time therefore means few T2 effects on the image (Fig. 1.**7**).

Which Repetition Time TR for a T2-Weighted Image?

On a T2-weighted image T1 effects (saturation effects) should be minimal.

Conclusion: The T1 effect is minimal when T1 relaxation has completely finished. A long TR

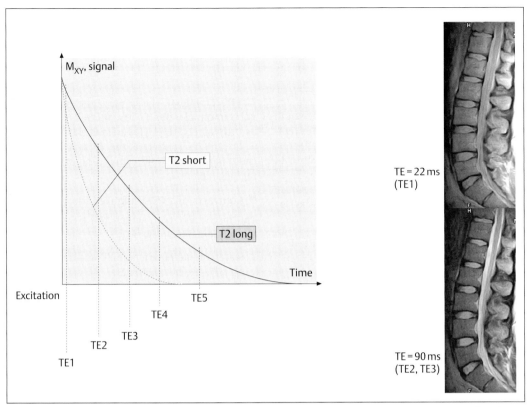

TE = 22 ms
(TE1)

TE = 90 ms
(TE2, TE3)

Fig. 1.6 TE time and T2 contrast. Depending on the echo time TE, various T2 weightings can be generated on the MR images. With a short TE time (TE < 22 ms) dephasing of all the tissues, and thus also the T2 contrast on the image, is slight. With a longer TE time (TE = 90 ms) dephasing in tissues with a short T2 time increases to a larger degree and the signal is less than in tissues with a long T2 time. The contrasts of the image represent qualitatively the T2 differences of the tissues. With an even longer TE time (TE > 200 ms) dephasing increases so much that the image quality is affected as a result of the low signal.

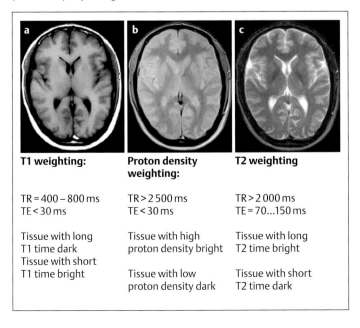

Fig. 1.7 Summary of the acquisition parameters TR and TE and the contrasts for T1, PD, and T2 image weighting.

T1 weighting:	Proton density weighting:	T2 weighting
TR = 400 – 800 ms	TR > 2 500 ms	TR > 2 000 ms
TE < 30 ms	TE < 30 ms	TE = 70...150 ms
Tissue with long T1 time dark	Tissue with high proton density bright	Tissue with long T2 time bright
Tissue with short T1 time bright	Tissue with low proton density dark	Tissue with short T2 time dark

time (usually 4 times the T1 of the tissue) is the precondition for little T1 effect on the image (Fig. 1.**7**).

Proton Density (PD)

The PD indicates how many protons are present in a certain amount of tissue. The tissues differ relatively little in their PD values, so that the effect of PD on image contrast is less than the effect of T1 or T2.

A high PD results in a stronger signal because more protons are present to contribute to the signal. Tissues with low PD are more hypointense.

■ Parameters TR and TE for a PD-Weighted Image

PD weighting is achieved when the contrast effects from both relaxation processes T1 and T2 are minimal:

T1 effect minimal. There is no T1 effect on the image when T1 relaxation has elapsed completely. This is the case with a long TR time (usually four times the T1 time of the tissue) (Fig. 1.**5**).

T2 effect minimal. The T2 effect on the image signal is minimal when T2 relaxation has progressed as little as possible. This means that only when echo time TE is short is the T2 effect small because there is still only a small amount of dephasing (Fig. 1.**6**).

■ Contrasts of a PD-Weighted Image

The brightness with which the tissues are displayed depends on the PD:

● water and fat have a high PD and appear bright on a PD-weighted image,
● PD is low in bone tissue (compact bone) and in calcifications: they appear dark.

Fundamental Scanning Sequences

Preliminary Comments on Two- and Three-dimensional Acquisition Methods

In MR imaging two different acquisition techniques are used:

● two-dimensional technique,
● three-dimensional technique.

Because with the *two-dimensional* technique each imaging slice of the slice package is excited separately and successively within the TR interval, the echo signal is a summation signal of all the protons in the excited layer.

In contrast to this, with the three-dimensional technique all the layers (partitions) of the imaging volume (slab) are excited together, and the echo signal is the sum of the signals from all slice acquisitions. This is the great advantage of the three-dimensional technique because the intensity of the echo signal is no longer dependent on the thickness of each slice in the three-dimensional volume but rather on the thickness of the entire three-dimensional volume.

With the two-dimensional technique the signal intensity from one slice is directly proportional to the slice thickness; the thinner the slice,

the smaller the signal, because the number of protons in the slice decreases with decreasing slice thickness. The result is that, with thin slices, the ratio between useful signal and background noise (the signal-to-noise ratio) is poor and the quality of the image suffers. A remedy is found by increasing the data acquisitions, although this consequently prolongs scanning time.

With very thin slices, therefore, use of the three-dimensional technique is preferred.

Especially when images with a different alignment are to be reconstructed secondarily from the primary slice images, or when MR angiographic reconstructions are to be performed, the three-dimensional technique is indispensable because of its very thin slices.

In principle, all sequences can be combined with the two-dimensional and the three-dimensional technique.

The acquisition time TA for a two- and three-dimensional scan is calculated as follows:

two-dimensional scanning: $TA = m \times TR \times AC$
three-dimensional scanning: $TA = m \times TR \times AC \times PA$
m = number of raw-data lines
TR = TR time
AC = number of data acquisitions [1]
PA = number of partitions (slices in the three-dimensional sample volume)

[1] In some MR scanning processes the raw data are measured several times and subsequently averaged to improve image quality. The number of scans corresponds to the data acquisitions AC. With several acquisitions the scanning time is prolonged accordingly.

Gradient Echo Sequence

Modern MR devices use a large number of GRE sequences. Many of these sequences are optimized for certain applications, e.g., for MR angiography.

For this reason only the most universal GR sequence, the FLASH sequence, will be addressed here. Other expressions are also used for the term FLASH sequence (FLASH = fast low angle shot): spoiled GRASS (GRASS = gradient recalled acquisition in steady state) or fast-field echo.

Advantages of the FLASH sequence
- short scanning time,
- few motion artifacts due to short scanning time,
- wider range of diagnostic possibilities, e.g., sensitivity to susceptibility effects,
- three-dimensional scanning with the highest resolution in a short scanning time.

Disadvantages of the FLASH sequence
- no T2, but T2* contrast with long TE time, depending on the quality of the magnetic field,
- susceptibility artifacts.

■ Basic Remarks on FLASH Sequence

GRE sequences have no 180° RF rephasing pulse. Instead, fast gradient fields generate the rephasing of the signal. The lack of an RF rephasing pulse causes a high sensitivity to field inhomogeneities, which have a strong effect on the GRE, especially with a long TE echo time. The contrast of these images is therefore not T2 contrast but T2* contrast. Apart from the inhomogeneities of the magnetic field, the patient's own field distortions play a large role.

These field distortions occur at interfaces between substances with very different magnetizability, e.g., between air and tissue, and lead to spatially limited inhomogeneities that result in signal cancellations. These effects are referred to as *susceptibility artifacts*. They increase with longer echo time so that they are most pronounced in T2*-weighted FLASH sequences. (A more precise explanation of susceptibility artifacts is provided on p. 24.)

These effects are usually undesirable because they destroy image information. On the other hand, e.g., in the diagnosis of cerebral hemorrhage, they provide valuable details about the extent and age of the hemorrhage.

■ Reduction of Scanning Time with the FLASH Sequence

An obvious way to reduce scanning time is to shorten the repetition time TR. However, this results in an increase in saturation and alters image contrasts.

A way must therefore be found to reduce TR time without at the same time intensifying saturation effects.

To optimize signal and contrast in GRE sequences an excitation pulse that is smaller than 90° can also be used. The angle at which the magnetization is rotated from the Z direction into the XY plane is called the flip angle α.

The subsequent T1 relaxation is faster after an α pulse because the magnetization does not have to relax the whole 90°-angle from the XY plane back into the Z direction but only the lower α angle.

In practice this means we can compensate for the increasing saturation effects of a shorter TR time by using a lower flip angle (Fig. 1.**8**).

■ FLASH Sequence and T2* Weighting

Especially with T2 weighting, the T1 effect and saturation should be as small as possible. With the aid of low-angle shot imaging we have a means of reducing TR time yet still keep the T1 effects low.

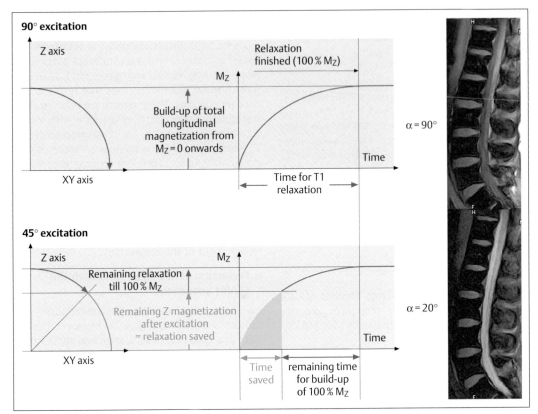

Fig. 1.**8** **GRE sequence.** To optimize contrast with GRE sequences excitation pulses are used that rotate the longitudinal magnetization M_Z by less than 90°. With an excitation of less than 90° not the all the magnetization is flipped from the Z direction into the XY plane, but rather a residual magnetization remains in the Z direction, which, does not need to be built up again. Thus the time for building up the total longitudinal magnetization ($M_Z = 100$ %) will be shorter. In this way (with the TR time constant) the T2 image contrast of the images can be intensified by reducing the flip angle.

■ FLASH Sequence and T1 Weighting

The following applications are foremost when using T1-weighted FLASH sequences:

- demonstration of contrast agent inflow with a high temporal resolution,
- fast acquisition for agitated or critical patients and for abdominal examinations in breath-holding technique,
- enhancement of T1 contrasts (Table 1.1).

■ In-Phase/Opposed-Phase Contrast

The in-phase/opposed-phase technique is often used to increase contrast in GRE sequences.

The opposed-phase image displays tissue containing water and fat components with reduced signal intensity because the opposed-phase image shows the difference between the signals of fat and water. The signal in the opposed-phase image is the sum of this difference, i.e., always positive, regardless of the sign of the difference.

This means that when the signal components of fat and water are approximately the same, they almost cancel each other out and the tissue is displayed with a low resultant signal. If one component increases (e.g., the water component due to edema), the resultant signal also increases, and a greater contrast results as compared with the surrounding tissue, which is displayed with less intensity. The acquisition of an opposed-phase image can, therefore, result in a gain in contrast.

Table 1.1 Sequence parameters for T2*- and T1-weighted FLASH acquisitions using high-field systems

T2*-weighted			T1-weighted	
TR	TE	Flip-angle α	TE	Flip-angle α
(ms)	(ms)	(degrees)	(ms)	(degrees)
1000	15–30	35°	< 15	90°
800	15–30	30°	< 15	90°
600	15–30	25°	< 15	90°
400	15–30	15°	< 15	90°
200	15–30	10°	< 15	80°
100	15	7°	< 15	70°
50	–	–	< 15	60°

T2 weighting:*
With decreasing TR time the flip angle α is also set lower in order to reduce saturation effects.

T1 weighting:
α is generally larger than with T2*-weighted FLASH acquisitions. With relatively long TR times (more than 300 ms) a 90° pulse is used, as with SE. A reduction of α is only necessary when the TR time of the FLASH acquisition falls below 300 ms in order to prevent too much saturation.

Which Processes Result in an In-Phase and Opposed-Phase Image?

Fat and water protons precess in the magnetic field with a slightly different frequency; this frequency difference is also referred to as chemical shift (see also p. 25).

The difference amounts to 3.5 ppm and is:
- approximately 150 Hz for 1 tesla
- approximately 220 Hz for 1.5 tesla.

Apart from dephasing due to T2 relaxation, this also results in an additional dephasing of the protons of the fat and water components after excitation.

Other than with T2 dephasing, where the effects of the protons on each other are variable over time, the effect of chemical shift is constant. For this reason, the precise point of time at which fat protons (because of their slower precession) are lying exactly opposite the water protons in the XY plane can be calculated. At this point fat and water protons have a difference in phase of 180°; this is the opposed phase condition, in which the resultant signal is once again the difference between the signals of water and fat. After twice the time, the water protons have once again caught up with the fat protons and both types of protons precess in phase for a brief period. This is the in-phase condition. In this state the signals of fat and water combine to produce a large resultant signal.

Opposed and in-phase states alternate continually in a fixed time pattern.

Using the echo time TE, GRE sequences can be set with regard to whether data acquisition is to occur in the opposed-phase or in the in-phase condition (Fig. 1.9).

Spin Echo Sequence

The 180° rephasing pulse generates an SE and reduces susceptibility and inhomogeneity effects in comparison with GRE so that with long echo times the images show true T2 contrast.

Advantages of the SE sequence
- low susceptibility to inhomogeneities,
- few susceptibility artifacts,
- strong T2 contrast is possible.

Disadvantages of the SE sequence
- long scanning time.

■ T1 Contrast with SE Sequence

Because SE sequences usually use 90° excitation pulses, a TR time of 400–800 ms is required to yield a good T1 contrast with good image quality. The echo time TE should be as short as possible, certainly below 15 ms.

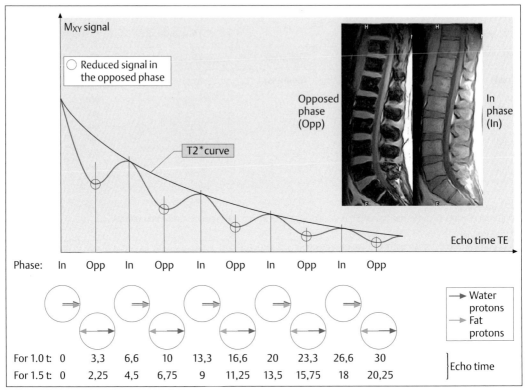

Fig. 1.**9 In-phase/opposed-phase contrast.** In-phase and opposed-phase scans are adjusted in GRE sequences with the aid of the echo time TE. In-phase and opposed-phase conditions recur in a fixed time pattern of 3.3 ms at 1.0 tesla and 2.25 ms at 1.5 tesla.

■ Proton Density and T2 Contrast with SE Sequence

With the aid of SE double-echo sequences, PD- and T2-weighted images can be reconstructed in one scanning process.

Since a long TR time is required for both weightings (> 2000 ms), only the echo time TE is the decisive factor as to whether the image is PD- or T2-weighted.

With a double-echo sequence both a PD- and a T2-weighted image can be acquired in one scanning process. Scanning two echoes does not prolong acquisition time for the sequence. The information content is increased, however, because two images with different weightings are available from each slice (Fig. 1.**10**).

Inversion-Recovery (IR) Sequence

In order to increase the contrast of the SE sequences further, there is the possibility of transmitting a 180° pulse before the SE sequence. An SE sequence preceded by a 180° pulse is referred to as an IR sequence. The preceding 180° excitation pulse inverts the longitudinal magnetization and alters the T1 effect on the image contrast, while T2 contrast is still only regulated by the echo time TE.

With IR sequences the time between the 180° pulse and the subsequent SE sequence serves to adjust the T1 contribution to image contrast. This time is also referred to as the *inversion time TI*.

T1 relaxation of the longitudinal magnetization M_Z occurs within the TI time, starting from a negative baseline value (Fig. 1.**11**).

Depending on the selected TI time and the T1 time of the tissue, three situations can arise after a 180° excitation:

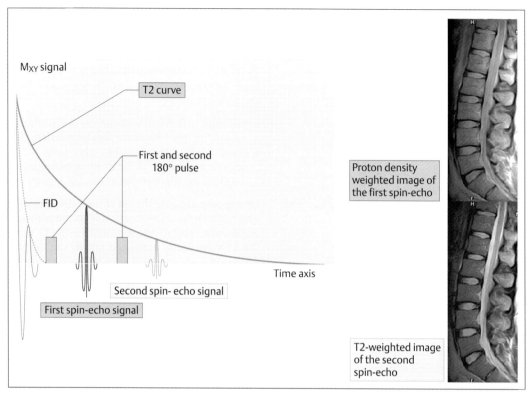

Fig. 1.**10** **Double-echo sequence.** With a double-echo sequence two 180° RF pulses rephase the signal so that two echoes arise at different echo times. The first 180° pulse rephases M_{XY} so that a short first echo is generated. Afterwards a second 180° rephasing pulse is applied to generate a second late echo.

1. TI time is so short that M_Z is still negative,
2. TI time is just long enough that $M_Z = 0$,
3. TI time is longer still so that M_Z has already become positive again.

The subsequent 90°-pulse rotates the M_Z formed during the TI interval into the XY plane where, as transverse magnetization M_{XY}, it emits a signal.

Thus there are also three different transverse magnetizations M_{XY} possible:

- If M_Z is still negative at the time of the 90° pulse (situation 1), M_{XY}, and with it the signal, is negative after the 90° excitation.
- If $M_Z = 0$ at the time of the 90° pulse (zero crossing of M_Z, situation 2), M_{XY}, and with it the signal, is negative after the 90° excitation.
- If M_Z is already positive at the time of the 90° pulse (situation 3), M_{XY}, and with it the signal, is positive after the 90° excitation.

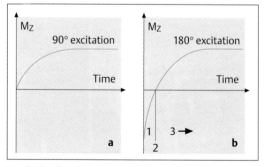

Fig. 1.**11 a, b** **IR sequence:**
a With a 90° excitation only positive signals occur.
b With a 180° excitation, M_Z is inverted so that shortly after the excitation negative signals can also be measured. For an explanation of situations labeled 1, 2 and 3 see text (p. 15).

In most MR systems there are two types of IR sequences, which differ in their presentation of the negative signal:

IR sequences that display the signal according to its sign (True IR). Negative signals are displayed with less intensity than the background (background = zero signal). To make this possible, the background usually has a gray level of 2048 in these images. Negative signals have a gray level <2048, positive signals a gray level >2048.

IR sequences that display the signal with its absolute value (modulus IR). Negative signals are displayed positively (modulus display). Tissues on the image that display the same absolute signal value, yet have a different sign, are indistinguishable from each other as a result of modulus calculation.

Example:
Signal of tissue 1 (with short T1) = +1000
Signal of tissue 2 (with long T1) = –1000
Both tissues are displayed with a signal of +1000.

The IR modulus sequence is of greater importance. It is used to suppress the signal of certain tissues. To do this, TI time is adjusted so that M_z is just passing through its zero crossing. The correct TI time for suppressing the signal of a specific tissue depends on its T1 time, which again varies with different field strengths.

To suppress the fat signal with high-field systems (1.0 tesla, 1.5 tesla) the TI time is approximately 150 ms, for the suppression of the signal of free water (cerebrospinal fluid) the TI time amounts to approximately 2300 ms. Because of their significance, these two IR sequences have their own names:

- STIR (Short TI IR): IR sequence with a TI time of approximately 150 ms for fat suppression.
- FLAIR (fluid attenuated IR), dark-fluid IR: IR sequence with a TI time of approximately 2300 ms for suppression of the CSF signal.

Fat suppression with the aid of the STIR technique also has its risks. In association with the administration of a contrast agent to shorten the T1 time, the T1 time in the enhanced region can drop to the T1 time of fat. A STIR scan following contrast administration can therefore cover up the diagnostic result (Fig. 1.**12**).

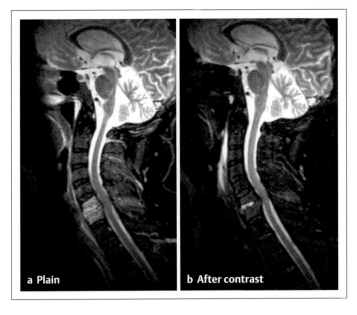

a Plain   b After contrast

Fig. 1.**12 a,b   Comparative STIR measurement**. Note the low contrast that develops after administration of contrast medium, due to the reduction of T1 time in the region of uptake. In this example the T1 time of the finding was reduced by the contrast medium to the T1 time of fat:
a Plain
b After contrast administration.

Ultrafast Imaging

One disadvantage of MRI in the early years of clinical use of this technique was the relatively long acquisition time for individual scans and subsequently for examinations as a whole. Since then very fast, frequently referred to as "ultrafast," scanning techniques have become available with acquisition times down to as low as 50 ms for imaging one single slice. The imaging techniques SE and GRE already described also form the foundations for ultrafast procedures.

The following procedures will be reviewed below:
- turbo spin echo (TSE),
- turbo gradient spin echo (TGSE, GRASE),
- echo planar imaging (EPI).

(Various manufacturers of MR tomographs offer the techniques described here under a variety of names.)

Turbospin Echo

Whereas with single-contrast SE sequences or GRE sequences one echo is generated with each excitation pulse and stored in one line of the raw-data set, with TSE sequences several echo signals are generated with one excitation pulse. This is achieved by the use of multiple 180° pulses. Each of these echoes is position encoded with variably strong phase-encoding gradients and arranged in different areas of the raw-data set. This results in the raw-data set being filled, for example, seven times more quickly with a 7-echo pulse sequence. With this procedure, signals with different echo times, and consequently with different T2 weightings, are combined in one image. The echoes that are stored in the center of the raw-data set, however, largely determine contrast on an MR image. A suitable scanning and sorting schema can therefore determine contrast in the resultant image. The echo time of the central raw-data lines is usually referred to as the *effective echo time* TE_{eff} (Figs. 1.**13** and 1.**14**).

The saving of scanning time can now be put to use in various ways:

- to reduce examination time,
- to improve image quality (signal-to-noise ratio) by averaging the data several times, yet maintaining the same scanning time,

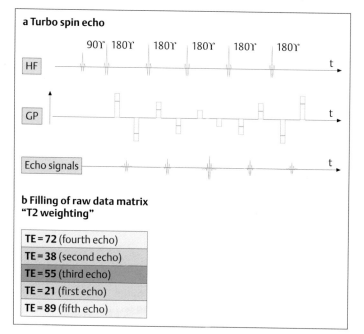

a Turbo spin echo

b Filling of raw data matrix "T2 weighting"

| TE = 72 (fourth echo) |
| TE = 38 (second echo) |
| TE = 55 (third echo) |
| TE = 21 (first echo) |
| TE = 89 (fifth echo) |

Fig. 1.**13 a,b   TSE sequence.** Several echo signals are generated with one excitation pulse (each being separately phase-encoded, **a**). These are filled in different areas of the raw-data set (**b**). The raw-data set is completed more rapidly according to the number of echoes. For reasons of simplicity not all gradient pulses appear on the pulse-sequence diagram.
GP = phase-encoding gradient
HF = high-frequency pulse

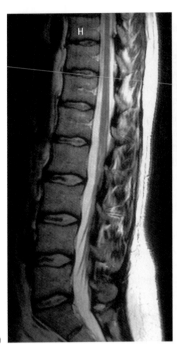

a

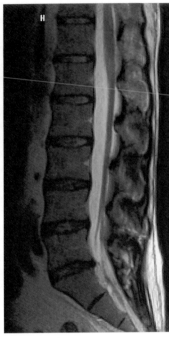

b

Fig. 1.**14 a, b** **TSE sequence:**
a Example of a T2-weighted, sagittal section of the lumbar spine (TR = 4000 ms, TE$_{eff}$ = 120 ms, matrix 512, scanning time 4.52 mins).
b Image scanned in about 30 s. The sequence generates 29 echo signals after one excitation pulse. The acquisition matrix was reduced to 203 x 256.

● to obtain higher resolution of and to compensate for the lower signal-to-noise ratio by additional data averagings; the practical clinical use of scans with a matrix size of 512 or 1024 has been made possible with the introduction of these techniques.

The number of SEs that can be measured after one excitation and stored in the raw-data set can be increased to the extent that the whole raw-data set can be acquired in a " single shot." These techniques are called RARE (rapid acquisition with relaxation enhancement) or, in a modified form, HASTE (half Fourier single shot turbospin echo technique). They allow a fast scan of very heavily T2-weighted images in single slices. In this way, for example, the entire liver can be scanned during one breath-hold phase.

Turbo IR sequence. An interesting extension of the TSE sequences described here is the turbo IR sequence. As with the SE IR sequence, the magnetization used in the turbo IR technique is also inverted with the aid of a 180° pulse before the actual generation of the signal. The magnetization is allowed to relax for a certain (selectable) time TI before the prevailing longitudinal magnetization is flipped into the transverse plane with a 90°

pulse. By selecting the correct TI time one will achieve suppression of fat or water.

From a clinical point of view it should be pointed out that signal enhancement with contrast medium, e.g., in a tumor, displays less contrast when fat saturation is achieved using IR sequences than when a frequency-selective suppression technique is used. Findings can thus be covered up, as it were. Nevertheless this form of fat suppression is of interest particularly with low-field systems.

In the example in Fig. 1.**15** a sagittal section of the spine is shown using fat-suppressed T2 weighting.

By applying the 180° pulse with a time lag TI, a relatively large amount of time is initially "lost" with the IR technique. This means that the number of slices that can be acquired simultaneously per unit of time is comparatively small. Until the introduction of turbo IR sequences, therefore, the IR technique was hardly ever used. However this has changed in recent years.

Turbo Gradient Spin Echo

A further development of the TSE sequence is the turbo gradient spin echo technique, also referred to as GRASE (gradient spin echo). Here, after a given excitation pulse, a train of 180° pulses are used to create a series of spin echoes. Apart from each SE, further switchings of gradient fields generate additional GREs, which are in turn assigned to different areas of the raw-data set. The raw-data matrix is filled by the mix of fast GREs and SEs more rapidly than with the TSE sequence. The gains in time can be used in the same way as those resulting from TSE. The contrast is T2-weighted and the overall appearance is very similar to that of the SE technique (Fig. 1.**16**).

Echo Planar Imaging

The fastest technique currently available for MR imaging is echo planar imaging (EPI) which is also a single-shot procedure. With EPI the whole raw-data set is acquired with a fast train of GREs after one RF excitation pulse. The scanning time for a single image amounts to a minimum of 50 ms. EPI images are usually T2-weighted.

Technical requirements for the EPI technique are:

- good magnetic field homogeneity
- a high-performance gradient system:
  - fast rise times,
  - sufficiently high peak amplitude,
  - a high duty cycle.

Even with optimized magnetic-field homogeneity, EPI images are often not quite free from distortions, so-called susceptibility artifacts, because the patient disturbs the local magnetic field. These cannot be corrected by simple means. This applies particularly to air–tissue interfaces where substances with different magnetizability (susceptibility) converge, resulting in local field distortions and signal cancellations.

By virtue of its imaging speed, EPI opens new avenues for diagnostics using MRI, especially with regard to functional studies. Furthermore, pulse sequences have been developed that are sensitive to differences in the diffusion behavior of water molecules. This allows the demonstration of early brain infarcts.

Because of the previously mentioned susceptibility effects that occur at tissue interfaces with different magnetizability, e.g., at bony structures, the EPI technique has proved of little use in the spinal region.

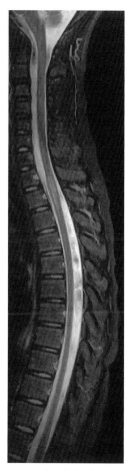

Fig. 1.**15 Turbo IR sequence.** Example of the thoracic spine taken with a spine array coil (TR = 5 s, TI = 150 ms, TE = 60 ms, matrix 512).

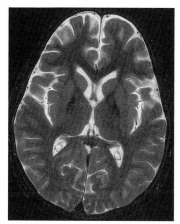

Fig. 1.**16 Turbo gradient spin echo.** T2-weighted image with a 1024 matrix (TR = 7400 ms, TE_{eff} = 115 ms; scanning time 4.04 mins).

Artifacts on MR Images

As with all other imaging techniques, MRI is also not free from image artifacts. Some of the most common artifacts, their physical backgrounds and possible corrective measures will now be addressed briefly:

- metal-induced artifacts,
- motion artifacts,
- aliasing,
- truncation artifacts,
- susceptibility artifacts,
- chemical-shift artifacts.

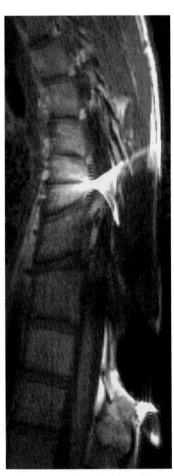

Fig. 1.**17 Metal-induced artifact.** Metal-induced artifact due to a ferromagnetic clip on the clothing in the region of the thoracic spine.

Metal-Induced Artifacts

Metallic objects in the field of view (in or on the patient, or in the field of examination near the patient) can distort the local magnetic fields. This applies to the RF field that is being irradiated with RF pulses as well as to the magnetic field—both the main field and the gradient fields. While the RF field interacts with any conducting material, the magnetic field becomes disturbed by ferromagnetic materials (i.e., iron-containing materials) producing spatial distortions on the image. The extent of the disturbances depends on the size of the metallic object and the strength of the main magnetic field.

Metal-induced artifacts (Fig. 1.**17**) can be caused by quite small objects, e.g.

- zip fasteners,
- hairpins,
- coins,
- buttons,
- as well as such "insignificant" objects as:
  - metallic threads woven into the labels of sweaters,
  - eye shadow containing metallic dust,
  - tattoos.

It is virtually impossible to correct these artifacts by image postprocessing. The patient should therefore be asked about metallic objects before the examination. This questioning is also essential for safety reasons with regard to any ferromagnetic objects that the patient is carrying because such materials can be strongly attracted by the magnetic field.

Motion Artifacts

Movement of the patient can result in blurs on the image. In addition, movements (e.g., breathing, blood flow, involuntary eye and swallowing movements) lead to misinterpretations of the signals received. This applies when a piece of tissue moves during the time between excitation and echo so that excitation pulse and signal emission subsequently occur at slightly different positions. The moving protons experience frequency changes and phase alterations while moving along magnetic field gradients, which the Fourier transform is then unable to assign correctly.

Various techniques are used to minimize these kinds of motion artifacts:

- data averaging,
- gradient motion rephasing,
- saturation ranges,
- breath-holding techniques,
- triggering.

Data averaging. Not only do data averagings improve the signal-to-noise ratio, but motion effects are also averaged. A certain degree of edge blurring due to motion is hardly avoidable.

Gradient motion rephrasing. Gradient motion rephasing technique refers to the use of special gradient pulses within the sequence (with SE sequences usually before and after the 180° pulse). The gradient pulses cause reversal of phase errors, e.g., due to flow in the scanning plane. (This is referred to as rephasing and refocusing.) (Fig. 1.**18**.)

Saturation ranges. Regional saturation pulses are often used, especially in examinations of the spine. Therefore, in sagittal scans of the cervical spine, for example, the laryngeal region signal is usually suppressed by a saturation area to avoid artifacts due to swallowing movements. The fundamental idea behind this technique is that image regions that are of no importance for the diagnosis are suppressed by saturation and can therefore no longer cause any more artifacts. For this purpose a 90° pulse is employed (in this example) in a thick coronal plane (saturation area) before the actual excitation of the sagittal plane. Gradient pulses follow this excitation pulse and dephase the magnetization in the saturation area. If the 90° excitation pulse is now applied in the sagittal plane, then there is no longitudinal magnetization in the saturation area that can be excited. The result is that no signal is emitted from this region—it remains dark on the image. Therefore the signals of these moving tissue parts do not contribute to the motion artifact (Fig. 1.**19**).

Breath-holding techniques. In the field of abdominal imaging the use of fast scanning methods in breath-holding technique has become popular in recent years. This is a very effective method of avoiding respiratory artifacts, but it does require appropriate scanning sequences and sensitive enough receiver coils (Fig. 1.**20**).

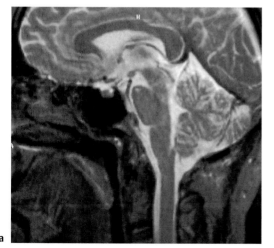 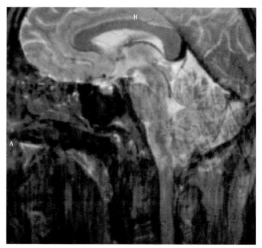

a

b

Fig. 1.**18 a, b** **Scan of the head and the craniocervical junction**:

a With motion rephasing

b Without motion rephasing.

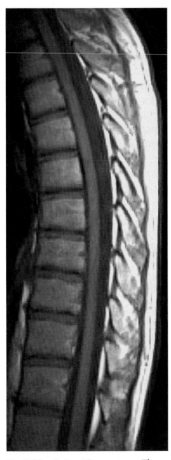

Fig. 1.**19** **Saturation range.** Thoracic spine using T1-weighting with coronal saturation range to suppress the signal from moving organs in the thorax.

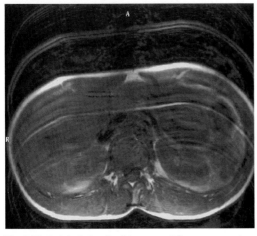

Fig. 1.**20 Axial abdominal image with gross respiratory motion-induced artifacts**.

Triggering. The final method of avoiding motion artifacts to be considered is ECG triggering. Both pulsating blood flow and pulsating CSF also result in image artifacts in the region of the spine. Now if the signal from the ECG or the peripheral pulse is recorded during MR imaging, scanning can be synchronized with the physiological signals—each individual acquisition is always performed at the same time during the cardiac cycle. The flow motion becomes virtually frozen. The disadvantage of this technique is that it prolongs scanning time and may alter contrast to some extent because the repetition time depends on the heart rate. That is why ECG triggering is only seldom used for examinations of the spine. Analogous to ECG triggering, a respiratory signal can also be used in principle to synchronize data acquisition.

Aliasing

Aliasing (also referred to as wrap-around, backfolding, or overlap) occurs when the region being imaged is larger than the selected field of view (FOV), yet is still located within the sensitive area of the receiver coil. This results in, e.g., the nose, which lies in front of and outside the FOV, reappearing at the back part of the skull in sagittal images of the head. On sagittal images of the spine, structures of the sacrum are folded back to the upper part of the spine.

The reason for this aliasing lies with the mechanism of image generation and image reconstruction using Fourier transform. The received signal is scanned with a predetermined grid of sampling points. With this grid a certain maximum signal frequency can be accurately displayed. Signals with even higher frequencies are also registered, but not correctly identified and processed further.

The effect can occur within the scanning plane along the frequency- and phase-encoding direction, as well as along the slice-selection direction in *three-dimensional* scans.

To avoid the occurrence of these wrap-around artifacts, most systems today offer the possibility of correctly recording even higher frequencies by oversampling the signals. Whereas *oversampling along the frequency-encoding direction* occurs without altering the scanning time, *oversampling along the phase-encoding direction* prolongs acquisition time proportionally to the number of additional phase-encoding steps. Since in this case the signal-to-noise ratio also increases, additional data averaging can be dispensed with where appropriate. Sometimes it may also be advisable to exchange phase and frequency encoding direction. In doing so, the parameters influencing potential motion artifacts, FOV size, signal-to-noise ratio and scanning time has also be taken into account (Fig. 1.**21**).

Truncation Artifacts

Truncation artifacts (also referred to as Gibbs artifacts, ringing, edge ringing) are the repeated appearance of image structures parallel to the true anatomic structures. This occurs particularly at structures with very abrupt contrast changes, e.g., CSF/brain matter in T2-weighted scans (Figs. 1.**22**– 1.**24**).

The basis of MR image reconstruction can also result in truncation artifacts occurring. A signal change from black to white from one pixel to the next can only be correctly reproduced by Fourier transform when an infinite number of sampling points and frequency components are taken into account. That is virtually impossible and the cutting off, or truncation, of data produces signal oscillations next to the areas of abrupt contrast change.

These artifacts can be avoided by performing the scans with larger matrices, particularly along the phase-encoding direction where matrices of reduced size are often used to save time (rectangular matrix).

The use of raw-data filters (e.g., a Hanning filter) helps reduce the degree of truncation artifact.

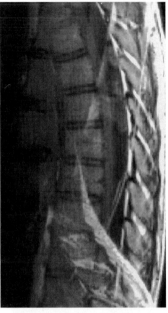

Fig. 1.**21 Example of aliasing in the thoracic spine.** The scan was taken with a long spine coil. The selected field of view was much smaller in the head-to-foot direction than the sensitive area of the receiver coil. Structures of both the neck and the lumbar spine are superimposed.

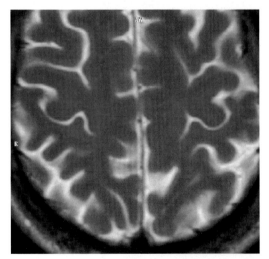

Fig. 1.**22 Truncation artifacts alongside the abrupt contrast change between the two cerebral hemispheres.**

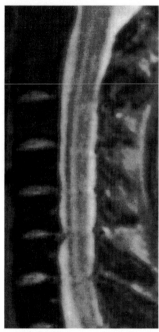

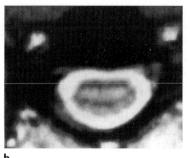

b

a

◁ Fig. 1.**23 a**, **b**   **Truncation artifacts within the spinal cord**:
a Sagittal section with evidence of truncation artifacts in the anterior third of the spinal cord (TR = 600 ms, TE = 20 ms, flip angle = 10°, matrix 180 x 256, FOV = 250 mm²).
b Transverse section through the cervical spine of the same patient. Truncation artifacts appear oval and wide within the spinal cord (TR = 600 ms, TE = 20 ms, flip angle = 10°, matrix 180 x 256, FOV = 240 mm²).

Susceptibility Artifacts

Susceptibility artifacts have a similar cause to that of the metal-induced artifacts described above. Different tissues and structures in the body exhibit a different magnetizability (magnetic susceptibility) when they are exposed to an external magnetic field. This applies particularly for air–tissue or bone–tissue interfaces. The different magnetization of contiguous tissues generates local static magnetic-field gradients, which are superimposed on the main field and the switched gradient fields. With the use of GRE sequences, these local field distortions result in signal dephasing that, as with SE sequences, are not refocused again. This is the cause of the local signal cancellation.

These dephasings can be avoided by using SE or TSE techniques. However, should GRE sequences be used (especially for *three-dimensional* techniques), attention should be paid to use as short an echo time as possible to allow the spins in the region of the local field distortions little time to dephase (Fig. 1.**25**).

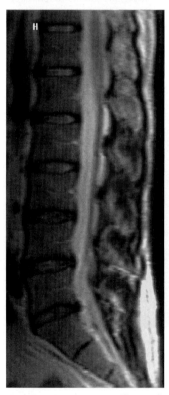

Fig. 1.**24**   **Truncation artifacts adjacent to and in the vertebrae**.

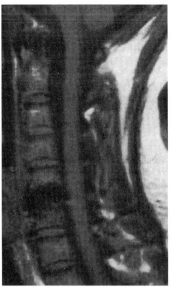
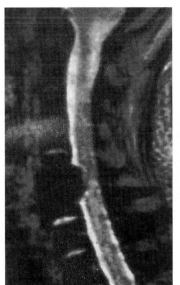
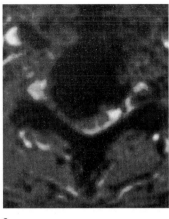

a   **b**

c

Fig. 1.**25 a–c   Example of a susceptibility artifact**:
a T1-weighted SE image at the C5/C6 level after an operation with the introduction of Pallocos^R (TR = 685 ms, TE = 20 ms).
b The image of the same patient using a GRE sequence (TR = 600 ms, TE = 20 ms, flip angle = 10°). Marked susceptibility artifacts are generated by the Pallocos^R

inlay giving the impression here of spinal cord compression.
c GRE sequence in transverse slice orientation (TR = 600 ms, TE = 20 ms, flip angle = 10°). The transverse image clearly shows the simulated compression of the spinal cord by the marked susceptibility artifacts. The "narrowing" of the entire spinal canal due to the artifact is clearly recognizable.

Chemical-Shift Artifacts

Protons in hydrogen atoms that are bound in water molecules (OH binding) experience a different local magnetic field than those in fat-like molecules (CH bindings). This is attributed to the different shielding effects of the molecular electron shell. In the MR frequency spectrum, this results in a difference in resonance frequencies of 3.5 ppm. For a 1.5 tesla system this means a frequency shift of about 220 Hz.

In the Fourier transform used for image reconstruction, frequency and phase information are used for position encoding. If the fat and water protons of a voxel have different frequencies, the fat signal appears shifted to a different site from the water signal. This displacement corresponds to an offset of 1–2 pixels in many of the commonly used scanning sequences. At interfaces between more water-containing and more fat-containing tissues, bright and, on the opposite side, dark contours give the image a relief-like impression (Fig. 1.**26**).

To avoid this artifact, the use of sequences with sufficiently wide readout bandwidths is recommended so that the signals of water and fat converge on one pixel. If the interest is only in the watery tissue anyway, these can just as well be used for imaging, either by selective excitation of the water protons or by fat suppression. This can be achieved by the IR technique described or by frequency-selective saturation techniques.

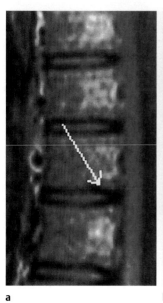 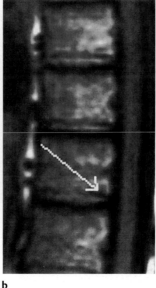

Fig. 1.**26 a**, **b** **Chemical shift:**
a Image in a craniocaudal phase-encoding direction. Chemical-shift artifact in the AP direction. There is a corresponding, somewhat unsharp contour of the dorsal vertebral component at its interface with CSF and a uniform display of the vertebral cortex in all sections (arrow).
b AP phase-encoding direction with chemical-shift artifact in craniocaudal direction. On this image the vertebral contours are unevenly displayed with accentuation of the superior end plate and thinning of the inferior end plate. The dorsal vertebral contour, on the other hand, is shown more clearly and is more sharply demarcated from CSF (arrow).

a   b

Future Perspectives

This introduction has presented the fundamental techniques of MRI. Based on these, more scan sequences and techniques have been developed over recent years that have further extended the diagnostic options of MRI. Apart from obviously accelerating the examinations and further increasing image resolution, new methods have also been developed for specific clinical objectives. The advances in MR angiography and in the depiction of early brain infarcts should be mentioned here as examples.

Especially in the region of the CNS, and here in particular in the spine, MR diagnostic imaging has become an indispensable tool.

Summary

- *Image contrasts* can be adjusted by the appropriate selection of TR and TE times, and in GRE sequences by the flip angle.
- The SE sequence, with short TR and TE times, and the GRE sequence, with a large flip angle and short TE time, are available for the *reconstruction of T1-weighted images*.
- *T2-weighted images* are generated with the aid of TSE sequences, or alternatively with GRE sequences that require a low flip angle and a TE time of 15–30 ms.
- An important sequence for obtaining water-sensitive images is the *STIR sequence*, which is based on a short inversion time of about 150 ms.

- Information about the fat and water content of the tissue can be obtained with the *in-phase and opposed-phase method*.
- Various artifacts can affect image quality:
  - metal-induced artifacts,
  - motion artifacts,
  - aliasing,
  - truncation artifacts,
  - susceptibility artifacts,
  - chemical-shift artifacts.
- Furthermore, flow artifacts can be caused by blood flow in the major vessels and heart as well as by CSF flow in the spinal canal.
- There are means for suppressing these artifacts, which in the majority of cases, however, is done at the expense of imaging time.

■ References

Edelman, R. R., P. Wielopolski, F. Schmitt: Echo-planar MR Imaging. Radiology 192 (1994) 600–612

Feinberg, D. A., B. Kiefer, A. W. Litt: High resolution GRASE MRI of the brain and spine: 512 and 1024 matrix imaging. J. Comput. assist. Tomogr. 19 (1995) 1–7

Lissner, J., M. Seiderer: Klinische Kernspintomographie. Enke, Stuttgart 1990

Morneburg, H.: Bildgebende Systeme für die medizinische Diagnostik, 3. Aufl. Publicis MCD, München 1995

Reimer, P., P.M. Parizel, F.-A. Stichnoth; A Practical Approach to Clinical MR Imaging. Springer, Berlin, Heidelberg, New York 1999

Uhlenbrock, D.: Kernspintomographie des Kopfes. Thieme, Stuttgart 1990

■ Acknowledgements

We should like to thank the following hospitals for providing the image examples: Josef's Hospital, Dortmund, Germany; Yamaguchi University Hospital, Lund University Hospital, Tokyo Metoro; Ebara Hospital.

2 MRI and Spinal Surgery - Indications Based on the Spectrum of Surgical Therapeutic Options

R. Schultheiss

Contents

General Comments on Preoperative Diagnostics and Planning Strategy

In almost all the cases of spinal lesions amenable to surgery, spinal MRI currently allows a very *precise diagnosis* and *guidelines for preoperative planning* to be established without direct contact between the patient or examiner and the prospective surgeon. The main indication for spinal MRI is usually to secure a diagnosis.

Any question directed to the examiner regarding the possible level and nature of the lesion must be formulated as precisely as possible and include an *exact neurological classification* of the clinical findings. This is particularly helpful when no pathological finding has been noted on MRI despite unequivocal clinical symptoms. A disturbance of gait, for instance, can be caused by cervical myelopathy, lumbar spinal canal stenosis, normal pressure hydrocephalus, Parkinson's disease, disseminated encephalitis, polyneuropathy, an intramedullary tumor or a bone metastasis to the spine, or a spinal AV fistula—only an exact analysis of the patient's history and the clinical findings will in this case provide the examiner with the necessary data on which to focus the examination technique. It should be borne in mind that an exclusion diagnosis, in particular, can sometimes be technically very demanding.

In addition, information from the surgeon's point of view regarding operative strategy, which may not necessarily have been offered for a routine examination, might nevertheless become important. In order to make optimal use of the imaging equipment, thoughts about preoperative planning or additional information on how the indication was reached should, if possible, be available for consideration at the initial diagnostic MRI scanning.

The following aspects are of particular interest when a pathological finding amenable to surgery is noted on MRI:

- topographic assignment,
- specific diagnostic classification.

Documentation of *level* and *expansion* of the lesion must be precise, i.e., it must be possible for the surgeon to take responsibility for counting off each vertebral segment from the spinal sections depicted on the MR image and to transfer the findings on to plain x-rays and intraoperative fluoroscopy. The neck and upper thoracic spine will therefore require depiction of the vertebral landmarks of the craniocervical junction, and inclusion of the sacrum is necessary for the lower thoracic and lumbar spine. For the mid-thoracic spinal region, it is always obligatory to provide a sagittal reference image that includes the sacrum or the craniocervical junction.

Assigning and labeling the level of individual vertebrae on the image are only helpful when done electronically by the examiner, thus converting it into a permanent document and rendering it legally binding. Otherwise the image must be repeated in order to assure the necessary reliability of the assigned level. Labels on the film may be accurate, but they do not provide any legally binding basis for the site of the operation because it will never be certain with hindsight whether the labeling was done authentically by the examiner or later—and possibly incorrectly—by some other observer. The operative strategy of the much cited minimally invasive surgery requires, in the first instance, an exact localization—a lateralized spinal meningioma, for example, already demonstrated earlier during laminectomy, which had included the adjacent segments, can only be removed microsurgically by a stability-maintaining hemilaminectomy if it is possible during surgery to locate exactly which hemi-arch is to be removed.

It is always compulsory to *display spinal disorders in the sagittal and transverse plane*, and often preferably in the *frontal plane*, even though the information value of this frontal slice orientation is limited because kyphosis or lordosis requires an adjustment of the scanning plane for depiction of the spinal canal. It can, however, facilitate orientation in paravertebral lesions of the thoracic and retroperitoneal cavities. Because the plethora of image sections will sometimes require limitation of the final amount of image documentation, it is important that a *continuous image series* is taken to provide the surgeon with some form of spatial orientation. Omitting seemingly irrelevant images can lead to confusion and faulty assignment of location. Anatomical considerations also play a decisive role when planning the operative approach so that the documented images should allow additional anatomical information to be gleaned as comprehensively as possible and recorded in three dimensions.

The choice of slice thickness and of the interval between individual sections will depend on the dimensions of the lesion in question. For example, thin slices in the region of the tumor are decisive for preoperative planning, particularly with intramedullary tumors. With spinal metastases, on the other hand, it is important that virtually the entire spine is depicted to avoid overlooking tumor formations additional to the metastasis responsible for the symptoms. In case surgical stabilization is required, portrayal of the vertebrae adjacent to the lesion will provide enough assurance that these are not affected by the tumor and can be used for supporting the instrumentation. Since, in this case, priority lies more in including contiguous regions, it is advisable to use thicker slicing. It can be helpful if the relevant images of the various scanning planes are combined on one or a few films. However, this is no substitute for the information value provided by a complete series with regard to anatomical considerations relating to preoperative planning.

With the increasing significance of *neuronavigation* in spinal surgery, it will presumably be wise in future, when a finding requiring surgery is noted, to electronically store image data sets for later use by the respective neuronavigation systems after consultation with the potential surgeon. Digital documentation of the image data would be ideal, allowing appropriate evaluation at any time. Paper radiographs would then probably suffice for an overview assessment in cases of more complex lesions, where they might otherwise be limited in their informative value.

In view of the number of sections in different planes and sequences, it is helpful if the *relevant images* are *marked* with self-stick dots or the like. This can save a considerable amount of time during the overview assessment.

The *specific diagnostic classification of the observed findings* by the examiner is considerably more relevant than with other imaging techniques. While with CT, for example, an interpretation of the images by others poses no problem as a rule, the appreciation of why a particular MR imaging sequence was selected obviously requires additional diagnostic information that is not always available to those foreign to the matter. It is therefore of utmost importance that the examiner specify the degree of differential-diagnostic certainty of a finding.

MRI is becoming increasingly important for the *emergency diagnostics of acute spinal cord paralysis* so that attempts should be made whenever possible to widen the availability of this diagnostic procedure, at least on a regional basis, by allowing examinations to be also performed outside regular office hours. A spinal empyema, an epidural hematoma and a central cervical cord lesion are often difficult, or even impossible, to detect with other techniques; the density of information in a case of metastatic disease of the spine can be enlarged rapidly so as to allow well-founded indications to be defined and, perhaps, even considerations regarding an overall oncological concept to be taken into account. Routine diagnostics of spinal trauma using MRI is still certainly a problem because there are only very limited possibilities of monitoring vital signs during the diagnostic work-up. Nevertheless, it should be remembered that, e.g., the diagnostics of traumatic vascular dissection of the cervical spine, a problem area which up to now has been difficult to diagnose despite its primary importance, could be considerably better addressed in the future; a similar widening of the diagnostic spectrum can also be expected for other spinal regions.

The *timing of the examination* in spinal diagnostics can be decisive for the further course of the disorder. It should, therefore, always be ensured that, for example, when admitting patients with incipient paralysis or disturbance of bladder function as a sign of a transverse spinal lesion, a top-priority emergency appointment for the examination is given. The urgency depends here on the severity of the symptoms so that in the presence of marked neurological deficits an immediate examination should be performed.

Should a *space-occupying mass of the spine* be identified, it is wise to contact the surgeon immediately in order to make urgent arrangements for surgery. This can be indicated in the presence of neurological deficits as well as for instability of the spine. Depending on the clinical picture, the examiner will often be required to save time by arranging for immediate and specific referral of the patient. Once the necessity of emergency surgery has been established, it is extremely helpful to tell the patient to remain fasting as a precaution until a final decision on this has been made. It is most important for psychological reasons that patients with malignant tumors in particular are only informed that the opinion of the surgeon should be sought and not that surgery will be necessary. The decision to operate can often only be reached after unraveling a complex array of factors that will eventually define the indication. Especially in the case of oncological patients, hopes of a "still possible" operation can be dashed by the fundamental disappointment that surgery is "no longer feasible"—unnecessarily sometimes if other therapeutic alternatives are to be given priority anyway.

Where the diagnosis automatically dictates the indication for surgery, it is often extremely comforting for the patient to receive *information about treatment options* from the examiner first. It helps the surgeon if, when introduced, the patient is already informed about this, yet not necessarily about a specific therapeutic procedure. The patient can only reach a decision for or against possible therapeutic measures, which often include a considerable range of variations, after close discussion with the person who will actually perform the operation. Considering the multitude of factors influencing the decision to recommend a specific operative strategy, a discussion unaffected by any previous statements should, in the interests of the patient, be all the more specific. The surgeon is certainly just as grateful to the examiner for his advice in favor of surgery as for his measured restraint regarding concrete remarks on type, extent and time frame of a possible operation.

Surgical Management of Spinal Diseases with Reference to MRI

Objectives underlying operative management can include:

- Removal of a pathological lesion (intervertebral disk prolapse, tumor, empyema, angioma, and the like).
- Stabilization of the either primarily unstable spine or the spine having become unstable after resection of the lesion.

Stabilizing surgery sometimes forms an integral part of a primary decompressive operation, e.g., in surgery for cervical disk prolapse. On the whole there is a general tendency with regard to stabilizing operations towards *instrumented spondylodesis*, with titanium finding increasing use as an implant system because of the imaging problems otherwise associated with MRI. *Reconstructive procedures* for maintaining joint function ("disk replacement") are still undergoing clinical trials.

Cervical Intervertebral Disk Prolapse

MRI is optimal for detecting a soft-disk prolapse and anterior narrowing of the spinal canal or intervertebral foramina by marginal osteophyte formation in the form of a "hard" disk prolapse. The aim of surgery is decompression of the nerve root(s) or the spinal cord. Even if the main feature of the clinical picture is a radicular lesion or cervical myelopathy, equal attention should be paid during surgery not only to sufficient radicular but also medullary decompression.

Anterior diskectomy has become an extremely standardized operation, free of complications, particularly for a "soft" or sequestrated disk prolapse. The removal of bony ridging in a dorsal and, above all, lateral direction (Fig. 2.1) in the form of an *uncoforaminotomy* is technically more difficult, but the consequential use of this procedure has ultimately optimized treatment results.

The use of (high-speed) burrs, however, often produces *metal abrasion* from the burr or the metal suction probes, which is highly apparent *in situ* as artifacts on postoperative MRI follow-up studies. For this reason a CT scan may be preferable in some cases for a reliable postoperative confirmation of adequate decompression. Interposition material used for interbody spondylodesis can also give rise to further artifacts. The use of a round *Cloward bone dowel* has been largely abandoned for reasons of stability in favor of the Smith and Robinson horseshoe-shaped *tricortical iliac crest bone graft* (Fig. 2.2), with the implants secured by an *anterior metal plate* (e.g., the methods of Caspar, Orozko) (Fig. 2.3).

Screw fixation systems where the *screws are rigidly fixed to the plate* (Morscher plate, ACP plate, Atlantis plate) are also enjoying increasing use. However, these plates are thicker and therefore produce artifact effects. This technique has been modified by the interposition of *polymethyl-*

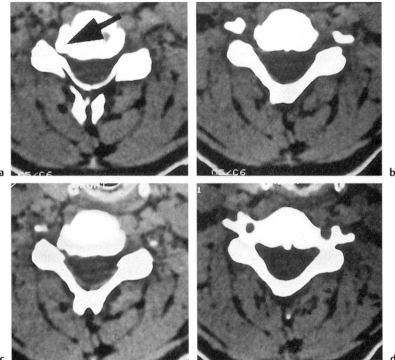

Fig. 2.**1 a–d   Small osteophyte of the cervical spine
(arrow) located exactly in
the intervertebral foramen
and giving rise to radicular symptoms**. Removal
was made via a so-called
anterior uncoforaminotomy.

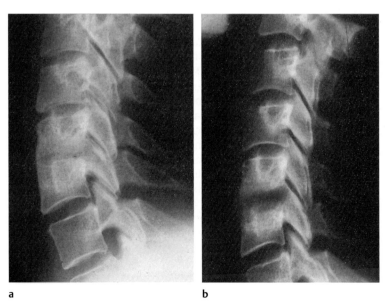

Fig. 2.**2 a, b   Solid bony fusion of the C4/C5 seg-
ment:**
a Postoperative film after
  nucleotomy and insertion
  of an autologous Smith-
  Robinson bone dowel.
b Preoperative state.

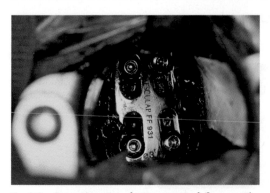

Fig. 2.3 **Operative site during cervical fusion.** The Caspar plate is seen deep down, stably fixed to the cervical spine by screws.

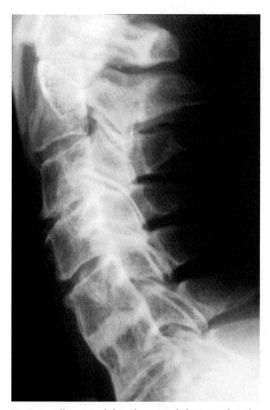

Fig. 2.4 **Fully consolidated cervical fusion of C5/6.** Here polymethylmethacrylate (PMMA) was used as a spacer, often referred to clinically as a "dowel." Final fusion is not complete until years after surgery when the PMMA beads are covered on all sides by bone.

methacrylate (PMMA, e.g., Palacos or Sulfix) (Fig. 2.**4**), *titanium* and *carbon fibers* and, albeit rarely, is even used without fusion (with the risk of later kyphosis formation of the cervical spine). Interposition materials can also give rise to artifacts on postoperative follow-up scans (Figs. 2.**5** and 2.**6**).

For long-segment stenosis of the cervical spinal canal associated with myelopathy, *vertebral replacement* is increasingly preferred as a technically simpler operation that facilitates extensive decompression of the spinal canal. An iliac crest bone graft, Harms titanium cage (Fig. 2.**23**) and, less frequently, carbon fibers can be used as interposition materials. The procedure is being increasingly employed for the management of OPLL syndrome (ossification of the posterior longitudinal ligament), which occurs frequently, and primarily in Japan, but less often in Germany where it will sometimes be seen as a diagnostic pitfall.

It is essential to establish a diagnosis because of the marked adhesions present between this calcified longitudinal ligament and the dura. Dural tears can appear during resection of the space-occupying mass, so the occurrence of CSF accumulations should be looked for after surgery.

Adequate documentation is important after diagnosing any cervical spine deformity (kyphosis?) or its correction after surgery. For technical reasons the width of the spinal canal can be underestimated on T2-weighted images so that T1-weighted sections should be used for an anatomically correct assessment. Because MR imaging is generally insufficient in depicting bone, the extent of the stenosis can be better assessed on a supplementary CT scan. Dorsal narrowing of the myelon by infolded ligamenta flava is only detectable by MRI on sagittal sections. This narrowing can be surgically corrected by holding the motion segment apart with some form of interposition material, which will require monitoring on follow-up scans after surgery. At times, only MRI will allow the diagnosis of marked diskoligamentous stenoses of the cervical spinal canal on inclination, so that with clinically unequivocal symptoms, but initially inadequate findings, only a view of the cervical spine in maximum anteflexion will provide the exclusion diagnosis of stenosis of the cervical spinal canal.

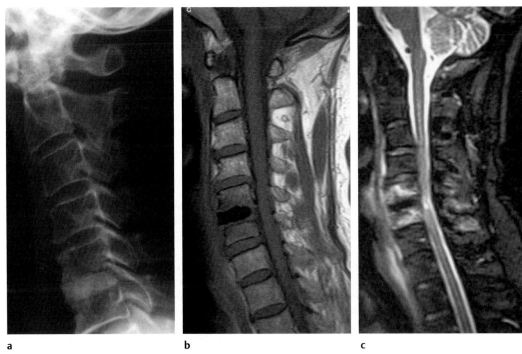

a   b   c

Fig. 2.**5 a–c** **Implantation of a Sulfix dowel:**
a Finding after implantation of a Sulfix dowel as a re-placement for the removed disk C5/6.
b Note the typical signaling on the T1-weighted image.

c The changes on the T2-weighted image are typical for long-term reactions in the adjacent vertebrae, which can demonstrate marrow edema and fatty marrow formation and cause local symptoms.

Fig. 2.**6 a–e** **Formation of artifacts after implanta-** ▷ **tion of titanium spacers in the intervertebral cavity during surgery for stenosis of the cervical spinal canal secondary to osteochondrotic ridging at the C5/6/7 level:**
a The spinal canal can still be assessed despite the arti-facts.

Fig. 2.**6 b–e**   p. 37

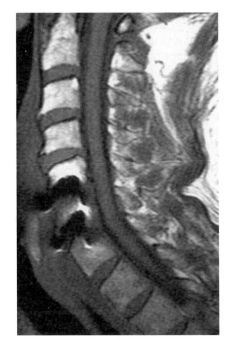

Operative technique of anterior operations on the cervical spine

Since most pathological changes associated with degenerative disorders of the cervical spine lie anterior to the spinal cord and nerve roots, an anterior procedure is more efficient and less hazardous than a posterior operation in the vast majority of cases. Nearly every patient dreads the risk of spinal cord paralysis during surgery, an unjustified fear given the performance statistics from experienced surgeons. Even in extreme spinal stenosis, deterioration secondary to surgery is exceedingly rare provided the correct operative technique is used, and when it does occur then obvious risk factors are most likely involved (angiopathy, cardiopulmonary decompensation).

A transverse median skin incision is placed two-thirds off midline towards the side of the operative site. The side of approach is often merely a question of the surgeon's handedness rather than one of, for example, the location of the prolapse. After dividing the platysma longitudinally, blunt dissection is carried down, displacing the trachea and esophagus medially (*take care*: there is risk of injury; watch for air collections after surgery as an indication of infection secondary to perforation) while the neurovascular bundle (carotid artery, jugular vein, vagus nerve) is displaced laterally. After division of the deep cervical fascia, access is gained to the anterior aspect of the cervical spine; the longus colli muscle is detached on either side and then the actual procedure on the cervical spine is performed:

For diskectomy, the intervertebral disk is incised and the disk space cleared, taking care to remove all cartilage remains from the adjacent end plates of the cervical vertebrae. Expansion screws are inserted into the adjoining vertebral bodies to assist in distracting the vertebrae. Under magnification, diskal tissue is now removed completely, after which the dorsal marginal rims are undercut with a spherical burr. After this, disk sequesters can be removed if this has not already been done during the initial clearance of the interspace. The longitudinal ligament is now resected with foot-plated bone punches, which should have no space-occupying effect. The vertebral margins are also removed if they are compromising the spinal canal. In cases of

sequestered disk protrusion, the sequesters are removed during resection of the longitudinal ligament. Here exploration by palpation is sometimes necessary far laterally into the intervertebral foramen (Fig. 2.**7**).

If compressive infraforaminal ridges are present, they must be carefully removed in a lateral direction while strictly protecting the roots. This allows complete decompression of the roots far laterally along the entire extent of the root canal (so-called uncoforaminotomy). This part of the operation can be technically very demanding, but it is the only possible way of immediately and effectively restoring normal width to the neuroforamen (Fig. 2.**8**). This method allows decompression of the nerve roots over several levels in the severely degenerative cervical spine. Usually an interpositional implant is then inserted to achieve fusion of the adjacent vertebrae. The following implants are used:

- autologous bone,
- titanium spacer (Figs. 2.**9** and 2.**10**),
- carbon fibers in various prefabricated geometric forms,
- synthetic materials (PMMA, e.g., Palacos or Sulfix), which cure *in situ*.

Treatment of cervical myelopathy can proceed in a segmental fashion using the technique already described (Fig. 2.**11**), although in cases of marked osteophytic ridging over several levels it may be less hazardous and more efficient to remove one or more vertebrae to eliminate the stenosis.

Vertebral body replacement is then performed using autologous bone, if necessary in combination with a Harms titanium mesh cage or a carbon-fiber spacer. Finally, plate fixation of the bridged segment is performed.

As a rule, dissection of the vertebral artery is not necessary, even if the vertebral canal has been opened during the uncoforaminotomy mentioned above. With severe osteophytic ridging, even laterally, resection of the uncus and its marginal osteophyte automatically results in decompression of the displaced vertebral artery. There is general disagreement over the likelihood of these marginal osteophytes actually compromising vertebrobasilar circulation.

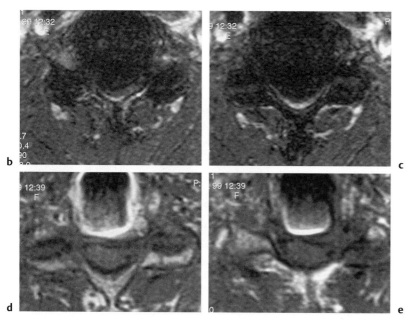

b

c

d

e

Fig. 2.**6 b–e** The extent of the artifact effect depends on the sequences selected and, particularly in the axial sequences, can have considerable influence (**b**, **c**) or hardly any at all (**d**, **e**).

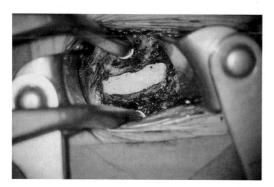

Fig. 2.**7** **Operative site during fusion of the cervical spine.** Note the exposed intervertebral space. The dura is covered by a thin strip of hemostatic agent.

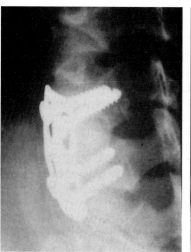

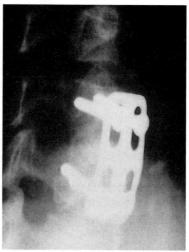

a

b

Fig. 2.**8 a, b** **Oblique views of the cervical spine after arthrodesis and fixation with a Caspar plate.** A burr was used to completely clear the foramina in the fused segment.

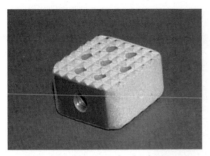

Fig. 2.**9** **Titanium interbody device.**

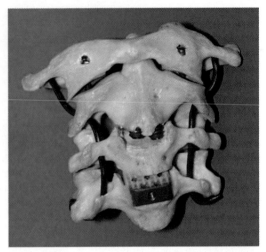

Fig. 2.**10** **Anatomical preparation of the upper cervical spine with titanium interbody device as a disk replacement between C3 and C4.** The heads of two titanium screws are seen at the inferior edge of C2, i.e. the base of the dens, which have been inserted from an anterior direction in a fashion similar to that of odontoid screw fixation. The lateral masses of C1 (the axis) have been perforated by the tips of the screws, as with Magerl's method of screw insertion for transarticular C1/C2 screw fixation.

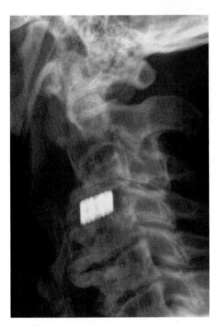

◁ Fig. 2.**11** **Titanium implant as an interbody spacer for cervical arthrodesis** (Cervidisk, made by Weber, Germany).

Lumbar Intervertebral Disk Prolapse/Degenerative Diseases of the Lumbar Spine

Soft intervertebral disk prolapse is usually the cause of lumbar radicular syndromes, with stenosis of the lateral recess and vertebral canal more frequently contributing to root compression. The diagnostic work-up is directed towards locating site and extent of the radicular compression. The management of disk protrusion or sequestered prolapse is not difficult if microsurgical technique is used; after a usually very limited *interlaminar foraminotomy*, removal of the sequester and sub-

sequent *nucleotomy* are performed with the intention of preventing recurrence by removing the degenerated disk elements as thoroughly as possible. By using as small a microsurgical approach as possible and replacing the epidural fat, an attempt is made to keep postoperative scarring to a minimum. One advantage is that this technique of open diskectomy allows the elimination of bony stenoses, often with only slight variations of the procedure as will be described later under stenoses of the spinal canal.

The procedure becomes technically more difficult if *extra- and intraforaminal prolapses* are present, in which case an intertransverse approach is used (i.e., also from a dorsal direction, but reaching further laterally as far as the transverse processes). Because the nerve is not protected by fat present in the epidural space to act as a gliding tissue after it enters the foramen, scar formation, which is detectable on MRI, is more likely to occur after these types of disk prolapse, subsequently giving rise to nerve root irritations. Only the administration of contrast medium will permit differentiation between scar tissue and recurrent prolapse with a fair amount of certainty in these cases.

The operation also becomes more difficult in the (very rare) presence of *intradural sequester formations* where the procedure is often similar to that for an intradural tumor. Endoscopic operative techniques are currently being tested with the aim of minimizing operative trauma. They can also be used for sequestered prolapses, but they hardly allow any additional bony decompression.

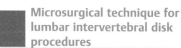

Microsurgical technique for lumbar intervertebral disk procedures

The patient is placed in the prone position, usually modified by a more or less pronounced knee-chest position. After confirmation of the correct level with an image intensifier a small, usually longitudinal, incision is made and the fascia split. The muscles are eased off the midline and a microsurgical self-retaining retractor is inserted (the approach is usually roughly finger-shaped). The ligamentum flavum is resected; at the level L5/S1 it can often be preserved. Bone is sparingly removed cranially and laterally, just enough to expose the root, which is usually displaced upwards by the prolapse. The procedure is referred to as interlaminar foraminotomy. The protrusion or sequester(s) is now identified below the root, i.e., anteriorly. Sequesters are removed first, the disk itself is incised and removed as completely as possible with the aid of grasping forceps. At the end of the operation the epidural fat, which was removed or displaced previously during root dissection, is replaced (for scar prevention).

Recess Stenosis and Spinal Canal Stenosis

Degeneration of the intervertebral disk results in the familiar loss of disk-space height. This collapse leads to increased joint degeneration and consequently to secondary stenosis of the spinal canal due to joint hypertrophy, culminating in a T-shaped narrowing. The collapse itself also gives rise to foraminal stenosis (Fig. 2.**12**).

If this process is monosegmental, it will result in the long-known *isolated disk resorption syndrome*, which is an almost regular occurrence, particularly after a diskitis. Apart from stenosis of the intervertebral foramina and the spinal canal, there is also disturbance in motility of the disk segment. Overloading of the adjacent vertebrae often leads to transformation of blood-forming bone marrow into fatty marrow in the areas immediately adjacent to the affected disk. Such segments are readily diagnosed from the increased signal intensity of fat; they are always a sign of a so-called instability which is basically the indication for performing spondylodesis, although this should not be confused with the type of instability as defined by traumatologists.

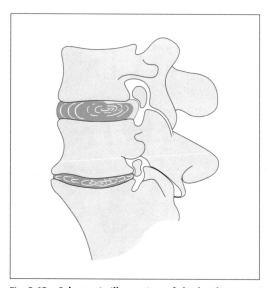

Fig. 2.**12   Schematic illustration of the lumbar spine showing root compression due to collapse of the interspace and subsequent degeneration of the joints secondary to the increased loading.**

Apart from the pathogenetic mechanism mentioned above, *spinal canal stenosis,* i.e., the pathological reduction in diameter of the lumbar spinal canal, is also enhanced even further by hypertrophy of the ligaments, most notably the ligamenta flava, which probably occurs as a reaction to the altered micromovements in the segment and results in a distinct additional narrowing of the spinal canal. Apart from the familiar radicular syndromes, claudicatio spinalis can develop secondary to the reduction in diameter of the spinal canal. This clinical picture presents with weakness of the legs during exercise and lumbar lordosis, or even with definite sensory symptoms, resulting in a reduced walking distance. Due to the postural kyphosis taken on when riding a bicycle, patients with claudicatio spinalis can usually cycle without restriction, which is not the case with intermittent claudication of vascular origin.

The therapy of choice is surgical decompression to widen the foramina or spinal canal. There are no therapeutic alternatives, with the exception perhaps of expectant observation of the spontaneous course supported by conservative treatment. Whereas years ago *laminectomies* where performed, often with the result of producing something similar to a "trough with straight walls," an attempt is made today to be as

least invasive as possible with regard to the stability of the spine. If at all, laminectomies are done very narrowly and centered on the midline, the vertebral arches are then undermined laterally in a trapezoid fashion. A technique better suited for maintaining stability, so-called *undercutting decompression,* involves preserving the spinous processes and the interspinous ligament so that the dorsal tension-band effect of the lumbar spine is not compromised (Fig. 2.**13**).

The vertebral arches are not resected but undercut. This is ideally done via several extended interlaminar foraminotomies. This procedure is ideal for maintaining stability, but unfortunately for this very reason it is most time-consuming if performed over several segments.

Technique of decompression for recess stenosis and undercutting decompression for lumbar spinal stenosis

Exposure of the spine is either monosegmental, as described under lumbar disk surgery, or multisegmental with bilateral retraction of the muscles and insertion of laminectomy retractors. The hypertrophied bony elements of the vertebral arch and joint overlying the ligamentum flavum can be removed with a spherical burr. The inner cortex of the vertebral arch is exposed by cutting out the cancellous bone, which is then removed with a very fine foot-plated bone punch without further narrowing the spinal canal. Then, using microscopy, the roots are dissected and decompressed laterally, alternating between a grinding and punching technique. This way, often considerable amounts of overhanging parts of the joint surfaces are removed. For this part of the dissection small dental chisels and curved sharp curets (for the ligamenta flava) are sometimes used; special curved bone punches allow decompression far laterally into the foramen. The areas of bone to be removed are shown in Fig. 2.**13**. The multisegmental use of this technique allows treatment of stenosis of the lumbar spine. The advantage of laminectomy lies in its faster operability and—particularly important with the elderly—little risk of injury to the dura with subsequent CSF leakage.

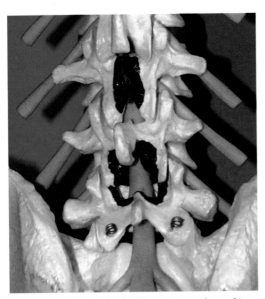

Fig. 2.**13 Model of the lumbar spine with markings indicating the removed bone after laminectomy (above) and after undercutting (below).**

Stabilizing procedures can also be used as an alternative or a supplement to this decompressive procedure, with *spondylodesis augmented by transpedicular instrumentation* having established itself as the method of choice (Figs. 2.**14**–2.**17**).

Bony bridging over the entire length of the fusion is necessary for a secure spondylodesis. Whereas in the past it was even more common to regard posterolateral sections of bone graft inserted intertransversally and in the joint region as sufficient, there is a preference nowadays for interbody fusion (Fig. 2.**18**).

This can be done from an anterior (ALIF = anterior lumbar interbody fusion) or a dorsal approach (PLIF = posterior lumbar interbody fusion), although there is a tendency towards the posterior technique because of the invasive nature of anterior approaches. Increasing use is being made of *cages*, i.e., hollow cylindrical devices made of titanium, carbon, or the like, filled with cancellous bone (or sometimes with bone-replacement material such as tricalcium phosphate or calcium hydroxylapatite), which are introduced into the disk interspace after nucleotomy (Fig. 2.**19**). Anterior approaches for endoscopic spondylodesis are also enjoying increasing use.

Chemonucleolysis and *PLDD (percutaneous laser disk decompression)* may also be regarded as

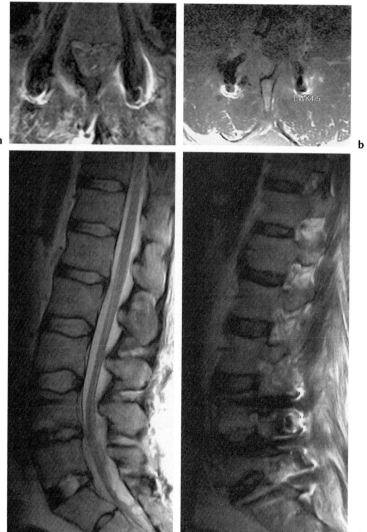

Fig. 2.**14 a–d Artifacts after implantation of a titan rod system with pedicle screws:**

a, b Sometimes the spinal canal appears assessable (**a**), while in (**b**) visibility is impaired by the formation of artifacts.

c, d Evaluation is usually also possible in the mid-sagittal section (**c**), not in the paravertebral slice orientation (**d**).

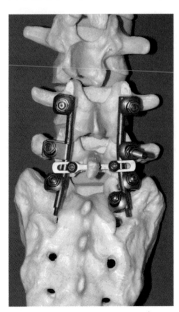

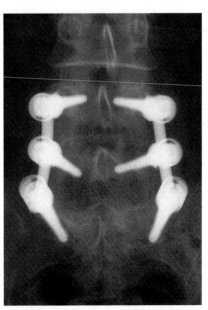

Fig. 2.**15 Model of the lumbar spine with transpedicular screwing of L4/5 and S1.** The pedicle screws are typically connected by longitudinal rods and both longitudinal rows connected by a transverse rod (Tenor-Titan-System, Sofamor-Danek company).

Fig. 2.**16 X-ray picture of instrumented spondylodesis of L4-S1 fixed with transpedicular titanium screws**. AP view (Diapason-System, Stryker corporation).

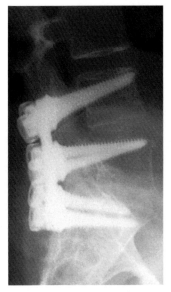

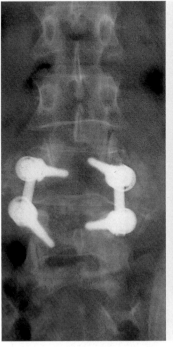

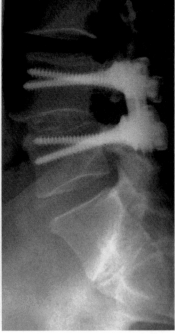

Fig. 2.**17 X-ray picture of instrumented spondylodesis of L4-S1 fixed with transpedicular titanium screws**. Lateral view (Diapason-System, Stryker corporation).

a

b

Fig. 2.**18 a, b** X-ray picture of monosegmental instrumented spondylodesis of L4/5. The bone material has been inserted from a dorsal approach (PLIF) and is easily recognized on the lateral projection (Diapason-System, Stryker corporation).

operative procedures, albeit less invasive. The aim of both techniques is to destroy the nucleus pulposus and thus reduce intradiskal pressure. The problem is that, although these procedures do not cause scar-tissue formation around the nerve root, the resorbed-disk mechanism can still progress at an accelerated rate. The indication for these procedures should therefore be defined as strictly as for the open operation. A major problem for postoperative MRI diagnostics is persisting and recurrent pain after disk surgery. Causes include recurrent prolapse, scar-tissue formation and stenosis (see above). Differentiation between recurrent prolapse and scar-tissue formation is possible using MRI supplemented by the administration of contrast medium, where contrast uptake is only seen with scar-tissue formation and not with recurrent prolapse. Apart from clinical signs (characteristic being above all tenderness on percussion of the heels), a spondylodiskitis will display distinct changes of the adjacent vertebrae on MRI.

Functional diagnostics of the lumbar spine using MRI is unfortunately still confined to experimental studies. In the long term, however, the option of assessing the lumbar spine while standing, during weight bearing and in a functional position without the need of myelography would certainly be enormously helpful in assessing segmental disturbances of motility and those stenoses otherwise only detectable during weight bearing.

Failed Back Surgery Syndrome (Post Diskectomy Syndrome)

The term post diskectomy syndrome is more frequently, yet not quite correctly, used to describe a clinical picture in which persistent symp-

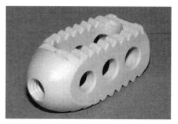

Fig. 2.**19** **Synthetic hollow device ("cage") designed to be filled with autologous cancellous bone as an interbody implant for fusion of two vertebrae.**

toms prevail after surgery of the lumbar spine. Failed back surgery syndrome is a more accurate description. With regard to MRI, it is not a diagnosis but a challenge:

Nowadays it is possible to secure the diagnosis of a whole array of these specifically treatable clinical entities and offer individual patients considerably better prospects of a positive therapeutic outcome for this symptom complex, which would otherwise be very difficult to address:

- persistent recess stenosis,
- recurrent prolapse—scarring, possibly with distortion of the dural tube (Fig. 2.**20**),
- synovial cysts with a space-occupying effect,
- resorbed disk with foraminal stenosis; CSF leakage and accumulation, spondylolysis, etc.

Spondylolisthesis

A cleft in the pedicles, or spondylolysis, usually results in *vertebral slippage*, or spondylolisthesis. If the intervertebral disk undergoes degeneration as a result of the increased load and prolapse occurs, *nucleotomy* alone can prove successful, depending on the age of the patient and the degree

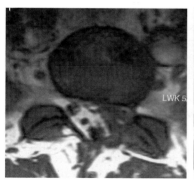
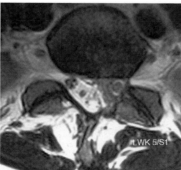

Fig. 2.**20 a, b** **Postoperative images of the L5/S1 segment after microsurgical interlaminar foraminotomy and removal of a sequestered disk prolapse.** "Normal" scarring, asymptomatic with regard to this segment.

a   b

of degenerative changes of the segment, but *primary spondylodesis* (with reduction of the spondylolisthesis performed for biomechanical reasons) appears safer in the long term. The technique is identical to that of transpedicular spondylodesis with interbody fusion (posterior or anterior approach) as outlined above. After solid bony fusion, the often large spondylolytic area of scar formation responsible for the sometimes immense compression of the nerve root will disappear and the segmental instability of the spine secondary to disruption of the joint chain is also removed.

Opinions remain divided regarding the timing of surgery, but it seems agreed that an immediate and more extensive approach is, in the long run, less invasive in terms of disease sequelae, particularly with young patients.

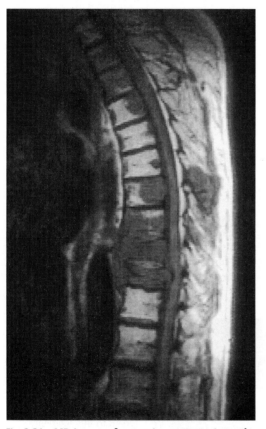

Fig. 2.**21** **MR image of extensive metastasis to the spine on the mid-sagittal section.** It is obvious here that a stabilization procedure will have to bridge four vertebrae, apart from the collapsed vertebrae responsible for the symptoms of a transverse spinal lesion. More vertebral metastases further cranially show the limitations of any possible measures.

Spinal Tumors

Here the most common lesions are metastases from malignant tumors. From an operative view, expeditious diagnostics is crucial once symptoms of a transverse spinal lesion have become apparent. Usually it is necessary to proceed on the assumption of an emergency situation because it is often difficult to assess how rapidly the symptoms will deteriorate once they have begun. Moreover, since a prudent decision on the indication for surgery can only be reached with full knowledge of the overall oncological situation, for which purpose supplementary diagnostic measures may be required, it is essential that no time is lost in reaching the primary diagnosis. Equipment-based diagnostics must be conducted under emergency conditions. Furthermore, even when the precise location of the lesion responsible for the clinical symptoms is known, comprehensive MRI examination of the axial skeleton is generally required to inform the decision about the indication for surgery. Should the whole spine reveal numerous metastases, instrumentation may no longer be possible or only feasible over a very long segment (Fig. 2.**21**).

Operative intervention is always indicated if it is considered prudent from an oncological view and decompression or stabilization is essential and practicable. After removal of one or several of the affected vertebrae, replacement is usually undertaken with an appropriate interbody device (Fig. 2.**22**). Dorsal rod systems with transpedicular fixation are usually used for stabilization in the region of the thoracic and cervical spines, as already outlined for operations of the lumbar spine. Modified plate systems are also used, but less frequently (Fig. 2.**22**).

An indication for surgery is less likely to be defined in the presence of *small-cell bronchial carcinoma* or *prostatic carcinoma*, where preference is given to other therapeutic procedures; only rarely is an operation performed with the aim of decompressing neural structures and thus gaining time for systemic or radiation therapy. It is important to have already differentiated *renal cell carcinoma* from similar disorders before surgery. Because of the marked hemorrhagic tendency of this type of tumor with the risk of massive intraoperative blood loss, it is imperative that preoperative embolization is performed. A parallel pre-contrast plane x-ray is always advisable for comparison in order to recognize *osteoplastic metastases* as such.

The use of *metallic implants* makes the post-operative assessment of MR images more difficult so that scout views should be obtained as a base-line for further follow-ups if, in the event of tumor recurrence, therapeutic consequences are to be expected from an oncological view (Fig. 2.**23**).

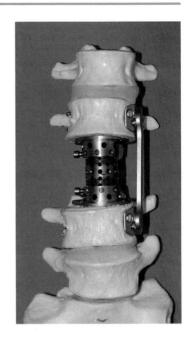

Fig. 2.**22   Model of the lumbar spine showing verte-** ▷
bral body replacement using an interbody spacer and fixation by a laterally mounted system (LID- and LIFT-Titanium System, Sofamor-Danek company).

Fig. 2.**23 a–d   Effects on imaging by titanium inter-** ▷
body devices in the cervical spine:
a   Metastasis to C4.
b–d Finding after stabilization using Harms titanium cage and a titanium plate (ACP system, Codman company).

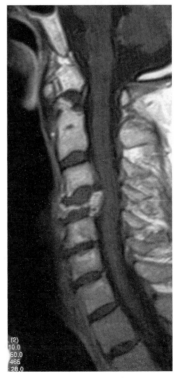

a

Fig. 2.**23 b–d** ▷

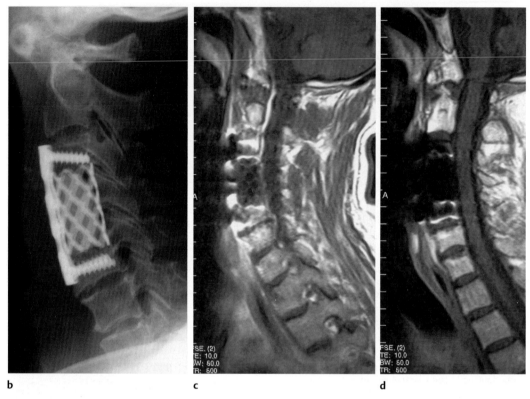

b   **c**   **d**

Fig. 2.**23 b–d**   Plain radiograph (**b**) and MR image (**c**, **d**) with different artifact formations.

Intraspinal Tumors

The operative technique to expose the spinal canal is different here. Approaches that maintain the anatomy are used more commonly in the form of *hemilaminectomies* or *laminoplasties*, where the resected arches are replaced and fixed with sutures, wirings or small titanium fixation plates. Metal implants must be applied sparingly, however, in order not to weaken the diagnostic reliability of postoperative follow-up imaging (Figs. 2.**24** and 2.**25**).

Extramedullary Tumors

Meningiomas and schwannomas (neurilem-momas, neurinomas) predominate in this tumor group. Their relation to the bony anatomy is decisively important for preoperative planning (see above).

Schwannomas must be assigned precisely to their nerve roots of origin in order to assess, in the case of clinically relevant nerve roots, the possible risk and consequences of producing a radicular lesion by resecting the tumor. Especially with large and predominantly extraspinal schwannomas (Fig. 2.**26**) it may also be wise to supplement the initial planning of the surgical approach by outlining the course of adjacent major arteries (e.g., vertebral artery in the region of the cervical spine) with the aid of MR angiographies. The paravertebral components of the schwannoma, which are often severely degenerated, can be removed easily via a purely dorsal paravertebral access, even if they do extend, sometimes far, into the thorax (Figs. 2.**27** and 2.**28**).

It is important, especially with *meningiomas*, to use CT imaging to gain some idea of their degree of calcification. A severely calcified tumor that can only be reduced in size instrumentally with great difficulty and where manipulation of the tumor is to be avoided due to contact with the compressed cord, can otherwise lead to unantici-

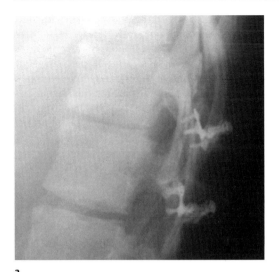

a

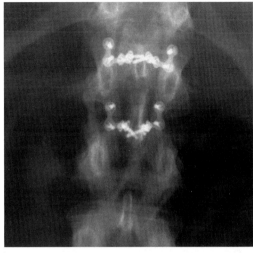

b

Fig. 2.**24 a, b X-ray findings after surgery of an ependymoma using two-level laminotomy and lami-** noplasty. The titanium interbody devices are used for refixation of the vertebral arch removed during surgery.

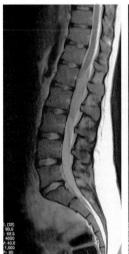

a

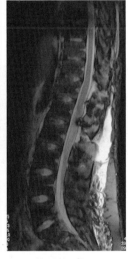

b

c

Fig. 2.**25 a–e Effect of the implants on postoperative follow-up MR images after laminoplasty:**

a   Depiction of the ependymoma at the level L1 and L2 before surgery.

b   Minor artifact forma-tion on the mid-sagit-tal section.

c   Frank artifact forma-tion from the titanium mini-plates in the sec-tion planes just lateral to it.

d, e   The artifacts have only a marginal effect on the axial sections.

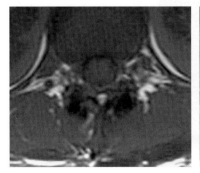

d

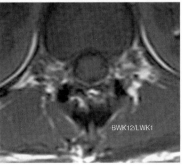

e

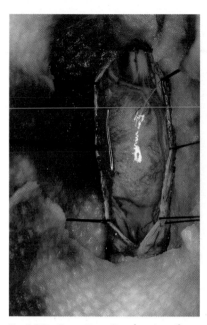

Fig. 2.26   Operative site showing the removal of a schwannoma at the level T10.   The tumor also extends far intraforaminally.

pated difficulties during removal. The characterization of a meningioma must always include an exact topographic description of any possible meningeal sign. In a significant percentage of cases, infiltrations of the meningioma are found in the dural regions displaying this signal behavior so that this information obtained from MRI must be taken into account when planning the operative approach.

Intramedullary Tumors and Syringomyelia

This tumor group, in particular, is considerably better detected nowadays during preoperative imaging than previously, and, for the first time, with the aid of MRI can be reliably and directly demonstrated. *Contrast medium administration* is an essential part of diagnostics, as is *obtaining sagittal and transversal sections*; the former for a reliable depiction of the tumor margins, the latter in order to appreciate intraoperatively the extent of the tumor in the cross-section of the spinal

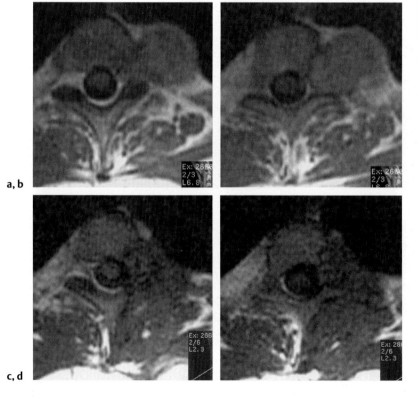

a, b

c, d

Fig. 2.**27 a–d   Thoracic hourglass schwannoma, partially extending into the thoracic cavity**:
a, b   Axial MRI sections before tumor extirpation.
c, d   Axial MRI sections after tumor extirpation.

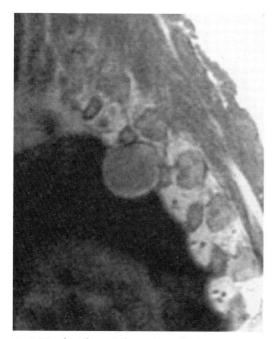 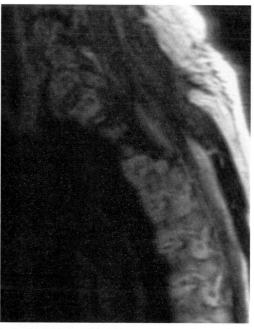

Fig. 2.28 a, b Thoracic hourglass schwannoma.
a Sagittal section before tumor extirpation from a dorsal approach.

b Sagittal section after tumor extirpation from a dorsal approach.

cord, because only this way is complete removal possible—provided of course that this is at all feasible as with, for example, an ependymoma.

After surgery, a *"baseline MRI"* is essential and should be performed about 3 months postoperatively after surgery-related changes on the image have settled. It will be used during tumor follow-up care as a baseline for comparisons with later images.

In the presence of *syringomyelia* it is mandatory, with the aid of contrast medium, to rule out an intramedullary tumor as its cause, particularly in the marginal areas of the syrinx. If an intramedullary tumor is not found as the cause of syringomyelia, then an active search must be made for malformations of the craniocervical junction (Arnold–Chiari malformation, basilar impression) or other stenosing processes in this area, if necessary, by widening the scope of the examination. The most common operative procedure for syringomyelia associated with an Arnold–Chiari malformation is decompression of the medulla in the foramen magnum by limited *occipital craniectomy* and resection of the arch of the atlas, followed by an *augmentation duraplasty*. If duraplasty is done using synthetic

material, then this material will easily show up on MRI. Successful drainage of the syrinx into the subarachnoid space via a very thin silicon tube can be monitored exclusively by MRI. Here it is important to demonstrate the correct position of the drain.

Changes at the Craniocervical Junction

Apart from malformations, tumors and sequelae of trauma (e.g., fracture nonunion of the dens), it is possible to optimally demonstrate rheumatic affects at the apex of the dens and, less frequently, at the atlanto-occipital joints. Dynamic imaging may be required in problematic cases to detect those stenoses that are purely motion-related. Especially in this region, MRI virtually has a diagnostic monopoly as regards the neural structures of the brain stem and upper cervical cord, so the use of titanium for instrumentation is almost obligatory—an assessment of the neural structures in the mid-sagittal plane of section is then usually still possible despite the sometimes larger implants.

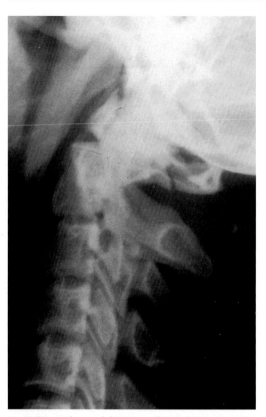

Fig. 2.**29** **Dislocated fracture of the dens**. Lateral X-ray film.

Among the special *stabilization techniques* used in the region of the craniocervical junction, mention should be made of:

- anterior odontoid screw fixation,
- posterior C1/C2 transarticular screw fixation supplemented with posterior cerclage wiring,
- craniocervical stabilization using a plate system fixed to the vertebral arches by cerclage wires or into the joint facets by screws.

Technique of anterior odontoid screw fixation

Type II dens fractures are the main indication for using this procedure. Once the patient has been positioned prone with head fixation, a conventional anterior approach is made to the cervical spine at approximately the C 5/C6 level. After exposing the inferior edge of C2, two guide wires are inserted into the dens before the fragment of the apex is fixed to the base of the dens with one or two screws. Several special-purpose instruments facilitate this technically complicated operation. (Figs. 2.**10**, 2.**29** and 2.**30**).

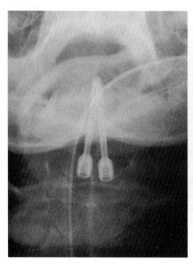

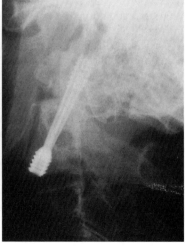

Fig. 2.**30 a, b** **X-ray spot film of the dens of the axis with anterior odontoid screw fixation after fracture**. Two double-threaded screws have been inserted into the dens of the axis:
a AP view.
b Lateral view.

a

b

Technique of posterior C1/C2 screw fixation and cerclage wiring

The oldest form of surgical C1/C2 stabilization is *cerclage wiring* with its many modifications. It is nowadays only rarely indicated as a sole form of instrumentation (Figs. 2.**31** and 2.**32**). The original variations, as described by Gallie and Brooks, proved to be mechanically too unstable, although they were used for many years, mainly for instabilities secondary to rheumatic destruction of the atlanto-occipital joints (Fig. 2.**33**). The most stable form according to biomechanical testing is the so-called *"BNI fusion" after Sonntag*, employing cerclage wiring of the C1 arch and passing the wire beneath the C2 spinous process (Fig. 2.**34**).

The *C1/C2 transarticular screw fixation* was first performed by *Magerl* and uses a dorsal approach with the patient positioned prone. The craniocervical junction is exposed, after which a drill hole is placed using a long twist drill, beginning at the inferior edge of the C2 arch directly medial to the joint surface and directed in a strictly sagittal alignment through the C1/C2 articular surface towards the anterior arch of the atlas which is recognizable on the lateral x-ray view. After placing a drill hole on the contralateral side, the wire is then substituted by an appropriately long cancellous screw. Supplementary cerclage wiring is performed, preferably using the BNI technique (Fig. 2.**34**). This combination produces the stablest form of fixation in this otherwise remarkably mobile spinal segment (Figs. 2.**35** and 2.**36**).

There are older techniques as alternatives to this procedure, using specially configured clamps for fixing the arches together. These include:

- the Halifax clamp (Fig. 2.**37**),
- the Roosen clamp (Fig. 2.**38**).

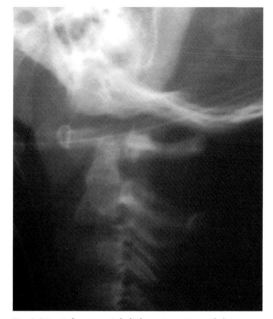

Fig. 2.**31** **Atlanto-axial dislocation.** Tear of the transverse ligament of the atlas and the alar ligaments due to trauma in a 3-year-old boy. Lateral x-ray view of the craniocervical junction.

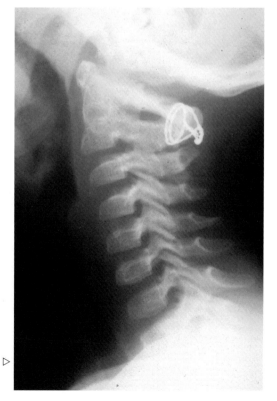

Fig. 2.**32** **Finding immediately after cerclage wiring** ▷ **to prevent secondary neurological deficits.** Only hemiparesis was present initially.

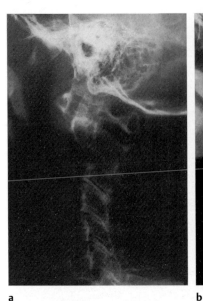
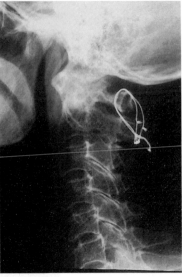

a b

Fig. 2.**33 a, b Rheumatoid atlanto-axial dislocation.** Stabilization with C1/C2 wiring. Lateral x-ray view.

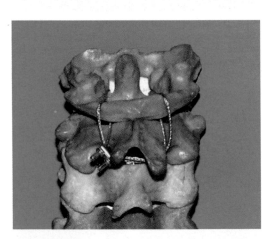

Fig. 2.**34 Model of the upper cervical spine with C1/C2 cerclage wiring as a "BNI fusion" according to Sonntag.** (BNI = Barrow Neurological Institute, Phoenix). The corresponding osseous interposition graft for completion of the arthrodesis has been omitted.

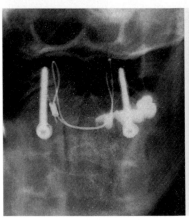
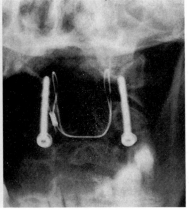

a b

Fig. 2.**35 a, b Transarticular C1/C2 screw fixation plus "BNI cerclage" for rheumatoid atlanto-axial instability with pannus formation dorsal to the axis of the dens.**
a Before transoral dens resection for complete decompression of the spinal cord.
b After transoral dens resection for complete decompression of the spinal cord.

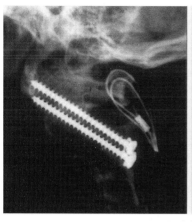 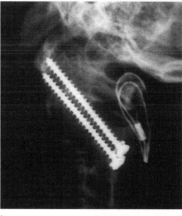

a   b

Fig. 2.**36 a, b** **Transarticular C1/C2 screw fixation plus "BNI cerclage" for rheumatoid atlanto-axial instability with pannus formation dorsal to the axis of the dens**.
a Before transoral dens resection for complete decompression of the spinal cord.
b After transoral dens resection for complete decompression of the spinal cord.

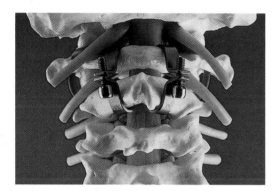

Fig. 2.**37** **Model of the upper cervical spine with C1/C2 fixation using Halifax clamps.**

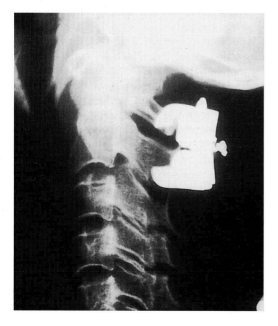

Fig. 2.**38** **Roosen clamp for fixation of C1/C2.** Lateral x-ray view of the craniocervical junction.

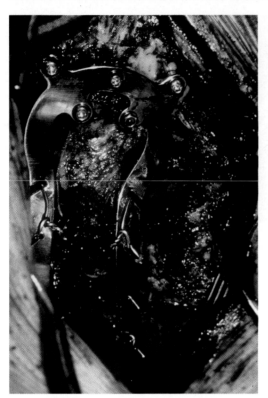

Fig. 2.**39** **Dorsal view of the operative site showing the dissected craniocervical junction with plate fixation for craniocervical stabilization** (Marburg plate according to Gschwend).

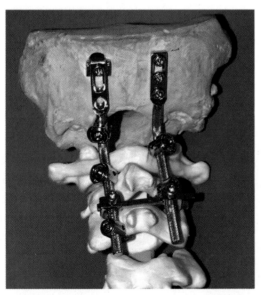

Fig. 2.**40** **Model of the craniocervical junction with fixation of a rod system to the occiput and vertebral arches of the upper cervical spine for arthrodesis.**

Technique of posterior craniocervical stabilization

After dissection of the occiput and the upper cervical spine, an omega-shaped metal plate or rod loop is fixed to the occiput with screws or cerclage wires (Fig. 2.**39**) and to the cervical spine using sublaminar wires. Because the wires which encroach on the spinal canal pose a direct threat to the spinal cord, instrument systems are now widely accepted in which a rod attached to the occiput by plates is fixed to the cervical spine by a screw driven through the joint facets and held by appropriately formed connecting pieces (Fig. 2.**40**).

Inflammatory Changes

In chronological order after clinical and then laboratory diagnostics, MRI is the first examination to enable the diagnosis of *diskitis secondary to disk surgery*. Because the pathogen is potentially less invasive, the clinical picture is not always diagnosed by the successful identification of an organism, particularly since abacterial diskitis is also possible in the form of an acute osteochondritis. Regeneration processes in the areas of the vertebral marrow adjacent to the disks are characteristic, while space-occupying abscess formations tracking anteriorly beneath the anterior longitudinal ligament are almost pathognomonic. Whereas the early stages of a diskitis are greatly amenable to conservative therapy, instrumented distraction spondylodesis is the method of choice for more advanced cases.

Primary inflammatory spondylodiskitis can be optimally diagnosed with the aid of MRI, particularly with regard to its anterior space-occupying effect. Eradication of the inflammatory focus is the primary goal of therapy, with operative relief and subsequent stabilization using autologous bone in a single session nowadays usually being the most promising therapeutic procedure, particularly for nonspecific changes that do not respond rapidly to antibiotics.

Tuberculous processes are more readily amenable to conservative treatment if there are no neurological disturbances and no relevant static changes threatening the spine. They can otherwise be rapidly and effectively treated by operative eradication of the focus, instrumented stabilization and implantation of autologous bone for spondylodesis.

Traumatic Changes

The diagnostics of trauma is still primarily the domain of radiographic techniques, given that fractured bony structures are optimally detected on plain radiographs and CT imaging. MRI is again the superior method for diagnosing space-occupying hematomas; it is unrivalled in diagnosing a *central cervical cord lesion* which is clinically seen relatively often in association with a pre-existing degenerative stenosis secondary to a relatively minor trauma. Even though the clinical picture of a distally accentuated motor and sensory disturbance of the upper, as opposed to the lower, extremities has a strong tendency to recover, disturbances of the dorsal column and relatively in-

tractable pain syndromes often remain. Initial diagnosis is very important, especially with regard to medicolegal questions. Because long-term sequelae are often difficult to demonstrate using imaging techniques, only documentation of the initial lesion will allow the specialist advisor to appreciate the later consequences of the injury. Therapy of this clinical picture is undergoing a process of change; until even recently, surgical intervention was considered contraindicated because subsequent neurological deterioration was often the result. The increasing and conscious use of atraumatic operative technique, with the application of vertebral body replacement where appropriate, allows prompt removal of the stenosis of the cervical spinal canal so that, ideally, postoperative edema only develops after decompression has been completed. Instrumented fusion should however be given preference, particularly in this situation.

Communication as a Problem of Diagnostics

Only an active exchange of information between those colleagues making the diagnosis and the surgeon will ensure that the "feed-back control system" of diagnostics and therapy really works. Rare findings must be passed on, including any special modifications of the operative technique if they could in any way have repercussions for

postoperative imaging. By using the simplest of means, cooperation in both directions of the dialogue between operative therapy and diagnostics will help in significantly optimizing the quality of the diagnostic process and consequently the quality of the result.

Summary

- For his operative planning, the neurosurgeon needs images that unequivocally allow a *topographic assignment* of the clinical findings.
- For this reason it must be possible to *count off each vertebral segment* on the images provided. This requires the inclusion on the image of either the craniocervical or the lumbosacral junction.
- It is imperative that *spinal lesions are displayed in two planes*, usually the sagittal and transverse planes, and in particular cases it will be necessary to provide additional images in a coronal scanning direction.
- The examiner should as far as possible provide a *specific diagnostic classification*.
- MRI has outstanding relevance in the emergency diagnostics of acute symptoms of a transverse spinal lesion, so that the imaging technique is required to be available at all times.
- In case a *spinal space-occupying lesion* is identified, the surgeon should be contacted immediately to make arrangements for, and to determine the urgency of, surgery.
- The examiner should be discreet about prognosis and exact details of therapy when informing the patient, but is called upon to explain the various *alternatives of treatment*.

- *Surgery of degenerative changes of the cervical spine* is usually performed using an anterior approach. Apart from clearing the disk space, including the cartilaginous elements of the end plates, the removal of any osteophytic bulges is also necessary. After that, fusion is undertaken, either with autologous bone, titanium or carbon fiber, less frequently with synthetic material.
- *Surgery of degenerative changes of the lumbar spine* is undertaken from a posterior approach, with removal of part of the ligamentum flavum and the posterior longitudinal ligament. This allows access to the disk space from which as large a portion as possible is removed.
- In the presence of *metastases*, the indication to operate is defined only after due consideration of the overall oncological situation.
- In the presence of metastases from a *small-cell bronchial carcinoma* or *prostatic carcinoma* there is less likely to be an indication to operate because alternatives are available in the form of chemo- and hormone therapy.
- *Changes at the craniocervical junction* may require a technically demanding anterior or posterior screw fixation.
- There may be an indication to operate in cases of *advanced spondylodiskitis*, with operative decompression and subsequent stabilization using autologous bone usually being the best procedure.

3 Malformations of the Spinal Canal

D. Uhlenbrock and D. Brechtelsbauer

Contents

This chapter will review disorders resulting from malformations of the midline. They can be associated with neurological, orthopedic and urological disturbances and sometimes require extensive surgery. Some of these patients will suffer permanent disability.

The majority of cases concern dysraphic malformations, although the slightly less common non-dysraphic malformations can also lead to disorders resulting from malformations of the midline. They too are classified under malformations of the spinal canal and will therefore also be dealt with here. Table 3.**1** provides an overview of the malformations.

Definition

Spinal dysraphism. Spinal dysraphism refers to disorders arising from a faulty development of the spine and spinal canal. Specifically they concern pathological connections of varying degrees of expression between bony structures, neuronal tissue and the subcutis or cutis. The spine itself usually exhibits disturbances of fusion as well as bony defects. Spinal dysraphism is classified into:

- open (spina bifida aperta) forms,
- closed (occult spinal dysraphism) forms.

Table 3.1   Malformations of the spinal canal

Dysraphic malformations:

Open spinal malformations
- myelocele
- myelomeningocele
- myelomeningocystocele
Closed spinal malformations
- meningocele
- spinal lipoma
- lipomyelomeningocele
- fibrolipomatosis of the filum terminal
- tethered cord syndrome
- split cord malformation types I and II
- dermal sinus
- split notochord syndrome

Non-dysraphic malformations:

- sacral agenesis
- congenital tumors (teratoma, dermoid, epidermoid)
- spinal cysts
- Arnold–Chiari types I and II malformations
- syringomyelia
- congenital spinal stenosis

Open spinal malformation (spina bifida aperta): This involves myelomeningocele (MMC), including its subforms (myeloschisis, hemimyelomeningocele, syringomyelomeningocele) and myelomeningocystocele.

The term "open" is supposed to express the fact that parts of the spinal canal are displaced dorsally through a bony defect of the spine and reach the level of the skin or protrude above skin level. There is direct contact between the spinal cord or the meninges or both, and the skin resulting in impending or manifest exposure of the spinal canal to the exterior.

Thus, in the presence of myelomeningocele, the spinal cord is exposed at the level of the skin and presents a direct risk of infection. Surgical intervention is therefore necessary during the first 24–48 hours after birth. After this time it is not uncommon for watchful waiting to lead to a rapid deterioration of the neurostatus. Such children also often present with hydrocephalus (Arnold–Chiari type II malformation), which will require shunt insertion after birth.

Closed spinal malformation (occult spinal dysraphism): A whole spectrum of clinical pictures are classified under this term whose common feature is that defects of the spinal canal are covered by skin and subcutaneous tissue. The neuronal structures do not herniate above skin level. When elevations do appear in the region of the back then they are characteristically caused by a large subcutaneous lipoma. At the level of the defect, however, skin changes may present in the form of hypertrichosis, pigment disturbances, angiomas, dimples or fistula tracts. In occult spinal dysraphism too, individual cases will present alterations in the form and function of the spinal cord with varying degrees of expression.

Spina bifida occulta. This merely refers to an incomplete fusion of the dorsal vertebral elements, especially the vertebral arch, without any changes within the spinal canal. The finding therefore bears no clinical significance.

> **Important information for the radiologist**
>
> Open spinal malformations are not normally examined using imaging techniques but undergo immediate surgery. This is done with the idea of preventing infections of the spinal canal at all

events. Imaging techniques are not usually used until the open malformations have been repaired and clinical problems arise after surgery.

Operations on closed spinal malformations on the other hand depend on the clinical picture. Here, there is usually no urgency, with the exception of a dermal sinus where surgery of this disorder is also done swiftly to avoid infections.

So in the other cases there remains enough time for an extensive and thorough examination, primarily using MRI and only seldom is myelography or CT myelography required. The latter are used above all for spinal cysts where the question of a communication between the subarachnoid space and the contents of the cyst can only be answered myelographically.

Understanding the pathogenesis of dysraphic malformations can only be gained with knowledge of their embryogenesis. The following chapter presents the embryogenesis in great detail and includes the various theories on the malformations of myelomeningocele and the Arnold–Chiari types.

Embryogenesis and Maldevelopments

Knowledge of embryogenesis and possible maldevelopments facilitates the understanding of congenital anomalies of the spine and spinal canal. The malformations can be explained by certain developmental disturbances occurring at various times during embryogenesis.

Development of the Central Nervous System

The development of the CNS is divided into different phases:

- the neurulation phase,
- the phase of caudal differentiation (canalization) and regression.

The Neurulation Phase

The neurulation phase covers the period of the development of the neural plate and the neural tube until their proximal and distal closure. This is reached by day 28 of embryonic development. After conception, a flat oval disk forms by cell division and is fully differentiated within 14 days into the two tissue layers—the *ectoderm* and the *endoderm*. On this disk, at its caudal end, ectodermal cells accumulate longitudinally to form a plate, the so-called *primitive streak*. At the cranial end of this streak a round pit forms, and around this pit cells proliferate to form a peripheral wall called *Hensen's node* (Fig. 3.**1**).

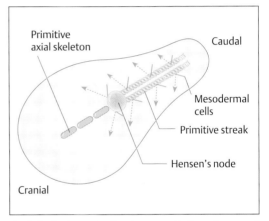

Fig. 3.**1** **Embryonic development before the onset of the neurulation phase.** Cells migrate from the primitive streak to form the mesoderm. The primitive axial skeleton is formed from the cells emanating from Hensen's node.

Along the primitive streak cells enter the disk and spread out in a cranial direction between ectoderm and endoderm to form the *mesoderm*. In addition, on days 15 and 16, cells migrate inward via Hensen's node and spread out cranially in the midline to form the primitive axial skeleton, the notochordal process (Fig. 3.**1**). The notochordal process develops a centrally open canal with a connection to the exterior via the primitive pit (Fig. 3.**2**).

The neurulation phase begins around 16–17 days after conception with the development of the neural plate. This process is induced by the notochordal process and begins with a thickening of the ectoderm along the notochordal process, cranial to Hensen's node. Formation of the neural groove occurs along the length of the notochordal process, the lateral margins of which thicken (Fig. 3.**3**).

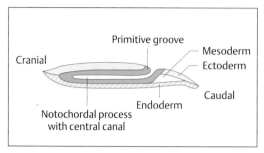

Fig. 3.**2** **Notochordal process with central canal.**

At this time the notochordal process is reorganized to form a plate, which is embedded into the endoderm. The central canal of the primitive axial skeleton thus degenerates and in its place an elongated groove develops in the midline. The primitive axial skeleton gains contact with the yolk sac by incorporation into the endoderm (Fig. 3.**4a**).

At the caudal end of the plate where the primitive groove merges into the axial skeleton, a communication now develops between the yolk sac and the amniotic cavity, the so-called *neurenteric canal* (Fig. 3.**4b**).

This canal degenerates again after 2–6 days due to separation of the notochordal plate from the endoderm, the endoderm once again forming a complete continuous covering and the cells of the primitive axial skeleton gathering to form a cylinder in the midline, the definitive *notochord* (Fig. 3.**4c**). Meanwhile the neural plate is further transformed. The neural groove deepens. The

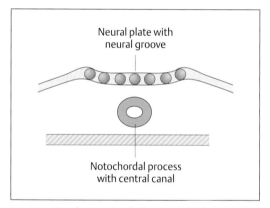

Fig. 3.3 **Development of the neural plate at the beginning of the neurulation phase.** The neural plate initially displays only a slight indentation. The notochordal process lies separated from both the endoderm and the ectoderm.

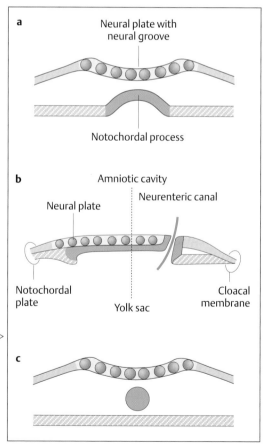

Fig. 3.4 a–c **Notochordal process:**
a The notochordal process embedding into the endoderm. The central canal degenerates, while the notochordal process forms a longitudinal groove. The neural groove displays a more marked indentation.
b Temporary communication between the amnion cavity and yolk sac.
c Division of the notochord from the endoderm and formation of a cylinder.

elevations on either side of the neural plate develop into the future neural crest. The neural plate is reorganized to form the neural tube by dorsal closure of the U-shaped plate, separation from the ectoderm and formation of an intact ectodermal surface, the future skin. Mesodermal tissue is formed between the ectoderm and the neural tube so that there is no longer any direct contact between the two tissues. The neural cells at either margin of the neural plate migrate downwards to accumulate dorsal to the neural tube where they form the *neural crest* (Fig. 3.5).

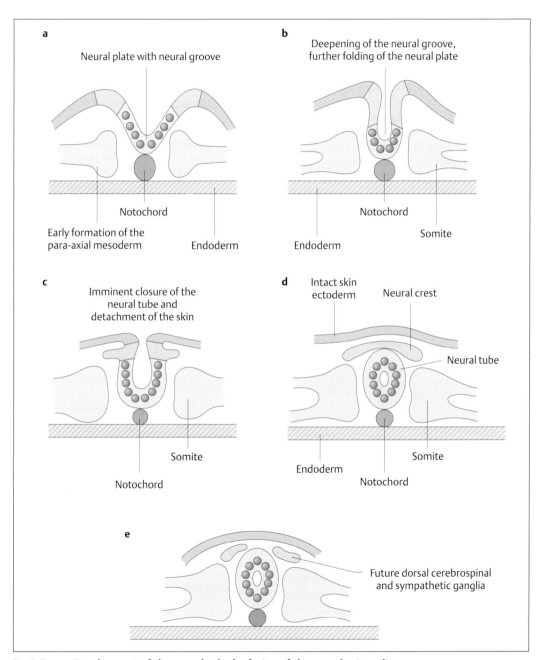

Fig. 3.**5 a–e** **Development of the neural tube by fusion of the neural primordium.**

At the same time mesodermal cells are transformed paraxially on either side of both the notochord and the neural tube to become the so-called *primitive segments*, the future somites, which flank the axial skeleton from around day 16–17. After 28 days, 30 of these original segments have already formed. They differentiate dorsomedially into the myotomes and eventually into the segmental paraspinal muscles. The anteromedial components develop into the sclerotomes and eventually into vertebral bodies, vertebral arches, ligaments and meninges, as well as into the ribs and intercostal muscles. The anterolateral elements develop into the dermatomes and form the skin, subcutaneous tissue and the muscles of the abdominal wall (Fig. 3.6).

The process of fusion of the neural plate begins in the mid portion and is continued in a caudal and cranial direction. The rostral end of the neural tube closes on day 24, the caudal end on days 26–28. The exact site of the caudal end is disputed, but most likely it is located in the distal lumbar region (Fig. 3.7).

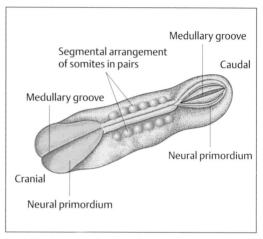

Fig. 3.**7** **Somites.** The neural primordium closes first in the mid portions. The somites are shown arranged in pairs along the midline.

Hensen's node and the primitive streak then undergo regression and migrate in a caudal direction to the future coccygeal region.

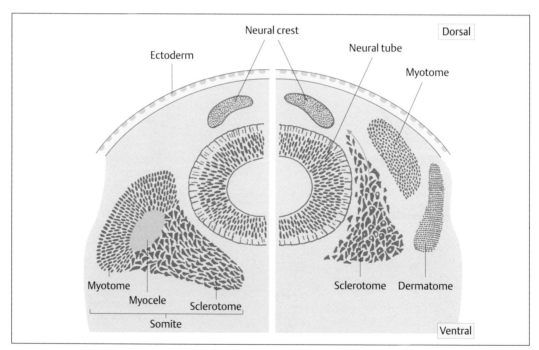

Fig. 3.**6** **Diagram of the formation of the somites with subsequent division into myotome, sclerotome, and dermatome.** The sclerotome itself divides into three major groups of mesodermal cells: the *dorsal group* forms the vertebral arches and the primitive meninges, the *medial group* the vertebral bodies, and the *ventral group* the ribs and intercostal muscles.

■ The Caudal Differentiation and Regression Phase

The formation of the spinal cord begins caudal to L4 with the cells of Hensen's node and of the primitive streak forming an undifferentiated cell mass beneath the intact ectodermal surface after their migration caudalward. Within this accumulation of cells, vacuoles are formed which coalesce, consequently leading to the formation of a tube surrounded by ependyma-like cells. This cell accumulation and its inner canal fuse with the *neural tube* (canalization). Around day 38 of embryonic development regression of this lumbosacral canal begins. The cell accumulation and the inner canal diminish in size, around days 44–48 cell necrosis occurs and the formation of the conus, ventriculus terminalis and filum terminale takes place. The filum is attached to the fifth coccygeal vertebra as a ligament. The vertebral column and the spinal cord grow at different rates resulting in the ascension of the conus medullaris. In the fourth week the conus is at about the L4/L5 level, in the second week at L3/L4, in the 40th week at L2/L3, and 10 weeks later reaches the adult level (L1/L2) (Barson, 1970; Di-Pietro, 1993).

Development of the Meninges

The meninges develop immediately after the formation of the neural tube, particularly after completion of its distal end. The caudal end of the dural sac reaches down to about S4 in the fetus and is situated at the S2 level in the adult. Thus the dural sac is subject to a less pronounced ascension compared with the conus medullaris.

Formation of the Vertebral Column

The vertebrae develop from the sclerotome cells, with one vertebra in each case being formed from the cells of the next higher and lower sclerotome. In addition, the cells of the right and left side merge to form one vertebra so that in total four groups of sclerotome cells are involved in the formation of one vertebra. The sclerotome cells lying between the vertebral bodies develop into the annulus fibrosus; the notochord is transformed into the nucleus pulposus. The notochord in the vertebral body undergoes complete regression. The dorsal components of the vertebrae are formed from paired sclerotome cells of the right and left side. The lumbosacral vertebrae develop in a less orderly fashion than the proximal vertebrae. Cells of the axial skeleton, the mesoderm and the caudal neural tube are transformed into somites (primitive segments), which in turn form the sacral and coccygeal vertebrae, and subsequently are then subject to regression, fusion and transformation. During this process a series of anomalies can develop, such as:

● lumbosacral lipoma,
● teratoma,
● sacral agenesis.

▌ Pathogenesis of Anomalies

Theories of the Pathogenesis of Myelomeningoceles and Arnold–Chiari Type II Malformation

There are a number of theories concerning the development of myelomeningoceles and Arnold–Chiari type II malformations, which will be outlined below. The individual ideas emanate in part from very different standpoints. For example, the question of whether spinal dysraphism develops before the completion of the neural plate and skin or afterwards is still disputed. The fact that myelomeningocele or myeloschisis is found only in the lumbosacral region might falsely suggest that, because the spinal cord and spine develop in this segment by canalization and regression beneath an intact ectoderm, this malformation usually develops underneath the intact skin which subsequently opens up.

■ Theory of Disturbed Cerebrospinal Fluid Circulation

Chiari (1891, 1895) and, later, Gardner (1973) considered the cause to lie in a disturbance of cerebrospinal fluid (CSF) circulation in the posterior cranial fossa. In the presence of maldevelopment of the CSF-containing spaces, CSF cannot drain sufficiently from the ventricles and disperses caudally via the neural tube. This results in dilation and disruption of the neural tube and consequently in the development of myeloschisis or myelomeningocele. According to this theory, Arnold–Chiari type II malformation develops from excessive pulsatile pressure of the supratentorial choroid plexus with a corresponding downward displacement of structures in the posterior fossa into the spinal canal.

Objections to this theory have been raised which point out that myeloschisis is already found before the development of the choroid plexus. Furthermore, this theory does not explain the small size of the posterior fossa, the upward herniation of the contents of the posterior fossa, the often slit-like formation of the fourth ventricle, and various other cerebral anomalies.

■ Traction Theory

According to this theory developed by Lichtenstein (1940, 1942) and Penfield and Coburn (1938), the Arnold–Chiari type II malformation is supposed to develop from traction occurring as a result of adherence of the spinal cord during myelomeningocele development. But this theory cannot explain why the dorsal components of the pons and medulla oblongata are mainly involved and the ventral elements less so. Traction does not explain the dorsal Z-shaped angulation of the medulla oblongata, so there must be pressure from above. Furthermore, myelomeningoceles also occur without Arnold–Chiari type II malformation, and Arnold–Chiari type II malformations are never present in occult spinal dysraphism despite tethering of the conus.

■ Theory of Maldevelopment of Segments of the Brain Stem

Cleland (1883) primarily suspected maldevelopment of the brain stem as the cause of the malformation. This theory was further developed by Daniel and Strich (1958) and

Peach (1965) who added that an insufficient or absent angulation of the pons, in particular, would result in maldevelopment with corresponding upward or downward displacement of parts of the brain. The question of why the angulation of the pons is absent remains unanswered, and also of how the other cerebral changes are to be explained.

■ Theory of Overgrowth or Underdevelopment of the Posterior Fossa

Based on the results of animal studies, Padget (1968, 1970, 1972) supported the theory of a reopening of the closed spinal cord in the course of the development of spina bifida aperta. According to this theory, fluid is supposed to collect at circumscribed sites within the closed neural tube and, through pressure, forces an opening in the myelon and the skin or, as in anterior spina bifida, contributes to the formation of a ventral cleft. The pathogenesis of Arnold–Chiari malformation is said to be associated with the development of the neural malformation, inasmuch as microcephaly and, consequently, reduction in size of the posterior fossa occur as a result of fluid escape at the level of the spina bifida aperta. The subsequent development of the cerebellum within the restricted posterior fossa is supposed to result in a downward displacement of parts of the midbrain and cerebellum. The theory of an embryonic microcranium of the posterior fossa as a cause of the Arnold–Chiari type II malformation gains support from the fact that, despite a pressure-producing hydrocephalus, these patients in fact demonstrate only a normal-sized skull and never develop a microcranium after shunt insertion.

Marin-Padilla and Marin-Padilla (1981) reached similar conclusions on the basis of results of animal studies. An underdevelopment of the occipital bone, especially the basal parts, was achieved by treating hamster embryos with vitamin A, which resulted in an insufficient development in the size of the posterior fossa. The fossa was unable to contain the cerebellum and brain stem within the predefined bony coverings so that parts were displaced caudally, toward the foramen magnum, yet were never seen within the cervical canal. For this reason, and due to the fact that further malformations associated with Arnold–Chiari malformation are not amenable to explanation by this theory, this concept has been regarded as unsatisfactory.

Theories originating from Barry (1957), and in a similar form from Brocklehurst (1969, 1971), also assume a disproportion between bony coverings and neuroepithelium in the posterior fossa. Barry suspected an excessive growth of neuroepithelial structures in the posterior fossa as a factor, while Brocklehurst assumed a disproportionate development of neural ectoderm and investing mesoderm.

■ Currently Accepted Theory

The theory that has enjoyed increasing acceptance over recent years was expounded by McLone and Knepper (1989) and is based on continuing animal studies. It differs only partly from the results obtained by Padget and Marin-Padilla in particular, while largely reaching similar conclusions. The animal studies yielded the result that the development of myelomeningocele, Arnold–Chiari malformation and the other cerebral malformations must be ascribed to a uniform pathogenesis according to which the regulation of their development is disturbed primarily on an enzymatic level—a development that is normally genome-induced and based on intra- and extracellular enzymatic processes. The starting point is the incomplete closure of the neural crest which, due to loss of CSF, leads to the collapse of the roof of the hindbrain (rhombencephalon) and thus to an inadequate expansion of the primitive ventricles. This results in an insufficient expansion of the posterior fossa. The development of the cerebellum and brain stem continues in the presence of the predetermined, yet insufficient, form of the bony coverings of the posterior fossa. The junction between brain stem and spinal cord is displaced below the foramen magnum. The angle of the brain stem is altered, parts of the cerebellum and the brain stem move cranially and caudally. A faulty development of the nuclei of the cerebral nerves results from this. The primitive ventricles become insufficiently filled with fluid, which results in disorganization of the cerebral cortex. The mechanical support of the primitive ventricles is a precondition for the normal organization of the cortex. The insufficient development of the cerebral hemispheres results in microgyria and ectopy as well as in dysgenesis of the corpus callosum. The third ventricle remains small, which

prevents the separation of the thalamic nuclei and leads to the formation of the intermediate mass. The inadequate expansion of the brain results in a disorganization of the collagen bundles of the cranial vault. Instead of radial lines the collagen forms winding and rounded collagen bundles, which are associated with the characteristic development of the lacunar skull (craniolacunia or Lückenschädel).

The hydrocephalus often associated with myelomeningocele can have various causes. On the one hand there may be a blockage of the basal cisterns and the subarachnoid space due to the downward displacement of parts of the cerebellum and brain stem or, alternatively, an occlusion of the aqueduct or of the foramina of the fourth ventricle can be the cause. Not least, a disturbance of circulation may be present, resulting from a blockage at the level of the tentorium. At the time of birth a large number of children present with microcrania that rapidly regress after closure of the sac (cele), so that the head circumference increases. With limited growth capacity of the bony coverings, hydrocephalus usually develops together with the increase in volume of the posterior fossa, which accompanies brain tissue growth. This leads to a blockage of the CSF pathways, particularly the CSF circulation at the level of the tentorium. Thus the development of hydrocephalus is also the result of the disproportionate growth of the cerebral structures and the cranial vault.

Theories of Pathogenesis of Closed Spinal Malformations

Pathogenesis of closed spinal malformations can arise from five different causes:

- failure of various tissues to separate,
- malformation of the neural tube,
- faulty development of the primitive axial skeleton,
- faulty development of the neurenteric canal,
- errors in canalization and regression at a lumbosacral level.

■ Lipoma and Lipomyelomeningocele

As a rule, the separation of ectoderm and neural tissue is a well-regulated process that proceeds in a bilaterally equal manner and during which the closure of the neural tube happens at the same time as the mesenchyme develops between the ectoderm and neural tube. Here the mesenchyme has no contact with the central canal. If the separation between ectoderm and neural tissue occurs prematurely or unilaterally, a disturbance of mesenchymal architecture can occur, possibly resulting in contact between mesenchymal cells and the central canal before the closure of the neural primordium.

Apparently mesenchymal tissue that gains contact with the neural groove and the future central canal is transformed into fat. This explains the development of lipoma and lipomyelomeningocele along the course of the spinal canal with the exception of the lumbosacral segments (Caram *et al.*, 1957; Emery and Lendon, 1969; Anderson, 1975; Bruce and Schut, 1979). In the lumbosacral region the pathogenesis can be explained by a faulty canalization and regression, inasmuch as the cell-tissue differentiation into a neural and mesenchymal component is inadequate and mesenchymal structures become enclosed in the spinal canal.

■ Dermal Sinus

The dermal sinus can be explained by absent or insufficient separation of ectodermal from neural tissue, resulting in a tract that connects the skin with the neural structures within the spinal canal. Epidermoids and dermoids can also arise from the ectodermal tissue and are often associated with a dermal sinus (Walker and Bucy, 1934).

■ Tethered Cord Syndrome

The process of canalization proceeds normally in the case of tethered cord syndrome, but errors of regression occur that consequently result in alterations of the filum terminale, such as fibrolipomatosis, a thickening or shortening, and in some cases the formation of connective-tissue bands that tether the spinal cord to the dura. This results in the fixed low-lying conus during the ascension phase (Jones and Love, 1956).

■ Split Cord Malformation, Neurenteric Cyst, Combined Anterior and Posterior Spina Bifida

These changes, which predominantly affect the thoracic and cervical regions and are frequently associated with malformations of the vertebrae,

can be regarded as different expressions of a uniform process of malformation.

During embryonic development, a canal is occasionally formed that connects the amnion cavity with the yolk sac. This canal only exists for a few days and then closes again. The cause of the malformation is not considered to be insufficient regression of this canal, however, but rather that an accessory neurenteric canal develops above the normal physiological canal (Pang *et al.*, 1992).

This accessory canal also develops in the midline and represents a communication between yolk sac and amnion cavity. It leads to a splitting of the neural plate and notochordal process, interfering with the development of the vertebrae and the neural tube in this segment.

The assumption that an accessory canal proximal to the proper physiological canal is the cause of the respective malformations is based on the fact that the physiological canal lies at the level of Hensen's node and during the caudal migration of Hensen's node comes to lie at the level of the coccyx. The resulting malformations, however, are always found above the coccygeal region.

The accessory canal is additionally surrounded by mesenchyme so that an endomesenchymal tract develops along the canal and occupies the space between the split notochordal process and the divided neural plate.

The final degree of expression of the malformation depends on three factors:

- the ability of the embryo to maintain the healing process along the endomesenchymal tract,
- the ultimately variable extent of the endomesenchymal tract,
- the final and definite development of the displaced mesenchyme and endoderm along the midline.

The split notochordal process is more able than the divided neural plate to initiate a process of healing along the fistula, resulting in the finding that clefting of the spinal cord is more often encountered than split vertebrae.

Although the entire endomesenchymal tract connecting bowel and skin can persist, it is more common for only parts of the tract to remain.

The endoderm can degenerate. Alternatively, it can form cysts lined with respiratory or gastrointestinal epithelium, both of which are derived from the endoderm.

Because the pluripotent mesenchyme is capable of transforming itself into fibroblasts, cartilaginous or bone cells as well as blood vessels, fat and myoblasts, the sagittal septum dividing the spinal cord can be composed of various tissues.

If the dorsal component of the endomesenchymal tract degenerates and the ventral portion persists, then this structure can connect the bowel with parts of the vertebra or spinal cord.

Inside this tract the endoderm can differentiate into intestinal epithelium, leading to an intestinal duplication that is connected to a vertebra or the spinal cord.

The development of this band can come to a standstill if no further endodermal differentiation takes place and can sometimes be the cause of intestinal malrotation inasmuch as the anticlockwise rotation of the bowel is prevented (McLetchie *et al.*, 1954; Beardmore and Wiglesworth, 1958; Bentley and Smith, 1960; Pang *et al.*, 1992).

Dysraphic Malformations

Open spinal Malformations

■ Myelocele and Myelomeningocele

Definition

In myelocele and myelomeningocele the spinal cord is exposed at a circumscribed site so that there is neither a bony nor cutaneous covering.

The spinal cord usually appears flat and stretched out (placode) and lies on a level with the skin.

The sac (cele) can extend far dorsally (myelomeningocele) or can lie almost on a level with the spinal canal (myelocele) (Fig. 3.**8**).

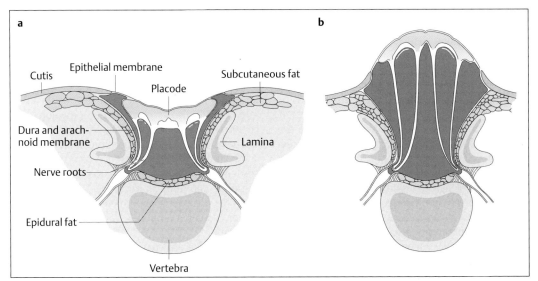

Fig. 3.8 a, b   Myelocele and myelomeningocele.
a Myelocele: The neural placode is a flat plate of neural tissue lying directly level with the skin. Dorsally the dura is non-existent. The pia mater and arachnoid membrane border on the ventral surface of the placode and dura, forming an arachnoid pocket or cyst, which is connected to the subarachnoid space proximally and distally. Both the dorsal and the ventral nerve roots arise from the ventral surface of the placode.
b Myelomeningocele: In contrast to myelocele, there is an expansion of the ventral subarachnoid space dorsally leading to a bulging protrusion of the placode above skin level.

Morphology

The skin generally forms the margin of the placode because in this type of malformation the neuroectoderm does not separate from the skin. Since the mesenchymal structures had no chance of occupying the region between skin and neural tissue they are not located dorsal to the neuroectoderm but are found anterolateral to the neural tissue. The skin is attached to the placode by a narrow strip of leptomeninx, which in turn is covered by epithelium (epithelial zone). The dura and arachnoid membrane do not invest the placode. Instead the meninges develop exclusively ventral to the placode.

The dura is contiguous with the skin on the lateral margin of the epithelial zone with the arachnoid membrane contributing to the formation of the epithelial zone.

The placode represents incompletely formed spinal cord in the sense that the lateral ends of the embryonic neural plate have not joined together. Consequently all the dorsal nerves enter and exit ventrally with the dorsal nerve roots lying lateral to the ventral roots. A central canal is either not recognizable at all or is incompletely formed and opens outwards so that CSF can escape freely.

The myelomeningocele is usually associated with severe bony defects. The dorsal vertebral components do not fuse, but instead the pedicles and laminae are displaced laterally and anterolaterally. This results in a distinct enlargement of the spinal canal. The craniocaudal dimensions of the bony defect extend beyond the skin defect. If the bony defect is situated at the level of the thoracolumbar junction, then a complete spina bifida develops from this point caudally and involves the whole lumbosacral space, regardless of the level at which the skin defect is located. At other sites the bony defect remains localized (Fig. 3.**9**).

The vertebrae can also have defects. Hemivertebrae, aplasias or wedge vertebrae are seen, as well as segmented block vertebrae, which are not infrequently encountered unilaterally. There are also malformations involving the ribs.

In the lumbar region, furthermore, ventral or ventrolateral displacements of the back muscles, including the psoas muscle, can be found. The paraspinal muscles subsequently act as flexors and not extensors. Together with the other bony malformations, this will result in the development of scoliosis.

Location

Myelomeningoceles are located at the following sites (French, 1990):

- 3 % cervical,
- 5 % thoracic,
- 26 % thoracolumbar,
- 25 % lumbar,
- 30 % lumbosacral,
- 10 % sacral.

Pathogenesis

About one-third of patients with myelomeningocele demonstrate an associated type II split cord malformation.

The clefting of the spinal cord can be above (approximately 45 %), below (approximately 30 %) or at the level of (approximately 25 %) the myelomeningocele (Emery and Lendon, 1973). Not infrequently there is also a hemimyelo(meningo)cele of the spinal cord present. It is seen in about 10 % of patients with myelomeningocele. In these cases one part of the spinal cord is developed in the form of a myelomeningocele, while the other part lies in a dural sac separated from the rest of the spinal canal by a fibrous or bony spur (type II split cord malformation). The normal spinal cord can, however, demonstrate tethering by a thickened filum terminale or, in rare cases, is also associated with a myelomeningocele lying caudal to the main finding.

There is also a form of hemimyelomeningocele associated with the occurrence of a type I split cord malformation, i.e. with the presence of a complete and uniform dural sac. In up to 20 % of cases the disorder is combined with an intradural tumor, usually a lipoma, rarely a dermoid or epidermoid.

About 11 % of patients present with syringo(hydro)myelia (Just *et al.*, 1990); in the study population of Emery and Lendon (1972, 1973) the rate was 43 %. Their extent and site vary considerably.

Syringomyelia is found both localized in the cervical region and directly above the myelomeningocele, but also as a complete lesion along the entire length of the spinal cord.

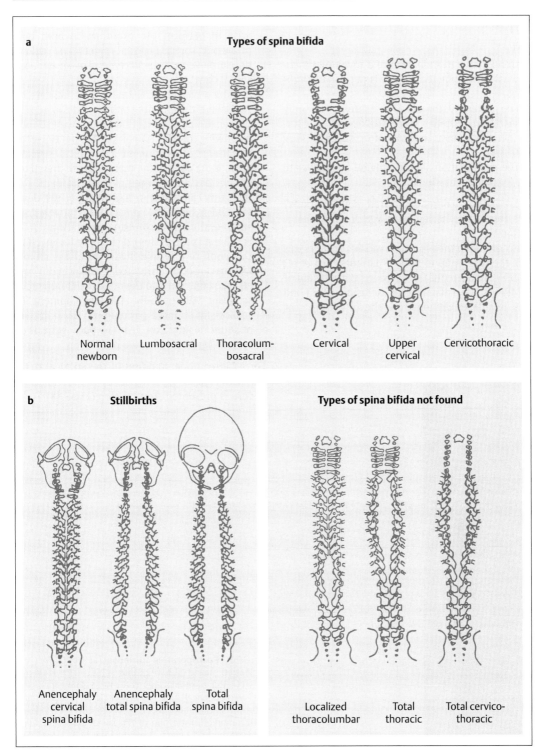

Fig. 3.**9 a, b Examples of the various types of spina bifida according to location of the defect with in-** volvement of the cranium (from Friede, R.L., *Developmental Neuropathology*, Springer, Berlin 1989).

Diagnostics

MRI

A preoperative examination of a myelomeningocele using imaging techniques is not usually indicated.

The necessity for an MRI examination only arises when, despite a successful operation, clinical deterioration is noticed after surgery (Figs. 3.**10**–3.**17**).

The examination should provide an answer to the following questions:

- Are there any other associated malformations?
- Is there re-tethering after a successful operation?

  According to the reports of various authors this is the case in up to 90 % of patients (Just *et al.*, 1990). Admittedly, the diagnosis with the aid of MRI is more a diagnosis of exclusion. Often MRI is unable to demonstrate the offending scar tissue directly. In particular cases it may be wise to perform the examination both in a prone and supine position to detect or exclude dorsal or ventral displacement of an exposed spinal cord.

- Is there an ischemic segment of spinal cord? An ischemic segment of spinal cord can be well demonstrated by a distinct and circumscribed narrowing of the spinal cord. The cause of ischemia can be due to a technical surgical error. If the ends of the meninges are drawn together too tightly when closing the dural sac, then this can result in narrowing of the dural sac, which keeps the spinal cord relatively constricted, thus compromising circulation.

- Is there a (progressive) syringo(hydro)myelia? Detection of a syringo(hydro)myelia is important because an untreated syringo(hydro)myelia can contribute to the rapid development of scoliosis. Alternatively, the development of scoliosis in shunted patients can be indicative of shunt dysfunction. (For the pathogenesis of syringo(hydro)myelia see p. 134).

For a better understanding of the surgical management of myelomeningocele, the operative procedure is presented step-by-step (Fig. 3.**18**).

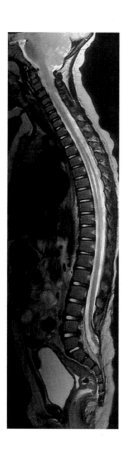

◁ Fig. 3.**10** **Postoperative lumbosacral MMC.** MRI examination using T2-weighting (TSE; TR = 4000 ms, TE = 112 ms) demonstrates the entire spine including the craniocervical junction. There is an Arnold-Chiari type II malformation and a syrinx at the T3–T9 level, with a marked distension of the spinal cord, and spina bifida at the L5/S1 level. The defect has been closed surgically. The spinal cord is elongated as far as S1; at the level of the bony defect there is a dorsal fixation of the conus to the dura (retethering).

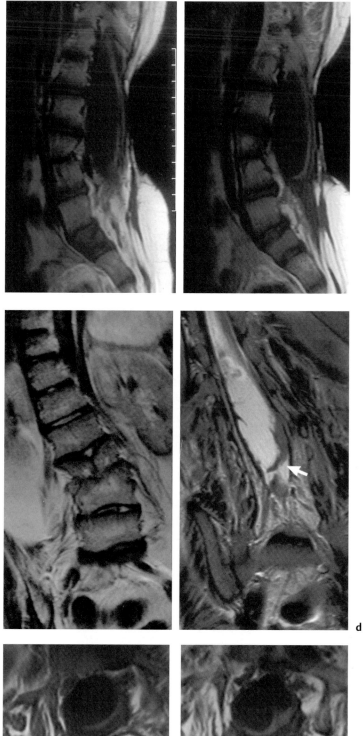

Fig. 3.**11 a–f** **Postoperative lumbar MMC.**
a, b T1-weighted sagittal section (TSE; TR = 800 ms, TE = 12 ms): The spinal canal is markedly enlarged in a dorsal direction at the level of the long-segment spina bifida. The spinal cord is flat and elongated, displaced dorsally, and exhibits caudal tethering in the lumbosacral region. The dorsal displacement is due to an arachnoid cyst, 8–9 cm in size. Note the vertebral dysplasia at the L3/L4 level.

c   T2-weighted coronal section at the level of the split vertebra L3. Marked right convex scoliosis of the thoracic and lumbar spine.

d   Slice 1.5 cm further dorsal: the lumbar enlargement of the spinal canal is easily seen together with the fixation of the spinal cord to the dura, particularly on the left (arrow). Apart from this, some band-like scarring is recognizable, which results in an additional fixation of the placode.

e, f Transverse section (SE; TR = 805 ms, TE = 14 ms): The image shows the dorsally very flattened and elongated placode at the level of the spina bifida with a broad fixation in the dural region, particularly towards the left.

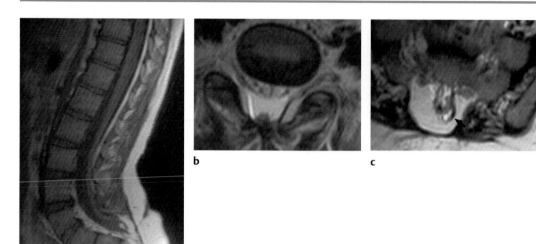

Fig. 3.**12 a–c Postoperative sacral MMC, now showing retethering:**
a T1-weighted sagittal section (TSE; TR = 800 ms, TE = 12 ms): Spinal cord elongated far sacrally and tethered to a small lipoma and the dura at the level of about S2/S3.
b Transverse image using T2-weighting (TSE; TR = 4800 ms, TE = 120 ms): The dorsal tethering of

the spinal cord is easily seen on this image. Note the spinal canal projecting slightly dorsally, although no bony interruption is recognizable here.
c Slice 1.5 cm further caudally. In this section the sacral bony interruption is well recognized. The small lipoma dorsolaterally on the left appears signal-intense (arrow). Tethering here of the spinal cord.

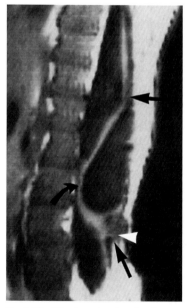

Fig. 3.**13 Meningomyelocele.** 3-year-old boy with a postoperative meningomyelocele. Note retethering of the spinal cord at two sites dorsally (straight arrow and arrowhead) and ventrally at about the L3 level (curved arrow). A dorsal arachnoidal cyst could be an additional cause of the ventral displacement of the spinal cord (SE; TR = 780 ms, TE = 25 ms).

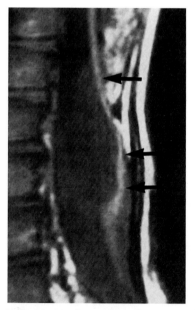

Fig. 3.**14 Myelomeningocele.** 5-year-old boy with a postoperative myelomeningocele. Note retethering with long-segment dorsal fixation of the spinal cord (arrow) (SE; TR = 780 ms, TE = 25 ms).

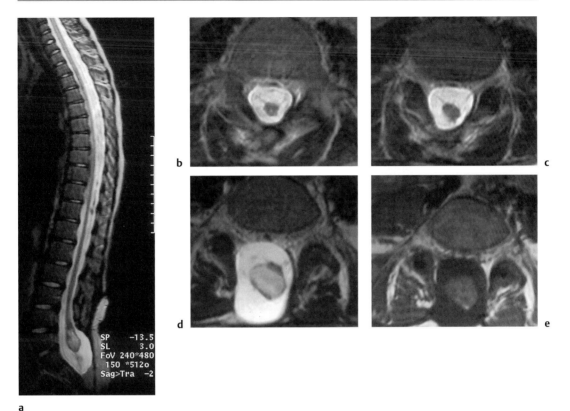

Fig. 3.**15 a–e** **Myelomeningocele.** 9-year-old boy with a postoperative lumbosacral myelomeningocele. The bony defect is at the L5 level and extends far down sacrally:

a T2-weighted sagittal section (TSE; TR = 5310 ms, TE = 112 ms): Long extended spinal cord reaching as far as L5/S1where it displays a cystic distension at the level of the conus in the form of a ventriculus terminalis. A definite fixation is not recognizable. There is no contact with the dorsal and ventral parts of the dura.

b, c Transverse images (TSE; TR = 5000 ms, TE = 120 ms): Distal parts of the spinal cord with a small punctiform syrinx. The band-like structures traversing in a ventral direction are most likely nerve roots, well recognizable from their alignment with the intervertebral foramina, as in **c** (5 mm caudal to **b**).

d Slice 15 mm further caudal from **c**. The cystic distension of the conus on this image is well recognizable. Here too there are no definite band-like attachments to the dura.

e Transverse T1-weighted section at the same level as **d** (SE; TR = 665 ms, TE = 14 ms): The cyst displays fluid with a relatively high signal intensity, most likely as an expression of its protein-rich composition.

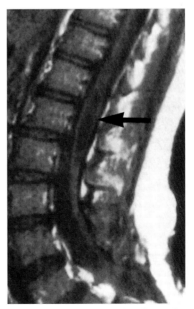

Fig. 3.**16** **Localized syringo(hydro)myelia above the operative region** (arrows). Note retethering of the spinal cord (SE; TR = 720 ms, TE = 20 ms).

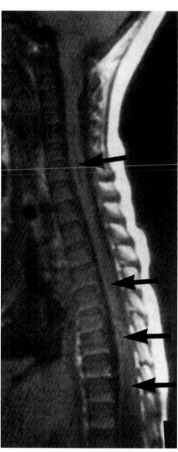

Fig. 3.**17** **Syrinx formation at multiple sites of the spinal cord** (arrow). These regions are not explicitly connected with each other (SE; TR = 650 ms, TE = 25 ms).

■ **Myelomeningocystocele**

Definition

The myelomeningocystocele (synonyms: myelomeningohydrocele, syringomyelomeningocele) represents a circumscribed herniation of the widened central canal and dysplastic membranous neural tissue dorsally through a bony defect between the dorsal columns of an otherwise correctly fused spinal cord. The sac (cele) is completely covered with skin.

Location

The finding is mainly seen in the cervical and thoracic regions (Figs. 3.**19** and 3.**20**). The spinal cord can taper off terminally into a cyst into which the often-widened central canal opens (Figs. 3.**21** and 3.**22**). There may be an only slight neurological defect.

Pathogenesis

The disorder is always associated with a caudally or proximally orientated syringomyelia and often with urogenital and anorectal defects.

Bladder exstrophy can develop. In addition scoliosis and partial or complete sacral agenesis are often present.

Fig. 3.**18 a–g** **Sectional diagrams of operative management of myelomeningocele** (from McCullough, D. C. Meningomyelocele. In Raimondi, A.J., M. Shoux, C. Di Rocco *The Pediatric Spine*, Vol. I, Springer, Berlin, 1989):
a First, the epithelial membrane is detached from the viable normal skin.
b After detachment, the membrane and neural structures are dissected down into the spinal canal.
c The epithelial membrane is dissected off the neural tissue.
d The placode is brought together dorsally and the dura mobilized on either side.
e The dura is closed dorsally.
f The fascia is mobilized, approximated medially, and closed with overlapping sutures.
g Subsequently skin and subcutaneous fat are closed.

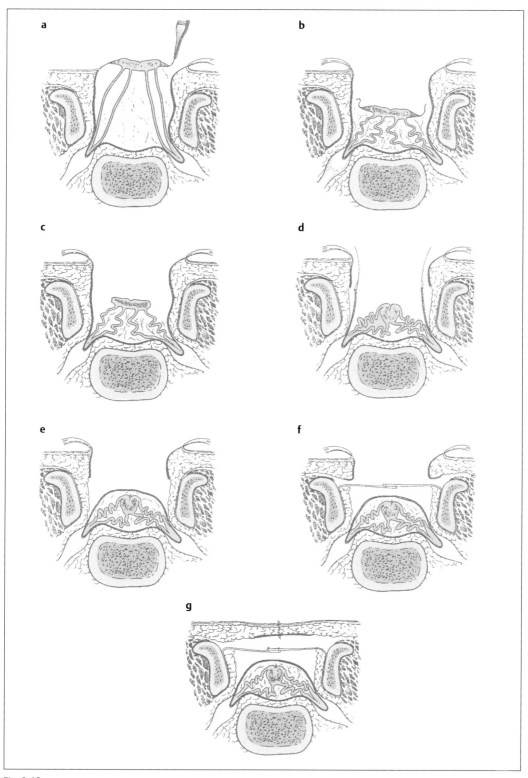

Fig. 3.**18 a–g**

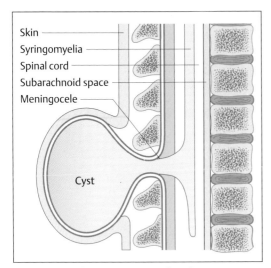

Fig. 3.**19** **Myelomeningocystocele.** The cyst is connected with the syrinx and is lined with ependyma. The cyst is larger than the meningocele.

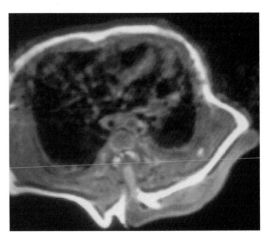

Fig. 3.**20** **Thoracic myelomeningocystocele.** Transverse section of a neonate showing a large sac (cele) formation, which extends far beyond the level of the skin and is connected to the spinal canal via a syrinx.

Fig. 3.**21** **Terminal myelomeningocystocele.** There is hydromyelia of the entire spinal cord. The central canal opens into a large cyst at the level of the conus. This cyst lies below the region of the bony spina bifida and, for the most part, below the clearly distended subarachnoid segments that surround the spinal cord distally.
SAS Subarachnoid segment

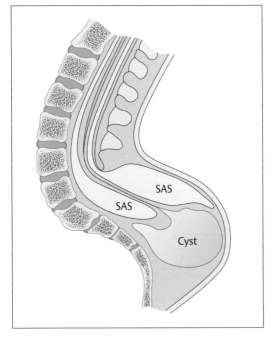

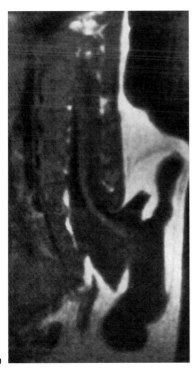

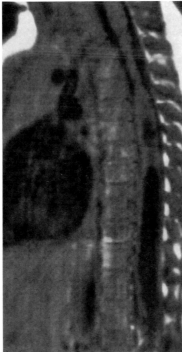

a

b

Fig. 3.**22 a, b** **Terminal myelomeningocystocele with severe malformations of the urogenital tract and sacral agenesis:**
a The spinal cord opens terminally into a large, irregularly bordered cyst that is covered by skin and extensive lipomatous components (SE; TR = 600 ms, TE = 20 ms). Normally cyst and subarachnoid space do not communicate, but this is not always discernible on MRI.
b Severe syringomyelia along the spinal cord (SE; TR = 600 ms, TE = 20 ms).

Closed Spinal Malformations

■ Meningocele

Definition

Meningocele consists of dorsal herniation of the dura and arachnoid membrane with a more or less distinct bulging protrusion of the skin.

Location and Pathogenesis

The bony defect tends to be small and can be confined to one vertebra. When more than one vertebra is involved, there is always an enlargement of the spinal canal. The sac (cele) does not usually contain any neural tissue, but in individual cases nerve roots can be found in the sac, especially when the bony defect is very wide. This can lead to tethering of the spinal cord. Arachnoidal adhesions can also lead to secondary fixations and closure of the sac. Normally the meningocele is covered by skin, but pressure necrosis can result in perforations. In this case there is an immediate indication for surgery.

Clinical symptoms, not usually present, are more likely to indicate a myelomeningocystocele.

Meningocele shows a different distribution pattern than that of myelomeningocele (French, 1990):

- 10 % cervical,
- 15 % thoracic,
- 4 % thoracolumbar,
- 37 % lumbar,
- 19 % lumbosacral,
- 15 % sacral.

Diagnostics

MRI

MRI serves the following purposes (Figs. 3.**23** and 3.**24**):

- identification of the lesion,
- exact definition of site and extent,
- verification or exclusion of further changes (e.g. myelomeningocystocele),
- demonstration of the conus medullaris and filum terminale.

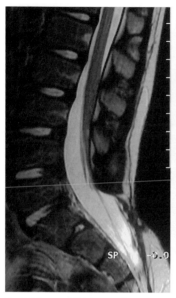
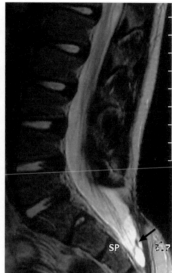
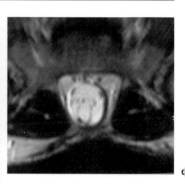

Fig. 3.**23 a–c** **Meningocele.** 6-year-old boy with postoperative sacral meningocele:

a T2-weighted sagittal section (TSE; TR = 5300 ms, TE = 120 ms): Bony defect at the S2/S3 level dorsally with herniation of the dural sac. Marked cutaneous and subcutaneous scar-tissue formation after surgery. The filum terminale appears band-like, seems shortened, and there is a corresponding low conus at the L3 level.

b Parasagittal section 3 mm lateral from **a**: In the sacral region band-like intradural changes are to be found,

which radiate both dorsally and ventrally into the dura. These can be aberrant neural structures, but also are more likely to be scar-tissue changes (arrow).

c T2-weighted transverse section (TSE; TR = 4600 ms, TE = 120 ms): Dorsal filum terminale, possibly tethered to the dura. On this image too, horizontally running structures are noticeable which possibly correspond to aberrant nerve roots. Marked extensive scarring of the skin.

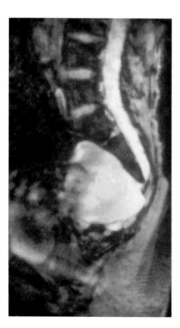

◁ Fig. 3.**24** **Large anterior sacral meningocele** (T2-weighted GRE sequence). Sagittal section showing an anterior meningocele in continuity with the sacral dural sac. Note the correspondingly typical signal iso-intense with CSF in the presacral parts.

Intradural Lipoma and Lipomyelomeningocele

Intradural Lipoma

Definition

The intradural lipoma is an accumulation of fatty tissue, which overlies the spinal cord in an extramedullary location, although it is also seen at extra- and intramedullary sites. The lipomas are, however, never completely intramedullary, but only demonstrate an expansion within the central canal, sometimes far cranially and originating from an extramedullary component.

If they are situated at the level of the conus or at a lumbosacral level, they are associated with a tethered cord syndrome and low-lying conus. However, two-thirds of all lipomas found do not demonstrate any spinal cord fixation. The lipomas account for 1 % of all primary intradural tumors (Giuffre, 1966). They are most commonly found at a thoracic level.

Incidence

The intradural lipoma and the lipomyelomeningocele are the most frequent forms of occult spinal dysraphism. In 30–45 % of all cases of occult spinal dysraphism it is a lumbosacral lipoma (Anderson, 1975; French, 1990; Tortori-Donati *et al.*, 1990). If the lipomyelomeningoceles are included, then approximately every second case of spinal dysraphism can be assigned to these two disorders.

Location

Out of 100 published cases of intradural lipoma (excluding lipomyelomeningocele) the following distribution was found:

- 12 % cervical,
- 24 % cervicothoracic,
- 30 % thoracic,
- 3 % thoracolumbar,
- 3 % lumbar,
- 5 % lumbosacral,
- 2 % confined to the filum terminale.

Eight percent of tumors involved almost the entire spinal cord, 6 % the cauda equina, and 7 % the cauda equina and the conus medullaris (Giuffre, 1966).

Intradural lipomas overlie the spinal cord dorsally in about 66 % of cases, less frequently dorsolaterally (24 %), and only in exceptional cases laterally and ventrolaterally (Giuffre, 1966).

Histology

Histologically intradural lipoma is an accumulation of mature lipid cells that is, at least partially, enclosed in a capsule.

A layer of collagenous connective tissue is found at the junction between the lipoma and neural tissue.

Lipomyelomeningocele

Definition

Lipomyelomeningoceles are complex lesions comprising spina bifida, a subcutaneous lipoma and a lumbosacral lipoma, which has contact with the dysplastic spinal cord and produces a low lying conus due to tethering of the conus. The subcutaneous lipoma is contiguous with the intradural lipoma by way of the bony defect.

At the junction between the correctly formed vertebrae and the bony defect there is always a strong fibrovascular band connecting the two vertebral arch components of the uppermost of those vertebra with a fusion defect of the arch. Those patients whose spinal canal caudal to the spina bifida is normal also demonstrate this band at the most distal of those vertebrae with a fusion defect of the arch. The band is attached to the vertebral periosteum. The meningocele and the spinal cord course dorsally below the proximal band to which the dura is sometimes firmly attached. The dorsal aspect of the spinal cord is compressed by this band and traction of the lipoma results in kinking at this point (Naidich *et al.*, 1983).

The spinal cord itself is dysplastic, its termination flat and elongated. As with myelomeningocele, the dorsal nerve roots lie laterally to the ventral roots. The dura is attached to the placode immediately lateral to the dorsal nerve roots. The lipoma is therefore extradural and, although attached to the placode, is not invested by the dura. The arachnoid membrane courses together with the pia mater ventral to the placode. The meningocele can vary in its degree of expression and is above all found as a ventral extension of the subarachoidal space due to the dorsal displacement of the intraspinal structures. It can however also extend dorsally, lateral to the spinal cord and lipoma behind the bony defect in the spine to reach far into the subcutaneous fat.

The central canal of the spinal cord tapers off into the lipomyelomeningocele. It is open dorsally where it is sealed off by fat. The fat can extend cranially within the central canal. The lipoma is often attached to the placode posterolaterally, thus causing the spinal cord to turn to the opposite side. This rotation can displace some of the nerve roots dorsally and others ventrally, which must be kept in mind during surgery (Naidich *et al.*, 1983).

Pathogenesis

Lipomyelomeningoceles and lumbosacral lipomas are not infrequently associated with a partial sacral agenesis (Dubowitz *et al.*, 1965). A scimitar sacrum may be noted on radiographs. A dermal sinus is found in about 10 % of cases (Bruce and Schut, 1979).

In 30–40 % of cases telangiectases, skin appendages, increased hair growth and small skin dimples are seen in the affected region (Naidich *et al.*, 1983).

Clinical Presentation

Not all patients show the condition clinically at the time of birth. Within their first 5 years of life about one-quarter of the patients present symp-toms; some 50 % show them during the second and third decade, and 15 % not until the fifth decade.

Trauma, pregnancy and physical exertion can initiate the onset of clinical symptoms (Giuffre, 1966).

Therapy

Today the generally accepted view is that the patients ought to be operated on, even if clinical symptoms are not yet apparent (Bruce and Schut, 1979; Chapman, 1982; McLone *et al.*, 1983). The aim of surgery is to decompress the spinal cord and remove parts of the lipoma. After successful surgery these patients have a better chance of remaining free of symptoms or experiencing only mild restrictions than patients who have not been operated upon and from whom surgery is withheld until symptoms occur.

Diagnostics

MRI

MRI displays signals specific for fat on all sequences. A concomitant edematous reaction is not found, nor is there enhancement with contrast. Images in two, and preferably in all three, planes are required. Thin slices and high-resolution images should be obtained for the examination in order to detect all concomitant malformations (Figs.3.**25**–3.**34**).

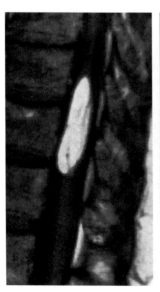
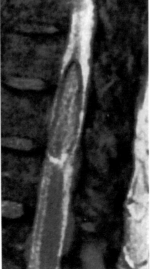

a b

Fig. 3.**25 a, b Lipoma**. 65-year-old patient with a thoracic lipoma overlying the spinal cord laterally. There is no tethered cord syndrome.
a T1-weighted image (SE; TR = 550 ms, TE = 20 ms): The lipoma shows a high signal intensity.
b T2-weighted sagittal section (SE; TR = 2100 ms, TE = 80 ms): Only slight signal intensity. Chemical shift artifact in the direction of the readout gradient (craniocaudal direction). There is a corresponding black, fringe-like stripe cranially and a bright stripe caudally outlining the lipoma.

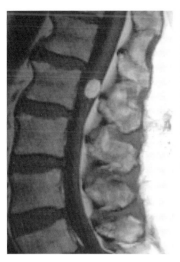

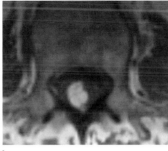

b

a

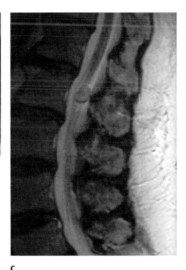

c

Fig. 3.**26 a–c Small dorsolateral lipoma at the L2 level:**

a T1-weighted sagittal image (TSE; TR = 588 ms, TE = 12 ms): The rounded small lipoma is situated at the level of the conus-cauda junction. Low-lying conus is not seen.

b T1-weighted transverse image (TSE; TR = 802 ms, TE = 12 ms): The dorsolateral location of the lipoma is easily seen on this image.

c T2-weighted sagittal image (TSE; TR = 5000 ms, TE = 112 ms): The lipoma demonstrates a signal intensity similar to that of fat.

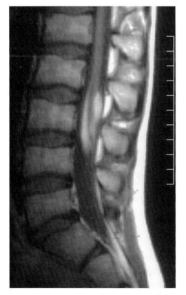

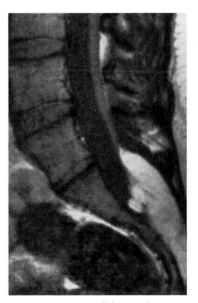

Fig. 3.**27 Lumbar lipoma with concomitant low-lying conus at the L3 level.** T1-weighted image (TSE; TR = 790 ms, TE = 17 ms): The lipoma envelops the spinal cord from the dorsal and ventral aspect and overlies the myelon over a long segment. It appears that there is fixation of the conus by the lipoma in the form of a tethered cord.

Fig. 3.**28 Lipoma of the cauda equina with tethered cord syndrome.** The spinal cord is elongated as far as S1. The spinal canal is markedly distended caudally (SE; TR = 680 ms, TE = 20 ms).

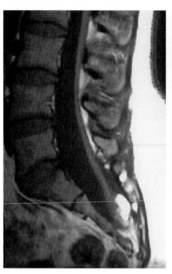

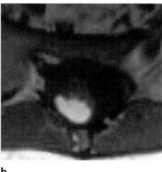

a

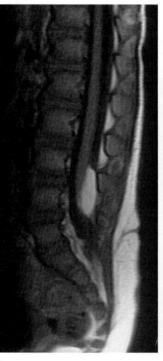

b

Fig. 3.**29 a, b** **Sacral lipoma with a concomitant finding corresponding to a caudal regression syndrome:**

a T1-weighted sagittal section (SE; TR = 450 ms, TE = 15 ms): The spinal cord is elongated as far as S2. The lipoma overlies the conus dorsally. The sacrum is markedly shortened in a caudal direction. The sacral canal appears enlarged.

b Transverse section (SE; TR = 580 ms, TE = 15 ms): The dorsal location of the lipoma is shown well in this slice orientation.

a

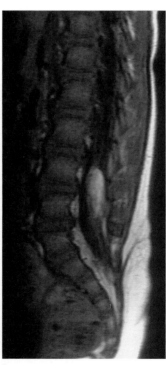

b

Fig. 3.**30 a, b** **Intradural lipoma at the level of L4 with associated malformation (dermal sinus):**

a T1-weighted sagittal section (TSE; TR = 800 ms, TE = 12 ms): The lipoma overlies the spinal cord dorsally at the level of L4. Note the concomitant dermal sinus traversing in a dorsal direction.

b Slice 3 mm parallel to **a**: The further course of the dermal sinus is well noted on this image. The sinus ends at the level of the bone, an intraspinal extension was not detectable, neither in the conventional images shown nor in the (not depicted) contrast-assisted images.

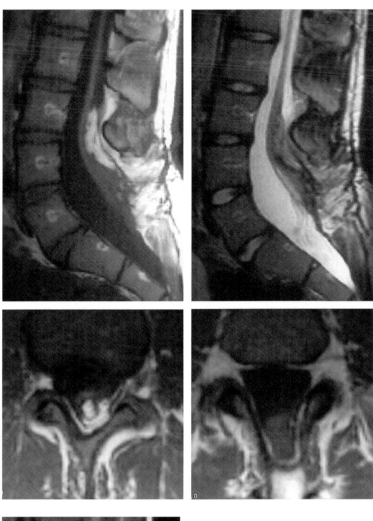

Fig. 3.**31 a–d** **Lipomyelo-meningocele:**

a T1-weighted sagittal section with evidence of an intradural lipomatous component at the level L3/L4. This lipoma communicates with the extradural part. Note the meningocele-like enlargement of the spinal canal, particularly dorsally. The spinal cord extends distally as far as L5/S1 where it exhibits a dorsal attachment to the dura.

b Corresponding T2-weighted image (TSE; TR = 5000 ms, TE = 112 ms): The lipoma is poorly delineated from the spinal cord components on this image. The nerve roots coursing ventrally at the level of L5/S1 can be seen easily.

c T1-weighted transverse image (SE; TR = 580 ms, TE = 15 ms): Dorsal lipoma with tethering of the spinal cord.

d Image 2 cm distal to **c**: Spina bifida with dorsal opening of the spinal canal. Meningocele-like enlargement. The spinal cord can be seen as a coarse structure in the dorsal segments of the spinal canal with attachment to the dura. Note the fringe-like epidural fat in the dorsal parts of the meningocele.

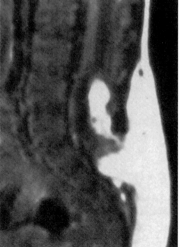

◁ Fig. 3.**32** **Lypomyelocele.** 3-week-old boy. Subcutaneous and intradural lipomas communicating with each other via the bony defect. Tethering of the spinal cord and low-lying conus at the level L4. No meningocele (SE; TR = 650 ms, TE = 25 ms).

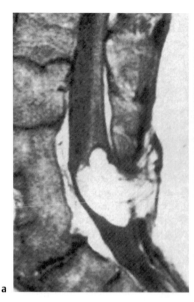
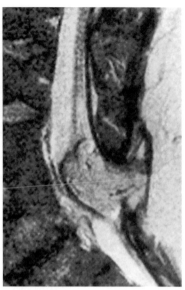

a

b

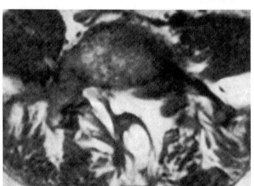

c

Fig. 3.**33 a–c** **Lipomyelomeningocele.**   41-year-old patient:

a Malformation of the distal three lumbar vertebrae with evidence of vertebral shortening and a considerable degree of fusion. Extensive subcutaneous lipoma communicating with the intradural component. Tethering of the low-lying conus. Enlargement of the spinal canal and evidence of a corresponding spinal bifida at the L4–L5 level (SE; TR = 750 ms, TE = 25 ms).

b T2-weighted image (SE; TR = 2100 ms, TE = 80 ms).

c Transverse section at the L5 level (SE; TR = 550 ms, TE = 25 ms).

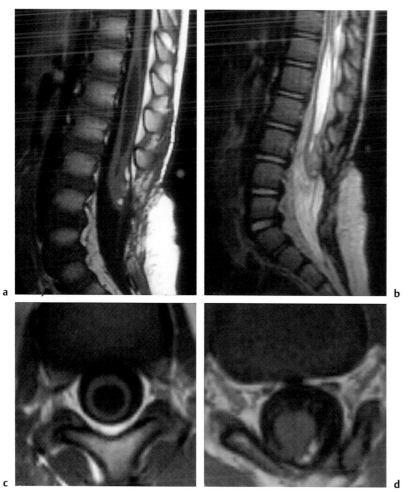

Fig. 3.**34 a–d** **Postoperative lipomyelomeningocele at the level of L3:**

a T1-weighted sagittal image (TSE; TR = 600 ms, TE = 12 ms): Extensive spina bifida reaching from L3 to S1. The caudal part of the spinal cord appears thickened at the level of L3. A small lipomatous remnant can be seen dorsally. The spinal cord appears dorsally attached to the dura. Large syrinx, in part with a distinct distension of the myelon.

b T2-weighted sagittal image (TSE; TR = 5000 ms, TE = 112 ms): The extent of the syrinx is easily identifiable due to its high CSF signal. The filum is seen as a thin linear structure, although it is evidently not stretched out.

c T1-weighted transverse section with T1-weighting at the level of the syrinx (SE; TR = 580 ms, TE = 15 ms): Marked ballooning of the spinal cord with corresponding pressure atrophy.

d Section at the level of a small lipomatous remnant (SE; TR = 580 ms, TE = 15 ms): The lipoma overlies the spinal cord with a fibrous component dorsally and extends laterally to the left. Note the nerve roots on either side evidently exiting atypically and dorsally from the spinal cord and also appearing slightly thickened.

■ Fibrolipomatosis of the Filum Terminale

The filum normally courses dorsally in the midline away from the conus in front of the dura, penetrates the dural sac and proceeds extradurally in the sacral canal, inserting on the dorsal aspect of the first coccygeal vertebra.

The filum is not infrequently divided into a second cord, which runs dorsally into the skin, giving rise to a small, circumscribed dimple (Emery and Lendon, 1969).

The filum is normally as much as 2 mm thick in diameter (measured at the level L5/S1).

Fibrolipomatosis of the filum terminale can develop from faulty regression at a lumbosacral level during the embryonic phase. This becomes evident from a thickening of the filum and can lead to shortening and consequently to a low-lying conus as a result of conus tethering. Oc-casionally however, the conus is found at a normal position despite the formation of fibrolipomatosis of the filum terminale. Fibrolipomatosis is found both in exclusively extradural and in-tradural-extradural locations, as well as exclusively extradurally.

The lipoma has a sausage-like configuration with intradural-extradural expansion and tapers at the site of penetration through the dura. The extradural component is not infrequently larger than the intradural part and can demonstrate a considerable expansion with infiltration of the surrounding tissue when occurring exclusively extradurally. The intradural lipoma normally has a capsule (Emery and Lendon, 1969).

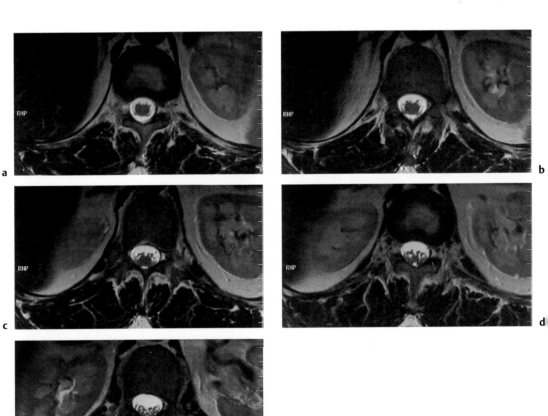

Fig. 3.**35 a–h Normal conus-cauda junction.** Transverse sections (TSE; TR = 6310 ms, TE = 120 ms):
a–e The transverse images show the nerve roots exiting from the conus and the junction to the cauda. The segmental spidery configuration is easily seen.

Diagnostics

MRI

The conus-cauda junction is well defined on T2-weighted transverse images. On T2- and T1-weighted images the filum is normally indistinguishable in its signal from the nerve roots, but delineation is clearly possible in the presence of fibrolipomatous transformation (Fig. 3.**35**).

Fibrolipomatosis is easily recognized on T1-weighted images by its characteristic fat signal.

Here sagittal and transverse images should be obtained to show its entire course.

For depiction of fibrolipomatosis, T2-weighted images should be taken using a GRE technique because the lipomatous components are well delineated from the cauda due to the complete loss of signal. The differentiation between cauda and fibrolipomatosis is often impossible using T2-weighted SE sequences (Figs. 3.**36**–3.**38**).

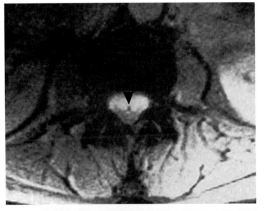

f

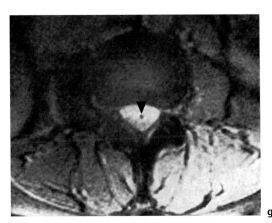

g

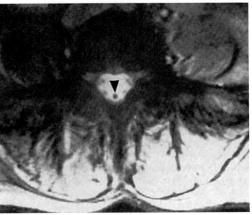

h

Fig. 3.**35 f–h** Depiction of the filum (arrowhead) which stands out well as a dark spot due to discrete fibrolipomatosis (GRE; TR = 680 ms, TE = 20 ms, flip angle α = 10°). No elongation of the conus. Due to the lack of lipomatosis the filum is demarcated neither on T2-weighted GRE images nor on T1-weighted images.

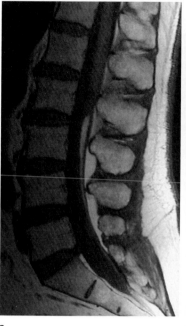

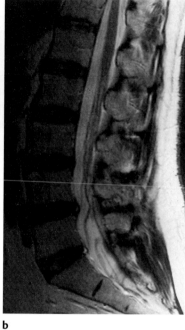

a

b

Fig. 3.**36 a, b** **Fibrolipomatosis with an obvious enlargement of the filum terminale at the level L3.**

a T1-weighted sagittal image (TSE; TR = 800 ms, TE = 12 ms): Well-defined filum with corresponding fibrolipomatous modification with a distinct thickening, recognizable particularly at the level L3. The caudal parts of the filum also appear somewhat thickened, albeit without deposits of fatty tissue. The conus is located at the level L1/L2 and is therefore not low-lying.

b Corresponding T2-weighted image using SE technique (TSE; TR = 4000 ms, TE = 120 ms): On this image the lipomatous modification is not recognizable.

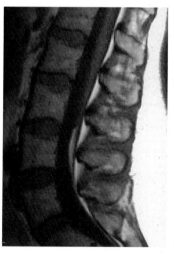

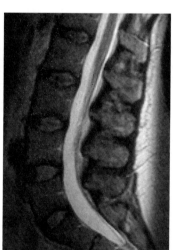

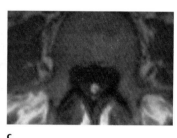

c

a

b

Fig. 3.**37 a–c** **Localized fibrolipomatosis at the level L4:**

a T1-weighted sagittal section (TSE; TR = 588 ms, TE = 12 ms): Fibrolipomatous modification of the filum with typical fat signal.

b Corresponding T2-weighted image using an SE technique (TSE; TR = 5000 ms, TE = 112 ms): The fibrolipomatosis is not clearly recognizable on this image.

c T1-weighted transverse section (SE; TR = 580 ms, TE = 15 ms): Well-defined fibrolipomatous structure.

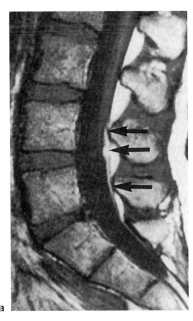

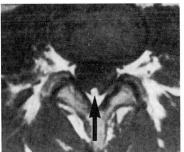

b

Fig. 3.**38 a, b** **Fibrolipomatosis with tethered cord syndrome.** 37-year-old patient:
a The sagittal section shows evidence of tapering of the conus with low-lying spinal cord at the level L4 (arrow) (SE; TR = 550 ms, TE = 20 ms).
b The transverse section also shows the lipomatous modification and thickening of the filum to a diameter of 4 mm (arrow) (SE; TR = 550 ms, TE = 20 ms).

▪ Tethered Cord Syndrome

Definition and Pathogenesis

In a broad sense, this term embraces all disorders that are associated with lumbosacral tethering of the spinal cord and result in a low-lying conus.

In these disorders, therefore, the conus does not reach its normal position at the level of L1/L2 that is found in healthy individuals about 8–10 weeks after birth.

The spinal cord, and especially the conus medullaris, demonstrates a change in form in these cases. The conus appears thin and elongated; the normal thickening of the spinal cord at the level of the conus is not found.

The tethered cord syndrome is caused by all disorders that result in this tethering of the conus:

- lumbosacral lipoma,
- lipomyelomeningocele,
- fibrolipomatosis of the filum terminale,
- split cord malformation,
- dermal sinus,
- intradural congenital tumors.

In a narrower sense, the tethered cord syndrome is a disorder brought about by an alteration of the filum terminale.

The filum is usually about 24 cm long and up to 2 mm thick. The tethered cord syndrome involves a shortening and thickening of the filum, which results in tethering of the conus in an abnormally low position distal to L2. The thickening of the filum is frequently associated with the formation of bands connecting the cauda equina and dura together in the lumbosacral space.

The clinical picture is very rare and is seen in only 2% of all patients with occult spinal dysraphism in large studies (Jones and Love, 1956).

Clinical Presentation

The patients often present with skin alterations as well as increased hair growth or a subcutaneous lipoma.

Bony alterations are not infrequently encountered, including:

- disturbances of vertebral fusion,
- enlargement of the spinal canal,
- scoliosis,
- malformation of the ribs,
- block vertebrae.

The patients develop clinical manifestations during childhood, rarely at the time of birth.

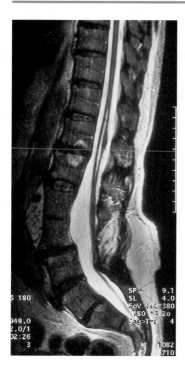

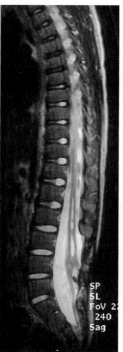

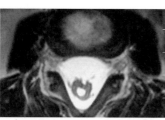

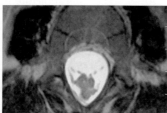

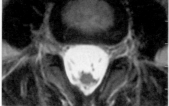

Therapy

The therapy of choice is the removal of the band-like adhesions and division of the shortened filum terminale (Jones and Love, 1956).

Diagnostics

MRI

Sagittal and transverse T1-weighted images demonstrate the thickening of the filum, displaying a signal typical for fibrous tissue. Lipomatous components are lacking. The spinal cord appears elongated, the conus stretched (Figs. 3.**39**–3.**41**).

◁ Fig. 3.**39**　**Thickened and shortened filum terminale with low-lying conus and corresponding thinning and elongation of the conus.** In addition, there is evidence of a syrinx in the region T12–L2 and incompletely fused vertebrae in the region L3/4 (TSE; TR = 3950 ms, TE = 112 ms).

Fig. 3.**40 a–d　Tethered cord syndrome.** Tethered cord syndrome in the presence of a complex malformation with evidence of spina bifida L3–S1, marked shortening and thickening of the conus at the L4 level, a syrinx in the region L1–L3 and an enlargement of the spinal canal in the region L3–S1:

a T2-weighted sagittal image (TSE; TR = 5310 ms, TE = 112 ms) with evidence of the extensive lumbosacral alterations.

b T2-weighted transverse section (TSE; TR = 5580 ms, TE = 120 ms): Syrinx at the level of the conus with obvious enlargement of the spinal canal dorsally. Well-defined nerve roots with ventral and dorsal exit points, although somewhat atypical, especially on the left side; anteriorly the root exits far interiorly, posteriorly it exits far dorsally.

c Slice 5 mm caudal to **b**: The syrinx now only extends into the right part of the spinal cord. Neurofibrous tissue overlies the spinal cord dorsally. On the left there is the impression that the nerve root exits from this tissue.

d Slice 5 mm further caudal to **c**: Spina bifida with lack of closure of the vertebral arch dorsally.

◼ Split Cord Malformation Types I and II

Definition

The split cord malformation is an occult spinal dysraphism associated with clefting of the spinal cord in a sagittal alignment. Clefting appears at a circumscribed site and is of variable length, being reported in the literature with values of between 1 and 10 cm. The two hemicords can develop both symmetrically and asymmetrically.

Each hemicord has its own central canal and normally supplies the ipsilateral dorsal and ventral nerve roots. In exceptional cases, however, contralateral nerve roots also develop within one hemicord, resulting in correspondingly fewer nerve roots being found on the opposite side. Each hemicord is invested by pia and has its own spinal artery.

> Two distinct forms can be differentiated, depending on how the arachnoid membrane and dura are separated

- The splitting of the spinal cord in *type I (diastematomyelia)* is associated with a fibrous or bony spur extending from the dorsum of the vertebral body in a sagittal direction dorsal to the vertebral arch. The arachnoid membrane and dura are laid down separately for each hemicord and each separately encloses the spinal cord. Hence each hemicord has its own subarachnoid space. Above the cleft and also, in the majority of cases, distal to it, the divided meninges reunite to form a uniform dura and arachnoid membrane with an appropriate normalization of the subarachnoid space (Fig. 3.**42**).
- In *type II*, each hemicord is invested separately by its own pia mater, but there is a common subarachnoid space. Both hemicords are therefore enclosed by a common arachnoid membrane and dura. Usually there is no fully developed spur but a fibrous septum between the hemicords.

Each of these two forms is seen in about 50 % of cases (Naidich and Harwood-Nash, 1983; Pang *et al.*, 1992).

Both types I and II can occur in the same patient at different levels, while the same form of spinal cord splitting has also been seen at multi-

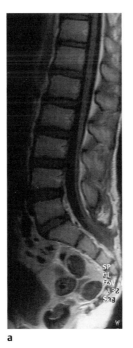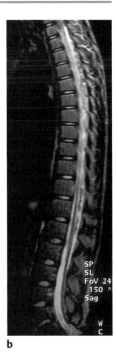

a   b

Fig. 3.**41 a, b** **Depiction of the filum terminale:**
a T1-weighted sagittal image (TSE; TR = 800 ms, TE = 12 ms): Thickened and shortened filum terminal with corresponding elongation of the conus, which terminates at the level of L3. The dural sac opens dorsally at the level of S2/S3, in which segment there is a large bony defect in the form of a spina bifida. In the sacral parts of the spinal canal the distinction between the CSF-containing dural sac and the extradural connective tissue is sometimes not possible.
b T2-weighted sagittal image (TSE; TR = 5310 ms, TE = 112 ms): The thickened and shortened filum terminal is well defined on this image. It courses in a dorsal direction following the lumbosacral curvature.

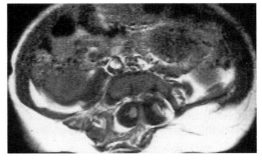

Fig. 3.**42** **Type I split cord malformation with spur.** Attachment of the left myelon to a lipoma that is contiguous with the subcutaneous fat. Vertebral and vertebral-arch dysplasia.

ple levels in the same patient. Apart from the dorsal and ventral nerve roots, which are typically situated laterally, paramedian roots are also seen along the spinal cord, although this duplication occurs more frequently dorsally and only very rarely ventrally. In type I the paramedian dorsal nerve roots course more horizontally from the medial contour of the hemicord and end blindly after a short distance. In type II they course away from the surface of the spinal cord dorsally and are longer than in type I.

Usually, the spinal cord is normal above the defect and reunites distal to it. Rarely does the cleft continue caudally in the form of a doubled filum terminale (Hilal *et al.*, 1974). In 76 % of cases the conus lies distal to L2, and frequently there is also a thickening of the filum terminale (Hilal *et al.*, 1974).

The spinal cord can be tethered to the dura by fibrous bands and dorsal nerve roots, although these structures can also course epidurally to reach the bone. These bands can additionally contribute to the low position of the conus. The fibrous band in type II always adheres to the medial side of the spinal cord. Sometimes these fibrous bands can be very thin so that they are not easily seen on MRI examination. The septum can be found exclusively ventral or exclusively dorsal to the split spinal cord and in these cases does not course entirely from ventral to dorsal. A complete septum is usually the exception.

Location and Clinical Presentation

According to the literature, 85 % of cases of diastematomyelia are found between T9 and S1. They are seen in an exclusively thoracic location in 21 % of cases, in a thoracolumbar one in 18 % of cases and in exclusively lumbar ones in 61 % of cases. Less than 1 % are found cervically (Hilal *et al.*, 1974).

The disorder is found more frequently in females than in males. In 33–40 % of cases it is combined with cutaneous alterations at the level of the spinal-cord malformation. Clinical alterations sometimes only present later and can become manifest as a result of physical exertion or pregnancy (French, 1990).

Meningocele manqué. A meningocele manqué is rarely seen in combination with a split cord malformation. It involves the formation of a mixed

bundle of nerve roots, fibrous structures and blood vessels extending from the dorsal surface of the spinal cord to the dura. Frequently the dura is infringed and this mixed fibroneurovascular bundle is tethered within the extradural tissue. In addition, the fibrous septum can contain fatty tissue as well as muscle cells.

Hydromyelia. In 30–40 % of cases hydromelia is also seen in these patients and can extend from a site cranial to the defect and reach caudal to the defect, embracing as it does one or even both hemicords.

Clinically the hydromyelia can become particularly manifest as a progressive scoliosis.

Myelomeningocele. In some cases the malformation is associated with the occurrence of a myelomeningocele. Three subtypes are differentiated.

Subtypes of myelomeningocele

- The placode represents the end of the spinal cord and the finding is identical with a classic lumbosacral myelomeningocele in the neonate. The placode is found immediately caudal to the spur or fibrous septum, both hemicords merge into the placode with the hemicords arising proximal to the bony defect.
- The placode does not represent the terminal end of the spinal cord, but rather a segmental section. It is situated immediately rostral to the bony spur or fibrous septum and the caudal part of the placode divides into the two parts of the spinal cord. The cleft of the spinal cord ends caudal to the spur or septum, which is situated in the midline, and the reunited spinal cord usually terminates in a caudal lipoma or a thickened filum terminale. In this subtype the split spinal cord is incorporated into the intact spinal canal caudal to the meningomyelocele.
- This type is predominantly found in a cervical location. There is no development of a placode, instead each part of the spinal cord displays a dorsal band containing glial-cell neurons, nerve roots and ganglion cells extending into a dorsally projecting pouch, which is usually completely embedded in thickened and impermeable membranes. These collateral dorsal neural band-like structures run parallel

to the fibrous septum, which is situated in the midline and similarly fixed in the pouch-like herniation of the meningocele.

In rare cases the two parts of the spinal cord can be formed asymmetrically with a strong as well as a very slender component. Alternatively the two hemicords can be situated in front of each other instead of in parallel, so that the septum assumes a course in a coronal direction. In addition, the occurrence of a threefold splitting has also been reported.

Bony malformations. Almost every case of split cord malformation is associated with malformations of the spine. The formation of block vertebrae occurs, as well as hemivertebrae ("butterfly" vertebrae). Kyphoscoliosis is often the result. Fusions between the arches of adjacent vertebrae are found, while diagonal fusions between contralateral vertebral arches as well as ipsilateral fusions between arches of the same side can also occur. The formation of a spina bifida nearly always occurs. The vertebral anomalies are usually concentrated on the region where the split cord malformation is found. During childhood the bony spur, which can divide the spinal cord, is only preformed in cartilage and can therefore be easily overlooked even on MRI images, depending on the degree of expression of the ossification center.

Diagnostics

MRI

On the whole MRI is well suited to confirm the diagnosis. It readily shows the dichotomy of the spinal cord and demonstrating hydromyelia creates no difficulties.

Difficulties of differentiation can arise regarding the portrayal of the fibrous or bony septum. Furthermore, the reliable depiction of the nerve roots and providing an answer to questions regarding the formation of arachnoid membrane and dura will not always be possible using MRI (Figs. 3.**43**–3.**50**).

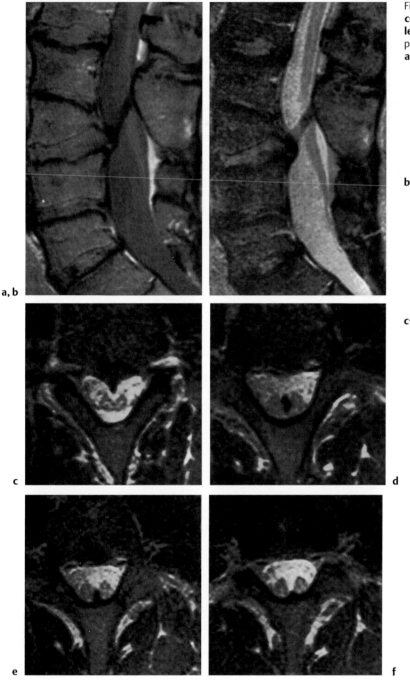

a, b

c

d

e

f

Fig. 3.**43 a–f   Type I split cord malformation at the level of L3.** 33-year-old patient:

a   PD-weighted sagittal section with evidence of a bony spur, which runs in a ventral-caudal to dorsal-cranial direction (SE; TR = 2100 ms, TE = 20 ms). The bony septum appears hypointense. Note dysplasia of L3.

b   On the T2-weighted sequence there is also a hypointense depiction of the bony spur. At the same time, there is also evidence of the low-lying conus at the level of L3/L4 due to tethering of the spinal cord (SE; TR = 2100 ms, TE = 80 ms).

c–f The transverse images confirm the splitting of the spinal cord (**c** caudal, **f** proximal) (SE; TR = 2100 ms, TE = 80 ms).

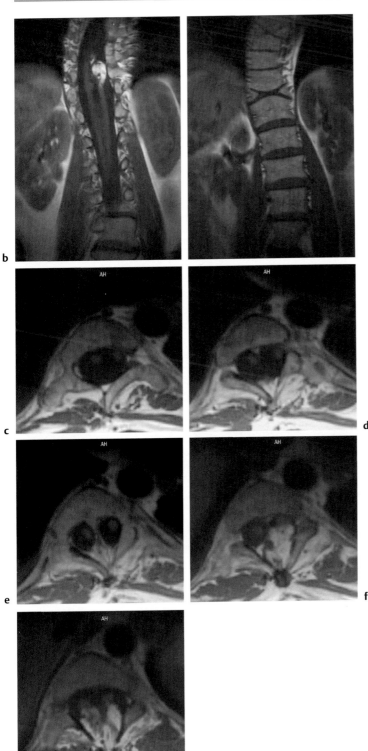

Fig. 3.44 a–l   Type I split cord malformation. Type I split cord malformation with complex malformation of the vertebrae at the thoracolumbar junction, an extensive intradural lipoma, a large bony defect in the form of a spina bifida at the level of T9 to L2, and an intra- and extradural epidermoid cyst.

a T1-weighted coronal section (TSE; TR = 600 ms, TE = 12 ms) with depiction of the clefting of the spinal cord and the partially adherent lipoma.

b Coronal section further ventrally with portrayal of marked vertebral dysplasias. Butterfly vertebrae, a partial block-vertebral formation and hemivertebrae can be delineated.

c–g T1-weighted transverse section with depiction of both hemicords and the spur. Note the large lipoma adherent to both hemicords, which is recognizable caudally.

Fig. 3.**44 h–l** ▷

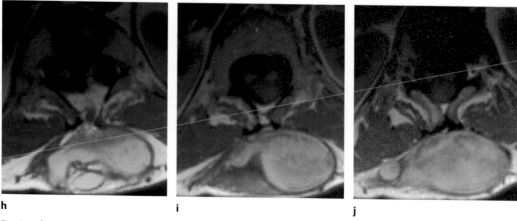

h   i   j

Fig. 3.**44 h–j** Slices further caudally with evidence of the large subcutaneous epidermoid cyst, clefting along the vertebral arch, and portrayal of a knotty structure dorsally overlying the spinal cord.

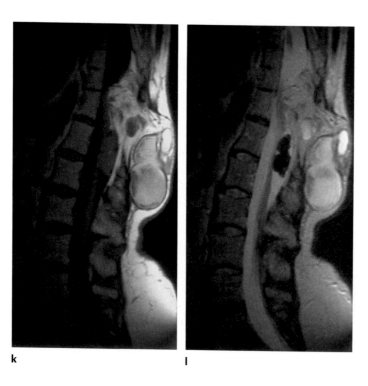

k   l

Fig. 3.**44**

k T1-weighted sagittal section with evidence of an extensive malformation in the region of the thoracolumbar junction, nodular structures dorsally overlying the spinal cord at the level of T12/L1 and the tethered cord with fixation of the conus at the level of L3.

l T2-weighted sagittal section. The epidermoid cyst shows a spotted inhomogeneous and overall very high signal; the intradural epidermoid components are dark.

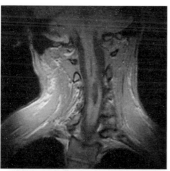

a

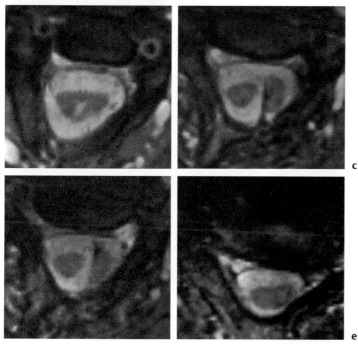

b

c

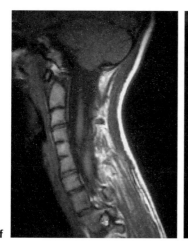

d

e

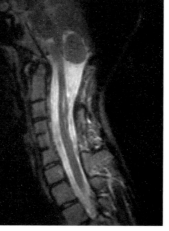

f

g

Fig. 3.**45 a–g** **Cervical type I split cord malformation (diastematomyelia):**

a   Coronal section (FLASH; TR = 500 ms, TE = 7 ms, flip angle α = 70°) with evidence of clefting of the spinal cord in the cervical canal.

b–e T2-weighted transverse section (FLASH; TR = 690 ms, TE = 24 ms, flip angle α = 25°): Delicate syrinx above the cleft, bony spur running from ventral to dorsal, renewed fusion of both hemicords distal to the bony spur.

Fig. 3.**45**

f   T1-weighted sagittal section at the level of the cleft (TSE; TR = 600 ms, TE = 12 ms): The interruption of the spinal cord is easily recognized. Furthermore there are dysplasias of the vertebrae C4 to C6 recognizable with partial fusions.

g   T2-weighted sagittal section (TSE; TR = 5000 ms, TE = 112 ms) with evidence of the proximal syrinx at the level of C2/C3.

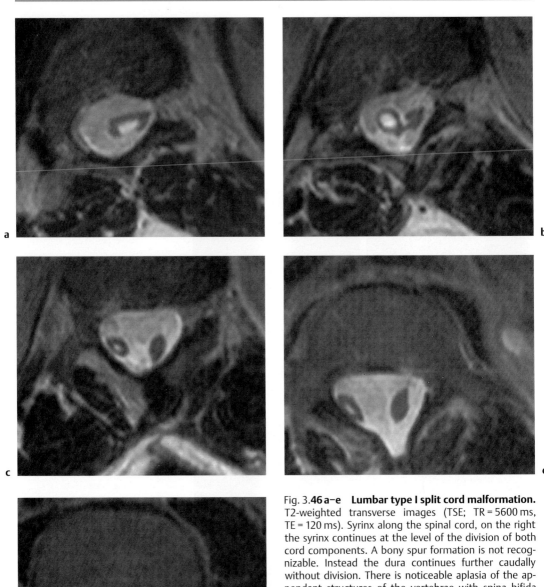

Fig. 3.**46 a–e   Lumbar type I split cord malformation.**
T2-weighted transverse images (TSE; TR = 5600 ms,
TE = 120 ms). Syrinx along the spinal cord, on the right
the syrinx continues at the level of the division of both
cord components. A bony spur formation is not recognizable. Instead the dura continues further caudally
without division. There is noticeable aplasia of the appendant structures of the vertebrae with spina bifida
and dorsal herniation of the spinal canal.

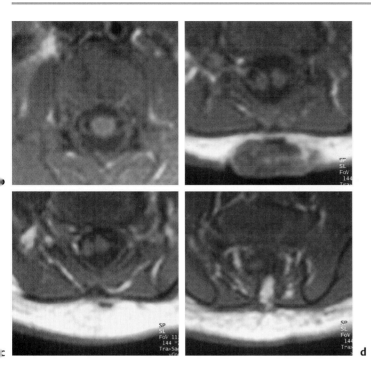

Fig. 3.47 a–d Type II split cord malformation and spina bifida.
Neonate with type II split cord malformation and spina bifida at the level of the lumbosacral junction plus the finding of an intradural lipoma:

a–c T1-weighted transverse images (SE; TR = 700 ms, TE = 14 ms): Clefting of the spinal cord without evidence of a septum or spur. Large cutaneous tag level with the dorsal skin.

d The distal section displays the lipoma bulging intradurally.

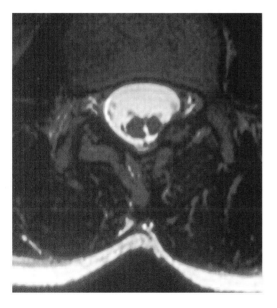

Fig. 3.48 Type II split cord malformation. Type II split cord malformation with adherence of the posterior component of the left myelon to the dorsal dura.

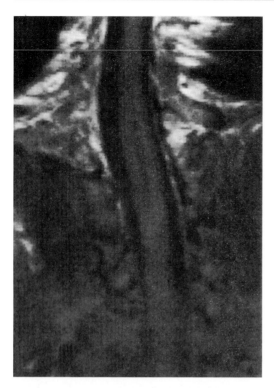

Fig. 3.49 a–c Cervicothoracic type II split cord malformation with meningocele manqué:

a Coronal section with evidence of clefting of the spinal cord. The two hemicords are divided neither by a bony spur nor by a fibrous septum.

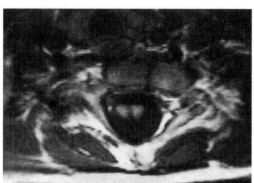

b T1-weighted transverse section with clefting of the myelon.

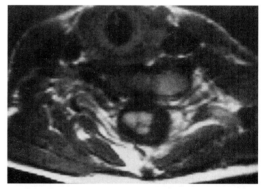

c Meningocele manqué: Intraoperative finding with convoluted tissue overlying both hemicords dorsally. A few thin nerve roots have their points of exit coming from this tissue.

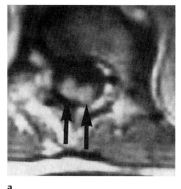 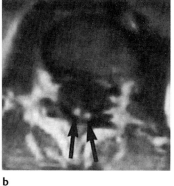 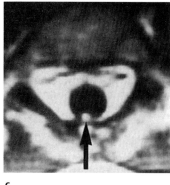

a   b   c

Fig. 3.**50 a–c Type II split cord malformation with tethered cord due to a thickened and shortened filum terminale:**

a Transverse section at the level of L2 with evidence of spinal cord clefting (SE; TR = 600 ms, TE = 30 ms).

b The two spinal cords taper caudally. Histological examination revealed both components to have alterations from scarring (SE; TR = 600 ms, TE = 30 ms).

c Short, lipomatous thickened filum terminale (SE; TR = 600 ms, TE = 30 ms).

■ Dermal Sinus

Definition

The dermal sinus is an epithelialized tract extending down from the skin in a dorsal direction. Usually the dermal sinus begins in the midline along the spine; less frequently the entrance is found parasagitally. Here a small dimple with an opening is found superficially, not infrequently combined with a capillary angioma, a hair nevus or a hyperpigmented area of skin. Hairs can grow out of the opening itself (List, 1941).

Extension

The depth to which it extends varies considerably. The tract can terminate subcutaneously, it can reach the bone, gain access to the epidural or subdural space, or even show contact with neural tissue, i.e. spinal cord, cauda equina, with individual nerve roots or with the filum terminale. An intradural connection to a dermoid, epidermoid or lipoma is not infrequently found. These tumors occur at both extra- and intramedullary locations.

The majority of cases present a mild form of dorsal spina bifida, although bony changes can be lacking completely. More pronounced bony defects are the exception. If the tract has a connection with neural structures, tethering of the spinal cord with inferior displacement can occur. During ascension of the conus medullaris, the tract itself can also be drawn up so that its course becomes aligned in a dorsal-caudal to ventral-cranial direction. It can also run horizontally, i.e. in a ventral-caudal direction, or even demonstrate a wavy course so that several thin cuts are required to demonstrate the tract on sagittal image sectioning.

Location

About 62–66 % of dermal sinuses are seen at a lumbosacral location and about 25 % are occipital. Only 10 % are found at a thoracic site and only a very small number are cervical (Wright, 1971).

Pathogenesis

This must be differentiated from the pilonidal sinus of the coccyx, which never has an intradural connection. An infection can develop via the dermal sinus immediately after birth, continuing into the subarachnoid space and resulting in arachnopathy. In the course of the inflammatory process, extradural inflammatory alterations can also occur, including the formation of an abscess.

Compression of nerve roots and the spinal cord from a dermoid or epidermoid can give rise to clinical signs and symptoms. With an intramedullary location of the tumor, the distension of the spinal cord can lead to corresponding symptoms.

The dermal sinus is always an indication for surgery, independent of the outcome of the MRI examination. MRI, therefore, only assists in preoperative planning.

Diagnostics

MRI

MRI should be performed with thin slices in two planes (transversal and sagittal). Images after administration of contrast agent are of particular significance because only then the extent of the inflammatory reaction, particularly intradurally, becomes apparent. In cases where the dermal sinus assumes an oblique course, attempts to acquire angled sagittal images should be made in order to visualize the whole course, preferably in one slice (Figs. 3.**51**–3.**53**).

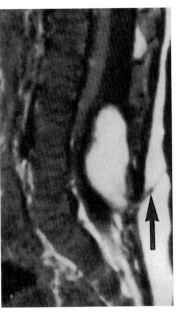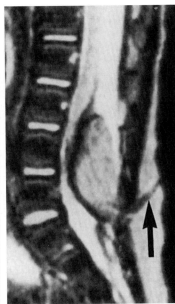

a   b

Fig. 3.**51 a,b**   **Dermal sinus.** 4-month-old infant:
a T1-weighted sagittal section (SE; TR = 660 ms, TE = 25 ms) with evidence of a dermal sinus at the level of L5/S1 running in a cranial-caudal direction and demonstrating contact with an intradural lipoma. The spinal cord is attached ventrally to the lipoma and is elongated caudally (arrow).
b T2-weighted section (arrow) (SE; TR = 2100 ms, TE = 80 ms).

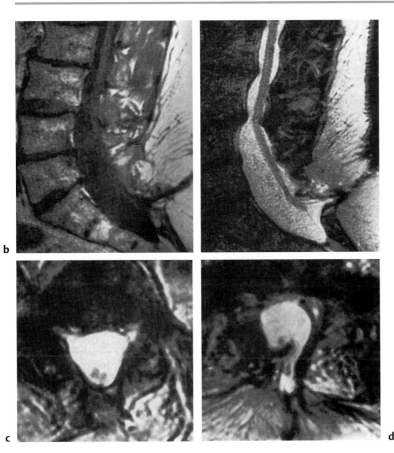

b

c

d

Fig. 3.**52 a–d   Dermal sinus.**
55-year-old patient in whom the dermal sinus was closed by surgery after birth:

a In the sagittal section evidence of the scarred and widened tract communicating with the spinal canal (SE; TR = 600 ms, TE = 25 ms).

b The spinal cord is elongated caudally and dorsally. A large bony defect and evidence of a small meningocele can be seen (SE; TR = 2100 ms, TE = 80 ms).

c In the transverse section, finding of diplomyelia in the form of a type II split cord malformation just above the bony defect (FFE; TR = 600 ms, TE = 20 ms, flip angle α = 25°).

d Caudal from here, the course of the spinal cord both ventral and dorsal to the bony spur (FFE; TR = 700 ms, TE = 20 ms, flip angle α = 25°).

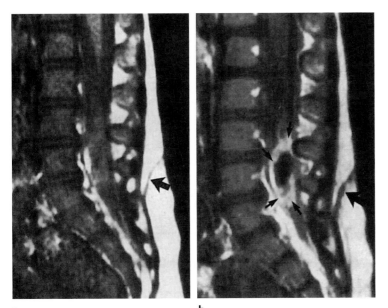

a

b

Fig. 3.**53 a,b   Dermal sinus.**
18-month-old girl:

a In the sagittal section the conus demonstrates a correct position at the level of L2. There is signal enhancement within the spinal canal at the level of L4/L5. The dermal sinus (arrow) runs from dorsal-cranial to ventral-caudal (SE; TR = 780 ms, TE = 25 ms).

b After application of contrast agent a strong intradural signal enhancement appears caudally at the level of L4/L5 (small arrow). Histological examination revealed extensive granulation tissue as an expression of the chronic inflammation.

■ Split Notochord Syndrome

Definition

The split notochord syndrome comprises a group of disorders that are characterized by a connection between parts of the intestines, spine, spinal canal and skin. Synonymous terms used include "combined anterior and posterior spina bifida," "dorsal enteric fistula," "spinal and cranial cysts" and "neurenteric cysts."

Pathogenesis

The pathological connection between mesodermal, neural and ectodermal structures evolves during embryogenesis. The theory of its development is summarized on pp. 66 and 67.

The finding is present at birth and displays very varied forms of expression, depending on the extent to which intrauterine healing of the defect was able to occur. In the most marked case there is a posterior cutaneous fistula in the midline communicating with parts of the intestine that lie anterior to the spine. There is therefore a direct connection between intestinal lumen and skin. Bowel contents can escape from the fistula. The spine displays a complete sagittal cleft along a circumscribed area. The following elements are therefore split:

- vertebral body,
- vertebral arch,
- dura,
- arachnoid membrane,
- spinal cord.

The spinal canal appears enlarged in the region of the anomaly and the finding can be combined with an anterior and posterior meningocele. The spinal cord can be fully developed on each side, with two anterior and two posterior nerve roots, although each spinal cord can also have two lateral nerve roots. Intestinal loops can bulge out at skin level via the fistula.

This form of split notochord syndrome with a posterior enteric fistula has only been reported in the literature 15 times (Hoffman *et al.*, 1993). In eight of these children the clinical picture was combined with a meningocele or myelomeningocele; five had an imperforate anus and two a rudimentary extremity, which resembled an arm with the bone extending from the spinal cleft. One of these patients had bladder exstrophy. There is possibly a connection between the split notochord syndrome and the occurrence of omphalocele, exstrophy, an imperforate anus and spinal defects.

If partial closing of the cleft occurs during intrauterine development then cysts, diverticula and blind-ending tracts form at various sites. The enterogenic cysts (intestinal duplications) can develop both anterior and posterior to the spine and connect with the vertebra via a fibrous band. Cleft vertebrae can be associated with a prevertebral location of the cyst, while cysts behind the spine can be combined with splitting of the vertebral arches and the spinous process. Prevertebral cysts are found at both thoracic and abdominal sites while intrathoracic cysts are situated in the posterior mediastinum. Enterogenic cysts tend to enlarge due to secretion.

The diverticula are parts of the intestine that appear elongated and are connected with the gut via fibrous bands. They can also have thoracic and abdominal locations, while intrathoracic sites are associated with a perforation of the diaphragm by the fibrous band. Cysts and diverticula can be lined with mucosa of the small intestine or even with esophageal or gastric epithelium.

Blind-ended tracts are found anteriorly. They originate from the skin and terminate in a sac-like cavity lined with skin or intestinal elements dorsal to the spine, sometimes with contact to bone.

Enterogenic cysts can also be found intraspinally. They are most frequently seen within the distal cervical and proximal thoracic segments of the spine (Agnoli *et al.*, 1984). They typically overlie the spinal cord anteriorly in the anterior subarachnoid space. They can be attached to the dura or leptomeninx and lead to compression and flattening of the spinal cord. Less frequently they can also have an intramedullary location. They are lined with mucosa, in particular cases by mucosa, submucosa and muscularis mucosae. The cyst epithelium can correspond to that of the stomach, small intestine or bronchus.

Enterogenic cysts are often combined with malformations of the spine. Hemivertebrae and cleft vertebrae have been reported. Intraspinal cysts can communicate with mediastinal or retroperitoneal lesions via bone defects.

The cysts are usually filled with a clear or milky fluid. They can rupture spontaneously, resulting in chemical meningitis. Intramedullary abscesses have been reported. Infections can spread from the bowel to the cysts.

Clinical Presentation

The majority of the cysts become clinically manifest within the first 6 months after birth. Symptoms are seen less frequently later on in life, when these tend to be smaller cysts with little compression. Males are affected three times more often than females.

Diagnostics

MRI

On MRI investigations the cysts predominantly display signal intensity that is somewhat higher than that of CSF. On T1-weighted images it can be lower or even higher than that of the spinal cord (Kantrowitz *et al.*, 1986; Aoki *et al.*, 1987; Geremia *et al.*, 1988; Pierot *et al.*, 1988; Kak *et al.*, 1990). They do not enhance with contrast material (Pierot *et al.*, 1988).

In particular, concomitant mediastinal and abdominal or retroperitoneal alterations should also be looked for with the aid of imaging techniques (Figs. 3.**54** and 3.**55**).

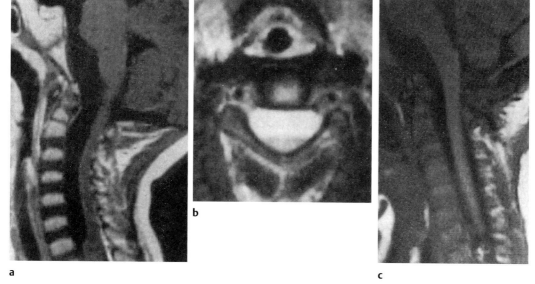

a

b

c

Fig. 3.**54 a–c Craniocervical neurenteric cyst:**
a MR image before surgery shows a ventral space-occupying cyst extending from the caudal base of the pons to C7.

b T2-weighted transverse image with a marked compression of the myelon.
c Image after surgical decompression of the spinal cord and brain stem components.

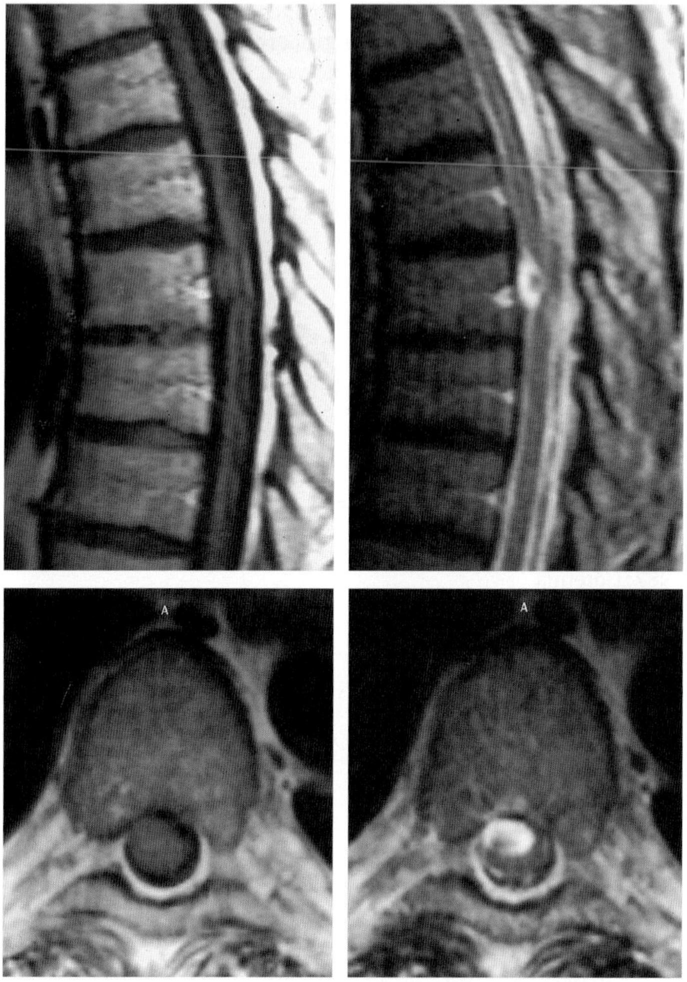

a, c

b

d

Fig. 3.**55 a–d   Small intradural cyst overlying the spinal cord ventrally at the level of T7:**

a   T1-weighted sagittal image. The cyst lying ventral to the spinal cord shows signal intensity similar to that of the myelon. Note the compressive effect (TSE; TR = 800 ms, TE = 12 ms).

b   T1-weighted transverse image (SE; TR = 805 ms, TE = 14 ms): The cyst is poorly defined on this image due to the relatively identical signal intensity.

c   T2-weighted sagittal image: The cyst displays a high signal intensity, but a small punctate hypodensity is apparent dorsally (TSE; TR = 5310 ms, TE = 112 ms).

d   T2-weighted transverse image (SE; TR = 5570 ms, TE = 120 ms): Well in accordance with the sagittal image, the ventral cyst is depicted showing a predominantly high signal intensity with a void in the dorsal component.

Non-dysraphic Malformations

Partial and Total Sacral Agenesis

Definition

Sacral agenesis is a clinical picture that occurs with most varying degrees of severity. Partial as well as complete forms of sacral agenesis are seen, sometimes with involvement of lumbar segments. Unilateral forms are differentiated from bilateral forms.

Pathogenesis

Sacral agenesis is frequently associated with disorders of the urogenital tract:

- unilateral renal agenesis,
- renal duplications,
- rectovesical fistulae,
- bladder exstrophy,
- cryptorchism,
- ovarian aplasia,
- partial aplasia of the uterus.

In addition, anomalies of the gastrointestinal tract are also found, including:

- omphaloceles,
- tracheoesophageal fistulae,
- Meckel's diverticula,
- rectal prolapse at the time of birth.

Neurogenic disturbances of the bladder and rectum are the rule.

Etiologically the clinical picture is considered to be teratogenically and genetically induced. A concentration of this disorder has been observed in insulin-dependent diabetic mothers, as well as in families. Furthermore, teratogenic damage during embryogenesis has been confirmed as a cause in animal studies.

Clinical Presentation

Apart from the symptoms arising from concomitant disorders, instabilities at the lumbosacral junction, scoliosis, contractures and deformities of the feet and knees, subluxations and disloca-tions of the hips predominate and are the result of skeletal changes.

Four types of sacral agenesis are differentiated (Fig. 3.**56**) (Renshaw, 1978):

> ### Types of sacral agenesis
>
> - *Type I* is defined as partial or total *unilateral* agenesis of the sacrum.
> - *Type II* comprises partial sacral agenesis occurring bilaterally and asymmetrically. There is a stable articulation between the ilia and the normal or hypoplastic first sacral vertebra.
> - *Type III* is associated with lumbar agenesis of varying degrees and a total sacral agenesis with the ilia articulating with the distal lumbar vertebra.
> - *Type IV* also comprises lumbar and total sacral agenesis, but in contrast to type III the ilia only interarticulate with each other or are fused.

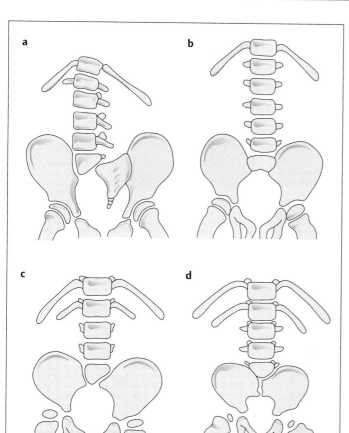

Fig. 3.**56 a–d   Various types of sacral agenesis** (classified according to Renshaw [1978]):

a Type I: Unilateral total or partial agenesis.

b Type II: Partial bilateral sacral agenesis. There is a stable articulation between the ilia and hypoplastic first sacral vertebra, as displayed here.

c Type III: Combination of a partial lumbar with a total sacral agenesis. Illustrated here is a hypoplastic L3 articulating with the ilia.

d Type IV: Partial lumbar and total sacral agenesis. The ilia themselves interarticulate with each other, the articulation with the lumbar spine is either partial or lacking.

Type I is not infrequently associated with the appearance of a so-called scimitar sacrum, a deformation of the unilaterally formed sacrum that resembles a curved sword. Further bony deformities can be present. A tethered cord syndrome can present intradurally, and intradural lipomas are not uncommon. The process can be associated with a meningomyelocele. Furthermore an anterior sacral meningocele can also be found.

The scimitar sacrum can sometimes develop in the course of follow-up investigations, its alteration in form being probably brought on by hydrostatic pressure and CSF pulsations (Holtzmann and Stein, 1985).

Lumbosacral lipomas are often associated with partial sacral agenesis. The incidence of this bony anomaly is as much as 50 % in some series, together with bony spina bifida. The finding is not infrequently combined with block vertebra formations of the cervical spine, similar to those found in Klippel-Feil syndrome.

Type II is the most common defect in some series. Here too, meningomyeloceles or lipomeningomyeloceles are often associated with it. This type is also combined with hip dysplasias and dislocations. The same applies for type III.

Type IV represents the most severe form of sacral agenesis. This form is normally associated

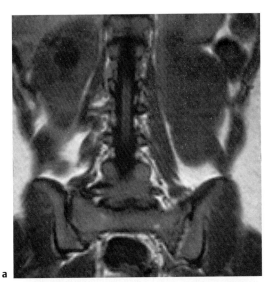

a

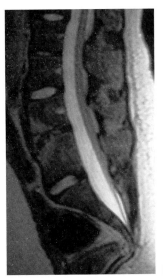

b

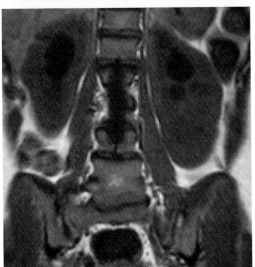

c

Fig. 3.**57 a–c Hypoplasia of the sacrum.** 12-year-old girl:
a T1-weighted coronal section (SE; TR = 500 ms, TE = 15 ms): L5 appears accentuated in height and slightly coarse in appearance, possibly having developed as a result of ankylosis. There is proper articulation with the sacrum. The iliosacral region appears normal.
b Slice 6 mm further ventrally.
c Sagittal section (TSE; TR = 5000 ms, TE = 112 ms): L5 can be recognized easily and is accentuated in height. The sacrum is hypoplastic and shortened. Tethered cord with a shortened filum terminale and a spinal cord elongated caudally as far as the region of the lumbosacral junction.

with a progressive pelvic kyphosis, which will subsequently require surgical fusion. Here too, thoracic meningomyeloceles are not unusual. Patients with type IV often present with foot deformities while the majority of patients with type III and type IV suffer from lumbopelvic instability.

The majority of patients without a meningomyelocele demonstrate a loss of motor innervation distal to the last vertebra. Sensory innervation is usually present far caudal to the last vertebra.

Diagnostics

MRI

The alterations of the sacrum can be clearly demonstrated, particularly in sagittal and coronal sections. The transverse scan orientation is suited for displaying intradural alterations. In principle, T1- and T2-weighted slices should be performed. T2-weighted images in particular succeed in showing the spinal cord, the cauda and the filum concisely. The routine administration of a contrast agent is not necessary (Figs. 3.**57**–3.**64**).

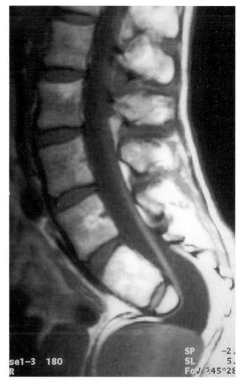

Fig. 3.**58** **Partial sacral agenesis, anterior meningocele with presacral dermoid, tethered cord attached to a lipoma.** T1-weighted sagittal section (SE; TR = 600 ms, TE = 12 ms).

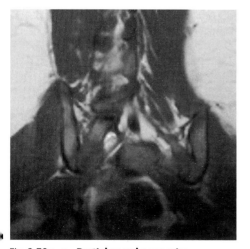

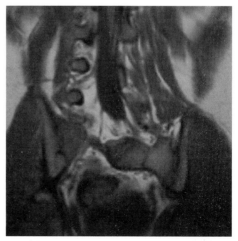

b

Fig. 3.**59 a–e** **Partial sacral agenesis:**
a Coronal section (TSE; TR = 644 ms, TE = 12 ms): Articulation of the dysplastic sacrum with appendant spi-

nal structures can be seen on the right. This type of articulation is not present on the left.
b Slice 1.5 cm further ventrally. Note dysplastic sacrum left laterally. Fig. 3.**59 c–e** ▷

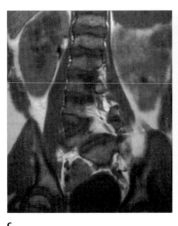
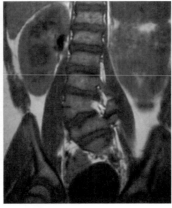
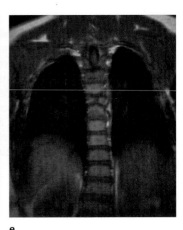

c   d   e

Fig. 3.**59 c–e**
  c Articulation of this component, which extends in a left-lateral direction, with the last lumbar vertebra. Severe deformity of the spine.
  d The failure of vertebral segmentation with asymmetric development of vertebral height can be seen on this image.

  e Coronal section of the thoracic spine (TSE; TR = 587 ms, TE = 12 ms): Vertical clefting of T6 in the form of a butterfly vertebra with corresponding deformity of T7. Evidence of a left-sided defect at the level of T5.

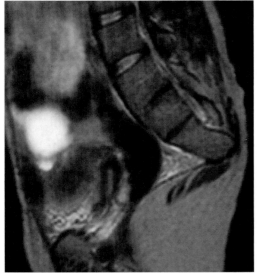

a

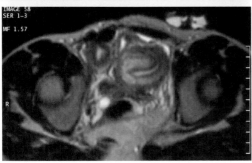

b

Fig. 3.**60 a, b Prediagnosed caudal regression syndrome, right-sided renal agenesis, uterus duplex primordium and primary anal atresia.** 24-year-old woman:
  a Sagittal T2-weighted section (TSE; TR = 4053 ms, TE = 112 ms): Partial agenesis of the sacrum with only S1 formed. Very narrow spinal canal. Dysplasia of the vertebral disks L4/L5 and L5/S1 with considerable loss of height and partial fusion of L4 and L5 ventrally.
  b Transverse section with evidence of the uterus duplex. Strongly developed uterus on the left with correct three-layered signal intensity; the high signal intensity within the cavum uteri corresponds to the endometrium, followed by a thin dark band as the inner layer of the myometrium, while the outer myometrium displays a moderate signal intensity.

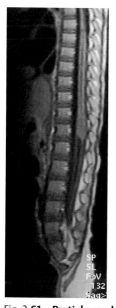

Fig. 3.**61**   **Partial sacral agenesis with spinal cord malformation.** Sagittal section using T1-weighting (TSE; TR = 900 ms, TE = 12 ms): The spinal cord shows a markedly coarse appearance and thickened form at the level of the conus medullaris. It is tethered dorsally. It tapers off into two band-like residual structures, which terminate in the lumbosacral lipomatous tissue. A syrinx is proximal to the thickened conus medullaris.

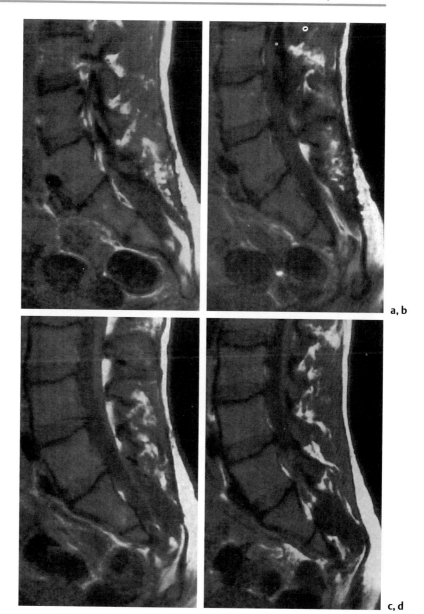

a, b

c, d

Fig. 3.**62 a–d**   **Type 1 partial sacral agenesis (scimitar sacrum).** The images show, from left to right, the shortened sacrum with an opening of the spinal canal ventrally and laterally into the presacral space on the right. Manifest enlargement of the spinal canal sacrally, particularly towards the right and laterally. The spinal cord tapers off caudally due to a shortening and tethering of the filum terminal in the lipomatous tissue.

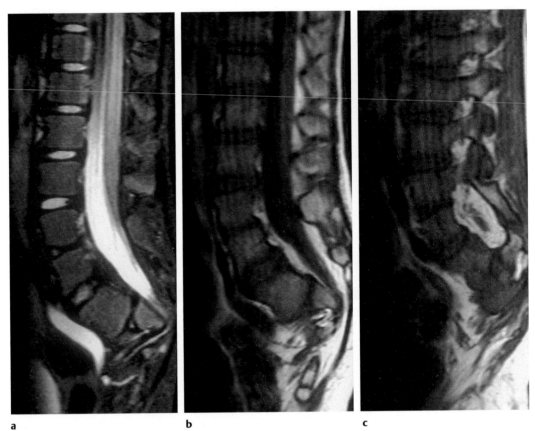

a   **b**   **c**

Fig. 3.**63 a–c** **Partial sacral agenesis**. 5-year-old boy:

a Sagittal section using T2-weighting (STIR sequence): Dysplasia of the sacral vertebrae and the disk L3/L4. Tethered cord with elongation of the conus as far as L3 due to shortening of the filum terminale.

b Sagittal T1-weighted section (TSE; TR = 800 ms, TE = 12 ms): On this image a small distal residual sacrum is recognizable.

c Parasagittal section using T1-weighting: Very marked epidural lipomatosis in the lumbosacral region with simultaneous absent primordium of the pedicles so that a broad communication exists between the foramina in the lumbosacral region.

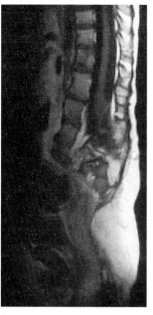

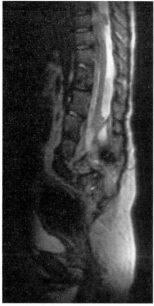

a   b

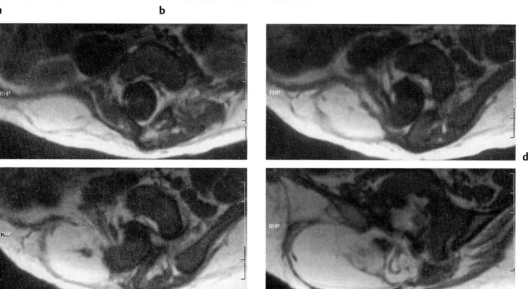

d

f

Fig. 3.**64 a–f   Partial sacral agenesis with absence of L5, type III according to Renshaw.** Failure of segmentation of the lumbar spine. Tethered cord with evidence of a lipomyelomeningocele and an additional large extradural lipoma:

a   Sagittal section using T1-weighting (TSE; TR = 644 ms, TE = 12 ms) with evidence of one element of the segmentation failures of the lumbar spine. The tethering of the spinal cord dorsally in the lipoma can be recognized easily.

b   Sagittal T2-weighted section (TSE; TR = 5000 ms, TE = 112 ms).

c–f Transverse images using T1-weighting (TSE; TR = 630 ms, TE = 15 ms): Tethering of the spinal cord in the large lipoma situated left laterally.

Congenital Tumors

■ Teratomas

Location

Teratomas can occur along the entire course of the spinal canal and are usually unilocular, rarely multilocular. An expansion reaching from the posterior cranial fossa to the cauda equina has also been reported. A lumbosacral occurrence is not infrequently associated with a tethered cord syndrome resulting from adhesions with the nerve roots of the cauda equina as well as from a shortening and thickening of the filum terminale.

Usually teratomas are found at an intradural-extramedullary location, although they can be intramedullary. The tumors can lead to an enlargement of the spinal canal, which can involve both the vertebral arches and the posterior contour of the vertebral bodies. A failure of vertebral fusion is possible; these patients present clinically with a scoliosis.

Histology

Histopathology reveals tissue elements from all three germinal layers, exhibiting an epithelial, mesenchymal and neuroectodermal differentiation. Thus dermal appendages, endodermal glands, and mesenchymal derivatives such as bone, cartilage, smooth muscle, as well as nerve and brain tissue can be found. Macroscopically, solid as well as solid-cystic and purely cystic tumors can occur.

Intraspinal cystic teratomas can be lined with epithelial cells that resemble bronchial or gastrointestinal epithelium. For this reason they are not infrequently, yet wrongly, regarded as neurenteric cysts. The combination of teratomas with other germinal-cell tumors is common.

Pathogenesis

As regards the development of teratomas, it is assumed that pluripotent germinal cells that migrate from the yolk sac into the embryo form tumors there, before accumulating in the urogenital ridge. On the other hand, the view is also upheld that they are cells left behind during the migration of Hensen's node coccygealward, which exhibit pluripotency and can go on to form tumors.

Teratomas are classified according to their malignancy into three grades, with the majority of teratomas being assigned to grade I. These are encapsulated, slow-growing tumors. Secondary malignant transformation of benign teratomas is rare.

Diagnostics

MRI

MRI findings vary very strongly, depending on the composition of the tumors. Cystic elements can demonstrate signal intensity similar to that of CSF. On the other hand, fatty components can be well defined on T1-weighted images as signal-intensive regions. The differentiation of purely cystic tumors from other cysts can be difficult or even impossible.

The location can be of assistance in differential diagnosis; cystic teratomas are preferentially found dorsal to the spinal cord and principally at the level of the conus (Rewcastle and Francoeur, 1964) (Figs. 3.**65**–3.**67**).

■ Sacrococcygeal Teratomas

Sacrococcygeal teratomas occupy an exceptional position. These tumors can be transmitted as an autosomal dominant trait and are associated with other malformations. They have a presacral location and can extend out beyond the pelvic floor. In few cases these tumors demonstrate communication with the sacral canal.

> **Types of Sacrococcygeal Teratomas (Altman *et al.*, 1974)**
>
> - *Type I* (47%): Sacrococcygeal expansion with an, at most, minimal presacral component.
> - *Type II* (35%): Large presacral component in the region of the pelvic floor.
> - *Type III* (8%): Externally visible tumors with the main tumor mass being intrapelvic in location.
> - *Type IV* (10%): Entirely presacral tumors with involvement of the pelvic floor with no apparent external components.

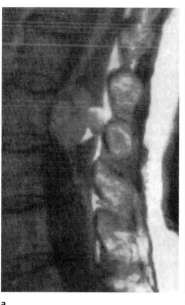

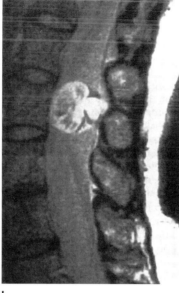

a

b

Fig. 3.**65 a, b**   **WHO Grade I teratoma.** 46-year-old female patient with long-standing symptomatic complaints:

a Teratoma at the level of L2. The spinal cord runs into the tumor to which it is attached. The spinal canal is distended. The tumor displays fatty components communicating with the epidural space (SE; TR = 600 ms, TE = 20 ms).

b Signal enhancement of most of the tumor components on the T2-weighted image (SE; TR = 1600 ms, TE = 16 ms).

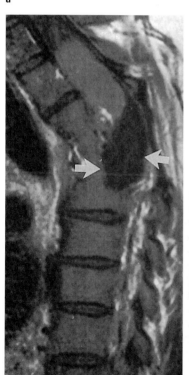

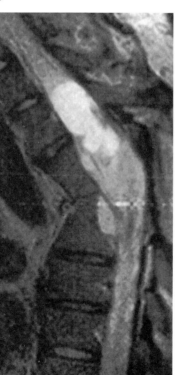

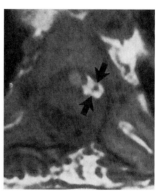

c

a

b

Fig. 3.**66 a–c**   **Solid cystic teratoma.** 37-year-old male patient:

a Congenital vertebral fusion T6/T7. Large cystic tumor component leading to a dorsal vertebral erosion (arrow). A solid tumor component is demonstrable proximal to this (SE; TR = 600 ms, TE = 25 ms).

b On the T1-weighted image the solid tumor component shows a clear signal enhancement (SE; TR = 2100 ms, TE = 80 ms).

c Note fat components ventrally in the area of the tumor (arrows).

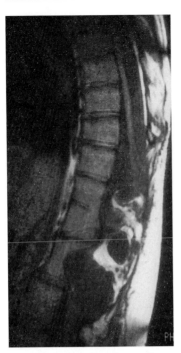

Fig. 3.**67 Large complex malformation tumor with mesenchymal and neuroectodermal elements.** The tumor is associated with a considerable distension of the spinal canal. The spinal cord tapers off into this tumor and is fixed by the tissue in the form of a tethered cord. The T1-weighted sagittal image shows extensive lipomatous, solid and cystic tumor components. Partial vertebral fusion and evidence of scalloping by cystic elements can be seen.

Diagnostics

MRI

The tumors frequently demonstrate a very inhomogeneous picture, explainable by their heterogeneous composition. Larger fatty elements are mostly found with a correspondingly high signal, particularly with T1-weighting. Calcifications can lead to signal attenuations. Individual cases will reveal large cysts. Solid components in the cyst wall can be made visible by the administration of contrast medium.

■ Dermoids and Epidermoids

Definition

Dermoids are derived from cells of the superficial skin layers and their appendages, i.e. hair or sebaceous glands. The *epidermoids* arise exclusively from cells of the superficial skin layers.

Epidermoids occur more frequently than dermoids. On the whole, their occurrence within the spinal canal is very rare. About 1–2 % of all intraspinal tumors are dermoids or epidermoids.

Location and Distribution

Epidermoids are slightly more uniformly distributed over the entire spine than dermoids, which are predominantly lumbosacral in location and are virtually never found at a cervical site. In 5 % of cases a multiple occurrence has been observed.

The tumors have a predominantly extramedullary location, although an intradural, intramedullary occurrence has been reported. In the thoracic region epidermoids are more often seen at an intramedullary location. Most of these tumors develop on the posterior aspect of the spinal cord.

Epidermoids are seen more frequently in males; dermoids demonstrate a uniform sex distribution.

Pathogenesis

Dermoids and epidermoids are not infrequently associated with spinal dysraphism. They therefore commonly occur concomitant with diastematomyelia. In about 20 % of cases they are associated with a dermal sinus (List, 1941). The combination with a dermal sinus is particularly seen in the upper thoracic cavity and in the distal part of the cauda equina (List, 1941).

As regards their development, ectodermal cellular inclusions are thought to be involved during the development of the neural tube. Whether a dermoid or an epidermoid develops depends on when the cell inclusion actually occurs. If the cell inclusion occurs at a later phase of development, the cells are already partially differentiated and only an epidermoid can develop.

Epidermoids and dermoids can also be of iatrogenic origin. Accumulations of epidermal or dermal cells can be dispersed within the spinal canal during lumbar puncture where they develop into tumors (Visciani *et al.*, 1989).

Clinical Presentation

It is possible for clinical symptoms not to occur until late. Not infrequently the condition will only become clinically conspicuous during patients' second and third decades of life, unless the tumor is associated with a dermal sinus. The clinical symptoms can vary; long intervals without symptoms are also observed.

The clinical picture depends on the location. An acute exacerbation of the clinical symptoms can develop from rupture of the cyst with scattering of cholesterol crystals throughout the subarachnoid space, resulting in acute chemical meningitis.

Diagnostics

MRI

At MRI epidermoids are frequently iso-intense with CSF and are only detectable indirectly from signs of a space-occupying lesion (Fig. 3.**68**).

Dermoids more often have a signal intensity that follows that of fat (Figs. 3.**69** and 3.**70**).

Contrast material administration is useful because it can sometimes demonstrate concomitant alterations. In case of an infection in the region of the cyst, enhancement of granulation tissue is seen, sometimes with involvement of the cyst wall or even the cyst contents. Besides that, the administration of contrast material can possibly provide evidence of further alterations present in the spinal canal.

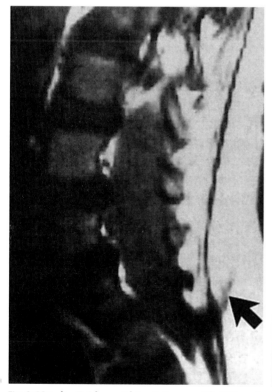 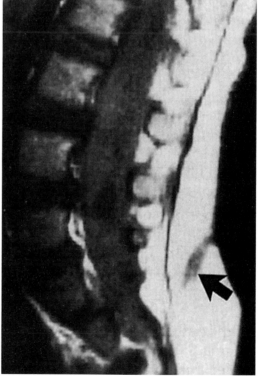

b

Fig. 3.**68 a, b** **Epidermoid iso-intense with CSF and dermal sinus entering into this tumor.** T1-weighted sagittal section: The tumor is not definable within the spinal canal due to the signal being iso-intense with CSF.

The dermal sinus traverses in a craniodorsal to caudoventral direction. Even the administration of contrast medium failed to achieve a better delineation of the dermoid (arrows).

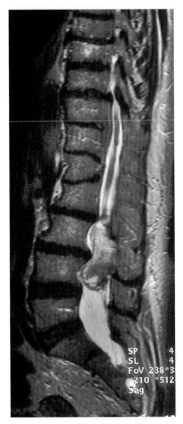

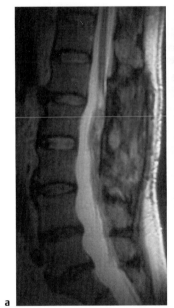

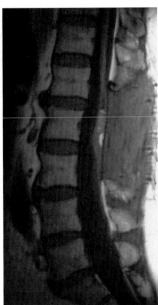

a

b

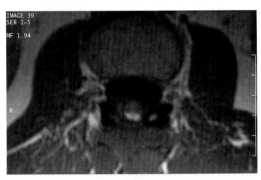

Fig. 3.**69**   **Intraspinal dermoid.** T2-weighted sagittal image (TSE; TR = 4500 ms, TE = 112 ms): Situated at the level of L3/L4, the tumor shows an inhomogeneous signal intensity, which partly matches that of fat. The spinal cord runs into this tumor and is tethered at the level of L3. The dorsal vertebral body contours of L3 and L4 demonstrate scalloping with a convex alteration in configuration. There are also segmental changes of the vertebrae with disk dysplasias, partial fusions, and incomplete development of the vertebral structures.

Fig. 3.**70 a–c**   **Postoperative situation after partial removal of an intraspinal dermoid:**
a Sagittal T2-weighted section (TSE; TR = 5000 ms, TE = 112 ms): The small tumor remnant lies dorsal to the cauda equina at the level of L2. It shows moderate signal intensity. Delineation against the neural structures is poor. There is a large postoperative defect in the region of L1–L3.
b Sagittal T1-weighted section (TSE; TR = 588 ms, TE = 12 ms): The dermoid demonstrates a moderate signal intensity. In addition there are signal enhancements equivalent to fat.
c Transverse section using T1-weighting (SE; TR = 620 ms, TE = 15 ms): On this image the tumor is well defined in the dorsal sections. The fat equivalents appear signal-intensive.

Spinal Cysts

Pathogenesis

Depending on their location, spinal cysts are classified as extra- and intradural lesions. With the extradural cysts the distinction is made as to whether they involve the nerve roots or lie outside a nerve root (Nabors *et al.*, 1988).

> ▬▬▬ **Classification of spinal cysts** ▬▬▬
>
> - *Type I:* Extradural meningeal cyst without nerve root involvement.
> - *Type Ia:* Extradural meningeal cyst.
> - *Type Ib:* Occult sacral meningocele.
> - *Type II:* Extradural meningeal cyst with nerve root involvement (Tarlov cyst)
> - *Type III:* Spinal intradural cyst.

Type Ia is also referred to in the literature as an "extradural cyst," "extradural pocket" or "extradural diverticulum" and type Ib as a "meningeal diverticulum" or "sacral arachnoid cyst." Type II includes the perineural (Tarlov) cyst.

The terms "spinal arachnoid cyst" and "meningeal diverticulum" are also found in the literature to describe intradural cysts.

Fig. 3.**71** provides an overview of the positional relationships of the various cysts relative to the nerve root and the accompanying membranes.

The type Ia extradural cysts can be described as congenital diverticula of the dura. It is assumed that a dural defect, usually situated in the region of the posterior nerve roots, is the starting point for the cyst. However, they can also arise from the midline.

The typical case comprises a posterior, extradural, compressive cyst lying flat on the dura

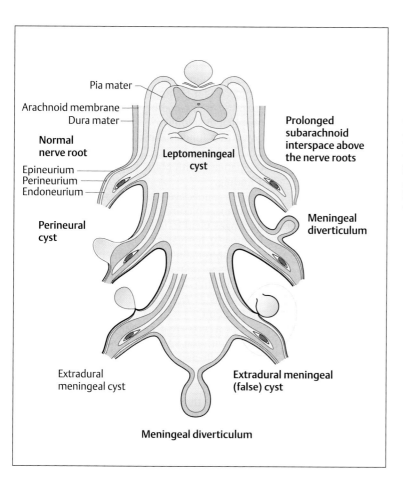

Fig. 3.71 Schematic drawing of some types of spinal intra- and extradural cysts. The type Ia cyst (extradural meningeal cyst), the type II cyst (perineural cyst), and the type III cyst (meningeal diverticulum) are shown. In addition, the relationship between the nerve roots and the endoneurium, perineurium, and epineurium are illustrated. The drawing is based on Tarlov's original work.

Pia mater

Arachnoid membrane
Dura mater

**Normal
nerve root**

Epineurium
Perineurium
Endoneurium

Leptomeningeal
cyst

Prolonged
subarachnoid
interspace above
the nerve roots

**Perineural
cyst**

**Meningeal
diverticulum**

Extradural
meningeal cyst

**Extradural meningeal
(false) cyst**

Meningeal diverticulum

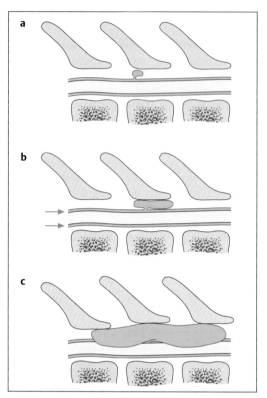

Fig. 3.72 a–c   Development of a type Ia cyst. The diagram shows the development of an extradural cyst through a dural defect in the spinal canal:

a First a small extradural herniation develops with an epidural expansion. At this time there is a pressure difference between the extradural cyst and the intradural space. The pressure within the dura is higher than the extradural pressure.

b Due to these pressure conditions the cyst begins to grow, expanding as a proximal and distal elongation. This can lead to partial compression of the connection between the intradural space and the cyst. This causes pressure to build up inside the cyst because backflow of cystic fluid into the intradural space is hindered or even impossible. Transitory increases in intradural pressure can cause the further leakage of CSF into the cyst.

c By the late phase, a multisegmental extradural cyst has developed whose pressure conditions now produce compression of the dural sac. Pressure inside the cyst is higher than outside because backflow is impossible. A significant compressive effect develops with possible impairment of myelon function. Thus bony absorption and rarefaction, particularly of the lamina, are found, even in the late phase.

and extending across several segments (Figs. 3.72–3.74).

They can produce pressure atrophy of the bone, which accordingly becomes thin, especially the vertebral arch and the vertebral pedicle. A more or less pronounced compression of the spinal cord can develop with corresponding clinical symptoms. The symptoms can already occur during adolescence. Under certain circumstances, communication of the extradural cyst with the subarachnoid space is only detectable using CT myelography because contrast-material uptake by the cyst is sometimes very delayed and thus only slight differences of density are manifest that can escape detection by conventional myelography.

Type Ib cysts are identical with the classic occult sacral meningocele. They are more or less large extradural cystic formations in the sacral space, which can produce substantial thinning of the bone (Figs. 3.75–3.79).

In the typical case, this meningocele or cyst communicates with the dural sac, with the connection always being in the form of a narrow duct. The cyst displaces the sacral nerves anteriorly. The assumption that this meningeal cyst is of congenital origin is supported by the fact that they are often found together with changes in the form of spinal dysraphism. Sacral cysts can extend far down in a lumbar direction. Sacral meningocele can also be an acquired lesion. Thus two-thirds of the patients with Marfan syndrome present such a finding.

The connective-tissue weakness underlying the clinical picture is regarded as the cause. The meninges yield to CSF pressure, which results in meningeal herniation and bone erosions. Sacral cysts can remain clinically silent for a long time and not become clinically manifest until an advanced adult age. They can produce radicular symptoms as well as severe bladder and rectum dysfunction.

Type II cysts are principally found in a sacral location with the S2 and S3 roots being most commonly affected. The cyst wall consists of arachnoid and dura with the cyst itself occupying the space between perineurium (arachnoidal covering of the roots) and the endoneurium (external layer of the pia mater which surrounds the nerve roots).

In contrast to meningeal cysts or diverticula, type II perineural cysts contain, at least in part,

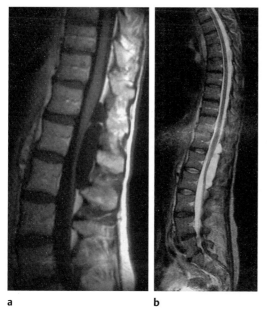

a   b

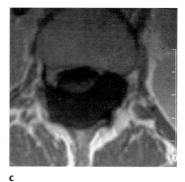

c

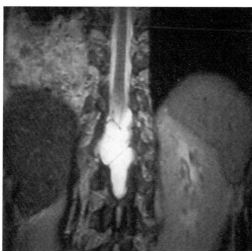

d

Fig. 3.**73 a–d** **Large extradural type Ia cyst at the level of T12 to L2:**

a Sagittal T1-weighted section (SE; TR = 450 ms, TE = 15 ms): Dorsal septated extradural meningeal cyst with an enhanced CSF signal. Marked compression of the spinal cord and the cauda equina by the cyst. Furthermore, there is pressure erosion of the appendant structures of the dorsal vertebrae.

b Sagittal T2-weighted section (TSE; TR = 5000 ms, TE = 112 ms): An enhanced CSF signal intensity is also present on this image. Note the clearly recognizable septations.

c Transverse T1-weighted section (SE; TR = 580 ms, TE = 15 ms): The dorsal extradural cyst herniates far into the intervertebral foramen on the left. The excavation of the bony structures is particularly well recognizable on this image. There is significant compression of the dural sac.

d Sagittal section using T2 weighting (TSE; TR = 5000 ms, TE = 112 ms): The septation of the cyst is particularly well demonstrated on this image. The components projecting far laterally to the right and left are also visible.

nerve fibers and also occasionally ganglion cells. In individual cases the entire cyst can be lined by neural structures. Destruction of nerve fibers by the cyst has also been noted.

The cysts most frequently arise at the connection between the dorsal nerve root and the dorsal ganglion. They often have a multiple occurrence (Figs. 3.**80**–3.**82**).

Type II cysts have a broad connection with the subarachnoid space so that usually they are uniformly filled with contrast material at myelography or CT myelography.

The connection with the subarachnoid space is occasionally interrupted by connective-tissue structures, preventing the cysts from taking up contrast material.

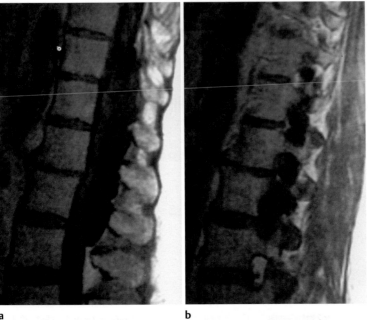

a

b

Fig. 3.**74 a, b** **Large dorsal extradural cyst in the region T10 to L1 with significant compression of the spinal cord and the cauda equina, as well as pressure erosion in the region of the bony structures dorsally:**
a Sagittal T1-weighted image (SE; TR = 500 ms, TE = 20 ms): The cyst shows an enhanced CSF signal. The pressure effect in the region of the bony structures is easily recognizable dorsally.
b Parasagittal section using T1-weighting: The cystic elements extending far intraforaminally are well demonstrated on this image.

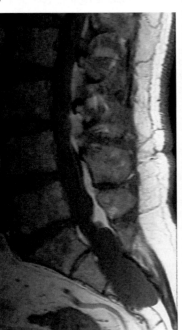

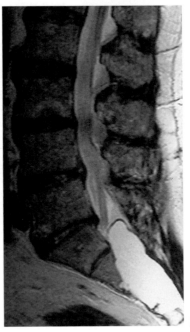

a

b

Fig. 3.**75 a–e** **Large sacral meningocele (type Ib):**
a Sagittal T1-weighted image (TSE; TR = 800 ms, TE = 12 ms): The cyst extends sacrally from S1–S5. It demonstrates marked bony erosion. The cystic contents show an enhanced CSF signal.
b T2-weighted section (TSE; TR = 3635 ms, TE = 120 ms): On this image the relation of the sacral meningocele to the dura is well recognizable. Note how the nerve roots are displaced ventrally.

Type II cysts are associated with bone erosion and enlargement of the spinal canal or, in particular, the intervertebral foramina. They can also lead to a convex change in the form of the dorsal contour of the vertebrae. These bony alterations most likely arise as a result of liquor pressure, possibly in association with a valve mechanism that causes the cysts to become increasingly filled with fluid. They are usually clinically asymptomatic, although they can cause complaints, especially in

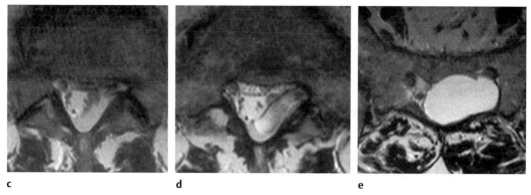

c   d   e

Fig. 3.75 c–e Transverse T2-weighted sections (TSE; TR = 4460 ms, TE = 120 ms): The images show distally the relation of the meningocele to the dura. Note that the meningocele develops dorsal to the dura and occu- pies a large part of the sacral canal in the caudal regions, resulting in distinct pressure erosion and widening of the sacral canal. The compression of the S2 root on the left can be easily seen.

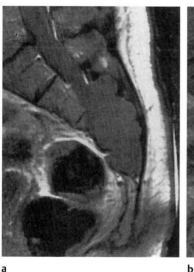
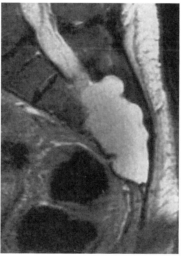

a   b

Fig. 3.76a, b Type Ib sacral meningocele:
a Sagittal T1-weighted section (SE; TR = 2100 ms, TE = 80 ms): Extensive bony erosions due to the extradural sacral cyst. En- hanced CSF signal.
b Enhanced CSF signal also on the T2-weighted image (SE; TR = 2100 ms, TE = 80 ms).

the form of sciatica. In their study, Paulsen *et al.* (1994) found type II perineural cysts in 4.6 % of all patients examined in the region of the lumbar spine, with the cysts being regarded as the cause of symptoms in 22 %. Hence, less than 1 % of per- ineural cysts are the cause of pain back or neuro- logical symptoms. Depending on the clinical symptoms, there is an indication for surgery even for small type II cysts if they are the cause of radicular complaints.

Intradural type III cysts most commonly arise posterior to the spinal cord, less often anterior to it. These cysts also display a more or less dis- tinct communication with the subarachnoid space, which can be interrupted by adhesions. They can lead to bone erosions because here too a valve mechanism is assumed to lead to fluid uptake by the cyst. Like the type II cysts, intradural cysts often have a multiple occur- rence.

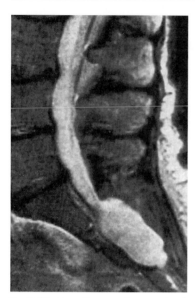

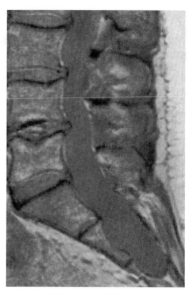

Fig. 3.**77** **Type Ib cyst.** The extradural cyst reveals distinct bony erosion with an enlargement of the sacral canal. The signal intensity corresponds to that of CSF (SE; TR = 2100 ms, TE = 80 ms).

Fig. 3.**78** **Type Ib sacral meningocele with broad-based connection to the dural sac.** (SE; TR = 2100 ms, TE = 20 ms).

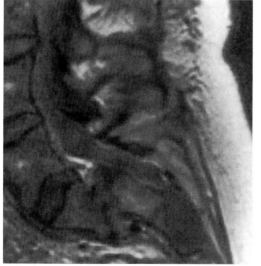

a

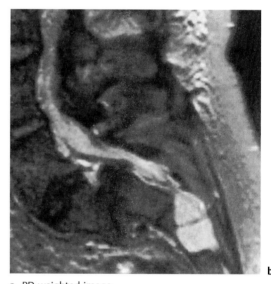

b

Fig. 3.**79 a, b** **Sacral meningocele in a patient with Marfan syndrome.** PD- and T2-weighted images with a sacral extradural cyst. Subluxation between S1 and S2 in the form of a spondyloptosis (SE; TR = 2120 ms, TE = 80 ms).

a PD-weighted image.
b T2-weighted image.

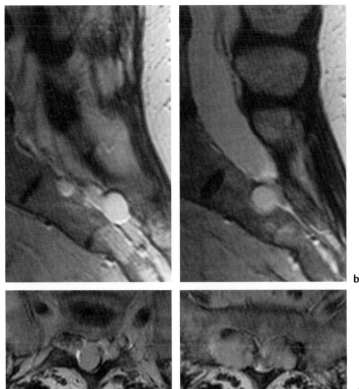

a

b

c

d

Fig. 3.80 a–e   Sacral and thoracic type II cysts:

a, b Sagittal section of the sacral region with evidence of several small parasagittal perineural cysts, both on the right and on the left (TSE; TR = 4000 ms, TE = 120 ms).

c, d Transverse section of the same patient: The cysts have in part caused a distinct distension of the foramina. The nerve roots are incorporated in the wall of the cyst.

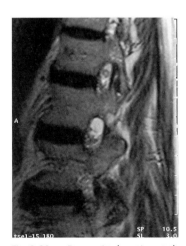

Fig. 3.**80 e**   Parasagittal section at the level of the distal thoracic spine in the same patient showing an infraforaminal perineural cyst. Contact between the cyst and the nerve root is clearly shown (TSE; TR = 4000 ms, TE = 120 ms).

Intradural meningeal cysts most commonly become clinically symptomatic between the third and fourth decades of life; they are principally thoracic in location between T3 and T7, rarely lumbar and extremely rarely cervical. Apart from their congenital development, a post-traumatic and postinflammatory genesis is considered possible.

Diagnostics

MRI

Even if meningeal cysts or diverticula differ from type II perineural cysts in their pathology, they have identical appearances on MRI examination and on myelography. The cysts are easily recognized by their typical CSF signal present on all sequences. Principally, images should be taken in two planes, preferably transverse and coronal, in order to record their full extent. The exact portrayal of their positional relationship relative to the nerve roots poses problems. Their connection with the dural sac cannot always be unequivocally documented (Figs. 3.**73**–3.**82**). In individual cases myelography or CT myelogra-phy will be required to assess the exact extent and communication with the subarachnoid space.

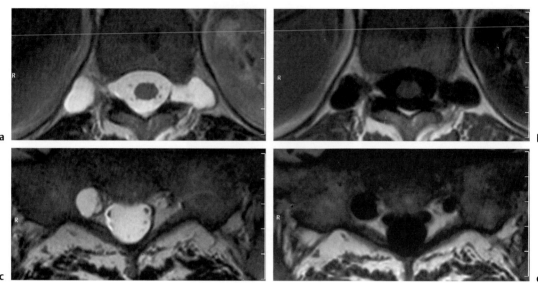

a

b

c

d

Fig. 3.**81 a–d   Multiple thoracic and sacral perineural cysts:**

a Transverse T2-weighted image with evidence of bilateral perineural cysts at the level of T12/L1 (TSE; TR = 6300 ms, TE = 120 ms).

b T1-weighted image. The connection between the perineural cyst and the nerve root is well shown on the right (SE; TR = 630 ms, TE = 14 ms).

c Transverse image of the same patient with evidence of a right-sided sacral perineural cyst (TSE; TR = 6300 ms, TE = 120 ms).

d T1-weighted image corresponding to Fig. **c** (SE; TR = 630 ms, TE = 14 ms).

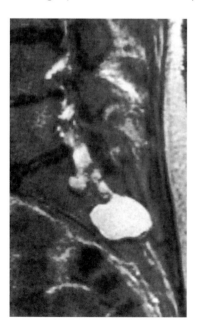

◁ Fig. 3.**82   Multiple sacral type II cysts, partly with marked bony erosion** (SE; TR = 2100 ms, TE = 80 ms).

Arnold–Chiari Malformation

■ Arnold–Chiari Type I Malformation

Definition

This disorder is defined by an inferior location of the cerebellar tonsils, which extend through the foramen magnum caudally into the cervical canal. A caudal displacement of 2–3 mm is usually of no clinical relevance. There is no caudal displacement of the cerebellar vermis and usually no alteration of the brain stem, even though mild protrusions of the medulla can occur in a caudal and dorsal direction (Friede, 1976).

As with type II, an ascending course of the C1 and C2 roots is possible. The clinical picture is commonly associated with occipital dysplasia presenting in the form of platybasia and basilar invagination.

Between 25 % (Friede, 1976) and 50 % (Banerji and Millar, 1974) to 65 % (Appleby *et al.*, 1969) of patients present with syringomyelia.

Pathogenesis

As regards the development of the malformation, it is generally assumed that it is a congenital and not an inherited disease resulting from an occipital and suboccipital dysplasia. Although only a small number of patients presents with severe forms of platybasia and basilar invagination, exact morphological studies revealed signs of occipital dysplasia in two-thirds of patients (Hertel *et al.*, 1974; Schady *et al.*, 1987).

The posterior cranial fossa is flatter and smaller in volume than in unaffected people. The clivus is shortened and Chamberlain's line is reduced. The foramen magnum is often enlarged. Basilar invagination and platybasia can result in a further reduction of the capacity of the posterior fossa. Why the cerebellar tonsils and not the cerebellar vermis herniate is unclear. The development of the vermis precedes that of both hemispheres and their tonsils. At the time of development of the tonsils, the midline is already occupied by the cerebellar vermis. Older theories postulating that Arnold–Chiari type I malformation arises from an intracerebral hydrocephalus based on an obstruction of the foramina of the fourth ventricle have not been proven valid (Gardner and Goodall, 1950).

The majority of patients do not demonstrate hydrocephalus or even remnants of one. The foramina of the fourth ventricle are often open but not infrequently occluded due to arachnoid adhesions.

The malformation can also be acquired. Welch *et al.* (1981) were able to demonstrate the development of tonsillar herniation in patients with a lumbo-ureteral shunt. Diverting CSF into the ureters produces relative spinal hypotension as compared with intracranial CSF pressure.

Clinical Presentation

The Arnold–Chiari type I malformation does not usually become clinically symptomatic until adulthood. The frequency peak is between 31 and 40 years of age (35 %), followed by the 41–50 years (27 %) and the 21–30 years (19 %) age groups. Complaints as early as during adolescence or after 50 years are rarely encountered (Appleby *et al.*, 1969; Banerji and Millar, 1974).

The patients often present with headaches and cervical pains related to movement, combined with an atactic gait, nystagmus and lower cranial-nerve signs. A para- or tetraparesis may also be noted. Extensive disturbances of sensation are often found in the presence of syringomyelia.

Diagnostics

MRI

Sagittal images of the craniocervical junction using T1 weighting are particularly suitable. The slice thickness should not exceed 3 mm (Figs. 3.**83**–3.**86**).

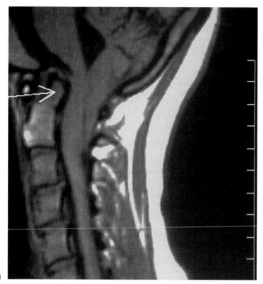

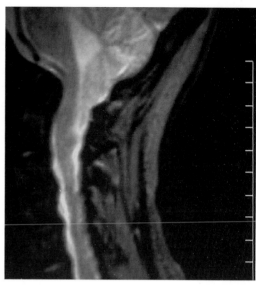

a

b

Fig. 3.**83 a, b   Arnold-Chiari type I malformation:**
a Sagittal T1-weighted section with evidence of extensive caudal displacement of the cerebellar tonsils into
the cervical canal, mild thickening of the cervical spinal cord proximally, and an incipient impression on
the medulla oblongata by the dens (arrow) (SE;
TR = 500 ms, TE = 15 ms).

b Corresponding T2-weighted image (two-dimensional
FLASH; TR = 688 ms, TE = 24 ms, flip angle α = 25°):
The anatomical positional relationships are well
depicted. The impression on the medulla by the dens
is especially well demonstrated.

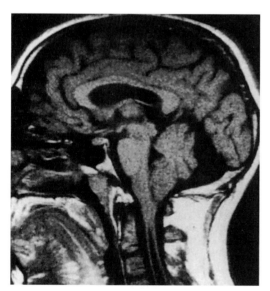

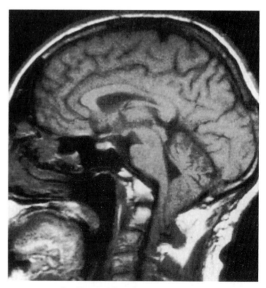

Fig. 3.**84   Arnold-Chiari type I malformation with
distinct syrinx**. 38-year-old patient.

Fig. 3.**85   Platybasia, basilar invagination, and low
position of the cerebellar tonsils.** Marked compression
of the medulla and pons by the inversion of the skull
base. 40-year-old patient.

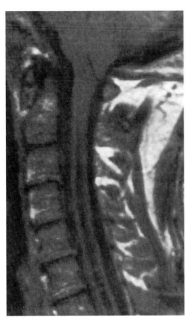
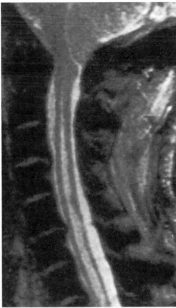

a   b

Fig. 3.**86 a, b** **Low position of the cerebellar tonsils and syringomyelia from C2 onwards.** 57-year-old patient:
a SE; TR = 680 ms, TE = 20 ms.
b FFE; TR = 600 ms, TE = 20 ms, flip angle α = 10°.

■ Arnold–Chiari Type II Malformation

Definition

The Arnold–Chiari type II malformation is a complex deformity mainly involving the craniocervical junction and including the hindbrain. It is virtually always combined with a myelomeningocele.

Cerebellum. The posterior fossa is obviously and markedly reduced in size with the cerebellum appearing proportionately smaller than normal. Parts of the vermis and the cerebellar hemispheres are displaced caudally through the enlarged foramen magnum into the cervical canal. Apart from the pyramids, uvula and nodules of the vermis, severe cases also demonstrate downward herniation of the biventral lobules, the superior and inferior semilunar lobules of the cerebellar hemispheres and the tonsils (about 18 % of cases; Variend and Emery, 1976). Whereas that part of the cerebellar hemispheres which is displaced caudally can be restricted to the tonsils, larger sections of the cerebellar vermis are virtually always involved. The cerebellar components can reach far down into the spinal

canal, in rare cases even as far as C7/T1. They then demonstrate a configuration that is pointed and tapered caudally.

No correlation has been noted between the degree of caudal displacement of cerebellar elements and the clinical picture.

Patients with symptoms arising from the brain stem or the long tracts display more marked displacements as compared with patients without these signs. In individual cases this can require surgical enlargement of the posterior fossa (Curnes *et al.*, 1989).

The cerebellum also exhibits proximal changes. The grooves of the cerebellar vermis are absent or only mildly expressed. The fissures do not assume a curved course but are V-shaped, in the most severe case almost parallel to one another in the AP direction, and are associated with a separation of the cerebellar hemispheres (Variend and Emery, 1979). The frequently associated hypoplasia of the tentorium results in a high location of the proximal cerebellar components, especially after shunt surgery for hydrocephalus. Parieto-occipital gyri can fold into the supracerebellar cisterna, which is often enlarged, as are the cisterna laminae tecti, the cisterna veli interpositi and the cisterna ambiens. Ventrally the cerebellum is wrapped around the brain stem. Cerebellar components can be found in front of the medulla and the cerebellopontine-angle cisterns can be obliterated.

Medulla oblongata. The medulla oblongata is also elongated caudally. Parts of it can lie dorsal to the cervical cord, with this protrusion taking on a bead-like or Z form.

The cause of this configuration is the tethering of the proximal cervical cord by the dentate ligaments at the level of the foramen magnum. The displacement of the medulla occurs dorsal to the ligaments with the result that the medulla accordingly extends in a caudal direction dorsal to the cervical cord.

The proximal part of the spinal canal has an enlarged sagittal diameter, which increases with age and appears principally as an enlargement of the subarachnoid space ventral to the spinal cord.

Fourth ventricle. The fourth ventricle is also usually elongated caudally. In the majority of cases the walls lie flat and parallel to each other; the lateral recesses are absent. The largest sagittal diameter is at the level of the foramen magnum. The foramen of Magendie (median aperture) can be absent.

A classification of the Arnold–Chiari malformations has been devised based on the alterations of the fourth ventricle and the medulla oblongata (Wolpert *et al.*, 1987).

Classification of the Arnold–Chiari malformation

- *Stage I*: Medulla oblongata and fourth ventricle do not extend below the level of the foramen magnum; only the inferior vermis is elongated caudally beyond the foramen.
- *Stage II*: The fourth ventricle extends below the level of the foramen magnum; the medulla oblongata has a slight recess dorsally. The fourth ventricle lies in the axis of the central canal in front of the tapered vermian peg.
- *Stage III*: There is a noticeable elongation of the medulla dorsal and caudal to the cervical cord with the fourth ventricle tapering off into this elongation, being either collapsed (*stage IIIa*) or dilated (*Stage IIIb*).

Pons and midbrain. The pons is hypoplastic and flattened. As a consequence of this, the clivus has a concave alteration in form. The mamillopontine distance is lengthened and can amount to as much as 3 cm (El Gammal *et al.*, 1988). The aqueduct often appears shortened, its course angled and convoluted. It is usually patent, but due to its course it is functionally blocked and exposed to compression from outside as a result of the dilation of the lateral ventricles.

The positional change of the aqueduct results from an alteration of the quadrigeminal plate, which is thickened and often elongated beak-like in a dorsal direction. The course of the aqueduct follows this protrusion (Emery, 1974).

The colliculi can be fused together. The third ventricle is not infrequently slightly enlarged and reveals diverticulum-like extensions. The intermediate mass of the thalamus is thickened; the hypothalamus can be elongated.

Cerebrum. The tentorium has a low occipital attachment and is often hypoplastic. It courses almost vertically and, correspondingly, so does the straight sinus. As a result of the positional change of the tentorium, the occipital lobes enter the posterior fossa far caudally.

The cerebral hemispheres can also be included in the alteration. The gyri often appear narrowed, an appearance that is sometimes referred to in the literature under the term "microgyria" (Cameron, 1957).

Histologically there is a regular six-layered architecture to the cortex. The term "stenogyria" has therefore been used by other authors to distinguish between these alterations and those resulting from a disturbance of migration (Wolpert *et al.*, 1987). Partial aplasia and hypoplasia of the corpus callosum are often noted. The anterior horns can be drawn downwards and show typical lateral flattenings on transverse sections.

Hydrocephalus. The hydrocephalus can be explained in various ways. Apart from obstruction of the aqueduct, disturbances of circulation at the level of the foramina of the fourth ventricle or cisterna ambiens are also considered possible causes (Yamada *et al.*, 1982).

Lacunar skull (craniolacunia or Lückenschädel). Bony alterations of the cranial vault are observed and are circumscribed by the term craniolacunia or Lückenschädel, the German term that has also found its way into English medical language. It refers to thinned-out areas distributed throughout the vault and attracting attention as round structures with increased radiolucency on x-ray.

Diagnostics

MRI

MRI has established itself as the method of choice. It allows the extent of alterations to be shown on a survey view, especially using sagittal sections.

T1-weighted sequences will usually suffice. T2-weighted sequences are better able to demonstrate possible disturbances of CSF circulation. PD- and T2-weighted sequences are required especially for proof of periventricular CSF diapedesis, with the FLAIR sequence being an alternative recommendation (Figs. 3.**87**–3.**90**).

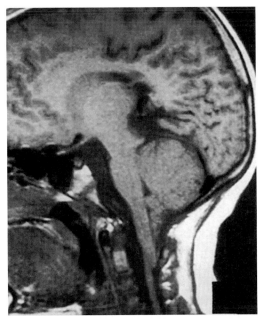

Fig. 3.**87** **Arnold-Chiari type II malformation.** 2-year-old boy. Postoperative myelomeningocele. The cerebellar components protrude plait-like into the spinal canal. Z-like kinking of the medulla oblongata. Hypoplastic tentorium with a very steep course. Microgyric pattern of the parieto-occipital gyri. Beak-like elongation of the quadrigeminal plate. Pons hypoplastic with concave form of the clivus. Dilation of the prepontine cisterns. Increase of the mamillopontine distance.

Fig. 3.**88** **Arnold-Chiari type II malformation and myelomeningocele.** 9-month-old child. Postoperative image after valve placement. Distinct elongation of the cerebellum down to C3. Parts of the occipital lobes extend far caudally. Beak-like elongation of the quadrigeminal plate. Accentuated elongation of the hypothalamus. Moderate dilation of the prepontine cisterns. Hypoplastic corpus callosum.

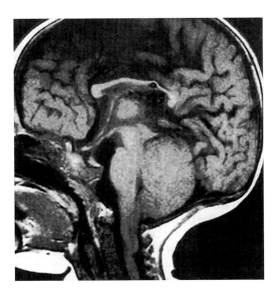

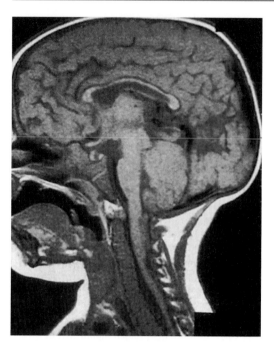

Fig. 3.**89 Arnold-Chiari type II malformation.** 15-month-old child. Postoperative meningomyelocele. Elongation of the cerebellar components and the medulla oblongata down to C4. The fourth ventricle is slightly shortened. Hypoplastic tentorium, parts of the occipital lobes displaced far into the posterior fossa. Distinct enlargement of the supracerebellar cisterns. Flattening of the quadrigeminal plate and thickening of the lateral mass. Increase of the mamillopontine distance. Slightly hypoplastic pons. Distinct hypoplasia of the entire corpus callosum.

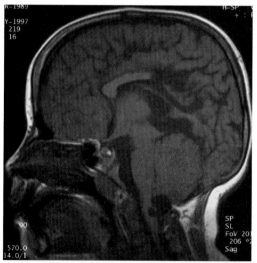
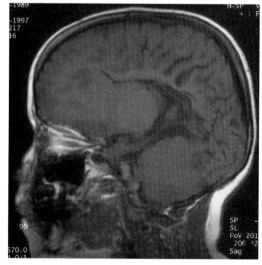

Fig. 3.**90 a–e Arnold-Chiari type II malformation.** 7-year-old boy.

a Sagittal section using T1-weighting (SE; TR = 570 ms, TE = 14 ms): Parts of the cerebellum and medulla oblongata protrude to approximately C3 with additional cystic structures being obvious at the level of the foramen magnum. Very smooth contouring of the cerebellar vermis with absent patterning of the folia. Flat fourth ventricle appears as if collapsed. Very low-lying, hypoplastic and, in most parts, absent tentorium with vertical course. Microgyric structure of the occipital lobes. Large supracerebellar cistern. Beak-like elongated quadrigeminal plate. An aqueduct is not recognizable. Partial agenesis of the corpus callosum, especially along the splenium.

b Parasagittal section with distinct depiction of the microgyric patterning, particularly along the occipital lobe.

Fig. 3.**90 c–e** ▷

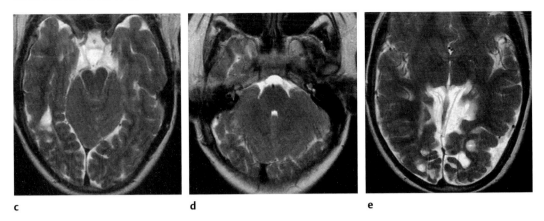

c   d   e

Fig. 3.**90**

c, d T2-weighted sections (TSE; TR = 4465 ms, TE = 120 ms): The folds of the cerebellar vermis are lacking completely; there is a V-shaped configuration of the fissures. The segments of the cerebellar hemispheres envelop the brain stem.

e Section at the level of both occipital lobes with evidence of the marked microgyric patterning of the cortex. Concomitant high-grade hypoplasia in the region of the occipital lobes. Very large supracerebellar cisterns communicating with the ambient cistern due to the absence of the posterior parts of the corpus callosum.

Syringomyelia

Definition

Syringomyelia is an intramedullary cavitation usually extending over several segments. The syrinx is filled with CSF and can result in an enlargement of the spinal canal. Syringomyelia is found outside the central canal and should be distinguished from hydromyelia, which is defined as a dilation of the central canal. In the majority of cases, however, MRI is not always able to make this distinction, nor is it always possible histologically.

Combinations are also possible. Thus the cavitation can course partly as a hydromyelia and partly lie outside the central canal. Syringomyelia can extend into the medulla oblongata, when it is known as syringobulbia. The syrinx very rarely expands far into the pons.

Location

In Arnold–Chiari type I malformation the cavitation is most commonly found at a cervical location. It can extend into the thoracic though rarely into the thoracolumbar region. At a cervical loca-

tion syringomyelia is often associated with a distinct enlargement of the spinal cord, while syringobulbia usually appears as a slit. It is mainly found unilaterally, although a bilateral occurrence is also possible.

In Arnold–Chiari type II malformation, syringomyelia is usually located above the placode. It often appears extended and reaching as far as the cervical cord, with the expansion not infrequently running discontinuously and the spinal cord appearing normal in parts.

In patients with postoperative myelomeningocele, the syringomyelia or hydromyelia is most commonly found at a thoracic location. It is typical for the cavitation to appear at several sites without noticeable connections. A long-segmented, continuous syringomyelia is therefore hardly ever seen, but appears rather as short-segmented distensions, each occurring at circumscribed cervical, thoracic and lumbar locations.

Adhesions in the region of the foramina of the fourth ventricle and of cysts in the posterior fossa are associated with a cervical syringomyelia, mostly in conjunction with a syringobulbia. The majority of patients with a connection between the syringobulbia and the fourth ventricle via the obex also have a hydrocephalus.

In the tethered cord syndrome, syringomyelia is commonly seen just above the fixation site with an expansion of only a few centimeters (Raghaven et al., 1989).

Histology

Histologically syringomyelia develops mainly in the gray substance and usually lies dorsal to the central canal. The lining of the cavity depends on the site of expansion and duration of the illness. The syrinx can demonstrate an irregular margin and be lined with neural structures. Myelinated fibers are found, and in long-standing findings there is a lining with a 1–2 mm-thick layer of astrocytes and glia fibers.

In hydromyelia the wall consists of ependymal cells that can, however, be destroyed by pressure atrophy.

Histologically, syringobulbia has no contact with the fourth ventricle. If there is communication of the syringobulbia with the fourth ventricle via the obex, then the majority of such patients present with hydrocephalus.

Apart from the slit-like form of syringobulbia, saccular cavitations are also seen, especially in trauma patients (Sherman et al., 1987).

Pathogenesis

Pathogenetically a distinction is made between syringomyelias, based on an impairment of CSF circulation in the region of the craniocervical junction, and the other forms. The group of syrin-gomyelias based on pathology of the craniocervical junction is referred to as *communicating syringomyelia*; all others are described as *non-communicating forms*.

Various causes underlie syringomyelia. A congenital form is distinguished from an acquired form. The most common causes are summarized in Table 3.2.

The cause of about 35–50% of all syringomyelias is attributed to an Arnold–Chiari type I malformation. Malformations in the posterior fossa, which can result in cysts, as in the Dandy-Walker syndrome, or in fibrous adhesions in the region of the foramina of Luschka and Magendie, are also common causes of syringomyelia (Banna, 1988).

The Arnold–Chiari type II malformation is associated with syringomyelia or hydromyelia in 11–43% of cases, though some authors suggest an even higher percentage (Cameron, 1957; Emery and Lendon, 1972, 1973; Just et al., 1990).

Intra- and extramedullary tumors are often associated with syringomyelia, which mostly develops above the tumor. The occurrence of syringomyelias has also been observed after the removal of an extramedullary tumor (Castillo et al., 1988).

Clinical Presentation

Patients normally become symptomatic between 20 and 30 years of age. This applies particularly for syringomyelias in combination with an Arnold–Chiari type I malformation. The most common symptoms are:

- paresis of the upper extremities,
- dissociated sensory loss,
- paresthesias,
- disturbances of depth perception.

Cranial nerve deficits are an infrequent presentation but when present are usually unilateral. The extent of the syrinx usually goes beyond the clinically conspicuous region and there is no correlation between clinical presentation and size of the cavity. Because of this fact it is assumed that the clinical symptoms are not caused directly by pressure damage, but indirectly by disturbances of arterial or venous circulation (Schroth and Palmbach, 1988).

Table 3.2   Causes of syringomyelia

Congenital form of syringomyelia
- Arnold–Chiari type I malformation
- Arnold–Chiari type II malformation
- cysts of the posterior fossa:
  - Dandy-Walker syndrome
  - arachnoid cysts
- fibrous adhesions in the region of the foramina of Luschka and Magendie
- tethered cord syndrome

Acquired form of syringomyelia/hydromyelia
- spinal trauma
- intra-/extramedullary tumors

Idiopathic syringomyelia

■ Communicating Syringomyelia

Increased Intraventricular Pressure Theory

This theory proposes that syringomyelia or syringobulbia arises from a maldevelopment in the region of the fourth ventricular floor with incomplete formation of the foramina. It is assumed that a craniocaudal communication between the fourth ventricle and the cervical canal results from an increase in intraventricular pressure (Gardner, 1965). According to this theory, the absence of foraminal openings in the region of the fourth ventricle is also supposed to be responsible for the development of Arnold–Chiari type I malformation with displacement of the tonsils into the cervical canal.

■ Differential Intraspinal and Intracranial Pressure Theory

A modification of the theory mentioned above considers that differences between intracranial and intraspinal CSF or venous pressure or both are responsible for the development of syringomyelia. The idea is that the inferior location of the tonsils in Arnold–Chiari type I malformation and other forms of obliteration (e.g. cysts) obstruct the free communication between spinal canal and intracranial CSF. A valve-like mechanism is attributed to the tonsils (or cysts). If transient increases in pressure arise in the spinal canal as a result of physical exertion, CSF is forced in a cranial direction, squeezes past the tonsils (or other cause of obliteration) and crosses into the intracranial cisterns. From there, however, it cannot flow freely back into the spinal canal due to the obstruction of the CSF pathways, but rather is pressed into the intraventricular space. Because an increase in pressure develops within the ventricular system, the craniocaudal pressure gradient causes the drainage of CSF out of the fourth ventricle into the spinal cord (Williams, 1970, 1980).

However, it appears that in the majority of cases this explanation for the development of communicating syringomyelia does not stand up to actual facts. In particular, communications between the fourth ventricle and syringobulbia or syringomyelia are not usually found, even in Arnold–Chiari type I malformation. In fact, syringomyelia often does not begin until the C2- or C3 level. In most cases there is no syringobulbia. Furthermore, syringobulbia is almost never seen in isolation but always in association with more or less long-segment alterations of the syringomyelic cervical cord, thus substantiating the presumption of a retrograde development in a caudal–cranial direction (Williams and Timperley, 1976).

CT examinations using intrathecal application of contrast material have been unable to prove that syringomyelia in patients with Arnold–Chiari type I malformations are demonstrated by contrast-uptake of the fourth ventricle alone. On the contrary, the passage of contrast medium into the syrinx must be assumed to be from subarachnoid contrast material in the spinal canal region (Aubin *et al.* 1981).

■ Theory of Direct Drainage of CSF into the Spinal Cord

According to the ideas of Aubin (1981) and Aboulker (1979), syringomyelia arises from an increase in pressure in the spinal canal as a result of changes in the region of the posterior fossa or the craniocervical junction, with the result that CSF drains into the spinal cord. The decisive factor for this is that, at least in animal studies, a not inconsiderable production of CSF has been demonstrated within the spinal canal (Sato *et al.*, 1972). This CSF drainage can be explained by the presence of enlarged Virchow-Robin spaces in the spinal cord as well as by an edematous softening of the spinal cord so that smaller gaps and fissures allow extracellular communication with the syrinx (Ball and Dajan, 1972; Aboulker, 1979; Ikata *et al.*, 1988).

■ Non-communicating Syringomyelia

The cause of syringomyelia in the presence of a non-communicating form (e.g. in association with a tethered cord syndrome or a spinal-cord tumor) is regarded to lie in chronic ischemia in the proximal part of the spinal cord. The ischemic reaction in the case of a tethered cord syndrome results from traction on the spinal cord; in the case of a spinal cord tumor it is secondary to circulatory pressure changes, with venous congestion being regarded primarily as the cause of the ischemia.

Syringomyelia occurs above the tethering of the spinal cord, although it can be found both above and below the fixation point in cases of compression secondary to tumor.

A cranial expansion up into the cervical cord is not infrequently found in tethered cord syndrome (Raghavan *et al.*, 1989).

Syringomyelias secondary to tumors can some-times experience a considerable degree of expansion.

Diagnostics

MRI

The MR image of syringomyelia is not dependent upon the genesis of the disorder. T1-weighted sequences are particularly suitable and should be used in sagittal and transverse slice orientation. The syrinx presents a hypointense signal, corresponding largely to that of CSF. The diagnosis should, however, be secured by additional T2-weighted sequences where a signal behavior equivalent to that of CSF should also be expected. The spinal cord can be markedly distended while, on the other hand, the cavity can be collapsed. Especially after surgery, the distension should visibly start to recede in comparison with preoperative images. If the syrinx collapses, then the cavity will become shortened, especially in the AP direction, while its right- and left-lateral diameter will essentially remain unchanged. This is explained by the right- and left-lateral tethering of the spinal cord in the region of the spinal canal by the denticulate ligaments, which maintain the form of the spinal cord in its transverse plane, while there is a larger margin for movement in the AP direction, allowing a reduction in cavity size (Schroth and Palmbach, 1988).

A distinct signal enhancement of the spinal cord is not infrequently found on T2-weighted images at the cranial and caudal ends of the syrinx, corresponding histologically to a reactive gliosis. Turbulences can cause the fluid in the syrinx to appear very hypointense in signal on T2-weighted images. The canal is not always uniform in its extension; it can have a lobular appearance of varying diameter. These lobules can also display septations, which prevent communication of the syrinx fluid throughout the entire cavity. This has consequences when planning the surgical approach, since false placement of the syringo-subarachnoid shunt can obviate a positive surgical outcome because the septations separate the cavitations from one another.

The syringo-subarachnoid shunt is not always well defined on MRI imaging. Usually scarring of the spinal cord can be detected at the point of drainage between spinal cord and subarachnoid space. Because the shunt is usually only inserted when the syrinx is under strong pressure, and therefore displays a round or ellipsoid configuration, this distension should have disappeared on postoperative examination. If not, the surgery must be regarded as ineffective.

Contrast medium should be administered in all equivocal cases of syringomyelia to ensure that any tumor within the syrinx is found. The tumor may be located at the end of the syrinx; it can also be found at an eccentric location. It should be noted that the syrinx can expand discontinuously so that an apparent end of the syrinx may be identified although it is in fact further caudal. In these cases complete examination of the spinal cord from cervical to lumbar is therefore essential (Figs. 3.**91**–3.**100**).

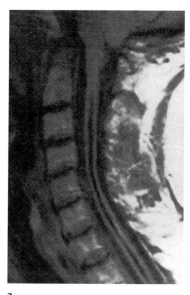
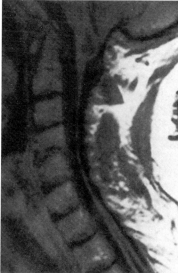

a   b

Fig. 3.**91 a–c** **Arnold-Chiari type I malformation and long-segment syringomyelia and syringobulbia.** 69-year-old female patient:
a, b Transverse PD-weighted sections (SE; TR = 1600 ms, TE = 30 ms).

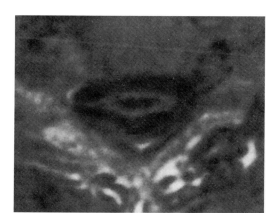

c Well-demonstrated collapse of the syrinx in the transverse section; distinct atrophy of the spinal cord (SE; TR = 550 ms, TE = 30 ms).

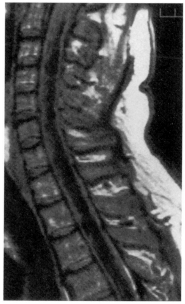

Fig. 3.**92** **Syringomyelia with Arnold-Chiari type I malformation.** 44-year-old patient. The syrinx exhibits a distinct space-occupying effect with pressure atrophy of the spinal cord; it extends cranially as far as C2 (SE; TR = 2100 ms, TE = 20 ms).

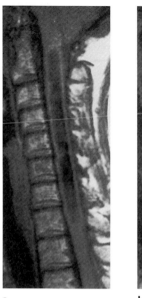
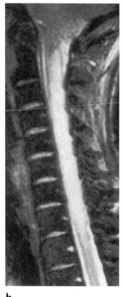

a   b

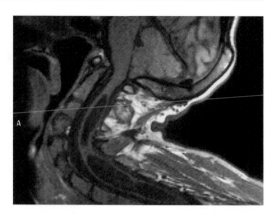

Fig. 3.**94 Incipient Arnold-Chiari type I malformation.** 25-year-old patient. Sagittal section with marked syrinx, partly with cavitation. Massive distension of the myelon with corresponding pressure atrophy. Considerable enlargement of the spinal canal with an obvious reduction in the diameter of the cervical and thoracic vertebrae. Marked lordotic deformity of the cervical spine.

Fig. 3.**93 a, b   Arnold-Chiari type I malformation and syringomyelia from C2–D1.** 27-year-old woman. Clearly distended syrinx with corresponding pressure atrophy of the spinal cord.
a SE; TR = 650 ms, TE = 25 ms.
b FFE; TR = 520 ms, TE = 20 ms, flip angle α = 10°.

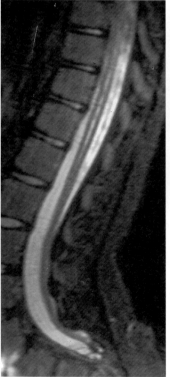

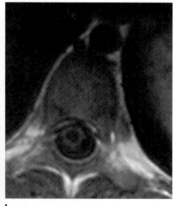

b

Fig. 3.**95 a, b   Syrinx in a patient with postoperative myelomeningocele:**
a Sagittal T2-weighted section (STIR; TR = 4890 ms, TE = 60 ms): The spinal cord is tethered at level S2–S3. A syrinx is present which is definable down to L1/L2.
b Transverse section with characteristic and distinct distension of the spinal cord due to the central syrinx (SE; TR = 430 ms, TE = 14 ms).

a

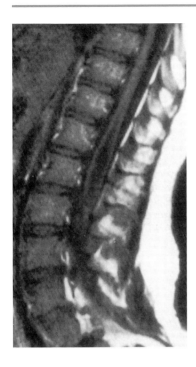

◁ Fig. 3.**96** **Postoperative myelomeningocele.** Re-tethering of the spinal cord. Circumscribed thoracolumbar syrinx (SE; TR = 720 ms, TE = 20 ms).

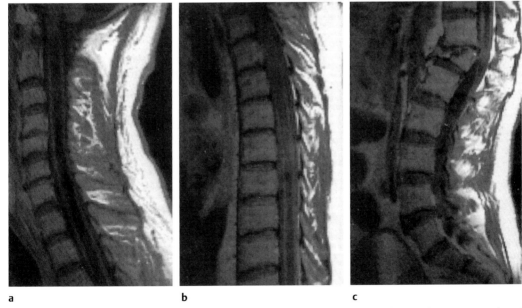

a   **b**   **c**

Fig. 3.**97 a–c** **Post-traumatic syringomyelia secondary to a compression fracture of L1.** 55-year-old patient. The syrinx extends over the entire spinal cord up to C1 (SE; TR = 500 ms, TE = 15 ms).

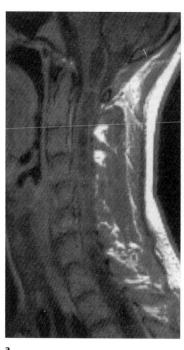
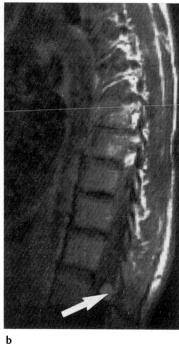

a   b

Fig. 3.**98 a, b** **Syringomyelia in the presence of a small hemangioblastoma at level of T11 (arrow).** The syrinx extends over the entire spinal cord as far as the medulla oblongata (SE; TR = 500 ms, TE = 15 ms). The views were taken after application of contrast. The hemangioblastoma node displays a strong enhancement; without contrast, there was no differentiation from the spinal cord (images by Prof. Gürtler MD, Bielefeld, Germany).

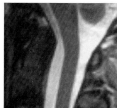
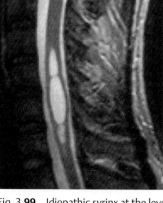

Fig. 3.**99** Idiopathic syrinx at the level C4–C7. A distinct distension of the spinal cord is evident in this section with massive atrophy. Septations are demonstrated within the syrinx (TSE; TR = 4600 ms, TE = 112 ms).

Congenital Spinal Stenosis

The causes of congenital spinal stenosis can be very varied. A few, very rare, congenital disorders exist that are associated with severe malformations of the whole skeletal system, including the spine, and mostly lead to hyposomia and disproportionate development of the skeletal system. These include:

- Kniest dysplasia,
- mucopolysaccharidosis,
- spondyloplasias of varying degrees,
- chondrodysplasias, above all chondrodysplasia punctata and achondroplasia.

■ Kniest Dysplasia

Kniest dysplasia represents a congenital maldevelopment of the skeletal system with severe hyposomia for which a series of skeletal changes have been reported. As regards the spine, radiology reveals platyspondylies associated with anterior wedging of the vertebrae. It is an autosomal dominant disorder with the defect lying in the degree of expression of type II collagen.

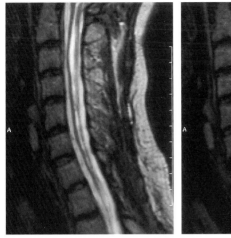 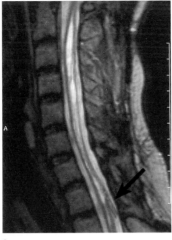 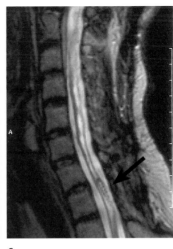

a   b   c

Fig. 3.**100 a–c** **Idiopathic syringomyelia and syrin-gobulbia with extension from the medulla oblongata to the thoracic cord:**
a Sagittal section with depiction of the syrinx over the entire course of the cervical cord. Atrophy of the spinal cord is present, while distension is absent.

b,c The views show the syringo-subarachnoid shunt inserted into the syrinx at the level of T1. Shunt position and course are well defined on both images (arrows). Note how the syrinx extends far into the thoracic cord.

■ Mucopolysaccharidosis

The various forms of mucopolysaccharidosis are associated with vertebral dysplasias of varying degrees, including hook-shaped vertebrae, ovoid deformities of the vertebral bodies, as well as platyspondylies with hypoplasias of the anterior parts of the vertebral body. Typical for the mucopolysaccharidosis type IV (Morquio disease) are alterations at the atlantodental junction. An inadequate ossification of the os odontoideum of C2 is seen which results in an atlanto-axial instability.

■ Spondyloplasia

The *spondylar chondrodysplasias* (e.g. spondyloenchondrodysplasia, Wiedemann–Spranger type spondylometaphyseal chondroplasia, Koslowski type spondylometaphyseal dysplasia) result in the development of often dorsally accentuated platyspondylies of varyingly severity, or even butterfly vertebrae, due to coronal cartilaginous clefting of the vertebral body, which results in narrowing of the spinal canal.

■ Chondrodysplasia

The chondrodysplasias also exhibit platyspondylies or irregular deformations of the vertebrae as their characteristic feature. Narrowing of the spinal canal has been reported as a frequent characteristic of achondroplasia. Here the spinal cord compression begins in the region of the craniocervical junction due to a too narrow foramen magnum and continues along the course of the cervical and thoracic cord (Figs. 3.**101** and 3.**102**). It is an autosomal dominant hereditary disorder.

■ Other Forms of Congenital Spinal Stenosis

Apart form the disorders already described, which are associated with dwarfism, there are known forms of congenital spinal stenosis that are seen more frequently. In particular, these include:

● Down syndrome (trisomy 21),
● congenital basilar impression.

Down syndrome: Down syndrome is the most common genetic cause of mental retardation and is due to a trisomy of chromosome 21 with its associated characteristic phenotype. The changes in the region of the spinal canal particularly affect the atlantodental interval, resulting in an atlantoaxial instability and subsequent spinal cord

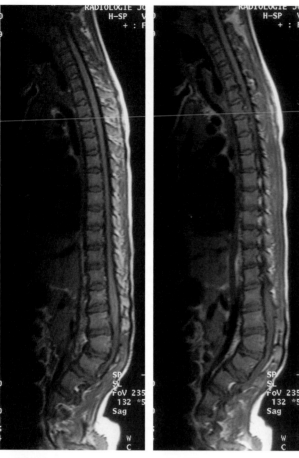

a   b

Fig. 3.**10 1a, b** **Known achondroplasia.** 9-year-old boy with a long-segment narrowing of the spinal canal. T1-weighted images (TSE; TR = 800 ms, TE = 12 ms). Long-segment narrowing of the spinal canal, mainly in the thoracic region. The cervical cord appears normal with no definite stenosis identifiable at the craniocervical junction either. Definite deformity in the region of the dorsolumbar junction.

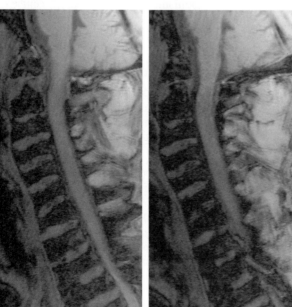

a   b

Fig. 3.**102 a–e** **Chondrodysplasia.** 53-year-old patient:

a, b T1-weighted sagittal image (FLASH two-dimensional; TR = 375 ms, TE = 11 ms, flip angle α = 90°): Distinctly coarse appearance of vertebrae in the cervical region, looking accentuated in the vertical diameter. Relative constriction of the spinal canal. Persistent os odontoideum.

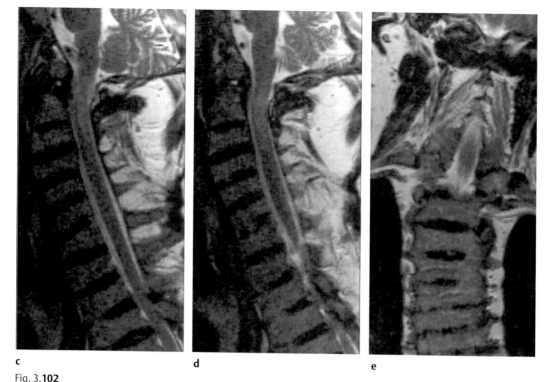

c   d   e

Fig. 3.102

c, d Corresponding T2-weighted images (TSE; TR = 4140 ms, TE = 128 ms): The images show the fibrous bridge between the os odontoideum and the axis. The spinal cord displays signal enhancement at the level of the craniocervical junction as an expression of edema secondary to compression.

e Coronary section using T2-weighting (TSE; TR = 4140 ms, TE = 128 ms): In this slice orientation the coarse appearance and widening of the vertebrae can be seen easily. Noticeable deformity of the spine, notably with a right convex scoliosis at the cervicodorsal junction.

compression. In addition, other bony changes also exist which are regarded as characteristic of Down syndrome, such as:

- hypoplastic wide pelvis with reduced iliac and acetabular angles,
- brachiocephalus,
- hypoplasia to aplasia of the frontal, maxillary and sphenoidal sinuses (Figs. 3.**103** and 3.**104**).

Congenital basilar impression: The congenital form of basilar impression is associated with a high position of the dens combined with a flattening of the middle cranial fossa. In severe cases spinal cord impression occurs even with the head in a neutral position; in milder cases only with ventral flexion of the head. The syndrome is not infrequently combined with an Arnold–Chiari type I malformation with a corresponding inferior displacement of the cerebellar tonsils. This is often associated with syringomyelia or syringobulbia (Figs. 3.**105** and 3.**106**).

Basilar impression can be acquired, in which case vitamin D deficiency with a bony deformation in the region of the skull base is the cause (Fig. 3.**107**).

The syndrome must be differentiated from acquired forms secondary to inflammation, often seen in long-standing cases of rheumatoid arthritis.

■ Idiopathic Spinal Stenosis

Apart from the forms of spinal canal stenosis already described, an idiopathic form should be mentioned that is associated with a congenital shortening of the vertebral pedicles and subsequently with a noticeable reduction of the ventrodorsal diameter of the spinal canal. The finding is more frequently seen in the lumbar than the cervical region (Fig. 3.**108**).

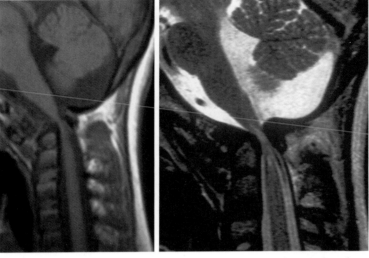

a

b

Fig. 3.**103 a, b   Trisomy 21.** 10-year-old girl. Atlantoaxial instability with marked spinal cord compression.
a Sagittal T1-weighted section (SE; TR = 570 ms, TE = 14 ms): Ventral displacement of the atlas with concomitant anterior dislocation of the dens axis, which no longer has contact with the base of the axis.

The spinal cord compression is due to the posterior arch of the atlas and due to the axis.
b Corresponding image using T2-weighting (TSE; TR = 3290 ms, TE = 120 ms): Development of edema of the myelon secondary to spinal cord compression.

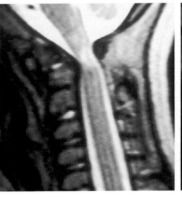
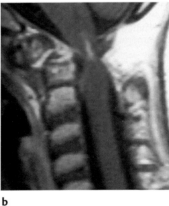

a

b

Fig. 3.**104 a–f   Trisomy 21 with atlantoaxial instability.** 4-year-old boy:
a Sagittal T2-weighted section (TSE; TR = 4600 ms, TE = 112 ms): Spinal cord compression due to displacement of the dorsal arch of the atlas anteriorly with concomitant dislocation between dens and body of axis. Distinct edema of the myelon.
b Sagittal T1-weighted image (SE; TR = 500 ms, TE = 12 ms): Intramedullary contrast enhancement at the level of the compression.

Fig. 3.**104 c–f** ▷

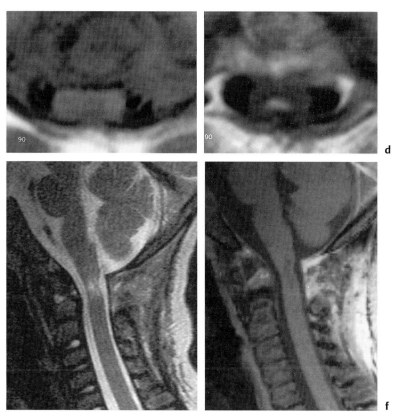

Fig. 3.**104**

c Transverse T1-weighted section (SE; TR = 385 ms, TE = 14 ms): Compression of the spinal cord is easily identifiable on this image from the flattening of the myelon.

d Transverse T1-weighted section after contrast medium administration: Disturbance of the blood-brain barrier is evident centrally with corresponding contrast enhancement.

e View after surgery to remove the posterior arch of the atlas. The T2-weighted image shows decompression of the spinal cord. The CSF-containing space appears normal, both ventrally and dorsally. Constriction of the myelon is seen dorsally. Signal enhancement still remains (TSE; TR = 4600 ms, TE = 112 ms).

f T1-weighted image after contrast application: There is signal attenuation within the spinal cord due to scarring. Disturbance of the blood-brain barrier is no longer present.

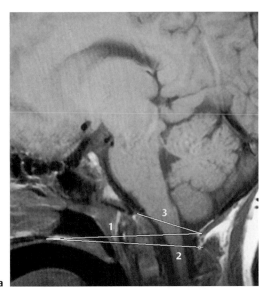

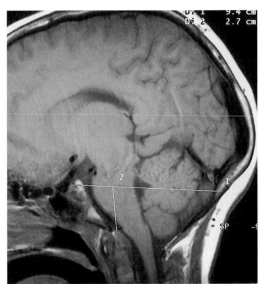

Fig. 3.**105 a, b Mild form of basilar impression.** Sagittal T1-weighted images with depiction of a superior location of the dens:

a The dens projects above Chamberlain's line (1) by about 1 cm and above McGregor's basal line by a good 1.5 cm. McRae's line (3) is not crossed. In normal individuals Chamberlain's line (palato-occipital line) should not be exceeded by more than 4 mm, McGregor's line (basal line) by not more than 5 mm.

b The Klaus height index is illustrated here. This determines the distance between the tip of the dens and the tuberculocruciate line (connection between the tuberculum of the sella and the cruciform eminence of the internal occipital protuberance; average 40–41 mm, from 36–30 mm equivocally pathological, below 30 mm evidence of basilar impression). In this case the value is reduced to 27 mm.

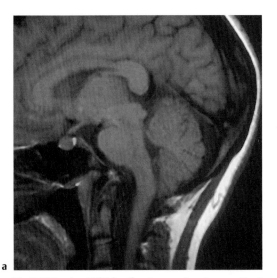

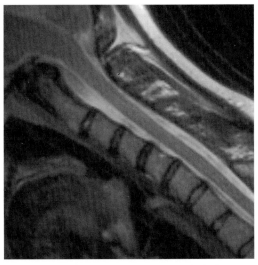

Fig. 3.**106 a, b Mild basilar impression in a patient with Arnold-Chiari type I malformation:**

a Sagittal T1-weighted section (SE; TR = 570 ms, TE = 14 ms): Note the low position of the tonsils, which extend approximately 1 cm into the cervical

canal. Superior location of the dens, which does not, however, reach the medulla oblongata.

b Functional study in anteflexion (TSE; TR = 2700 ms, TE = 120 ms): Even in anteflexion, there is no compression of the medulla by the dens.

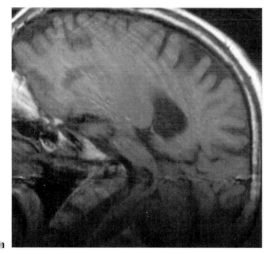

Fig. 3.**107 a–e Basilar impression secondary to vi-
tamin-D deficiency with marked bony deformity in
the area of the skull base.**

a Sagittal section using T1-weighting (SE; TR = 570 ms,
TE = 14 ms): Severe flattening of the skull base at the
level of the middle fossa with marked compression of
the pons and medulla by the dens.

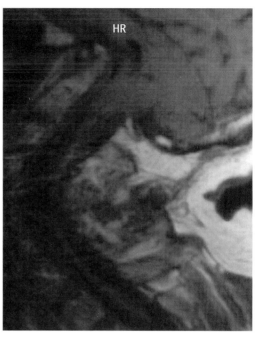

b Supplementary view of the cervical cord (SE;
TR = 350 ms, TE = 12 ms): High-grade atrophy of the
cervical myelon.

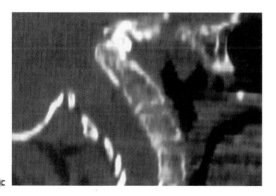

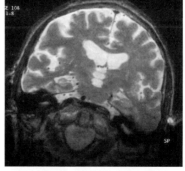

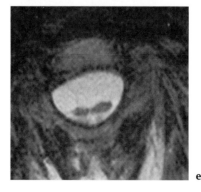

c Corresponding CT reconstruction with evidence of
flattening of the skull base and corresponding superior location of the dens.

d Coronal section using T2-weighting (TSE;
TR = 3100 ms, TE = 96 ms): Marked compression of
the midline structures due to flattening of the skull
base. Basilar artery is well shown to the right of the
midline.

e Transverse T2-weighted section at the level of the
cervical cord (TSE; TR = 4600 ms, TE = 120 ms): High-
grade spinal cord atrophy. The cord appears merely
as a flat disk.

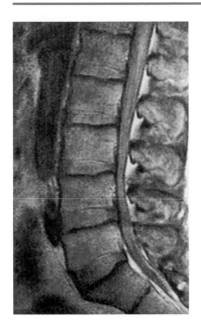

And not least, mention should be made of congenital bony malformations in the region of the craniocervical junction as isolated disorders associated with stenosis of the spinal canal. These include the os odontoideum, in particular, as well as other forms of bony malformation of the upper cervical spine, which can present in a large range of variations at the atlas (anterior or posterior atlas arch missing) or axis (absence of parts of the dens or axis in unilateral or bilateral forms) (Figs. 3.**109**–3.**111**).

◁ Fig. 3.**108** **Idiopathic lumbar stenosis of the spinal canal.** Congenitally narrow spinal canal. The spinal canal clearly tapers caudally in contrast with its diameter at L1. Minimum width of 10 mm at L4 (SE; TR = 2100 ms, TE = 20 ms).

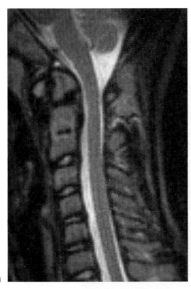
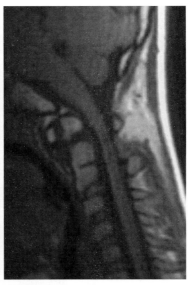

a

b

Fig. 3.**109 a–d** **Os odontoideum.** 12-year-old boy:

a Sagittal T2-weighted section (TSE; TR = 5000 ms, TE = 112 ms): Centers of ossification fail to unite between the tip of the dens and its neck or base. Instead, there is only a loose fibrous bridge. There is no compression of the spinal cord, but the subarachnoid-space reserve appears narrow on its anterior aspect. No indications of an Arnold-Chiari malformation.

b Sagittal T1-weighted section in anteversion (TSE; TR = 450 ms, TE = 12 ms): In anteversion there is a slight anterior displacement of the os odontoideum with a corresponding anterior displacement of the entire atlas. Corresponding narrowness at the level of the craniocervical junction.

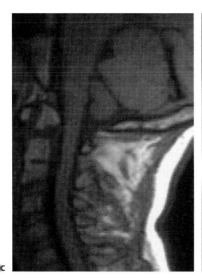
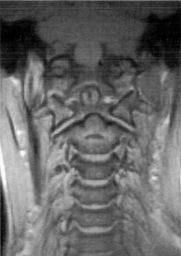

Fig. 3.**109**

c View in reclination. In reclination there is dorsal
sliding of the os odon-
toideum as well as the
atlas arch.

d Coronal section with evidence of the bony inter-
ruption between the tip
of the dens and its base.

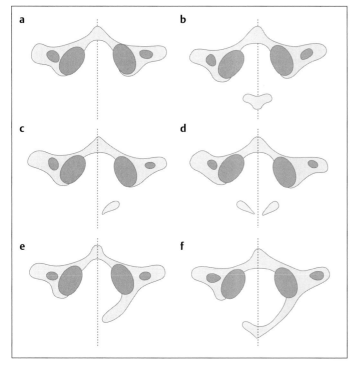

Fig. 3.**110 a–f Various types of
partial and complete aplasia of
the dorsal arch of the atlas** (from
von Torklus, D., W. Gehle *Die obere
Halswirbelsäule*, Thieme, Stuttgart
1975):

a Total aplasia.
b Keller type with persistent posterior tubercle (intercalary bone).
c Brocher type with paramedian
unilateral arch remnant.
d Bilateral remnant of the posterior
hemiarch with cleft.
e Hemiaplasia.
f Partial aplasia of one half of the
arch.

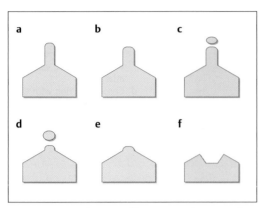

Fig. 3.**111 a–f Schematic illustration of various degrees of hypoplasia of the dens** (from von Torklus, D., W. Gehle: *Die obere Halswirbelsäule*, Thieme, Stuttgart 1975):
a Normal finding.
b Moderate hypoplasia of the dens.
c Hypoplasia of the dens and persistent terminal ossicle.
d High-grade hypoplasia of the dens with os odontoideum.
e High-grade hypoplasia of the dens.
f Aplasia of the dens.

■ Klippel–Feil Syndrome

This represents a shortening and malformation of the cervical spine. Fusion and hypoplasia of segments of the upper cervical spine are noted; sometimes hemivertebrae with consecutive torticollis are found. The disorder can be associated with cervical myelomeningocele and syringomyelia. In most cases a sporadic, non-hereditary occurrence is seen. Individual cases, however, do demonstrate an autosomal dominant inheritance.

Clinically the patients are remarkable for their short, wide neck with limited range of motion. The hairline lies low on the nape of the neck, redundant skin folds are apparent over the neck. The neck muscles attaching to the cervical spine sometimes demonstrate hypoplasia or an abnormal course. Cases have been reported with a concomitant heart disease or unilateral renal agenesis. Severe neurological disturbances are sometimes found associated with hemi- or paraplegia and paralysis of the lower cranial nerves, deafness, convergent strabismus, nystagmus, hyperreflexia and mental retardation (Fig. 3.**112**).

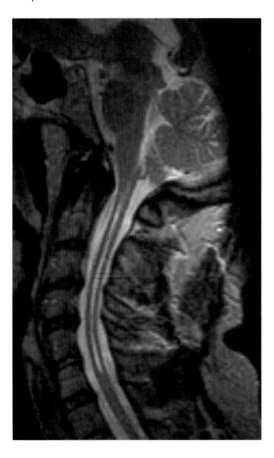

Fig. 3.**112 Incomplete Klippel-Feil syndrome, Arnold-Chiari type I malformation with syringomyelia.** Sagittal T2-weighted section (TSE; TR = 5000 ms, TE = 112 ms): Hypoplasia of the fifth and sixth cervical vertebrae. Mildly low position of the cerebellar tonsils with long-segment syrinx.

Summary

- A distinction is made with dysraphic malformations between the open and closed forms. The *open forms* involve:
  - myelocele,
  - myelomeningocele,
  - myelomeningocystocele.
- The *closed forms* comprise:
  - meningocele,
  - spinal lipoma,
  - lipomyelomeningocele,
  - fibrolipomatosis of the filum terminale,
  - tethered cord syndrome,
  - types I and II split cord malformation,
  - dermal sinus,
  - split notochord syndrome.
- *Combinations* between the open and closed forms of spinal dysraphism are seen not infrequently. A myelomeningocele therefore is often combined with a split cord malformation. Basically, almost every combination is possible, both between open and closed forms as well as among the closed forms. A combination with non-dysraphic changes (e.g. congenital tumors) is also seen.
- The *malformations of the spinal canal* arise during embryogenesis from a faulty differentiation of the spinal cord and its coverings. *Myelomeningocele* develops from an incomplete closure of the neural crest, leading to loss of CSF and collapse of the CSF-containing spaces of the posterior cranial fossa.
- *Lipomas and lipomyeloceles* develop from failure of the neural structures to detach themselves from the mesenchymal tissue during the formation of the neural tube.
- In the *tethered cord syndrome* the detachment of the neural tube from the mesenchyme proceeds normally, but an erroneous formation of intradural structures is noted during the development of the lumbosacral space.
- *Split cord malformation* and *split notochord syndrome* are regarded as residual conditions of a faulty cleft formation of the spinal canal. This splitting occurs physiologically for a short period during the embryonic phase and normally corrects itself completely.
- The open malformations are operated upon immediately after birth without prior imaging.

- Among the closed malformations, the dermal sinus requires an immediate diagnostic work-up and treatment to avoid inflammations of the spinal canal.
- The remaining closed malformations are frequently not diagnosed until late because they can remain asymptomatic for a long time.
- Imaging is used for the open malformations when clinical problems arise after surgery. The radiologist will be confronted with the following questions:
  - are there any other associated malformations?
  - has retethering occurred after successful surgery?
  - is there an ischemic segment of the spinal cord?
  - is there (progressive) syringomyelia?
- The commonest form of spinal dysraphism is the *lipoma* or *lipomyelocele*. The diagnosis is easily reached because of its characteristic signal, which follows that of fat. A lipoma is not always associated with an inferior displacement of the conus.
- *Fibrolipomatosis of the filum terminale* is a lipomatous distension of the filum terminale, frequently associated with shortening and a tethered cord syndrome. Normal thickness of the filum terminale: 2 mm. Shortening is also seen without lipomatosis.
- The *type I split cord malformation* is a clefting of the spinal cord associated with a fibrous or bony spur and subsequent division of the subarachnoid space.
- In *type II split cord malformation* there is clefting of the spinal cord, although a common subarachnoid space is maintained.
- The *dermal sinus* is an epithelialized tract, which can extend intradurally. It can also end extradurally. Diagnostic MR imaging must be performed at an appropriately adjusted sagittal angle. The application of contrast medium is required for the assessment of any possible meningitis.

Summary

- The *split notochord syndrome* can find expression in a variety of very different forms. The mildest form is an intradural cyst situated mainly at the cervicothoracic junction ventral to the spinal cord. Differentiation from a subarachnoid cyst is often only possible by histological examination.
- The *non-dysraphic malformations* comprise:
  - partial and complete agenesis of the sacrum,
  - congenital tumors (teratoma, dermoid, epidermoid),
  - spinal cysts,
  - Arnold–Chiari malformation,
  - syringomyelia,
  - congenital stenosis of the spinal canal.
- The *partial or complete agenesis of the sacrum* is often associated with intraspinal lipomas or a tethered cord syndrome. In addition, combinations with Klippel-Feil syndrome and other forms of vertebral body dysplasia are common.
- The *congenital tumors* often contain fat tissue components. The distinction between dermoid and epidermoid is usually only possible by histological examination. Cysts iso-intense with CSF can be present.
- *Spinal cysts* are differentiated according to their positional relation to the nerve root and dura. They always appear iso-intense with CSF. The cysts can have a considerable space-occupying effect.
- *Arnold–Chiari type I malformation* is often not diagnosed until adulthood. It is defined as an inferior displacement of the cerebellar tonsils and is not infrequently associated with syringomyelia or syringobulbia.
- The *Arnold–Chiari type II malformation* is associated with myelomeningocele. It is a complex malformation, mainly of components of the posterior cranial fossa. Hydrocephalus is often present.
- *Syringomyelia* can have very different causes. The radiologist must attempt to reach a conclusion on the pathogenesis. The whole spinal canal must be examined for clarification. After taking plain films, serial images must be made after contrast application.
- A whole variety of disorders can underlie *congenital stenosis of the spinal canal*, the commonest being:
  - Down syndrome,
  - congenital basilar impression,
  - Klippel-Feil syndrome,
  - idiopathic stenosis of the spinal canal.

References

Aboulezz, A. O., K. Sartor, C. A. Greyer, M. H. Gado: Positions of cerebellar tonsils in the normal population and in patients with Chiari malformation: a quantitative approach with MR imaging. J. Comput. assist. Tomogr. 9 (1985) 1033–1036

Aboulker, J.: La syringomyelie et les liquides intra radudiens. Neurochirurgie 25, Suppl. 2 (1979) 1–44

Agnoli, A. L., A. Laun, R. Schönmayr: Enterogenous intraspinal cysts. J. Neurosurg. 61 (1984) 834–840

Altman, P., J. G. Randolph, J. R. Lilly: Sacrococcygeal teratoma: American Academy of pediatrics surgical section survey – 1973. J. pediat. Surg. 9 (1974) 389–398

Anderson, F. M.: Occult spinal dysraphism: a series of 73 cases. Pediatrics 55 (1975) 826–835

Aoki, S., T. Machida, Y. Sasaki, K. Yoshikawa, M. Iio, T. Sasaki et al.: Enterogenous cyst of cervical spine: clinical and radiological aspects (including CT and MRI). Neuroradiology 29 (1987) 291–293

Appleby, A., J. B. Foster, J. Hankinson, P. Hudgson: The diagnosis and management of the Chiari anomalies in adult life. Brain 91 (1969) 131–142

Arredondo, F., V. M. Haughton, D. C. Hemmy, B. Zelaya, A. L. Williams: The computed tomographic appearance of the spinal cord in diastematomyelia. Neuroradiology 136 (1980) 685–688

Aubin, M. L., J. Vignaud, C. Jardin, D. Bar: Computed tomography in 75 clinical cases of syringomyelia. Amer. J. Neuroradiol. 2 (1981) 199–204

Babcock, D. S., B. K. Han: Cranial sonographic findings in meningomyelocele. Amer. J. Neuroradiol. 1 (1980) 493–499

Baleriaux-Waha, D., M. Osteaux, G. Terwinghe, A. de Meeus, L. Jeanmart: The management of anterior sacral meningocele with computed tomography. Neuroradiology 14 (1977) 45–46

Ball, M. J., A. D. Dayan: Pathogenesis of synringomyelia. Lancet II (1972) 799–801

Banerji, N. K., J. H. D. Millar: Chiari malformation presenting in adult life. Its relationship to synringomyelia. Brain 97 (1974) 157–168

Banna, M.: Syringomyelia in association with posteiror fossa cysts. Amer. J. Neuroradiol. 9 (1988) 867–873

Barnes, P. D., P. D. Lester, W. S. Yamanashi, J. R. Prince: Magnetic resonance imaging in infants and children with spinal dysraphism. Amer. J. Neuroradiol. 7 (1986) 465–472

Barnett, H. J. M., J. B. Foster, P. Hudgson: Syringomyelia. Saunders, Philadelphia 1973

Barry, A., B. M. Patten, B. H. Stewart: Possible factors in the development of the Arnold-Chiari malformation. J. Neurosurg. 14 (1957) 285–301

Barson, A. J.: Radiological studies of spina bifida cystica: The phenomenon of congenital lumbar kyphosis. Brit. J. Radiol. 38 (1965) 294–300

Barson, A. J.: Spina bifida: The significance of the level and extent of the defect to the morphogenesis. Develop. Med. Child Neurol. 12 (1970a) 129–144

Barson, A. J.: The vertebral level of termination of the spinal cord during normal and abnormal development. J. Anat. 106 (1970b) 489–497

Beardmore, H. E., F. W. Wiglesworth: Vertebral anomalies and alimentary duplications. Pediat. Clin. N. Amer. 5 (1958) 457–474

Bell, J., A. Gordon, A. F. J. Maloney: The association of hydrocephalus and Arnold-Chiari malformation with spina bifida in the fetus. Neuropathol. appl. Neurobiol. 6 (1980) 29–39

Bentley, J. F. R., J. R. Smith: Developmental posterior enteric remnants and spinal malformations: the split notochord syndrome. Arch. Dis. Childh. 35 (1960) 76–86

Boston, V. E., A. J. Wilkinson: A retrospective analysis of conservative versus active management in severe open myelomeningocele. Z. Kinderchir. 28 (1979) 340–346

Breningstall, G. N., S. M. Marker, D. E. Tubman: Hydrosyringomyelia and diastematomyelia detected by MRI in myelomeningocele. Pediat. Neurol. 8 (1992) 267–271

Brocklehurst, G.: A quantitative study of a spina bifida fetus. J. Pathol. Bacteriol. 99 (1969) 205–211

Brocklehurst, G.: The pathogenesis of spina bifida: a study of the relationship between observation, hypothesis, and surgical incentive. Develop. Med. Child Neurol. 13 (1971) 147–163

Brocklehurst, G.: Spina bifida for the Clinician. Heinemann, London 1976

Bruce, D. A., L. Schut: Spinal lipomas in infancy and childhood. Child's Brain 5 (1979) 192–203

Burrows, F. G. O., J. Sutcliffe: The split notochord syndrome. Brit. J. Radiol. 41 (1968) 844–847

Busse, O.: Nachweis einer kommunizierenden Syringohydromyelie mit öligem Kontrastmittel. Fortschr. Röntgenstr. 128 (1978) 764–766

Cameron, A. H.: Malformations of the neuro-spinal axis, urogenital tract and foregut in spina bifida attributable to disturbances of the blastopore. J. Pathol. Bacteriol. 73 (1957a) 213–221

Cameron, A. H.: The Arnold-Chiari and other neuro-anatomical malformations associated with spina bifida. J. Pathol. Bacteriol. 73 (1957b) 195–211

Caram, P., G. Scarcella, C. A. Carton: Intradural lipomas of the spinal cord. J. Neurosurg. 14 (1957) 28–42

Carstens, C., E. Schneider: Zur Kenntnis der partiellen Wirbelsäulenaplasie. Z. Orthop. 127 (1989) 569–574

Castillo, M., R. M. Quencer, B. A. Green, B. M. Montalvo: Syringomyelia as a consequence of compressive extramedullary lesions: postoperative clinical and radiological manifestations. Amer. J. Roentgenol. 150 (1988) 391–396

Chapman, P. H.: Congenital intraspinal lipomas, Child's Brain 9 (1982) 37–47

Chiari, H.: Über Veränderungen des Kleinhirns infolge von Hydrocephalie des Grosshirns. Dtsch. med. Wschr. 17 (1891) 1172–1175

Chiari, H.: Über Veränderungen des Kleinhirns, der Pons und der Medulla oblongata infolge von congenitaler Hydrocephalie des Grosshirns. Denkschr. Akad. Wiss. Wien 63 (1895) 71–115

Cleland, J.: Contribution to the study of spina bifida, encephalocele and anencephalus. J. Anat. Physiol. 17 (1883) 257–292

Cloward, R. B.: Congenital spinal extradural cysts: Case report with review of literature. Ann. Surg. 168 (1968) 851–864

Coria, F., F. Quintana, M. Rebollo, O. Combarros, J. Berciano: Occipital dysplasia and Chiari type I deformity in a family. J. neurol. Sci. 62 (1983) 147–158

Curnes J. T., W. J. Oakes, O. B. Boyko: MR imaging of hindbrain deformity in Chiari II patients with and without symptoms of brainstem compression. Amer. J. Neuroradiol. 10 (1989) 293–302

D' Almeida, A., D. H. Stewart: Neurenteric cyst: case report and literature review. Neurosurgery 8 (1981) 596–599

Daniel, P. M., S. J. Strich: Some observations on the congenital deformity of the central nervous system known as the Arnold-Chiari malformation. J. Neuropath. exp. Neurol. 17 (1958) 255–266

Davis, P. C., J. C. Hoffman jr., T. I. Ball, J. B. Wyly, I. F. Braun, S. M. Fry et al.: Spinal abnormalities in pediatric patients: MR imaging findings compared with clinical, myelographic, and surgical findings. Radiology 166 (1988) 679–685

De Baecque, C., D. H. Snyder, K. Suzuki: Congenital intramedullary spinal dermoid cyst associated with an Arnold-Chiari malformation. Acta neuropathol. 38 (1977) 239–242

De Saunders, R. L. Ch.: Combined anterior and posterior spina bifida in a living neonatal human female. Anat. Rec. 87 (1943) 255–278

Di Pietro M. A.: The conus medullaris: normal US findings throughout childhood. Radiology 188 (1993) 149–153

Doran, P. A., A. N. Guthkelch: Studies in spina bifida cystica. 1. General survey and reassessment of the problem. J. Neurol. Neurosurg. Psychiat. 24 (1961) 331–345

Du Boulay, G., S. H. Shah, J. C. Currie, V. Logue: The mechanism of hydromyelia in Chiari type 1 malformations. Brit. J. Radiol. 47 (1974) 579–587

Dubowitz, V., J. Lorber, R. B. Zachary: Lipoma of the cauda equina. Arch. Dis. Childh. 40 (1965) 207–213

Duncan, A. W., R. D. Hoare: Spinal arachnoid cysts in children. Radiology 126 (1978) 423–429

Emery, J. L.: Deformity of the aqueduct of Sylvius in children with hydrocephalus and myelomeningocele. Develop. Med. Child Neurol. 16, Suppl. 32 (1974) 40–48

Emery, J. L., R. K. Levick, The movement of the brain stem and vessels around the brain stem in children with hydrocephalus and the Arnold-Chiari deformity. Develop. Med. Child Neurol. 8, Suppl. 11 (1966) 49–60

Emery, J. L., D. Naik: Spinal cord segment lengths in children with meningomyelocele and the "Cleland-Arnold-Chiari" deformity. Brit. J. Radiol. 41 (1968) 287–290

Emery, J. L., R. G. Lendon: Lipomas of the cauda equina and other fatty tumours related to neurospinal dysraphism. Develop. Med. Child Neurol. 11, Suppl. 20 (1969) 62–70

Emery, J. L., R. G. Lendon: Clinical implications of cord lesion in neurospinal dysraphism. Develop. Med. Child Neurol. 14, Suppl. 27 (1972) 45–51

Emery, J. L., N. MacKenzie: Medullo-cervical dislocation deformity (Chiari II deformity) related to neurospinal dysraphism (meningomyelocele). Brain 96 (1973) 155–163

Emery, J. L., R. G. Lendon: The local cord lesion in neurospinal dysraphism (meningomyelocele). J. Pathol. 110 (1973) 83–96

Feetham, S. L., H. Tweed, J. S. Perrin: Practical problems in selection of spina bifida infants for treatment in the USA. Z. Kinderchir. 28 (1979) 301–306

Florez, G., S. Ucar: The occult intrasacral meningocele. Neurochirurgia 19 (1976) 46–53

French, B. N.: The embryology of spinal dysraphism. Clin. Neurosurg. 30 (1982) 295–340

French, B. L.: Midline fusion defects and defects of formation. In Youmans, R.: Neurological Surgery. Saunders, Philadelphia 1990 (pp. 1081–1235)

Friede, R. L., U. Roessmann: Chronic tonsillar herniation. An attempt at classifying chronic herniations at the foramen magnum. Acta neuropathol. 34 (1976) 219–235

Friede, R. L.: Developmental Neuropathology. Springer, Berlin 1989

Gammal, T. E., E. K. Mark, B. S. Brooks: MR imaging of Chiari II malformation. Amer. J. Roentgenol. 150 (1988) 163–170

Gardner, W. J., R. J. Goodall: The surgical treatment of Arnold-Chiari malformation in adults. J. Neurosurg. 7 (1950) 199–206

Gardner, W. J.: Hydrodynamic mechanism of syringomyelia: its relationship to myelocele. J. Neurol. Neurosurg. Psychiat. 28 (1965) 247–259

Gardner, W. J.: The Dysraphic States from Syringomyelia to Anencephaly. Excerpta Medica, Amsterdam 1973

Gelmers, H. J., K. G. Go: Intrasacral meningocele. Acta neurochir. 39 (1977) 115–119

Geremia, G. K., E. J. Russell, R. A. Clasen: MR imaging characteristics of an neurenteric cyst. Amer. J. Neuroradiol. 9 (1988) 978–980

Giuffre, R.: Intradural spinal lipomas. Acta Neurochir. 14 (1966) 69–95

Goldstein, F., J. J. Kepes: The role of traction in the development of the Arnold-Chiari malformation: an experimental study. J. Neuropathol. exp. Neurol. 25 (1966) 654–666

Gonzales-Crussi, F., R. F. Winkler, D. L. Mirkin: Sacrococcygeal teratomas in infants and children. Arch. Pathol. Lab. Med. 102 (1978) 420–425

Gray, L., W. T. Djang, A. H. Friedman: MR imaging of thoracic extradural arachnoid cysts. J. Comput. assist. Tomogr. 12 (1988) 646–648

Grivegnee, A., P. Delince, P. Ectors: Comparative aspects of occult intrasacral meningocele with conventional X-ray, myelography and CT. Neuroradiology 22 (1981) 33–37

Gross, R. H., A. Cox, R. Tatyrek, M. Pollay, W. A. Barnes: Early management and decision making for the treatment of myelomeningocele. Pediatrics 72 (1983) 450–458

Guidetti, B., F. M. Galiardi: Epidermoid and dermoid cysts. J. Neurosurg. 47 (1977) 12–18

Gupta, D. K., M. C. Deodkar: Split notochord syndrome presenting with meningomyelocele and dorsal enteric fistula. J. pediat. Surg. 22 (1987) 382–383

Gupta, R. K., A. Sharma: MR demonstration of paravertebral lumbar meningomyelocele with diastematomyelia. Neuroradiology 31 (1990) 554

Herren, R. J., J. E. Edwards: Diplomyelia (duplication of the spinal cord). Arch. Pathol. 30 (1940) 1203–1214

Hertel, G., M. Nadjmi, J. Kunze: A statistical comparative study of the basilar impression in syringomyelia. Europ. Neurol. 11 (1974) 363–372

Hilal, S. K., D. Marton, E. Pollack: Diastematomyelia in children: radiographic study of 34 cases. Radiology 112 (1974) 609–621

Hoffman, C. H., R. B. Dietrich, M. J. Pais, D. S. Demos, H. F. W. Pubram: The split notochord syndrome with dorsal enteric fistula. Amer. J. Neuroradiol. 14 (1993) 622–627

Holtzmann, R. N. N., B. M. Stein: The Tethered Spinal Cord. Thieme, Stuttgart 1985

Howieson, J., H. A. Norrell, C. B. Wilson: Expansion of the subarachnoid space in the lumbosacral region. Radiology 90 (1968) 488–492

Ikata, T., K. Masaki, S. Kashiwaguchi: Clinical and experimental studies on permeability of tracers in normal spinal cord and syringomyelia. Spine 13 (1988) 737–741

James, C. C. M., L. P. Lassman: Spinal Dysraphism: Spina bifida occulta. Butterworths, London 1972

Jones, P. H., J. G. Love: Tight filum terminale. Arch. Surg. 73 (1956) 556–566

Just, M., M. Schwarz, B. Ludwig, J. Ermert, M. Thelen: Cerebral and spinal MR-findings in patients with postrepair myelomeningocele. Pediat. Radiol. 20 (1990) 262–266

Kak, V. K., R. K. Gupta, B. S. Sharma, A. K. Banerjee: Craniospinal entereogenous cyst: MR findings. J. Comput. assist. Tomogr. 14 (1990) 470–472

Kantrowitz, L. R., M. J. Pais, K. Busnett, B. Choi, M. B. Putz: Intraspinal neurenteric cyst containing gastric mucosa: CT and MRI findings. Pediat. Radiol. 16 (1986) 324–327

Keiller, V. H.: A contribution to the anatomy of spina bifida. Brain (1922) 31–103

Kendall, B. E., A. R. Valentine, B. Keis: Spinal arachnoid cysts: clinical and radiological correlation with prognosis. Neuroradiology 22 (1982) 225–234

Kirsch, W. M., F. J. Hodges: An intramedullary epidermal inclusion cyst of the thoracic cord associated with a previously repaired meningocele. Case report. J. Neurosurg. 24 (1966) 1018–1020

Lamas, E., R. D. Lobato, T. Amor: Occult intrasacral meningocele. Surg. Neurol. 8 (1977) 181–184

Lassman, L. P., C. C. M. James: Meningocele manqué. Child's Brain 3 (1977) 1–11

Lee, B. C. P., M. D. F. Deck, J. B. Kneeland, P. T. Cahill: MR imaging of the craniocervical junction. Amer. J. Neuroradiol. 6 (1985) 209–213

Lerma, S., J. M. Roda, F. Villarejo, A. Perez-Higueras, M. Gutierrez-Molina, M. G. Blazques: Intradural neurenteric cyst: Review and discussion. Neurochirurgia 28 (1985) 228–231

Levy, L. M., G. Die Chiro, D. C. McCullough, A. J. Dwyer, D. L. Johnson, S. S. L. Yang: Fixed spinal cord: diagnosis with MR imaging. Radiology 169 (1988) 773–778

Lichtenstein, B. W.: Spinal dysraphism, spina bifida and myelodysplasia. Arch. Neurol. Psychiat. 44 (1940) 792–810

Lichtenstein, B. W.: Distant neuroanatomic complications of spina bifida (spinal dysraphism); hydrocephalus, Arnold-Chiari deformitiy, stenosis of the aqueduct of Sylvius, etc., pathogenesis and pathology. Arch. Neurol. Psychiat. 47 (1942) 195–214

List, C. F.: Intraspinal epidermoids, dermoids and dermal sinuses. Surg. Gynecol. Obstet. 73 (1941) 525–538

Lorber, J.: Results of treatment of myelomeningocele. An analysis of 524 unselected cases, with special reference to possible selection for treatment. Develop. Med. Child Neurol. 13 (1971) 279–301

Marin-Padilla, M.: The tethered cord syndrome: developmental considerations. In Holtzman, R. N. N., B. M. Stein: The Tethered Spinal Cord. Thieme, Stuttgart 1985

Marin-Padilla, M., T. M. Marin-Padiulla: Morphogenesis of experimentally induced Arnold-Chiari malformation. J. neurol. Sci. 50 (1981) 29–55

McCrum, C., B. Williams: Spinal extradural arachnoid pouches. J. Neurosurg. 57 (1982) 849–852

McLaughlin, J. F., D. B. Shurtleff, J. Y. Lamers, J. T. Stuntz, P. W. Hayden, R. J. Kropp: Influence of prognosis on decisions regarding the care of newborns with myelodysplasia. New Engl. J. Med. 312 (1985) 1589–1594

McLetchie, N. G. B., J. K. Purves, R. L. de Ch. Saunders: The genesis of gastric and certain intestinal diverticula and enterogenous cysts. Surg. Gynecol. Obstet. 99 (1954) 135–141

McLone, D. G., T. P. Naidich: Spinal dysraphism: experimental and clinical. In Holtzman, R. N. N., B. M. Stein: The Tethered Spinal Cord. Thieme, Stuttgart 1985a

McLone, D. G., T. P. Naidich: Terminal myelocystocele. Neurosurgery 16 (1985b) 36–43

McLone, D. G., S. Mutluer, T. P. Naidich: Lipomeningoceles of the conus medullaris. Concepts pediat. Neurosurg. 3 (1983) 170–177

McLone, D. G., P. A. Knepper: The cause of Chiari II malformation: a unified theory. Pediat. Neurosci. 15 (1989) 1–12

Menezes, A. H., J. C. van Gilder: Anomalies of the craniovertebral junction. In Youmans, R.: Neurological Surgery. Saunders, Philadelphia 1990a (pp. 1359–1420)

Menezes, A. H., W. R. K. Smoker, G. N. Dyste: Syringomyelia, Chiari malformation, and hydromyelia. In Youmans, R.: Neurological Surgery. Saunders, Philadelphia 1990b (pp. 1421–1459)

Merx, J. L., S. H. Bakker-Niezen, H. O. M. Thijssen, H. A. D. Walder: The tethered spinal cord syndrome: a correlation of radiological features and peroperative findings in 30 patients. Neuroradiology 31 (1989) 63–70

Mirich, D. R., J. T. Hall, C. H. Carrasco: MR imaging of traumatic spinal arachnoid cyst. J. Comput. assist. Tomogr. 12 (1988) 862–865

Monajati, A., R. M. Spitzer, J. L. Wiley, L. Heggeness: MR imaging of a spinal teratoma. J. Comput. assist. Tomogr. 10 (1986) 307–310

Nabors, M. W., T. G. Pait, E. B. Byrd, N. O. Karim, D. O. Davis, A. I. Kobrine et al.: Updated assessment and current classification of spinal meningeal cysts. J. Neurosurg. 68 (1988) 366–377

Naidich, T. P., D. C. Harwood-Nash: Diastematomyelia: hemicord and meningeal sheaths: single and double arachnoid and dural tubes. Amer. J. Neuroradiol. 4 (1983) 633–636

Naidich, T. P., R. M. Pudlowski, J. B. Naidich, M. Gornish, F. J. Rodriguez: Computed tomographic signs of the Chiari II malformation. Part I: Skull and dural partitions. Radiology 134 (1980a) 65–71

Naidich, T. P., R. M. Pudlowski, J. B. Naidich: Computed tomographic signs of the Chiari II malformation. Part III: Ventricles and cisterns. Radiology 134 (1980b) 657–663

Naidich, T. P., R. M. Pudowski, J. B. Naidich: Computed tomographic signs of Chiari II malformation. Part II: Midbrain and cerebelum. Radiology 134 (1980c) 391–398

Naidich, T. P., D. G. McLone, K. H. Fulling: The Chiari II malformation. Part IV: The hindbrain deformity. Neuroradiology 25 (1983a) 179–197

Naidich, T. P., D. G. McLone, S. Mutluer: A new understanding of dorsal dysraphism with lipoma (lipomyeloschisis): Radiologic eveluation and surgical correction. Amer. J. Neuroradiol. 4 (1983b) 103–116

Noseworthy, J., E. E. Lack, H. P. W. Kozakewich, G. F. Vawter, K. J. Welch: Sacrococcygeal germ cell tumors in childhood: an updated experience with 118 patients. J. pediat. Surg. 16 (1981) 358–364

Nyland, H., K. G. Krogness: Size of posterior fossa in Chiari type 1 malformation in adults. Acta neurochir. 40 (1978) 233–242

O'Rahilly, R., F. Müller: The normal and abnormal development of the nervous system in the early human embryo. J. pediat. Neurol. 2 (1986) 89–94

Osaka, K., T. Tanimura, A. Hirayama, S. Matsumoto: Myelomeningocele before birth. J. Neurosurg. 49 (1978) 711–724

Padget, D. H.: Spina bifida and embryonic neuroschisis – a causal relationship. Definition of the postnatal conformations involving a bifid spine. Johns Hopk. med. J. 128 (1968) 233–252

Padget, D. H.: Neuroschisis and human embryonic maldevelopment: new evidence on anencephaly, spina bifida and diverse mammalian defects. J. Neuropathol. exp. Neurol. 29 (1970) 192–216

Padget, D. H.: Development of so-called dysraphism, with embryologic evidence of clinical Arnold-Chiari and Dandy-Walker malformations. Johns Hopk. med. J. 130 (1972) 127–165

Palmer, J. J.: Spinal arachnoid cysts. Report of six cases. J. Neurosurg. 41 (1974) 728–735

Pang, D., M. S. Dias, M. Ahab-Barmada: Split cord malformation: Part I: A unified theory of embryogenesis for double spinal cord malformations. Neurosurgery 31 (1992) 451–480

Patten, B. M.: Embryological stages in the establishing of myeloschisis with spina bifida. Amer. J. Anat. 93 (1953) 365–395

Patten, B. M.: Fusion of notochord to neural tube in a human embryo of the sixth week. Anat. Rec. 95 (1946) 307–311

Patten, B. M.: Overgrowth of the neural tube in young human embryos. Anat. Rec. 113 (1952) 381–393

Paul, K. S., R. H. Lye, F. A. Strang, J. Dutton: Arnold-Chiari malformation. Review of 71 cases. J. Neurosurg. 58 (1983) 183–187

Paulsen, R. D., G. A. Call, F. R. Murtagh: Prevalence and percutaneous drainage of cysts of the sacral nerve root sheath (Tarlov cysts). Amer. J. Neuroradiol. 15 (1994) 293

Peach, B.: The Arnold-Chiari malformation. Morphogenesis. Arch. Neurol. 12 (1965) 527–535

Penfield, W., D. F. Coburn: Arnold Chiari malformation and its operative treatment. Arch. Neurol. Psychiat. 40 (1938) 328–336

Pierot, L., D. Dormont, S. Queslati, P. Cornu, M. Rivierez, J. Bories: Gadolinium-DTPA enhanced MR imaging of intradural neurenteric cysts. J. Comput. assist. Tomogr. 12 (1988) 762–764

Quencer, R. M., B. M. Montalvo, T. P. Naidich, M. J. D. Post, B. A. Green, L. K. page: Intraoperative sonography in spinal dysraphism and syringohydromyelia. Amer. J. Roentgenol. 148 (1987) 1005–1013

Raghavan, N., A. J. Barkovich, M. Edwards, D. Norman: MR imaging in the tethered spinal cord syndrome. Amer. J. Roentgenol. 152 (1989) 843–852

Raimondi, A. J., M. Choux, C. Di Rocco: The Pediatric Spine I. Development and the Dysraphic State. Springer, Berlin 1989

Ray, B. S.: Platybasia with involvement of the central nervous system. Ann. Surg. 116 (1942) 231–250

von Recklinghausen, F.: Untersuchungen über die Spina bifida. Virchows Arch. pathol. Anat. 105 (1886) 243–373

Renshaw, T. S.: Sacral agenesis. A classification and review of twenty-three cases. J. Bone Jt Surg. 60 (1978) 373–383

Rewcastle, N. B., J. Francoeur: Teratomatous cysts of the spinal canal. Arch. Neurol. 11 (1964) 91–99

Roth, M.: Cranio-cervical growth collision: another explanation of the Arnold-Chiari malformation and of basilar impression. Neuroradiology 28 (1986) 187–194

Rozen, M. J.: Pathophysiology and spinal deformity in myelomeningozele. In Mc Maurin, R. L.: Myelomeningocele. Grune & Stratton, New York 1977 (pp. 565–579)

Sato, O., T. Asai, Y. Amono, M. Hara, R. Tsugane, M. Yagi: Extraventricular origin of the cerebrospinal fluid: formation rate quantitatively measured in the spinal subarachnoid space of dogs. J. Neurosurg. 36 (1972) 276–281

Scatliff, J. H., B. E. Kendall, D. P. E. Kingsley, J. Britton, D. N. Grant, R. D. Hayward: Closed spinal dysraphism: analysis of clinical, radiological and surgical findings in 104 consecutive patients. Amer. J. Roentgenol. 152 (1989) 1049–1057

Schady, W., R. A. Metcalfe, P. Butler: The incidence of craniocervical bony anomalies in the adult Chiari malformation. J. neurol. Sci. 82 (1987) 193–203

Schey, W. L., A. Shkolnik, H. Wente: Clinical and radiolgraphic considerations of sacrococcygeal teratomas. An analysis of 26 new cases and review of the literature. Radiology 1977 (125) 189–195

Schlesinger, A. E., T. P. Naidich, R. M. Quencer: Concurrent hydromyelia and diastematomyelia. Amer. J. Neuroradiol. 7 (1986) 473–477

Schroth, G., M. Palmbach: Syringomyelie: Korrelation kernspintomographischer und klinischer Befunde vor und nach Operation. Fortschr. Röntgenstr. 149 (1988) 587–593

Schwartz, H.: Congenital tumors of the spinal cord in infants. Ann. Surg. 136 (1952) 183–192

Scotti, G., D. C. Harwood-Nash, H. J. Hoffman: Congenital thoracic dermal sinus: Diagnosis by computer assisted metrizamide myelography. J. Comput. assist. Tomogr. 4 (1980) 675–677

Sherman, J. L., A. J. Barkovich, C. M. Citrin: The MR appearance of syringomyelia: new observations. Amer. J. Neuroradiol. 7 (1986) 985–995

Sherman, J. L., C. M. Citrin, A. J. Barkovich: MR imaging of syringobulbia. J. Comput. assist. Tomogr. 11 (1987) 407–411

Shulman, K., M. D. Ames: Intensive treatment of fifty children born with myelomeningocele. N. Y. Med. 68 (1968) 2656–2659

Smith, J. R.: Accessory enteric formations: A classification and nomenclature. Arch. Dis. Childh. 35 (1960) 87–89

Stark, G. D.: Spina bifida, Problems and Management. Blackwell, Oxford 1977

Starshak, R. J., G. A. Kass, R. N. Samaraweera: Developmental stenosis of the cervical spine in children. Pediat. Radiol. 17 (1987) 291–295

Suneson, A., H. Kalimo: Myelocystocele with cerebellar heterotopia. J. Neurosurg. 51 (1979) 392–396

Taviere, V., F. Brunelle, J. Baraton, M. Temam, A. P. Kahn, D. Lallemand: MRI study of lumbosacral lipoma in children. Pediat. Radiol. 19 (1989) 316–320

Thron, A., G. Schroth: Magnetic resonance imaging (MRI) of diastematomyelia. Neuroradiology 28 (1986) 371–372

Tortori-Donati, P., A. Cama, M. L. Rosa, L. Andreussi, A. Taccone: Occult spinal dysraphism: neuroradiological study. Neuroradiology 31 (1990) 512–522

Träger, D.: Beitrag zum kaudalen Regressionssyndrom. Z. Orthop. 127 (1989) 566–568

Vade, A., D. Kennard: Lipomeningocystocele. Amer. J. Neuroradiol. 8 (1987) 375–377

Variend, S., J. L. Emery: The pathology of the central lobes of the cerebellum in children with myelomeningocele. Develop. Med. Child Neurol. 16, Suppl. 32 (1974) 99–106

Variend, S., J. L. Emery: Cervical dislocation of the cerebellum in children with meningomyelocele. Teratology 13 (1976) 281–290

Variend, S., J. L. Emery: The superior surface lesion of the cerebellum in children with myelomeningocele. Z. Kinderchir. 28 (1979) 327–335

Visciani, A., M. Savoiardo, M. R. Balestrini, C. L. Solero: Iatrogenic intraspinal epidermoid tumor: myelo-CT and MRI diagnosis. Neuroradiol. 31 (1989) 273–275

Walker, A. E., P. C. Bucy: Congenital dermal sinuses, a source of spinal meningeal infection and subdural abscesses. Brain 57 (1934) 401–421

Warkany, J.: Morphogenesis of spina bifida. In McLaurin, R. L.: Myelomeningocele. Grune & Stratton, New York 1977 (pp. 31–39)

Welch, K., J. Shillito, R. Strand, E. G. Fischer, K. R. Winston: Chiari I "malformation" – an acquired disorder? J. Neurosurg. 55 (1981) 604–609

Williams, B.: Current concepts of syringomyelia. Brit. J. Hosp. Med. 4 (1970) 331–342

Williams, B.: On the pathogenesis of syringomyelia: a review. J. roy. Soc. Med. 73 (1980) 798–806

Williams, B., W. R. Timperley: Three cases of communicating syringomyelia secondary to midbrain gliomas. J. Neurol. Neurosurg. Psychiat. 40 (1976) 80–88

Wippold, F. J., C. Citrin, A. J. Barkovich, J. S. Sherman: Evaluation of MR in spinal dysraphism with lipoma: comparison with metrizamide computed tomography. Pediat. Radiol. 17 (1987) 184–188

Wolpert, S. M., M. Anderson, R. M. Scott, E. S. K. Kwan, V. M. Runge: Chiari II malformation: MR imaging. Amer. J. Roentgenol. 149 (1987) 1033–1042

Wolpert, S. M., R. M. Scott, C. Platenberg, V. M. Runge: The clinical significance of hindbrain herniation and deformity as shown on MR images of patients with Chiari II malformation. Amer. J. Neuroradiol. 9 (1988) 1075–1978

Woo, P. Y. C., M. M. Sharr: Childhood cervical enterogenous cyst presenting with hemiparesis. Postgrad. med. J. 58 (1982) 424–426

Wright, R. L.: Congenital dermal sinuses. Progr. neurol. Surg. 4 (1971) 175–191

Yamada, H., S. Nakamura, Y. Tanaka, M. Tajima, N. Kageyama: Ventriculography and cisternography with water-soluble contrast media in infants with myelomeningocele. Radiology 143 (1982) 75–83

Yu, Y. L., I. F. Moseley: Syringomyelia and cervical spondylosis: a clinicoradiological investigation. Neuroradiology 29 (1987) 143–151

Zumpano, B. J., R. L. Saunders: Lumbar intradural arachnoid diverticulum with cauda equina compression. Surg. Neurol. 5 (1976) 349–354

4　Degenerative Disorders of the Spine

D. Uhlenbrock

Contents

Definition

Degenerative processes of the diskovertebral and synovial joints as well as degenerative changes of the ligamentous system are all included under the term "degenerative disorders of the spine."

Pathogenesis

Degenerative disorders are basically the consequence of the normal ageing process, resulting in damage to the intervertebral disks, the adjacent bony structures, the other joints, and the ligamentous system.

The factors promoting degeneration are the morphological changes that affect the biomechanics of the axial skeleton and include e.g.

- scoliosis,
- lumbosacral assimilations,
- other congenital vertebral anomalies.

Instabilities, e.g. due to laxity of the ligamentous system, spondylolisthesis or disorders of the joints, can also accelerate a degenerative process. In individual cases, continual bad posture or bearing abnormally heavy weights, as can happen with occupational overloading or sports activities, are of clinical relevance. Other causes such as genetic factors and autoimmune processes are also under discussion. In the majority of cases there are several factors that determine the pathogenesis of degenerative disorders of the axial skeleton.

The clinical relevance of the degenerative changes found can vary considerably in individual cases. Clinical symptoms may be completely lacking in one patient, while their clinical presentation in another may be more striking despite only the slightest sign of a degenerative process.

The Ageing Process of the Intervertebral Disk

A major factor in the pathogenesis of degenerative disorders of the spine is the ageing process of the intervertebral disk involving a biochemical and histological remodeling; this is the cause of a large proportion of clinically relevant symptoms. A great number of radiological and, in particular, MRI examinations are focused on the state of the intervertebral disk.

Structures of the Intervertebral Disk

Cartilaginous end plate. The cartilaginous end plate is the morphological, and also in a sense the metabolic, connection between the nucleus pulposus and the vertebral body end plate. Degenerative processes of the disk spread to the vertebral body via the end plate. Because the end plate in the adult no longer contains blood vessels, metabolic exchange between the structures is by diffusion.

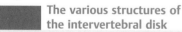

The various structures of the intervertebral disk

- cartilaginous end plate
- annulus fibrosus
- nucleus pulposus

Annulus fibrosus. The annulus fibrosus forms the anterior and posterior margins of the intervertebral disk. Its fibers are firmly attached to the bone via Sharpey's fibers. The fibers of the annulus are also attached to the anterior and posterior longitudinal ligaments.

Nucleus pulposus. The nucleus pulposus is composed of a gelatinous matrix with a high water-binding capacity. About 85–90% of the nucleus consists of water while the water content of the annulus fibrosus is around 80%. Elasticity is a characteristic of the nucleus pulposus (Modic *et al.*, 1988; Ho *et al.*, 1988; Yu *et al.*, 1988).

Histology

Histologically the nucleus pulposus and annulus fibrosus are composed of fibrocartilaginous ground substance and collagen. Protoglycans are the principal macromolecules found, and are present in larger numbers in the nucleus pulposus than in the annulus. The periphery of the annulus fibrosus (Sharpey's fibers) consists of dense collagen (type I) with lower water content. Collagen fibers with a higher water-binding capacity are found towards the center (type II collagen fibers)

(Modic *et al.*, 1988). In the normal disk, the MR signal represents the difference between the low signal intensity of the collagen and the high signal intensity of the fibrocartilaginous ground substance of the intervertebral disk.

During the ageing process and in the course of the degeneration of the intervertebral disk, the disk loses water. This process is more pronounced in the nucleus pulposus than in the annulus fibrosus. The water content is reduced in both structures to about 70 % overall. The reduction of the water-binding capacity of the nucleus pulposus is mainly due to the loss in molecular weight of the proteoglycan complexes, which is explained by shifts within their individual biochemical components. Furthermore, there is an increase in the fibrous structures of the nucleus pulposus, which grow towards the center of the intervertebral disk from the anterior or posterior margin.

In the final stage, nucleus pulposus and annulus fibrosus are no longer sharply demarcated from one another. In fact, a uniform amorphous fibrocartilaginous tissue with only slight elasticity and a clear reduction in height is found (Aguila *et al.*, 1985; Modic *et al.*, 1988; Yu *et al.*, 1988).

Degeneration of the Intervertebral Disk

Changes of the Cartilaginous End Plate

The degeneration of the intervertebral disk is associated with changes of the cartilaginous end plate. The chondrocytes situated near the vertebral body calcify and become degraded by the bone. The end plate consequently becomes reduced in thickness; its attribute of separating the vertebral body from the nucleus pulposus is lost. *Fissures* and microfractures develop that are partly lined with granulation tissue. In addition, *regenerating chondrocytes* are also found.

Nucleus pulposus material can penetrate into the fissures; intravertebral hernias can develop and are found together with disk degeneration. At this stage the vertebral end plates show signs of subchondral sclerosis on plain films and are sometimes interrupted and in parts irregularly contoured. Herniations within the cancellous bone are bordered by marginal sclerosis, which can be quite pronounced. In severe cases the subchondral sclerosis can involve large portions of the vertebral body. In rare instances complete eburnation of the vertebrae is found (Resnick and

Niwayama, 1978). The development of gas, which is found within the disk but can also leak out into the spinal canal via cracks and fissures, is typical for disk degeneration. This gas is nitrogen oxide.

Degenerative Changes at the Apophyseal Joints

Degenerative changes at the apophyseal joints can occur in conjunction with degeneration of the intervertebral disks. Disk degeneration leads to a *reduction in height of the intervertebral space*, which results in a caudal posterior *dislocation* of the vertebra situated proximal to the intervertebral disk. This leads to *subluxation* of the apophyseal joints, which alters articular load bearing and can result in reactive bony changes at the facets, particularly in the form of hypertrophy. Furthermore, disk degeneration also directly leads to additional load bearing. The loss of disk elasticity exposes the small vertebral joints to increased motion, particularly torsion movements. In addition, the loss of the nucleus pulposus displaces the center of rotation during movements within the spine further dorsally, even as far as the vertebral joints if the changes are pronounced. Instead of sliding motions, jerking movements occur which, in particular, lead to *instability of the vertebral joints*; this instability can be demonstrated on conventional functional views. In turn, as a result of the instability, increased tractive forces develop at the capsule-ligament complex of the joints with corresponding secondary bony reactions in the form of *osteophyte formations*. Instabilities can also be the *result of surgery* involving generous clearing of the intervertebral space. They can also occur secondary to chemonucleolysis or spondylolisthesis. Conversely, infectious or traumatic and, ultimately, also tumor-related processes, all of which result in instability of the small vertebral joints, can be the initiating cause of intervertebral disk degeneration (Resnick and Niwayama, 1988).

Degenerative Changes at the Ligament and Joint-Capsule Insertions onto the Bone

Degenerative changes are also found at the ligament and joint-capsule insertions onto the bone. These include, on the one hand, *deforming spondylosis*, which particularly develops anterior to the intervertebral space. Increased tractive forces are regarded as causative, originating from the annulus fibrosus, especially from Sharpey's fibers, and being transferred to the bone. These tractive forces are caused by ventral disk protrusions which, when extensive, can lead to partial ruptures of individual fibers and result in a progressive extrusion of the disk in an anterior direction. This results in additional traction on the anterior longitudinal ligament, which is transferred directly to the bone at those sites where the longitudinal ligament has its osseous attachments. It is at these attachment sites that *osteophytes* develop from the anterior margins of the vertebral body. The osteophytes first extend anteriorly, growing in a subligamentous fashion and spanning the protruding disk. In severe cases complete osteophytic bridging is found. A distinction should be made from *syndesmophytes*, which in the typical case display ossification and enclose the region of the annulus fibrosus. They grow in a vertical direction.

Calcifications

Calcifications are a further form of degeneration of the capsule-ligament complex. They are found in all segments of the vertebral ligamentous system and are of clinical relevance, especially when they occur in the region of the posterior longitudinal ligament and the ligamenta flava. Their development is promoted by instability associated with abnormal range of joint motion and thus by an increased traction on capsule and ligaments.

Because the ligaments contain abundant nerve fibers, these lesions can be the source of a considerable amount of pain in some cases (Resnick and Niwayama, 1988).

Classification of Intervertebral Disk Degeneration

Changes in the intervertebral disk have been further differentiated and classified by post-mortem MRI studies (Ho *et al.*, 1988; Yu *et al.*, 1988).

Types of nucleus pulposus

- *Type I:* in the neonate.
- *Type II:* in the child and juvenile.
- *Type III:* in the younger adult.
- *Type IV:* in the older adult.

■ Nucleus Pulposus Type I

The MR image of the intervertebral disk of the neonate differs completely from that obtained in the juvenile and adult.

On *T1-weighted SE images* the ossification center is demarcated and oval in shape. In the neonate it demonstrates slightly lower signal intensity than cartilage and intervertebral disk, though it becomes higher after a few weeks. There is no distinction between cartilage and the disk, which together display a structure of biconcave form with intermediate signal intensity. The annulus fibrosus too cannot be distinguished from the rest of the disk material, nor can the outermost fibers (Sharpey's fibers).

On *PD-weighted images* the ossification center appears relatively dark, while cartilage and disk are brighter, creating a contrast between these structures. Furthermore, disk and cartilage are demarcated on these images with the disk demonstrating the higher signal intensity and the cartilage appearing medium gray.

On the *T2-weighted image* the ossification center appears very dark, the cartilage dark gray and the disk very bright. Sharpey's fibers can be distinguished on T2-weighted images as a dark peripheral structure. The intervertebral disk appears very flat; the disk height is a maximum of 40 % of the vertebral body height (Figs. 4.1–4.4).

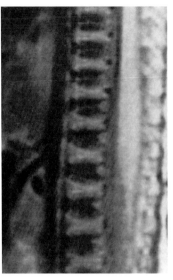

a

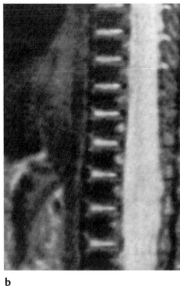

b

Fig. 4.**1a, b** **14-day-old child:**
a PD-weighted image (SE;
TR = 2100 ms, TE = 20 ms):
The ossification center is oval
in shape and dark. A mild,
band-like signal enhance-
ment is defined in part
within the ossification center.
The cartilage demonstrates
intermediate gray signal intensity, while the intervertebral disk appears relatively
bright. Cartilage and disk together give the impression of
a biconcave structure.
b T2-weighted image (SE;
TR = 2100 ms, TE = 80 ms):
On this image the bone appears black, the cartilage
dark gray and the disk bright.
The disk appears as a small
linear structure.

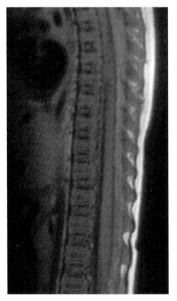

a

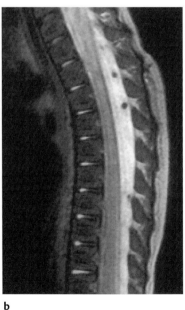

b

Fig. 4.**2a, b** **5-week-old child:**
a Sagittal T1-weighted section
(TSE; TR = 1120 ms,
TE = 12 ms): The bone ap-
pears dark but shows a small
signal-intense center, which
is depicted predominantly as
a band-like structure. Cartilage and disk cannot be
differentiated from each
other, but form a biconcave
structure with intermediate
signal intensity.
b T2-weighted image (TSE;
TR = 6130 ms, TE = 120 ms):
Bone and cartilage almost
form a unit. The bone ap-
pears as a central core
slightly darker against the
dark-gray cartilage. The intervertebral disk appears signal-
intense as a flat band.
Sharpey's fibers are de-
lineated as black structures,
as are the posterior and
anterior longitudinal ligaments. The confluence point
of the basivertebral vein is
well shown dorsally, in the
form of a wedge-shaped signal-intense structure in the
middle of the vertebral body.

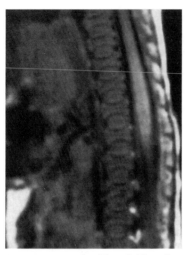

Fig. 4.**3** **3-month-old child.** (SE; TR = 650 ms, TE = 25 ms): The T1-weighted sagittal image now shows a slightly higher signal in the bone in comparison with the images in Figs. 4.**1** and 4.**2**, while the bone has an oval configuration. Intervertebral disk and cartilage appear with almost the same signal intensity. These two structures cannot be differentiated from each other; they form a biconcave structure of intermediate signal intensity, not differing significantly from that of the bone.

■ Nucleus Pulposus Type II

The bone demonstrates high signal intensity on *T1-weighted images*. The cartilage is well delineated as a dark gray stripe. The disk on the other hand appears bright. A differentiation between nucleus and annulus is not possible, whereas Sharpey's fibers are delineated as a thin black line.

On *T2-weighted images* the bone is medium gray, the cartilage very dark, the nucleus shows high signal intensity, annulus and Sharpey's fibers demonstrate a clear reduction in signal.

In the juvenile the structuring of the connective tissue of the nucleus begins with a band-like formation, which penetrates from a dorsal and ventral direction into the central core of the gelatinous tissue. The border between annulus and nucleus is sometimes rather ill defined. In addition, Sharpey's fibers are well differentiated due to their particularly low signal intensity. The core of the intervertebral disk gains in height and shows a rounded form (Figs. 4.**5**–4.**7**).

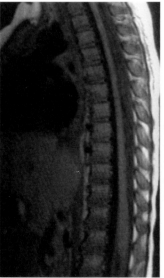

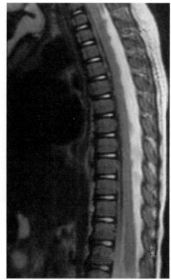

a b

Fig. 4.**4 a, b** **1-year-old child:**
a T1-weighted image (TSE; TR = 690 ms, TE = 12 ms): The vertebral body now demonstrates a higher signal intensity than the disk and cartilage. It has clearly gained in size. On the T1-weighted images the contour of the vertebral body is now already well differentiated with its almost rectangular form. Cartilage and disk are poorly differentiated; the cartilage shows lower signal intensity than the bone, as does the disk.
b T2-weighted image (TSE; TR = 3500 ms, TE = 120 ms): Intermediate signal intensity of the bone, very low signal intensity of the cartilage and high signal intensity of the intervertebral disk. Sharpey's fibers and annulus are demarcated as a black structure, both dorsally and ventrally.

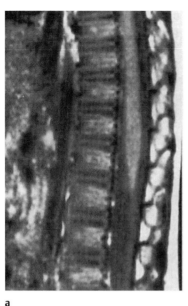
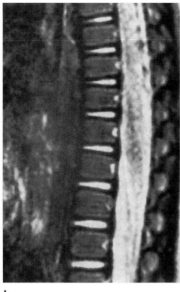

a b

Fig. 4.**5a, b** **2-year-old child:**
a T1-weighted image (SE; TR = 660 ms, TE = 25 ms): The bone has gained in height and demonstrates a relatively high signal intensity. In contrast to Fig. 4.**4**, intervertebral disk and cartilage are now well differentiated. The cartilage appears dark gray; the disk shows moderately high signal intensity. Annulus and Sharpey's fibers cannot be differentiated with certainty.
b T2-weighted image (SE; TR = 2100 ms, TE = 80 ms): On this image there is a high signal intensity for the nucleus pulposus. Annulus and Sharpey's fibers appear dark gray to black. The cartilage also demonstrates low signal intensity, appearing merely as a relatively thin band and only becoming slightly broader ventrally and dorsally. The bone reveals intermediate signal intensity. The entry points of the basivertebral veins are very well delineated as bright, rounded or wedge-like zones, each at the posterior margins of the vertebral bodies.

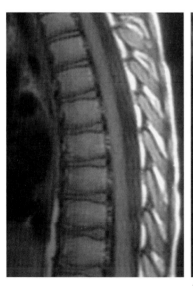
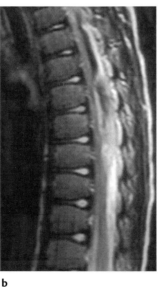

a b

Fig. 4.**6a, b** 7-year-old child:
a Sagittal section using T1 weighting (TSE; TR = 800 ms, TE = 12 ms): Essentially no significant change has occurred from the images from the 2-year-old child. The bone demonstrates moderately high, relatively homogeneous signal intensity. The cartilage is shown as a somewhat inhomogeneous, signal-reduced, circumferential zone. The disk material reveals slightly higher signal intensity than the cartilage. Neither the annulus nor Sharpey's fibers are sharply demarcated.
b T2-weighted image (TSE; TR = 4000 ms, TE = 120 ms): Intermediate signal intensity of the bone. Very high signal intensity of the nucleus pulposus which now begins to gain in height and therefore assumes an oval, almost rounded configuration. The cartilage is demonstrated as a very thin, narrow, dark-gray to black band. Sharpey's fibers and the annulus gain in thickness and show good delineation against the rest of the disk tissue because of their almost signal-free structure.

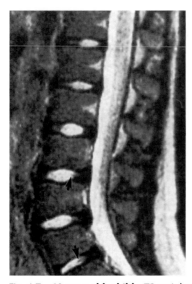

Fig. 4.**7** **10-year-old child.** T2-weighted image (SE; TR = 2100 ms, TE = 80 ms): The intervertebral disk gains further in height and the nucleus now appears demarcated with an ellipsoid form. In the distal lumbar spine it lies further anteriorly than in the proximal section of the spine. The annulus appears black. The caudal disks show initial horizontal stripes of connective tissue in the nucleus pulposus (arrows).

■ Nucleus Pulposus Type III

In about one-fifth of cases the type III intervertebral disk already demonstrates tears in the annulus fibrosus (Yu *et al.*, 1988).

On *T1-weighted images* the bone appears relatively hypointense due to its high proportion of blood-forming marrow. The disk demonstrates high signal intensity. Differentiation between nucleus and annulus is not possible. Sharpey's fibers can be delineated due to their lower signal intensity.

On *T2-weighted images* bone signal intensity remains low. The nucleus pulposus appears hyperintense. The central connective-tissue structures have expanded and now appear as a largely continuous hypointense line within the nucleus pulposus. The annulus is well differentiated from the nucleus due to its low signal intensity (Fig. 4.**8**).

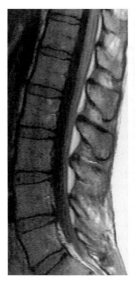 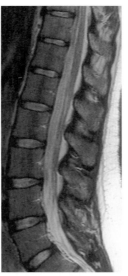

a   b

Fig. 4.**8 a, b   27-year-old woman:**
a T1-weighted sagittal section (TSE; TR = 800 ms, TE = 12 ms): The vertebral bodies demonstrate an intermediate signal intensity. Only dorsally, at the level of the entry point of the basivertebral vein, is there slightly higher signal intensity. The intervertebral disk shows signal intensity similar to that of the bone, leaving a relatively poor contrast between the structures. The annulus is not distinct, while Sharpey's fibers are demarcated as a thin black structure.
b T2-weighted image (TSE; TR = 5300 ms, TE = 120 ms): The bone has a low signal intensity. The intervertebral disk allows a good differentiation between nucleus and annulus. the horizontal stripes of connective tissue in the nucleus pulposus are continuous and appear very bold in part, which is typical for this age, and these changes have clearly increased in comparison with Fig. 4.**7**. The annulus and Sharpey's fibers appear normal, demonstrating respectively a low or absent signal. The posterior longitudinal ligament is not distinguishable in its course from the annulus.

■ Nucleus Pulposus Type IV

With type IV there is an evenly distributed reduction in signal from the intervertebral disk and usually a distinct reduction in height too. The nucleus pulposus can no longer be differentiated from the annulus fibrosus by signal intensity due to the dense connective tissue that is interspersed with the nucleus. Histologically, there is always a rupture of the annulus fibrosus present in these disks. A subchondral bony reaction in the adjacent vertebral body end plates is also typical, displaying a corresponding reduction in signal in the T1- and especially in the T2-weighted images (Fig. 4.**9**).

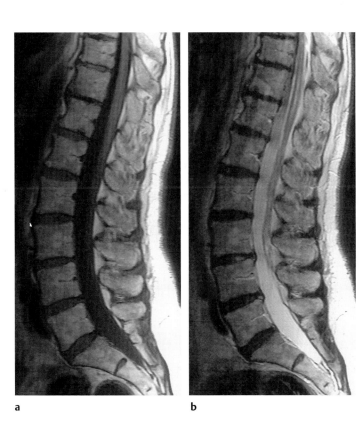

a   b

Fig. 4.**9 a**, **b** **61-year-old woman:**
a T1-weighted sagittal section (TSE; TR = 800 ms, TE = 12 ms): These images display a distinctly higher signal intensity in the bone in comparison with the intervertebral disk, in contrast to Fig. 4.**8a**. This results from the involution of the blood-forming bone marrow and its replacement by fatty bone marrow. The entry points of the basivertebral veins now make a hypointense impression. The bone marrow shows somewhat patchy signal intensity. The intervertebral disks have slightly lost height in total. The signal intensity of the disks is also becoming hypointense in the T1-weighted image as compared with Fig. 4.**8a**, recognizable from the low contrast between the CSF and disk signal. The annulus is poorly demarcated.

b T2-weighted sagittal section (TSE; TR = 5300 ms, TE = 120 ms): The vertebral bodies display an intermediate signal intensity, although a slightly higher signal can be seen at the level of the veins entering dorsally. The patchy delineation of the bone marrow is also conspicuous on this image. Overall the disks display an advanced stage of degenerative remodeling or a process of ageing and therefore show largely homogeneous signal attenuation. There are solitary signal enhancements in the region of the annulus, particularly in last three disks, which are signs of tears. Slight protrusions are present, although there is no distinction between annulus and nucleus.

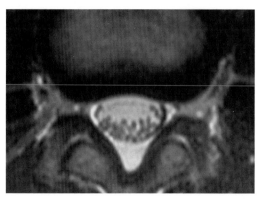

Fig. 4.10 Normal finding of the intervertebral disk.
T2-weighted transverse section (TSE; TR = 4465 ms, TE = 120 ms): Circumferential fibrous ring of the intervertebral disk, dark in appearance and looking completely intact in all sections. The nucleus pulposus is hyperintense and forms the core of the disk.

Types of Annular Tears

Fig. 4.**10** demonstrates the normal appearance of an intervertebral disk. The changes of the annulus have been classified with the aid of post mortem studies. Annular tears can be subdivided into four different types with regard to their form and location (Fig. 4.**11**) (Yu *et al.*, 1989).

Types of annular tears

- Concentric tear.
- Transverse tear.
- Radial tear.
- Complete tear.

■ Concentric Tear

A concentric tear results from disruption of the short transverse fibers connecting adjacent lamellae, but there is no interruption of the longitudinal fibers within the lamellae themselves. The tear extends vertically and lies within the transverse fibers of the annulus, although there is no connection with the nucleus pulposus. It frequently has an oval configuration (Fig. 4.**12**).

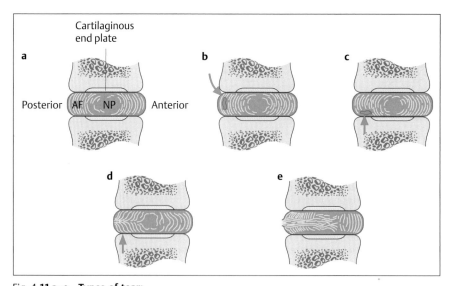

Fig. 4.**11 a–e Types of tear:**
a Normal finding.
    AF = Annulus fibrosus,
    NP = Nucleus pulposus
b Concentric tear.

c Transverse tear.
d Radial tear.
e Complete tear of the annulus fibrosus and the posterior longitudinal ligament.

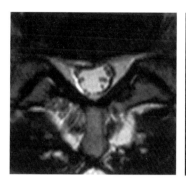
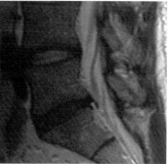

Fig. 4.**12 a, b** **Vertical tear (concentric tear):**
a Transverse image (TSE; TR = 4470 ms, TE = 120 ms): Signal enhancement within the outer transverse fibers of the annulus in the immediate vicinity of the posterior longitudinal ligament. This signal enhancement has no connection with the nucleus pulposus.
b Sagittal section displaying the vertical tear. Here too, there is no recognizable connection with the nucleus.

Histologically, fluid or a mucoid tissue is found is this fissure.

Since the intradiskal regions are not supplied with nerve fibers, this type of tear is not painful. It is therefore of no distinct clinical significance and is also seen without intervertebral disk degeneration.

A concentric tear can, however, develop into a radial tear. Histologically it is frequently located in the ventral part of the annulus. Usually the ventral tear is not detectable by MRI (Nowicki *et al.,* 1997).

■ Transverse Tear

The transverse tear is found in the outermost fibers of the annulus (Sharpey's fibers) near the marginal contour of the vertebral body. This type of tear is only found in the adult disk (type III) and in disks with degenerative changes (type IV). However, it is uncertain whether the tear should be regarded as the starting point of disk degeneration. It is assumed that the tear arises secondary to a particularly pronounced torsion involving the spine and disk tissue. These tears are depicted as transverse structures within the upper or lower parts of Sharpey's fibers, they contain mucoid material and sometimes even nitrogen oxide.

Pain can develop from a transverse tear. Since it can be well defined by MRI on T2-weighted images as a bright zone, it should also be taken into consideration when assessing intervertebral disks (Fig. 4.13).

After contrast administration, enhancement within the tear may appear as an expression of granulation tissue formation (Fig. 4.14).

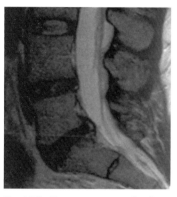

Fig. 4.**13** **Transverse tear in the penultimate disk.** There is also a vertical tear in the last disk. The sagittal T2-weighted image (TSE; TR = 4000 ms, TE = 120 ms) shows the small transverse tear near the marginal contour of the vertebral body in the lower part of Sharpey's fibers. The last disk displays a large vertical tear in the outermost parts of the fibrous ring.

■ Radial Tear

This type of tear is only seen in the degenerative disk (type IV). It represents fissures, which extend from the central parts of the nucleus pulposus to the periphery of the disk and are associated with a significant disruption of the integrity of the annulus fibrosus.

A high percentage of disk protrusions with an expansion of only a few millimeters will already show such radial tears of the annulus (Yu *et al.,* 1988). It is therefore a misconception that disk protrusions are associated with an intact annulus. Radial tears are subject to a remodeling process, which takes on the character of a repair mecha-

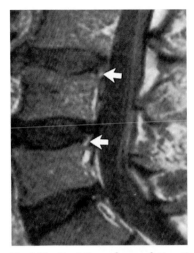

nism. Fibrovascular granulation tissue is formed that invades the fissures and can also develop along the annulus fibrosus (Yu *et al.*, 1988). Radial tears are the cause of pain (so-called diskogenic pain).

On T2-weighted images the radial tear displays high signal intensity within the annulus. Any granulation tissue possibly situated within this tear can contribute to the linear or globular appearance of a zone of contrast enhancement within the annulus fibrosus (Figs. 4.**15**–4.**17**) (Ross *et al.*, 1990).

Fig. 4.**14 Depiction of granulation tissue enhanced by contrast medium.** Sagittal section after administration of contrast (SE; TR = 780 ms, TE = 25 ms): Signal enhancement at the attachments of Sharpey's fibers on the posterior border of L3 and L4 as a sign of the tear undergoing reparative remodeling.

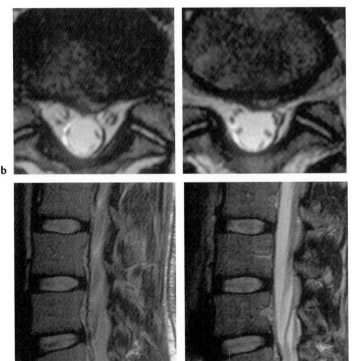

a, b

c   **d**

Fig. 4.**15 a–d   Radial tear:**
a   T2-weighted transverse image (TSE; TR = 4850 ms, TE = 120 ms): Oblique radial tear with subligamentous extension.
b   Image immediately cranial to **a**. On this image the radial tear merges into a vertical slit-like tear.
c, d Sagittal sections (TSE; TR = 5300 ms, TE = 120 ms) of a 29-year-old patient revealing a radial tear in the annulus at the level of L5/S1.

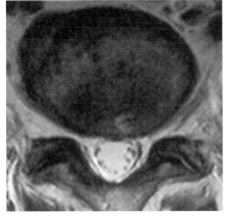

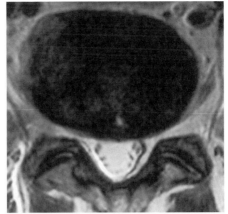

Fig. 4.**16 a**, **b** **Radial tear:**
a Fine radial tear running diagonally through the dorsal part of the annulus fibrosus and displaying a high signal intensity (TSE; TR = 4800 ms, TE = 120 ms).

b Caudal to **a**.

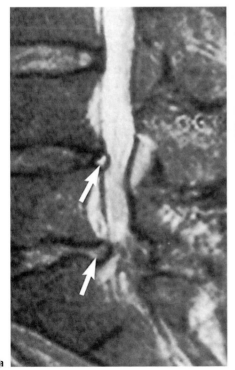

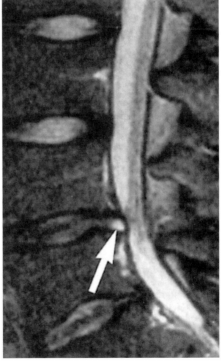

Fig. 4.**17a**, **b** **Tears of the annulus fibrosus and Sharpey's fibers:**
a Signal enhancement in the annulus and Sharpey's fibers on the T2-weighted image at L4 (arrows) as a sign of a tear (SE; TR = 2100 ms, TE = 80 ms):

Complete radial disruption of the annulus at L5 with subligamentous herniation of the nucleus.
b Signal enhancement in the annulus at L4 as a sign of a broad tear (SE; TR = 2100 ms, TE = 80 ms).

■ **Complete Tear**

This is a broad disruption of the annulus, usually associated with disk protrusion. As a result, more pronounced lumbago- or sciatic-type clinical symptoms are found (Fig. 4.18)

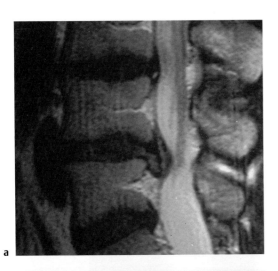

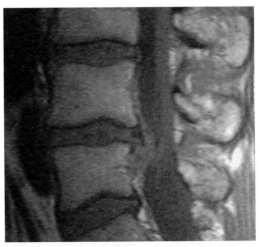

a

b

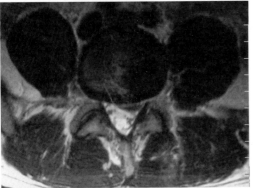

c

Fig. 4.**18 a–d** Complete tear of the L4/L5 annulus involving the posterior longitudinal ligament:
a T2-weighted sagittal image (TSE; TR = 3400 ms, TE = 120 ms): Broad annular tear with a large disk herniation displaced far caudally. On this image the posterior longitudinal ligament appears intact. The L3/L4 disk displays a small transverse tear near the contour of the posterior vertebral margin.
b T1-weighted sagittal image slightly off midline towards the left (TSE; TR = 800 ms, TE = 12 ms): On this image the wide annular tear is visible with an associated rupture of the posterior longitudinal ligament. The disk herniation extends far caudally resulting in a distinct compression of the dural sac.
c, d Transverse images with different window settings (TSE; TR = 5785 ms, TE = 120 ms): The wide tear runs obliquely in the region of the annulus and appears less rich in contrast using the standard window setting (**c**) than in the bone-windowed image (arrow) (**d**).

Contrast Enhancement Patterns of the Unoperated Intervertebral Disk, the Intraspinal Structures and the Vertebral Joints

In a systematic analysis, Geum-Ju Hwang *et al.* (1997) examined the contrast enhancement patterns of the degenerative intervertebral disk. Contrast enhancement displayed a particularly linear pattern along the posterior aspect of the annulus fibrosus and the bulging disk, less often a nodular pattern in the dorsal components of the disk. Apart from intradiskal contrast enhancement, nodular peridiskal enhancement is also seen, albeit less frequently (Fig. 4.**19**).

The frequency of a contrast-enhancement effect around the annulus fibrosus correlates with the degree of disk damage. Normal disks were enhanced in only 20 % of cases, bulging disks and protrusions in 55–95 % of cases, and sequestered disks with a sequestered herniation displayed peridiskal enhancement in all cases, with involvement of the sequester being an expression of the formation of granulation tissue. Zones of increased signal intensity (consistent with a concentric, transverse or radial tear) displayed a higher percentage of contrast enhancements as compared with disks without zones of increased signal intensity.

Granulation tissue formation usually corresponds histologically to the region of contrast enhancement (Figs. 4.**20**–4.**22**).

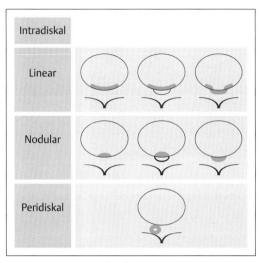

Fig. 4.**19 Diagram of enhancement patterns within the lumbar disk.**

The administration of contrast material can lead to reactions along the course of the nerve root (Jinkins *et al.*, 1993). In 25 % of patients with radicular symptoms there is nerve root enhancement after administration of contrast material without there having been any previous surgery. This enhancement pattern can be followed from

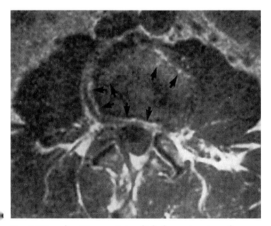

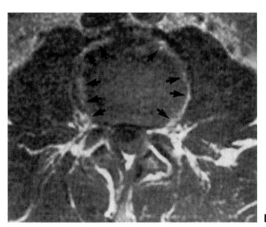

b

Fig. 4.**20 a, b Linear intradiskal contrast enhancement.** Transverse images of the L3/L4 disk after application of contrast material (SE; TR = 750 ms, TE = 25 ms): There is a distinct linear contrast enhancement along

the annulus fibrosus (arrow), involving not only the parts toward the spinal canal but also the more peripheral sections.

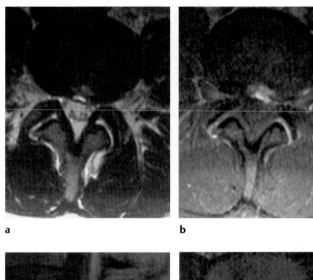

a

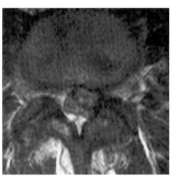

b

Fig. 4.21 a, b Nodular contrast enhancement:
a T2-weighted image of the L3/L4 disk (TSE; TR = 4465 ms, TE = 120 ms): Broad radial tear with a corresponding signal enhancement along the annulus.
b T1-weighted image with fat saturation after application of contrast material (SE; TR = 540 ms, TE = 20 ms): There is nodular, very strong contrast enhancement along the wide annular tear.

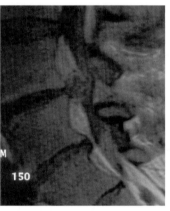

M

150

a

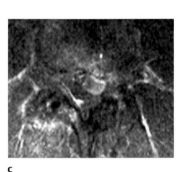

c

b

Fig. 4.22 a–c Peridiskal contrast enhancement with a large disk herniation:
a Sagittal section after administration of contrast material (TSE; TR = 921 ms, TE = 12 ms): Large disk herniation at the level of L4/L5 resulting in extensive compression of the dural sac. There is peridiskal, marginal signal enhancement.
b Transverse T2-weighted image of the disk herniation (TSE; TR = 6600 ms, TE = 120 ms): The large left mediolateral disk herniation displays marked compression of the dural sac.
c Image after administration of contrast material (TSE with fat saturation; TR = 539 ms, TE = 20 ms): The

disk herniation shows an apparently circumferential, peridiskal contrast enhancement. The part of the disk herniation projecting cranially appears in cross-section. The ventral section of the herniation is also surrounded by contrast material, as shown in **a**. Furthermore, there is relatively diffuse contrast enhancement along the annulus. In addition, there is distinct periarticular contrast enhancement, most notably along the right vertebral joint as an expression of an inflammatory reaction in the form of an activated osteoarthrosis.

an intra- to an extradural location and corresponds to the course of the nerve root. Whether it is an inflammatory irritation of the nerve root with a corresponding pial reaction or contrast enhancement of radicular veins remains a controversial issue.

Radicular veins are responsible for the drainage of venous blood from the conus medullaris and cauda equina into the epidural venous plexus. In doing so, these veins course in either a superior or inferior direction, depending on the level of the segment. At the L2 level, or above, drainage of the venous plexus proceeds into lumbar veins, which in turn reach the inferior cava vein or ascend to the azygos/hemiazygos vein. Below L2 there is a descending course, with radicular and foraminal veins draining into the iliolumbar veins from which, in turn, there is a connection with the common iliac veins. Radicular veins are present in the cauda equina in varying degrees. They can attain a diameter of 0.5–1.2 mm. Veins of this size are found primarily in the lower thoracic and upper lumbar region. In about one-quarter of all cases veins of this caliber are also found more distally and course along the filum terminale or one of the lumbosacral nerve roots (Fig. 4.23).

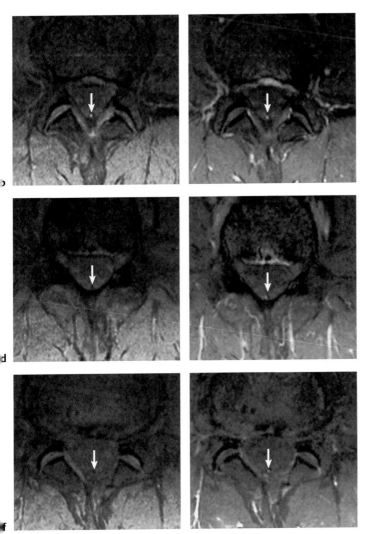

Fig. 4.**23 a–i** **Radicular vein coursing along the filum terminale** (arrows):
a Non-contrast scan of the spinal canal with fat saturation (SE; TR = 931 ms, TE = 20 ms): Flow-related enhancement in a radicular vein at the level of the filum terminale.
b The same slice, image after application of contrast material: The vein displays a slight increase in signal intensity.
c Slice 8 mm lower: On this image the vein shows loss of signal.
d Image after application of contrast material: Enhancement of the radicular vein.
e Image 1.2 cm further caudally: Here the radicular vein also displays slight signal loss, it lies somewhat further ventrally.
f Here too, clear enhancement after application of contrast material. In addition, a dorsal radicular vein also demonstrates circumscribed enhancement.

Fig. 4.**23 g–i** ▷

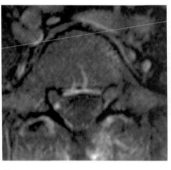
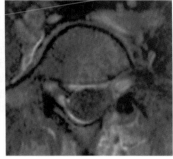
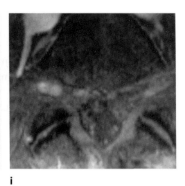

g   **h**   **i**

Fig. 4.**23 g–i**

g Another case with evidence of a larger radicular vein on the right side along the course of the L4 nerve root. Image after contrast material application (previously operated patient) with clear enhancement along the spinal process of the left side (SE with fat saturation; TR = 930 ms, TE = 20 ms). On the right, there is a strongly enhanced vein at the level of the L4 root.

h Slice 4 mm caudal to **a**: This vein courses towards the intervertebral foramen. On this image there is also a second, small, contrast-enhancing structure recognizable in the vicinity. Considering its size, it is presumably a collecting vein.

i Transverse image after application of contrast material (SE with fat saturation; TR = 686 ms, TE = 20 ms): On this image many small radicular veins are recognizable displaying a corresponding contrast enhancement.

Only small radicular veins are found in the remaining three-quarters of all cases. These small radicular veins (75–250 μm) are present in large numbers, are surrounded by endoneurium and overlie the nerve roots in each segmental region of the spine.

Enhancement of these veins by MRI depends primarily on contrast uptake by the larger radicular veins, although admittedly the limited resolving power of MRI does not allow a differentiation between vein and nerve root. In individual cases a flow-related increase of signal intensity in the vein is recognizable on transverse sections, applying above all to the first slice of a non-contrast axial T1-weighted SE sequence. The subsequent slices can demonstrate a reduction in signal (Fig. 4.**23**). A preceding saturation pulse can suppress the signal. The contrast-enhancing veins can be readily traced in a proximal direction on the transverse slices as far as their confluence with the larger radiculomedullary veins. This enhancement pattern is also seen in cases where asymptomatic patients have been examined. Should root compression subsequently occur, this will lead to impairment of venous drainage, and consequently to venous stasis, with the result that even small veins that are not normally visible will also demonstrate enhancement (Fig. 4.**24**).

These small veins do not usually allow detection of any flow-related enhancement either. The enhancement resolves after removal of the cause of the compression, e.g. within 6 months after surgery. Nor are these small vessels detectable by MR angiography, although larger radicular veins can be portrayed in individual cases during MR angiography.

In a study involving 227 patients presenting with low back pain or sciatica or both, Tyrrell *et al.*, (1998) reach the conclusion that nerve root enhancement with disk-caused compression of the nerve-root correlates in a high percentage of cases. The sensitivity for nerve root enhancement in the presence of disk prolapse is reported to be 23.5 % with a specificity of 95.5 %, which amounts to a positive predictive value of 76 % and a negative predictive value of 69.3 %.

In the presence of degenerative changes in the vertebral joints, marked effects of contrast enhancement can arise. Plain views will reveal the spondylarthrotic joints secondary to bony hypertrophy of the facets, disrelationship of the joint facets to one another even to the point of subluxa-

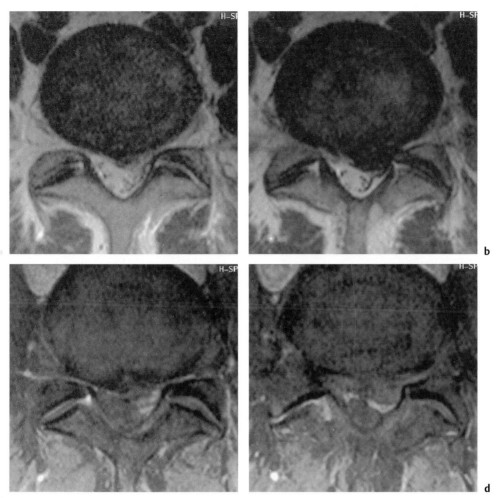

Fig. 4.24 a–d   Clear enhancement in the region of veins on the left side owing to a large left mid-lateral herniated disk:

a   T2-weighted transverse image (TSE; TR = 4500 ms, TE = 120 ms): The image shows the herniated disk with corresponding compression of the nerve root on the left in the immediate vicinity of the foramen.

b   Slice 4 mm caudal to **a**: The expansion of the herniated disk on this slice is greater mid-laterally

on the left. There is clear dorsal displacement and compression of the nerve root exiting on the left.

c, d   Corresponding slices to **a** and **b** after contrast administration (SE with fat saturation, TR = 930 ms, TE = 20 ms): Strong, in part very linear, enhancement at the level of the nerve root exiting on the left. A secondary finding of a clear enhancement in the vertebral joint on the right is also recognizable.

tion, and in individual cases joint-space widening and increased intra-articular accumulation of fluid. The capsule can be thickened. Clear enhancement of periarticular soft tissues, the facet joint and also of the bone can at times be seen after contrast application. Images with fat saturation are suited for the exact assessment of the ef-

fect of contrast enhancement (Figs. 4.**25**, 4.**103**, 4.**106**–4.**108**).

The clinical relevance of this contrast enhancement is not clear. It is possibly connected with the presence of a pseudoradicular syndrome.

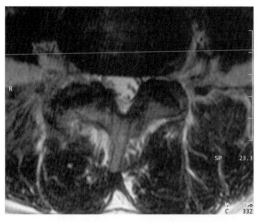
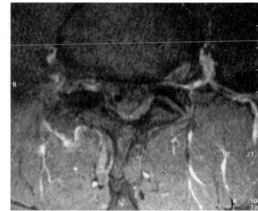

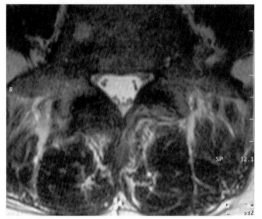

Fig. 4.**25 a–d Marked degenerative changes of the vertebral joints:**

a T2-weighted slice at the level of L4/L5 (TSE; TR = 5500 ms, TE = 120 ms): Conspicuous facet hypertrophy on the right, mild narrowing of the spinal canal from the right.

b Image with fat saturation after contrast application (TSE; TR = 930 ms, TE = 20 ms): Clear periarticular enhancement of the soft tissue and capsule on the right side.

c Slice 8 mm caudal to **a**: Clear sclerotic reaction of the inferior articular surface on the right side.

d Corresponding slice 8 mm caudal to **b**: Apart from a periarticular enhancement of the soft tissues, there is an additional enhancement of the bone at the level of the pedicle on the right.

Degenerative Changes of the Vertebral Body End Plates

Degenerative changes of the intervertebral disks often appear on MRI together with signal alterations of the bone marrow of the adjacent vertebral bodies. On MRI three types can be distinguished (Modic *et al.,* 1988):

▪ Type I Signal Change

Type I is the combination of low signal intensity on the T1-weighted image with high signal intensity on the T2-weighted image.

Edema and, in most cases, the formation of fibrovascular tissue within the bone in conjunction with a subsequent replacement of the bone marrow underlie this finding. A more or less pronounced trabecular thickening is also found (Fig. 4.**26**).

Plain radiographs will often reveal no signs of bony changes (Fig. 4.**27**).

In addition, this type is also found on MRI in the presence of radiologically detectable sclerosis of the vertebral body, in which case the signal enhancement on the T2-weighted image can be less pronounced and is at times found at the junctional region between sclerosed and normal bone. Hemispherical spondylosclerosis can also present changes of this type on MRI (Jensen *et al.*, 1989; Fig. 4.**28**).

Some authors have also implicated type I changes of the vertebral bodies with segmental instability. These signal changes have therefore been demonstrated in the presence of an unstable spondylodesis, while type II signal changes have been displayed in stable cases (Lang *et al.,*987). Type I MRI signal changes can develop into type II. Such signal changes can also be seen after disk surgery involving generous clearance of the interspace, possibly as a result of a postoperative segment instability, yet without there having been similar findings before surgery. They are probably the expression of an edematous (non-inflammatory) reaction of the bone and are therefore reversible (Fig. 4.**29**).

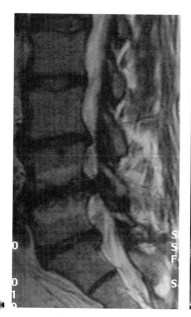
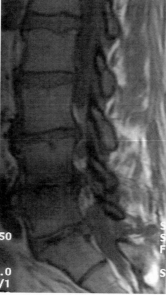

Fig. 4.**26 a–e   Type I reactive bone marrow changes:**
a T2-weighted sagittal section (TSE; TR = 3635 ms, TE = 120 ms): Wide signal-intense zone along the inferior and superior end plates of L4 and L5 in the presence of marked disk degeneration with osteochondrotic alterations.
b T1-weighted image (TSE; TR = 800 ms, TE = 12 ms): Altogether there is a relatively low signal intensity of the bone marrow. Additional reduction in signal is found subchondrally at L4/L5, corresponding to the signal enhancement on the T2 weighting.

Fig. 4.**26 c–e** ▷

b

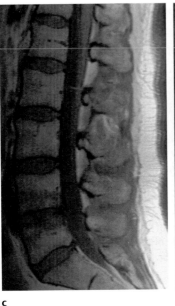
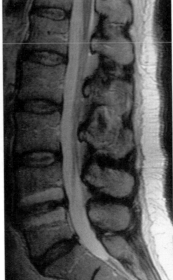
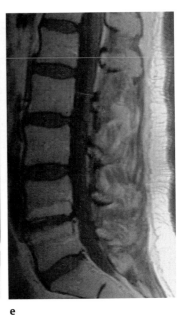

c   d   e

Fig. 4.**26 c–e**

c Another patient with a type I reactive bone marrow change. T1-weighted sagittal image (TSE; TR = 800 ms, TE = 12 ms): Clear subchondral reduction in signal in the L4/L5 region; the disk itself shows a slight loss of height.

d T2-weighted image (TSE; TR = 5300 ms, TE = 120 ms): Signal enhancement corresponding to the changes in Fig **c**. The disk shows a relatively high sig-

nal, loss of height and frank protrusion. This patient had undergone left-sided surgery of the L4/L5 disk.

e Post contrast image: Clear enhancement of the subchondral vertebral-body sections of L4 and L5. In addition there is contrast enhancement recognizable in the dorsal part of the disk consistent with granulation-tissue formation in this section.

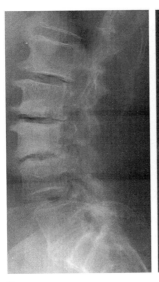
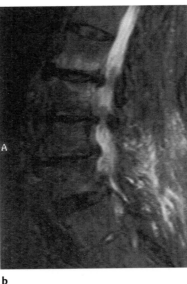

a   b

Fig. 4.**27 a–d** **Type I reactive bone marrow changes in a 77-year-old female patient who had undergone an extensive laminectomy of L3–L5:**

a The lateral radiograph demonstrates severe sclerosis with concomitant erosive osteochondrosis at the level of L3/L4 and slightly less marked at L2/L3. L1/L2 reveals disk degeneration with a vacuum phenomenon, alongside of which there is anterior spondylosis. There is no unequivocal finding in the vicinity of the inferior and superior end plates.

b T2-weighted sagittal image (STIR): Marked subchondral edema formation at L1/L2. Concomitant evidence of frank disk degeneration and protrusion.

Fig. 4.**27 c, d** ▷

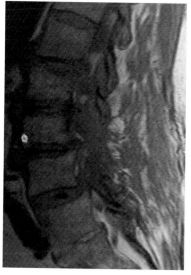

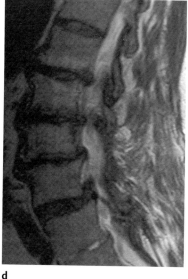

c

d

Fig. 4.**27 c, d**
c T1-weighted image (TSE; TR = 800 ms, TE = 12 ms) with reduction in signal.
d Corresponding subchondral signal enhancement with T2 weighting.

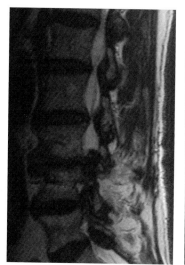

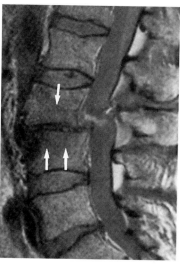

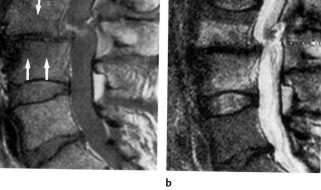

a

b

Fig. 4.28 Hemispherical spondylosclerosis in an 89-year-old man. T2-weighted sagittal image (TSE; TR = 3630 ms, TE = 120 ms) with a finding consistent with sclerosis-related reduction in signal in the inferior and superior end plates of L3 and L4. There is slight peripheral signal enhancement, particularly at the L4 level.

Fig. 4.29 a, b Spondylolisthesis at L3/L4 with instability in this segment. Type I change of the vertebral bodies:
a PD-weighted image (SE; TR = 2100 ms, TE = 20 ms): Reduction in signal of the bone marrow of L3 and L4. Extensive disk deterioration with severe loss of height.
b T2-weighted image (SE; TR = 2100 ms, TE = 80 ms): Clear signal enhancement of the bone marrow of L3 and L4 consistent with edema.

■ Type II Signal Change

A clear signal enhancement on the T1-weighted image and a mild signal enhancement on the T2-weighted image are seen with the type II signal change.

Histologically, transformation of the blood-forming bone marrow into fat marrow is noted, often accompanied by trabecular thickening.

This finding is not usually detectable on plain x-rays. Type II possibly precedes an osteochondrosis of the bone, which appears later on plain x-rays (Figs. 4.**30**–4.**32**).

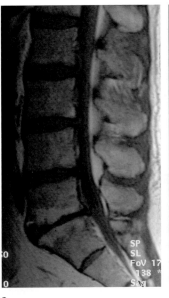
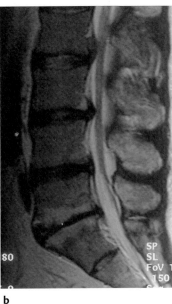

Fig. 4.30 a, b Fatty marrow degeneration (type II change of the vertebral-body end plates):
a T1-weighted sagittal image (TSE; TR = 800 ms, TE = 12 ms): Subchondral signal enhancement along L5 and S1 in the presence of disk degeneration.
b T2-weighted image (TSE; TR = 3635 ms, TE = 120 ms): The signal is enhanced against the other bone-marrow areas in the region of L5 and S1 due to fatty marrow. Concomitant evidence of a subligamentous disk herniation that has migrated cranially at the L2/L3 level, with a similar disk herniation at L3/L4. Protrusion with annulus tear at L4/L5.

a   b

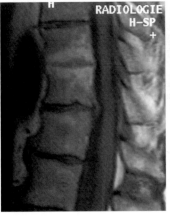
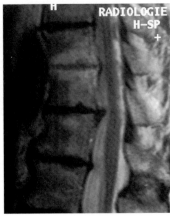

Fig. 4.31 a, b Type II changes of the vertebral-body end plates at the level of T10/11:
a T1-weighted sagittal image (TSE; TR = 800 ms, TE = 12 ms): Clear subchondral signal enhancement of the vertebral bodies projecting far dorsally with concomitant, extensive disk deterioration.
b T2-weighted sagittal image (TSE; TR = 3635 ms, TE = 120 ms): Using T2 weighting, considerable signal enhancement is also evident in this segment.

a   b

Fig. 4.**32 a, b** **Degeneration of fatty marrow in the region of the cervical spine at the level of C6/C7:**
a T2-weighted image (TSE; TR = 5300 ms, TE = 112 ms): Clear subchondral signal enhancement in the region of C6 and C7. Concomitant disk degeneration in this segment with protrusion and loss of disk height. The signal enhancement of the disk corresponds to loosely packed calcium deposits.
b GRE sequence using T1 weighting (TR = 90 ms, TE = 403 ms, flip angle α = 11°) with signs of clear reduction in signal of the subchondral bone.

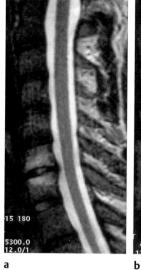
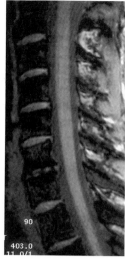

a   b

■ Type III Signal Change

This type shows low signal intensity both on T1- and T2-weighted images and corresponds to a dense sclerosis of the vertebral body. A corresponding finding of sclerosis can also be detected on plain radiographs (Fig. 4.**33**).

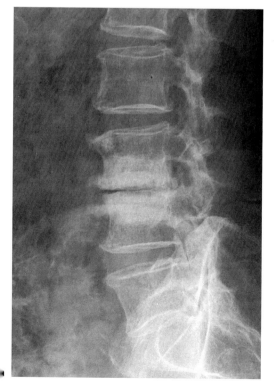

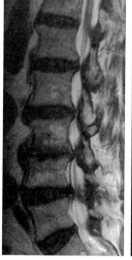
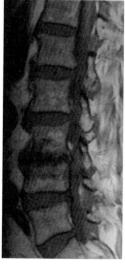

b   c

Fig. 4.**33 a–c** **Type III change of the vertebral bodies in the presence of hemispherical spondylosclerosis at the level of L3/L4:**
a Lateral radiograph of the lumbar spine with marked subchondral sclerosis of L3 and L4. Severe disk degeneration, erosive changes of the inferior and superior end plates. Marked spondylosis.
b T2-weighted sagittal MR image (TSE; TR = 3600 ms, TE = 120 ms): Reduction in signal in the region of L3 and L4 consistent with spondylosclerosis.
c T1-weighted image (TSE; TR = 800 ms, TE = 12 ms): The largely homogeneous reduction in signal with segmental degeneration in the periphery of the fatty marrow of the vertebral bodies can also be seen on this image.

■ Toyone Classification

Toyone *et al.* (1994) classify bone-marrow alterations solely according to T1-weighted images and differentiate between:

- Type A with decreased signal intensities on T1-weighted SE images,
- Type B with increased signal intensities.

The authors reach the conclusion that a high percentage of patients in group A present clinical symptoms of low back pain, while only a small proportion of patients in group B have clinical findings.

▌ Classification of Intervertebral Disk Herniation

There are a great many classifications of intervertebral disk herniations with no common central concept to be found either in the radiological literature or among radiologists, neurosurgeons and orthopedic surgeons. Classification of intervertebral disk herniation is often reduced to the question of whether or not the finding "merits surgery," thus prompting radiologists to incorrectly interpret "prolapse" as meriting surgery and "protrusion" as not meriting surgery.

The terms that have been adopted in the fields of CT and myelography do, indeed, go beyond what the radiologist can actually observe. In fact, the distinction of a prolapse from a protrusion requires delineation of the nucleus from the annulus, which is not possible using myelography or CT.

In the literature a *protrusion* is usually defined as an eccentric displacement of disk material in which the fibers of the annulus fibrosus are still essentially intact. Histological studies have shown that this is sometimes incorrect (Yu *et al.,* 1988), but the definition implies that nucleus pulposus material has not extruded through the annulus fibrosus. A special form of protrusion is "bulging" of the intervertebral disk, which has been particularly emphasized in the English literature. It involves a uniform, circumferential thinning of the annulus with a dorsal displacement of the nucleus pulposus.

Prolapse on the other hand is defined as a protrusion of the nucleus pulposus through the fibers of the annulus, involving a more or less extensive disruption of the annular fibers. A distinction can be made between a prolapse of nucleus pulposus tissue, which is still subligamentous in location and a prolapse that is already extraligamentous in location but is still in continuity with disk material (extraligamentous prolapse).

In contrast, the extraligamentous *sequester* has lost contact with the disk material and is epidural in location or, in extremely rare cases, intradural (intradural sequester) (Fig. 4.**34**).

Sometimes the literature will refer to a sequester if the disk herniation is already extraligamentous in location but still maintains connection with the nucleus pulposus (Modic *et al.,* 1989).

Computer tomography is unable to outline the posterior longitudinal ligament, and similarly there is no possibility of assessing the annulus fibrosus fibers. In this respect, attempts at distinguishing between protrusion and prolapse by CT are often not borne out by intraoperative observa-

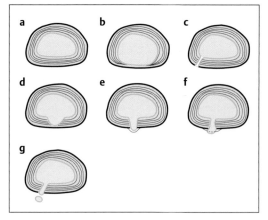

Fig. 4.**34 a–g** **Various forms of intraspinal disk displacement:**
a Normal disk.
b Bulging.
c Annular tear.
d Protrusion.
e Subligamentous disk herniation.
f Transligamentous disk herniation.
g Sequester.

tions. Radiological differentiation is based primarily on the form of the disk herniation:

- a protrusion is assumed if there is a uniform, broad-based dorsal displacement of disk material,
- a prolapse is assumed if there is a tongue-shaped displacement.

Studies have however shown that this differentiation contains a high margin of error (Haughton *et al.*, 1982).

MRI has the advantage over CT in as much as the annulus together with the posterior longitudinal ligament can be distinguished from the nucleus pulposus. With the exception of diskography, MRI allows a better differentiation between protrusion and prolapse in this respect than is the case with the other imaging techniques.

Examination Technique

MRI is being used increasingly for the examination of disk herniations. The option of obtaining a complete overview of a larger portion of the spine using sagittal sections is one of its advantages over CT. The images are richer in contrast, especially when delineating the disk from the surrounding structures. MRI allows assessment of the state of the nucleus pulposus and can detect incipient disk degenerations. The option of obtaining images in two planes allows a better assessment of the spinal canal and, in particular, of the foramina. MRI combines the clarity of myelography with the option of directly imaging the herniated disk.

The choice of sequence will depend on the region to be examined:

Lumbar Region

In the lumbar region, mainly T1- and T2-weighted SE sequences should be used. A T1-weighted sagittal TSE sequence, a T2-weighted sagittal TSE sequence and a T2-weighted transverse TSE sequence are recommended as basic examination techniques.

T1-weighted images. The T1-weighted sagittal SE sequence provides a good anatomical overview of the individual structures, although it does not provide for optimal contrast between disk tissue, dural sac and, in particular, the nerve roots. In this setting, bone marrow demonstrates intermediate signal intensity, depending on the age of the patient, with younger patients displaying a somewhat lower signal intensity due to a higher proportion of blood-forming marrow than older patients with a high proportion of fatty marrow. The contrast between bone-marrow signal and disk signal is usually only slight, with the age of the patient again playing an important role in the differentiation. In the young patient the bone-marrow signal equates approximately to that of the disk, while in old age the bone-marrow signal is higher.

The vertebral cortex is sharply defined as a thin dark peripheral margin, although the cortex can display a less sharp delineation in the direction of the readout gradient than in the direction of the phase-encoding gradient because of the chemical-shift artifact. The following therefore applies: if the phase-encoding gradient is switched in the craniocaudal direction, then an exact demarcation of the cortex along the contour of the posterior vertebral margin will be absent; conversely, if the phase-encoding gradient is switched in the AP direction, there will be a shift in the area of the cranial and caudal vertebral-body contour, e.g. with enhancement of the superior vertebral end plate and an ill-defined, reduced presentation of the inferior vertebral end plate (Fig. 4.**35**).

The intervertebral disk appears largely homogeneous, making differentiation between annulus and nucleus impossible. Sharpey's fibers, on the other hand, reveal a reduction in signal, although there is no delineation with respect to signal intensity between these fibers and the posterior longitudinal ligament.

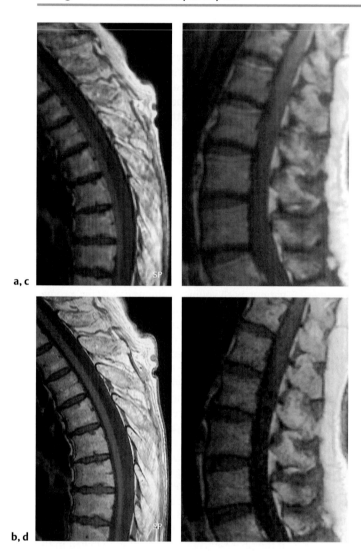

Fig. 4.**35 a–d Influencing the chemi-cal-shift artifact by altering the phase-encoding gradient:**

a Sagittal section using T1 weighting (TSE; TR = 800 ms, TE = 18 ms). Phase-encoding gradient switched in the craniocaudal direction: marked chemical-shift artifact in the dorsal direction. The posterior and the anterior peripheral margins of the vertebral bodies display a distinct double contour, resulting in an ill-defined delineation of the marginal strips (bandwidth: 78 Hz/pixel; one acquisition).

b Switching the phase-encoding gradient in the craniocaudal direction can give rather good image results if a not too narrow bandwidth is used (bandwidth: 195 Hz/pixel). Note the artifact-free reconstruction of the spinal canal on this image. The chemical-shift artifact along the posterior and anterior margins of the vertebral bodies is acceptable and does not impair assessment of the disks or the marginal contours of the vertebral bodies (same patient as in **a**). Admittedly, raising the bandwidth does increase image noise (S/N is proportional to $BW^{-1/2}$), but this can be compensated for, e.g. by a larger number of acquisitions. For this reason, **c** was generated with three acquisitions.

c Switching the phase-encoding gradient in the AP direction: the chemical-shift artifact now appears in the region of the inferior and superior end plates. The typical double contouring is recognizable in the area of the superior end plate. The inferior end plate appears widened. At the same time, the sometimes-disturbing motion artifacts now appear on the image as vertical lines, which contribute to a loss of detail at the boundary between cauda and spinal cord. Low bandwidth.

d Same slice as in **c**, merely with doubling of the bandwidth and unchanged number of acquisitions: clearly increased image noise, fewer chemical-shift artifacts.

The images are not suitable for assessing intramedullary lesions. Spinal cord edema is only rarely distinguishable. Disk protrusion or prolapse is usually poorly defined against the spinal canal because CSF only appears slightly dark in comparison with disk tissue.

T2-weighted images. Bone marrow appears dark on T2-weighted images, while the disk is dis-played bright or even dark, depending on the age of the patient. Annulus and nucleus are well-defined in the younger patient, but this delineation gradually disappears with degenerative remodeling of disk tissue, which becomes increasingly apparent with age. Nerve roots are usually well recognizable as thin black lines. Since CSF appears bright, there is high contrast between disk tissue and CSF (Fig. 4.**36**).

A T2-weighted TSE-image can by all means be obtained using a high turbo factor in order to achieve a contrast similar to that of myelography between disk tissue, CSF and nerve fibers. There is, in addition, sufficient differentiation between disk tissue and bone to allow a good distinction between fresh and older disk herniations with reactive bony bridging.

Axial T2-weighted images allow a particularly good differentiation of the nerve roots owing to the high signal intensity in CSF (Fig. 4.**37**).

They are also suitable for assessing arachnoid adhesions, thickenings of the nerve root, and inflammatory alterations of the nerve root. An inflammatory reaction will display thickening and signal enhancement of the nerve root.

Both the sagittal and the axial images allow a differentiation of annular tears, which usually appear signal-intense.

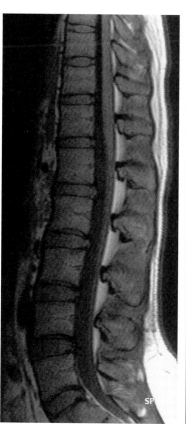
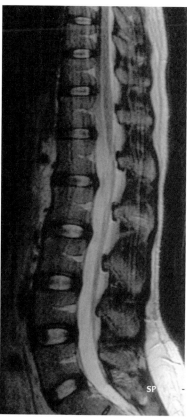

a
b

Fig. 4.**36 a, b   Normal finding of the lumbar spine in a 25-year-old female patient:**
a   T1-weighted sagittal section (TSE; TR = 800 ms, TE = 12 ms): This image provides a good overview of the anatomical structures. Relatively poor differentiation of the nerve roots along the cauda equina. The contrast between disk and dural sac is not good either. The bone-marrow signal in this young patient is low and differs little from the signal of the disk. Only dorsally, at the level of the exit points of the basivertebral veins, is there slightly higher signal intensity in the bone marrow. The disk displays intermediate signal intensity, while differentiation between nucleus and annulus is not possible. Only Sharpey's fibers are delineated dorsally as thin black lines. Differentiation of these structures from the longitudinal ligament is not possible. Good visualization of the conus medullaris.

b   T2-weighted sagittal section (TSE; TR = 5200 ms, TE = 120 ms): There is good differentiation of the cauda equina and individual nerve roots. The bone marrow displays a dark signal. Hence the disk is well demarcated, above all toward the nucleus. Nucleus and annulus are well differentiated. The annulus in this case is of normal thickness and shows no tears. There is high contrast between disk tissue and CSF.

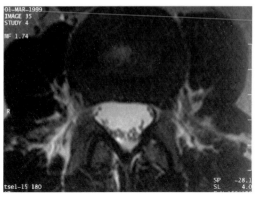

Fig. 4.37 Normal finding of the lumbar spine with axial slice orientation. Axial T2-weighted image of the lumbar canal at the level of L2/L3 (TSE; TR = 4465 ms, TE = 120 ms): The nerve roots appear dark and are well delineated due to the bright CSF signal. Anteriorly the posterior and anterior roots are each demarcated on the right and left. Both structures are situated at the level of their points of exit from the spinal canal.

Conclusion. T1- and T2-weighted images are usually sufficient for assessing bone-marrow changes (types I–III). If a particularly high-contrast reproduction of bone-marrow edema is required, T2-weighting with additional fat saturation or, alternatively, the use of a STIR sequence is useful.

It may be wise to supplement routinely used sequences with a T1-weighted GRE sequence if a particularly high-contrast differentiation between disk tissue and bony structures is required. This may be necessary in particular cases in order to highlight dorsal osteophytes, which is more successful with the GRE sequence than with the SE sequence. In doing so, these images should also be obtained using a sagittal slice orientation.

The application of a contrast agent for diagnostic confirmation, particularly in cases of degenerative changes of the lumbar spine, is not usually necessary. Contrast administration can, however, be considered in particular cases in order, for example, to differentiate a sequester from a tumor if the sequester has lost contact with the parent disk and therefore presents differential-diagnostic problems. In this respect it should not be overlooked that even old disk herniations can display peripheral enhancement due to scar-tissue formation. If the demonstration of even mild enhancements is required, then fat-saturated T1-weighted images using an SE or GRE technique are recommended.

In individual cases, subtraction of a plain from a contrast-assisted sequence may be useful, provided exactly identical examination parameters have been used.

Thoracic Region

Both SE and GRE sequences are suitable for the thoracic region.

T1-weighted images. As in the lumbar region, T1-weighted images do not allow an exact assessment of pathological intramedullary processes, unless they are space occupying or exhibit syringomyelic changes. Particularly a myelon edema secondary to compression of the spinal cord (e.g. due to a large disk herniation) is usually not assessable using a T1-weighted examination technique. The images do, however, show a sufficiently good contrast between bone and CSF, which appears dark, as well as the spinal cord, which displays light gray signal intensity. Even disk herniations are already definable on these T1-weighted images.

T2-weighted images. The T2-weighted GRE sequence is also suitable for detecting disk herniations since there is a high contrast between CSF and disk tissue. Alternatively, T2-weighted TSE sequences can be used, although here CSF flow artifacts are more strongly marked, which can make evaluation of the intradural space considerably more difficult in individual cases. The use of both techniques, i.e. a T2-weighted TSE technique together with a T2-weighted GRE technique, may be necessary in particular cases to provide more reliable information.

Both TSE and GRE sequences may be considered for transverse images, with T2-weighted sequences being particularly useful (Fig. 4.38).

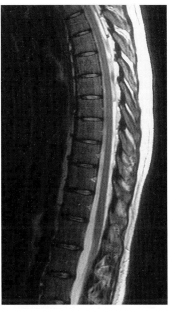
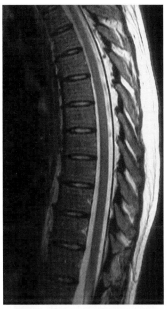
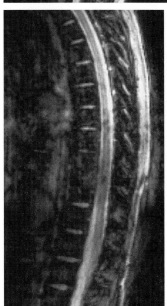
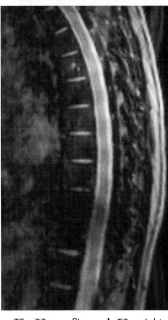

Fig. 4.**38 a–g** **Normal finding of the thoracic spine:**

a T2-weighted sagittal image (TSE; TR = 4800 ms, TE = 120 ms), phase-encoding gradient switched in the AP direction: The image displays a high signal intensity of the nucleus pulposus, allowing a good distinction between annulus and nucleus. The vertebral bodies show intermediate signal intensity. There is good differentiation between myelon and CSF. The image shows artifacts in the form of stripes resulting from breath excursions.

b Same patient as in **a**. T2-weighted sagittal image with phase-encoding gradient switched over to the craniocaudal direction (TSE; TR = 3400 ms, TE = 120 ms): The spine and the spinal canal are displayed without artifacts on this image. Truncation artifacts now appear in the region of the vertebral bodies with corresponding multiple horizontal hyper- and hypointense lines due to the switching of the phase-encoding gradient. There is also a good distinction on this image between nucleus and annulus. Chemical shift artifact in the AP direction, although there is a good delineation of the posterior margin. Artifact-free presentation of the spinal canal with good contrast between CSF and myelon. The myelon demonstrates homogeneous signal intensity. The image displays fewer CSF artifacts than in **a**.

c T2-weighted FLASH (TR = 714 ms, TE = 22 ms, flip angle α = 35°). Phase-encoding gradient switched in the AP direction: Artifacts very strongly interfering with the image, with not only motion artifacts but above all flow artifacts spoiling image quality. Very dark signal from the vertebral bodies. High signal intensity in the individual disks resulting in good contrast between these structures. The annulus is delineated as a very thin black structure, dorsally and ventrally. The contrast between CSF and myelon is poorer than on the SE images. Marked truncation artifact along the myelon.

d T2-weighted FLASH (TR = 714 ms, TE = 22 ms, flip angle α = 35°). Phase-encoding gradient switched in the craniocaudal direction: This image displays far fewer artifacts along the spine. The vertebral bodies are more easily delineated in this respect. The spinal canal is also more readily assessable along its entire course. The contrast between myelon and CSF remains as poor as on the SE sequence. Signal inhomogeneities along the myelon are also recognizable on this image.

Fig. 4.**38 e–g** ▷

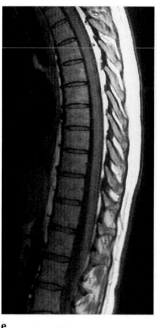
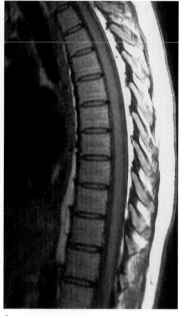

e f

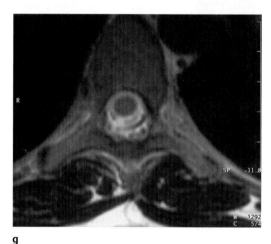

g

Fig. 4.**38 e–f**

e T1-weighted sagittal image (TSE; TR = 747 ms, TE = 12 ms), phase-encoding gradient switched in the AP direction: Intermediate signal intensity of the vertebral bodies with relatively poorer contrast in comparison with the disks. The annulus is delineated only ventrally and dorsally as a thin dark line. The spinal cord displays intermediate signal intensity with sufficient contrast against the CSF. The image shows mild streak artifacts due to respiratory movements. It is typical that these images display fewer flow artifacts than the images obtained using a GRE technique.

f T1-weighted SE image with the phase-encoding gradient switched in the craniocaudal direction (TSE; TR = 747 ms, TE = 12 ms): Overall, a very artifact-free reconstruction of the spinal canal. In comparison with **e** clear accentuation of the vertebral end plates, truncation artifacts along the direction of the phase-encoding gradient, and slightly ill-defined demarcation of the dorsal vertebral margins due to the chemical-shift phenomenon in the AP direction.

g T2-weighted transverse image of the spinal canal (TSE; TR = 3100 ms, TE = 120 ms): Most artifact-free presentation of the spinal cord, although CSF flow artifacts are recognizable, appearing dorsally as circumscribed, linear phenomena with reduction in signal along the course of the CSF.

Cervical Region

Sagittal images should be obtained using T1- and T2-weightings.

T1-weighted images. The use of a GRE sequence with T1 weighting has proven itself in achieving a better differentiation between bony structures and disk tissue. This distinction is far less possible with an SE sequence where the extent

of retrospondylosis can be underestimated in some cases.

T2-weighted images. Both GRE and TSE sequences are suitable for T2-weighted images. GRE sequences have the advantage of obtaining a high contrast between spinal cord and CSF, and the TSE sequence sometimes has the disadvantage of producing CSF flow artifacts, which could give cause for misinterpretation. Its advantage, on the other hand, lies in its otherwise lower susceptibility to artifacts as compared with the GRE sequence.

Transverse images should be obtained using T2 weighting, with GRE sequences being advantageous in this respect, although T1 weighting is useful in individual cases, particularly when contrast administration is intended (Fig. 4.**39**).

Imaging in two planes is necessary for the reliable detection of lateral herniations, which are more readily recognized on transverse than on sagittal slice orientations. Sagittal slices, on the other hand, are suitable for a broad survey of the entire cervical spine. They portray spinal cord alterations better than the transverse scan, particularly in the presence of compression-related spinal-cord atrophy. Slice thicknesses should be no more than 3 mm.

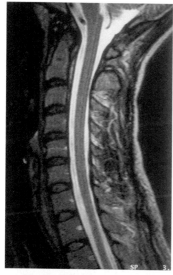

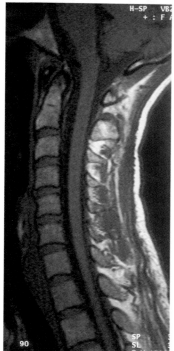

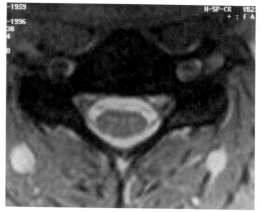

Fig. 4.**39 a–f Normal finding of the cervical spine:**

a T2-weighted sagittal image (TSE; TR = 4600 ms, TE = 112 ms): A somewhat decreased signal intensity in the disks of this 37-year-old patient. On the whole, however, differentiation between annulus and nucleus is still possible. The annulus appears as an intact structure dorsally. The bone-marrow signal is low. High contrast between disk tissue and CSF. Decreased signal intensity of the spinal cord with truncation artifacts visible as bright and dark lines along the spinal cord. Very good demarcation of the ligamenta flava and the interspinous ligamentous structures.

b Transverse slice orientation using T2 weighting (FLASH; TR = 703 ms, TE = 15 ms, flip angle α = 20°): High signal intensity of the CSF. Good delineation of the anterior and posterior roots. There is also a good presentation of the ganglion in the course of the right and left intervertebral foramina. Demarcation of the vertebral artery is possible on either side without difficulty.

c T1-weighted sagittal image (SE; TR = 351 ms, TE = 12 ms): The dorsal vertebral body margins are relatively poorly delineated. The differentiation between a retrospondylosis and CSF is often impossible on account of the dark CSF. The chemical-shift artifact is well recognizable in a craniocaudal direction after switching the phase-encoding gradient in the AP direction. The inferior end plate appears as a sharply defined dark line, the superior end plate displays a somewhat ill-defined border with the disk while signal cancellation by the cortex is lacking.

Fig. 4.**39 d–f** ▷

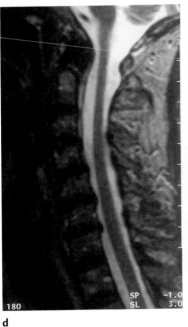
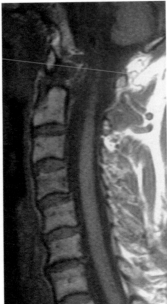
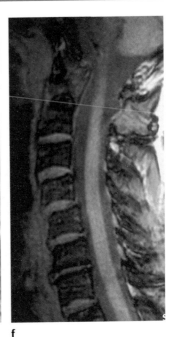

d e f

Fig. 4.**39 d–f**

d T2-weighted image (TSE; TR = 5300 ms, TE = 112 ms) of a 63-year-old female patient: The image shows an unremarkable finding of the myelon. Disk degeneration at C5/C6 and C6/C7. Evaluation of the dorsal structures is difficult because there is hardly any difference in signal intensity between bone and intervertebral disk.

e T1-weighted SE image of the same patient (SE; TR = 500 ms, TE = 12 ms): The image gives the impression of small disk prolapses at C5/C6 and C6/C7.

f GRE T1-weighted (FLASH two-dimensional; TR = 403 ms, TE = 11 ms, flip angle α = 90°): In contrast to the SE image, the reactive bony bridging around the C5/C6 and C6/C7 disks is now well demonstrated. In addition, this sequence readily displays the osteochondrosis with subchondral sclerosis at C6/C7, whereas this finding is recognizable neither on the T2-weighted TSE image nor on the T1-weighted SE image.

Clinical Symptoms

MR images not infrequently contain an abundance of pathological findings, which may, however, be of only slight clinical relevance in some cases. Alternatively, the finding responsible for the clinical symptoms may be unobtrusive or difficult to identify. This applies, for example, to lateral disk herniations or sequesters that have been extruded far into the spinal canal and have no connection with the disk of origin. These can elude the examiner if the clinical symptoms and their evaluation are not taken into account when planning the examination. It is therefore also important for the radiologist to become acquainted with the segmental innervation of the trunk and the extremities, to have an overview of the key muscles of the individual nerves, and to be able to interpret reflex patterns and their assignment to the individual spinal segments.

Various types of pain are differentiated according to its quality, origin and radiation:

Diskogenic pain. The region of a potential disk herniation, i.e. the posterior longitudinal ligament, the outermost components of the annulus fibrosus, parts of the periosteum and the vertebral body, as well as the meninges and blood vessels in the epidural space, has a direct somatosensory nerve supply. Therefore, changes in this region that are induced, for example, by a disk protrusion can lead to circumscribed, so-called diskogenic, pain. This pain syndrome is known by the term "*lumbago*."

Radicular pain. So-called radicular pain arising from irritation of the nerve root is different. Here the most common causes are disk protrusions or herniations, possibly combined with bony alterations of the vertebral end plates or the small joints between the vertebral bodies. Radicular pain is associated with pain radiation that corresponds to the respective dermatome.

The segmental innervation of the skin is summarized in Fig. 4.**40**.

This should not be confused with the innervation of peripheral nerves, which differs from the dermatomes. The peripheral nerve contains fibers from various segments of the spinal cord, as opposed to the dermatome, which has nerve fibers from only one segment of the spinal cord.

With root lesions, it is algesia that is foremost. Vegetative reactions on the part of the autonomic nervous system, such as sweating, vasomotor function, piloerection, are lacking. On the other hand, paresthesias can occur along the corresponding dermatomes. Sometimes there is a reduction in the power of the key muscles and, with more severe damage, muscular atrophy is seen. Reflex disturbances are characteristic and correspond to the damage.

Other pain symptoms. A completely different symptomatology is presented if there is direct compression of the spinal cord, e.g. secondary to disk herniation in the cervical or thoracic region. Apart from concomitant signs and symptoms of radiculopathy, these cases can present clinically with symptoms consistent with myelopathy. Myelopathy is characterized by:

- spastic paresis of the extremities,
- sensory deficit.

When the cervical region is involved, both the upper and lower extremities are affected, whereas only the lower extremities are affected with thoracic involvement. Reflexes can be increased. In the presence of very marked compression, there can be signs of bladder or rectal disturbances. The clinical picture is often indistinguishable from a tumor-related compression. Differential diagnostic considerations should also include multiple sclerosis, transverse myelitis and amyotrophic lateral sclerosis.

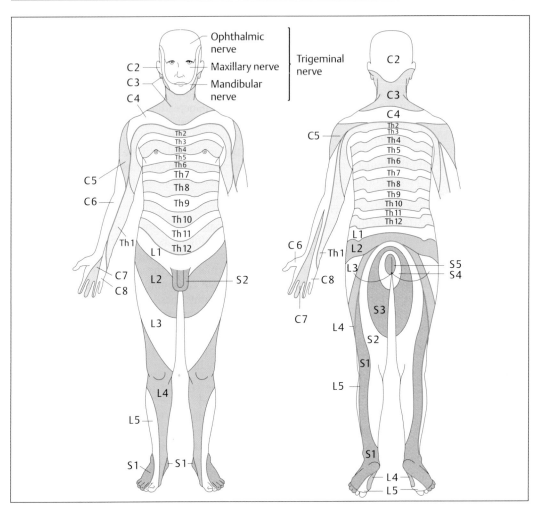

Fig. 4.**40 a–c** **Pain syndromes associated with root lesions:**
a Segmental innervation of the skin.

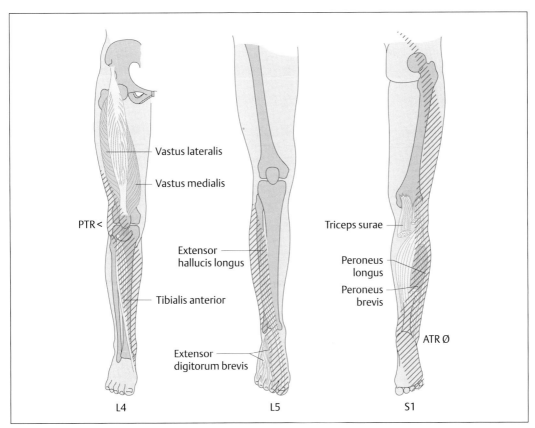

Fig. 4.**40 b**   Pain syndromes associated with L4, L5 and S1 root lesions with their key muscles and dermatomes.
ATR = Achilles tendon reflex
PTR = Patellar tendon reflex

Fig. 4.**40 c** ▷

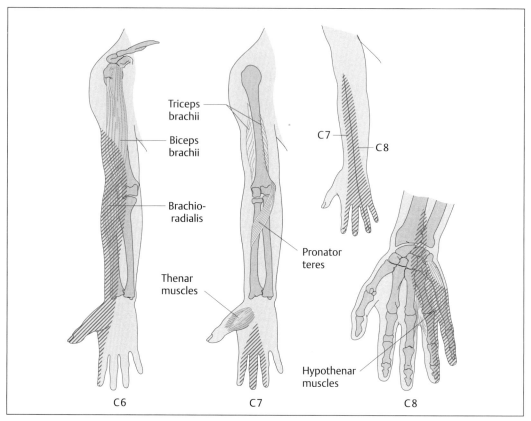

Fig. 4.**40 c**   Pain syndromes associated with C6, C7, and C8 root lesions with their key muscles and dermatomes.

Degenerative Changes of the Lumbar Spine

Protrusion and Prolapse

A protrusion appears on the MR image as a bulge in the tissue of the intervertebral disk that extends beyond the contour of the posterior vertebral margin. The annulus fibrosus is largely intact, thinned out, and sometimes associated with a concentric or transverse tear. It is possible that only the outermost Sharpey's fibers with their decreased signal intensity are recognizable on T2-weighted images. The nucleus pulposus has protruded far dorsally into the vertebral disk. The distinction between nucleus and annulus is usually reduced due to the presence of chondrosis. The protrusion can appear broad-based and even extend into the foramina, in which case only the lower part of the foramen is occupied by disk tissue and the disk can adjoin as far as the superior articular process of the next lower vertebra. On these lateral infraforaminal views the nerve root can be delineated above the protruded disk tissue, while compression of the infraforaminal structures, including fatty tissue, can lead to irritation of the nerve root. Normally the nerve root will appear rounded and is invested by fatty tissue. In the presence of compression it will assume a flat, disk-like form and can be pressed upwards against the marginal bony contours of the foramen. The disk protrusion can be associated with a slight caudal displacement, which is not uncommon particularly at the level of L5/S1 (Figs. 4.**41**–4.**43**).

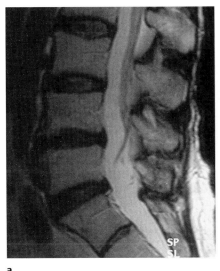
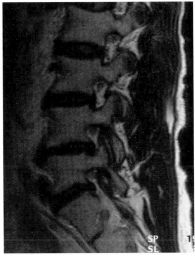

a   b

Fig. 4.**41 a, b**   **Disk protrusion in a 55-year-old female patient:**

a T2-weighted image (TSE; TR = 3635 ms, TE = 120 ms): The disks L4/L5 and L5/S1 show reduction in signal. At L4/L5 there is also loss of height and mild fatty-marrow degeneration, mainly in the anterior parts of L4. Both disks are displaced dorsally in the form of a protrusion. The annulus is intact, although L5/S1 does show a transverse tear along Sharpey's fibers at the transition with the bone in the area of S1.

b In the parasagittal slice, the expansion of the protrusion into the lateral recess and the foramen is easily recognizable. The nerve roots of L4 and L5 are not compromised by it, appearing rounded and encircled by fat. The other disks demonstrate a normal boundary with the foramen.

Fig. 4.**42** **Protrusions of disks L4/L5 and L5/S1.** ▷ Degeneration of disks L3–S1 with a corresponding loss of signal. Normal signal intensity in the more proximal segments. Sagittal section (TSE; TR = 3400 ms, TE = 120 ms): Largely unremarkable portrayal of the L3/L4 disk dorsally, no marked protrusion. Evidence of a Schmorl's node in the superior end plate of L4 with reactive bony bridging and fatty degeneration of the marrow. L4/L5 demonstrates a protrusion with a concomitant transverse tear. The posterior longitudinal ligament appears elevated. L5/S1 also reveals a mild protrusion.

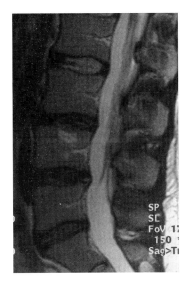

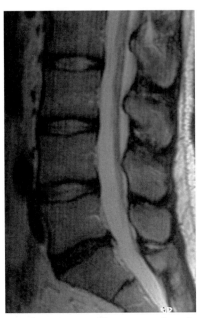

Fig. 4.**43** **37-year-old patient with evidence of frank disk degeneration of L5/S1 and a concentric tear.** Concomitant presence of mild disk protrusion (TSE; TR = 3635 ms, TE = 120 ms).

Extensive disruption of the annulus fibrosus fibers results in a prolapse of nucleus pulposus material, either in a subligamentous direction or in conjunction with a rupture of the posterior longitudinal ligament. MRI can delineate the anterior and posterior longitudinal ligaments. The anterior longitudinal ligament is always depicted more strongly than the posterior ligament. In either case, it is a black, band-like structure overlying the bone and annulus fibrosus. Detection of the posterior longitudinal ligament by MRI is best seen on PD- and T2-weighted images, although Grenier *et al.* (1989) also consider T1-weighted images suitable. Vascular structures are not infrequently recognizable dorsally between bone and posterior longitudinal ligament and usually represent the basivertebral veins. These vessels can be demonstrated with increased signal intensity on T1-weighted images after administration of contrast material. The posterior longitudinal ligament can be delineated on midsagittal sections as a uniform black band-like structure extending far laterally at the level of the disk. This gives the macromorphologic impression of a wasp-waist appearance of the posterior longitudinal ligament at the level of the vertebral body with spreading at the level of the disk (Figs. 4.**44** and 4.**45**).

Although in the presence of a subligamentous disk herniation the posterior longitudinal ligament can appear elevated from the bone and disk tissue, it does not display any interruption of contour. In contrast, extraligamentous herniations display a disruption of the posterior longitudinal ligament so that disk material is found between ligament and dura.

Regardless of the scanning sequences used, disruption of the posterior longitudinal ligament is frequently overlooked on MRI. In a comparison between MRI examinations and surgical findings, Silverman *et al.* (1995) achieved poor results when attempting a confident differentiation between a subligamentous and extraligamentous location of disk material. Sensitivity was clearly lower than specificity, thus confirming our experience that the detection of an extraligamentous herniation using MRI usually corresponds to surgical findings while many smaller extraligamentous herniations discovered at surgery are not demonstrated by MRI. This false-negative evaluation may be partially due to chemical-shift artifacts.

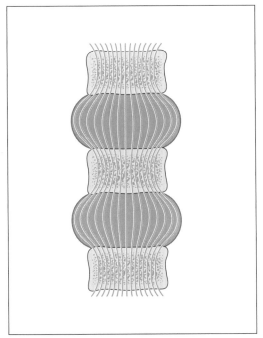

Fig. 4.**44** **Configuration and course of the posterior longitudinal ligament.**

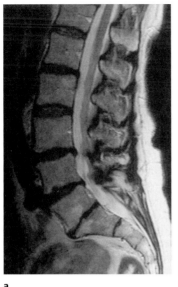 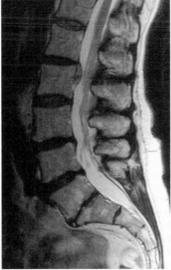 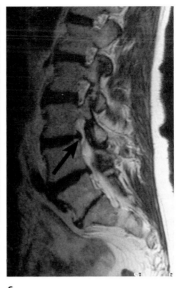

a   b   c

Fig. 4.**45 a–c** **Sagittal slices of the spine in a 64-year-old female patient** (TSE; TR = 3635 ms, TE = 120 ms):
a Depiction of the anterior and posterior longitudinal ligaments as uniform continuous dark lines in the midsagittal slice. The anterior longitudinal ligament is well shown as appearing thicker than the posterior one. The disks all demonstrate decreased signal intensity, L3/L4 with a somewhat dorsally projecting protrusion. Small protrusion also at L4/L5 with concomitant end plate discontinuity at L4. At the level of L5 the posterior longitudinal ligament is very poorly defined. Frank osteochondrosis of L5/S1.

b Slice 3 mm lateral to **a**. Large subligamentous disk herniation at L1/L2, which has migrated caudally. The posterior longitudinal ligament appears elevated.
c Slice 9 mm further lateral to **a**. Only parts of the longitudinal ligament are recognizable in the area of the disks, both in the ventral sections and dorsally. This applies particularly to L3/L4 (arrow). In the dorsal sections there is still also a longitudinal ligamentous structure present at the level L4/L5.

Extraligamentous herniations usually reach quite a considerable size and are not infrequently extruded far cranially or caudally. Subligamentous herniations have a noticeably flat delineation, despite the frequently substantially sized components of prolapsed disk material, and sometimes overlie the dorsal contour of the vertebral body in a band-like manner. In individual cases, very small extraligamentous sequesters can appear that are extruded far into the spinal canal and demonstrate no further attachment to the parent disk. Whereas these herniations can be overlooked on CT, with exact evaluation of the imaging material they are always detectable by MRI (Figs. 4.**46**–4.**51**).

Differentiation between a protrusion and a herniation is useful with regard to therapeutic consequences. Chemonucleolysis is usually only performed if the annulus fibrosus does not contain any larger tears through which the phar-

maceutical agent can leak. Protrusions and (with reservations) subligamentous flat herniations are amenable to percutaneous forms of therapy (e.g. laser nucleotomy) because the elasticity and resilience of the longitudinal ligament allow a certain degree of reduction of disk herniations once intradiskal relaxation has occurred. Extraligamentous herniations, on the other hand, are usually no longer susceptible to these techniques.

Herniated disks can display various degrees of signal intensity. At MRI, a fresh prolapse not infrequently shows high signal intensity on T2 weighting, appearing higher than that of the nucleus of the parent disk. In this case the herniation often demonstrates a somewhat rounded configuration with a considerable space-occupying effect. Herniations with high signal intensity exhibit a high water content that, as experience shows, decreases progressively and with it the size of the herniation. The signal intensity there-

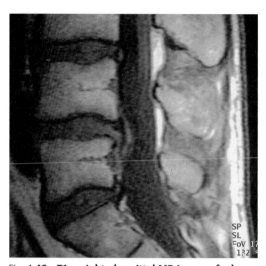

Fig. 4.**46** **T1-weighted sagittal MR image of a large, subligamentous disk herniation, which has migrated caudally at the level of L4/L5.** The wide perforation of the annulus fibrosus and extrusion of disk material caudally along the posterior border of L5 is well demonstrated, with the posterior longitudinal ligament appearing partly delineated and elevated. There is a protrusion at L3/L4 with a small subligamentous disk herniation projecting cranially at L5/S1.

fore allows conclusions to be drawn on likely future alterations in size that may be included in the overall therapeutic concept. Extraligamentous herniations and sequesters in particular display this high degree of signal intensity. There is no known reason for this (Fig. 4.**52**) (Masaryk *et al.*, 1988).

Disk herniations and sequesters can become enveloped by granulation tissue. In their study, Gallucci *et al.* (1995) discovered a correlation between the degree of granulation-tissue formation and the reduction in size of the disk herniation. Those patients who displayed a distinct formation of granulation tissue revealed a significant reduction in the size of the prolapse and a subsequent improvement in the clinical outcome. Cases that did not demonstrate granulation-tissue formation showed no modification of the size of the prolapse at follow-up MRIs and consequently demonstrated only a slight degree of clinical improvement.

The administration of a contrast agent during MRI can therefore help improve prognostic evaluation. In the typical case, the images will show a

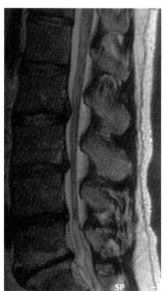

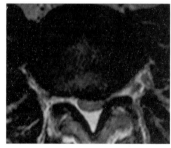

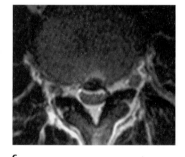

Fig. 4.**47 a–c** **Subligamentous disk herniation, which has migrated cranially:**
a T2-weighted sagittal image in a 44-year-old patient (TSE; TR = 3635 ms, TE = 120 ms): Large subligamentous disk herniation at L2/L3, which has migrated cranially with elevation of the posterior longitudinal ligament. A similar subligamentous disk herniation has migrated cranially at L3/L4. Protrusion at L4/L5. Osteochondrosis and protrusion at L5/S1 with concomitant evidence of fatty-marrow degeneration.

b T2-weighted transverse image at the level of L2/L3: The disk herniation appears somewhat accentuated toward the left midlateral side. There is compression of the dural sac. The annulus appears very thinned out dorsally.

c Slice 4 mm cranial to **b**: The subligamentous disk herniation is recognizable as a black structure of ellipsoid configuration in the region of the posterior margin.

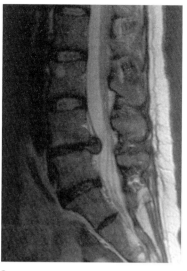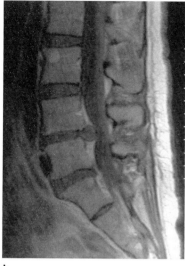

Fig. 4.48 a–c Massive subligamentous herniation at the level of L4/L5:

a T2-weighted sagittal image (TSE; TR = 3635 ms, TE = 120 ms): Massive subligamentous herniation at the lumbar segment L4/L5. The elevation of the longitudinal ligament is clearly visible.

b T1-weighted image (TSE; TR = 800 ms, TE = 12 ms): This image also demonstrates the displacement of the dura and the subligamentous location of the herniated disk.

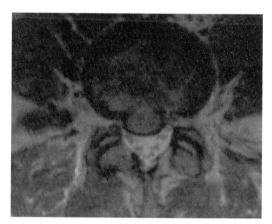

c T2-weighted transverse image (TSE; TR = 4465 ms, TE = 120 ms): The boundary of the disk herniation with the posterior longitudinal ligament is well shown on the transverse image.

clear signal enhancement around the prolapse, which can be even better demonstrated on fat-saturated images (Fig. 4.**53**).

Protrusions or herniations can lead to radiculopathy secondary to compression or even displacement of the nerve roots. This can occur within the dural sac along the course of the nerve root, although the nerve root is not infrequently compressed after exiting from the dural sac either lateral to the lateral recess or at the level of the intervertebral foramen (Fig. 4.**54**).

The extraforaminal part of the nerve root can be affected if a far lateral disk herniation is present. The nerve roots coursing within the dural sac are easily recognized on MRI using T2-weighted transverse images. Those parts outside the dural sac are well demonstrated on both T1- and T2-weighted images. In the acute phase, the nerve compression is not infrequently associated with a conspicuous swelling of the nerve root, which usually develops distal to the point of compression. The thickened nerve root demonstrates

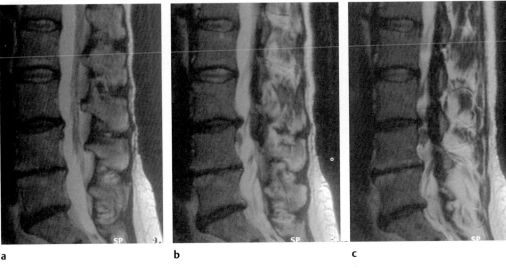

a   b   c

Fig. 4.**49 a–c   Small intraspinal sequester originating from the L3/L4 disk:**

a T2-weighted image (TSE; TR = 4400 ms, TE = 120 ms): The small sequester is identifiable immediately below the L3/L4 disk as a circumscribed small dark structure that is slightly elevating the dura.

b Slice 3 mm further lateral: The sequester appears elongated.

c Slice 6 mm further lateral to **a**: On this image the sequester is displayed as a slightly larger structure along the posterior margin of L4.

somewhat higher signal intensity on T1-weighted images than the non-irritated unaffected nerve root on the contralateral side. An edema can appear on T2-weighted images, leading to displacement of the nerve-root sleeve. This finding can be frequently followed further caudally for two or three slices (Fig. 4.**55**).

Fig. 4.**51 a–e   Massive herniation with a large intraspinally extruded component.** Smaller sequesters are recognizable alongside:

a T2-weighted sagittal image (TSE; TR = 4000 ms, TE = 120 ms): Large intraspinally extruded disk herniation as the cause of an obvious compression of the dural sac.

b Slice 3 mm further lateral: This image clearly demonstrates that both a subligamentous and an extraligamentous component are present. The displacement of the dura is well displayed.

c Slice 6 mm further lateral to **a**: Two small sequesters are recognizable on this image. The parent disk displays a distinct loss of height and reduction in signal. In addition there is a radial tear showing a corresponding signal enhancement.

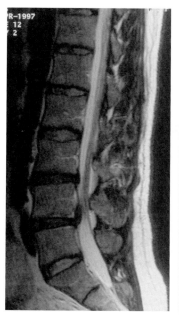
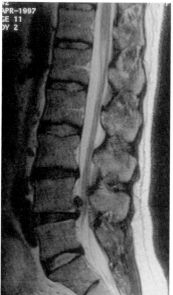
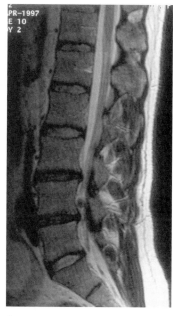

a

b

c

Fig. 4.**50 a–c** **T2-weighted sagittal images showing the presence of a sequester that has migrated cranially at the level of L4/L5:**

a Sagittal section (TSE; TR = 3635 ms, TE = 120 ms): Evidence of a disk herniation that has migrated slightly in a cranial direction and is mainly extraligamentous in location.

b Slice 3 mm lateral to **a**: The disk herniation displays a small, sequestrated fragment that is detached from the disk of origin at the level of the posterior margin of L4.

c Slice 6 mm lateral to **a**: A small sequestrated fragment recognizable here too at the level of the posterior margin of L4.

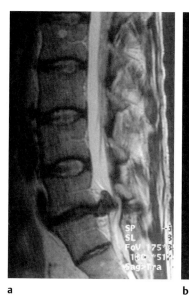
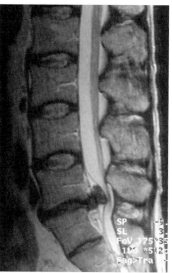
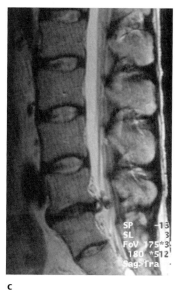

a

b

c

Fig. 4.**51 d, e** ▷

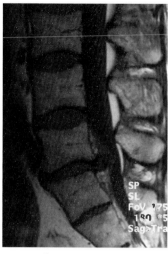
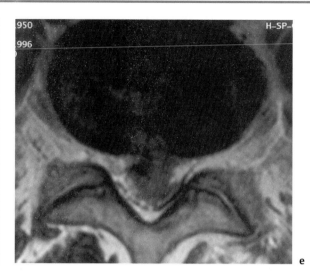

d

e

Fig. 4.**51 d, e**

d T1-weighted sagittal image (TSE; TR = 800 ms, TE = 12 ms): The subligamentous and extraligamentous components of the herniated disk are well differentiated. Furthermore, the wide opening in the area of the annulus is also recognizable on this image.

e T2-weighted transverse image (TSE; TR = 4800 ms, TE = 120 ms): The massive disk herniation has led to a marked compression of the dural sac. The wide interruption of contour in the central region of the annulus is well shown on this image.

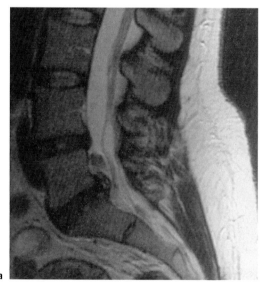
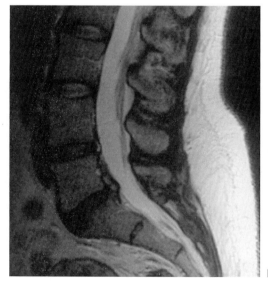

a

Fig. 4.**52 a–h   Images tracing the clinical course of a sequestered L5/S1 disk herniation:**

a T2-weighted sagittal image (TSE; TR = 4000 ms, TE = 120 ms) with evidence of a large, sub- and extraligamentous disk herniation that has migrated cranially plus an additional circumscribed sequester.

b Slice 3 mm lateral to **a**: This image shows a large subligamentous component. Both images demonstrate clearly higher signal intensity for the herniated part of the disk than for the parent disk itself.

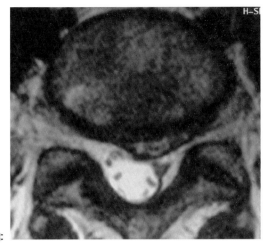

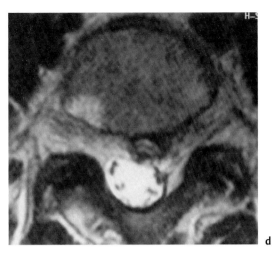

d

Fig. 4.**52 c, d**

c Transverse section (TSE; TR = 4846 ms, TE = 120 ms): The disk herniation is also well delineated on this image with the displacement of the posterior longitudinal ligament well recognizable in part. The disk herniation demonstrates high signal intensity.

d Slice 4 mm cranial to **c**: Here too, the high signal intensity of the herniated disk is well demonstrated.

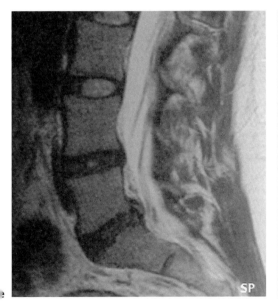

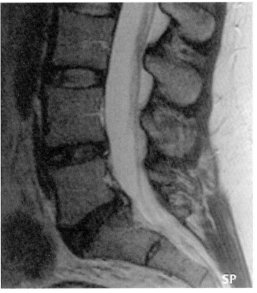

f

Fig. 4.**52 e, f**

e–h Follow-up scans 3 months later using the same slice orientation as **a** and **b**:

e T2-weighted sagittal image, largely identical to **a** as regards slice orientation: The disk herniation has clearly receded. All that remains of the sequester is a small circumscribed scar-like structure.

f Slice in an identical position to **b**: The regression of the subligamentous part of the prolapse is also well shown on this image.

Fig. 4.**52 g, h** ▷

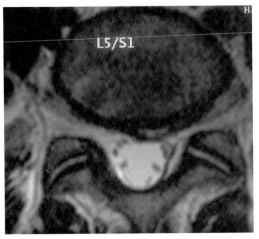

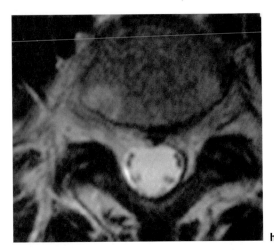

g

h

Fig. 4.**52 g, h**

g Slice position corresponding to **c** of the previous examination: Shrinkage of the disk herniation is also shown on this section.

h This slice corresponds to **d** of the previous examination: Considerable shrinkage of the disk herniation.

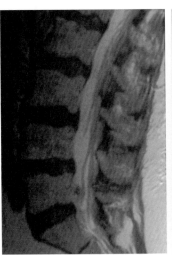

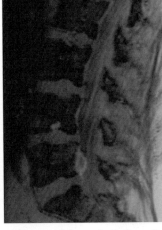

a

b

Fig. 4.**53 a–d Disk herniation with evidence of investing granulation tissue:**

a T2-weighted sagittal image (TSE; TR = 4000 ms, TE = 120 ms): disk herniation sequestered in a cranial direction, most probably originating from the L5/S1 parent disk.

b Post contrast sagittal image (FLASH; TR = 465 ms, TE = 11 ms, flip angle α = 90°): The T1-weighted GRE sequence obtained after administration of contrast material shows a very strong, almost circumferential signal enhancement and the disk herniation at the level of the posterior margin of L5.

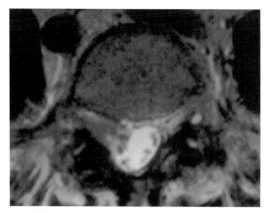

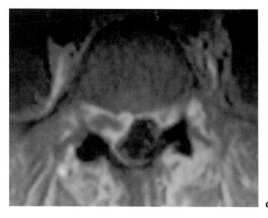

d

Fig. 4.**53 c, d**

c T2-weighted transverse image (TSE; TR = 6058 ms, TE = 120 ms): The disk herniation fills the lateral recess on the right, resulting in a conspicuous compression of the dural sac.

d Transverse image after application of contrast material (SE with fat saturation; TR = 572 ms, TE = 14 ms): On this image there is also a very well recognizable contrast enhancement along the disk herniation as an indication of granulation-tissue formation.

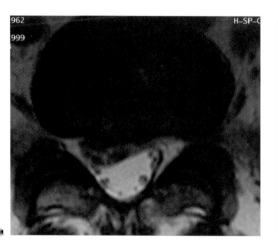

b

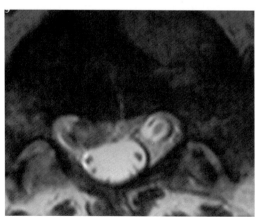

Fig. 4.**54 a–c   Frank compression of the right S1 root by a massive L5/S1 herniation mid-laterally to the right.** Each image 4 mm distal to the previous slice. The large disk herniation has led to compression of the S1 root on the right. Neither the anterior nor the posterior root is delineated on these images. The compression of the S1 root is particularly visible on the distal slices due to the signal loss along the course of the root sleeve. The sleeve on the left is filled with CSF. Here the anterior and posterior roots are both well outlined.

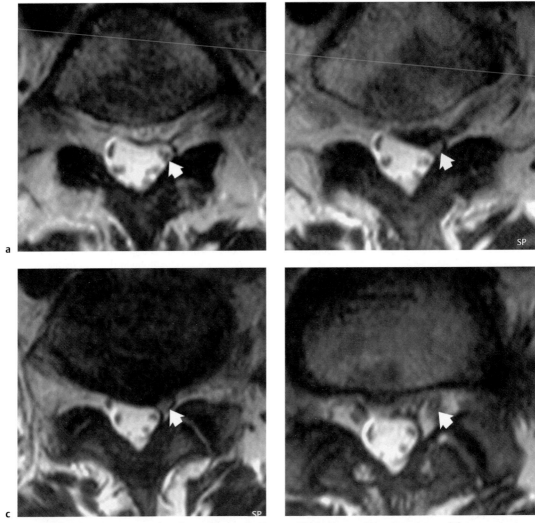

Fig. 4.**55 a–d** **Compression-related swelling of S1 root on the left:**

a Good delineation of the anterior and posterior roots of S1 on the left side (arrow).

b Herniation of the L5/S1 disk on the left with compression and displacement of S1. The root displays thickening and signal enhancement reflecting the edematous swelling (arrow).

c Thickening and reactive edema of the nerve root are also recognizable distal to the disk herniation.

d The next slice obtained further distally now demonstrates only a slight swelling of S1 on the left (arrow).

Lateral Disk Herniation

Lateral disk herniation is a special form of disk alteration. A distinction is made between:

- intraforaminal disk herniation,
- combined intra- and extraforaminal disk herniation,
- purely extraforaminal disk herniation located lateral to the foramen.

In contrast to medial and midlateral herniations, these lateral forms are particularly frequently found at L3/L4 and L4/L5 (approximately 90 % according to Bonneville *et al.*,1989). They principally arise when heavy objects are lifted and placed to the side while rotating the trunk with the legs stabilized in a fixed position and, conversely, when heavy objects are lifted from the side and placed in front of the body without moving the legs. The explanation for their frequent occurrence at L3/L4 and L4/L5 lies in the fact that especially these two levels are particularly mobile and are therefore principally loaded during the movements just described. In about 50 % of cases the total mobility of the spine in these patients is impaired by a re-duced mobility of one of the distal segments (e.g. L5/S1), secondary to, for example, osteochondrosis, sacralization or surgical fusion (Bonneville *et al.*, 1989). The average age of patients with a lateral herniation is usually slightly higher than in other patients with disk problems.

MRI has proven itself particularly superior in detecting lateral herniations. This comes from the possibility of obtaining sagittal slices of the foramina and the extraforaminal structures in addition to axial sections. A loss of fat signal on T1-weighted sequences is observed on the sagittal section, while intermediate signal intensity is found to emanate from the herniated disk. The disk herniation frequently extends proximally into the foramen, thus filling it entirely. The nerve root in this case is pressed against the bone and appears flattened (Grenier *et al.*, 1990).

However, detection is less easy on T2-weighted images; for this reason they should not be relied upon entirely for evaluation (Figs. 4.**56**–4.**58**).

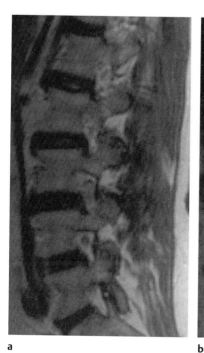
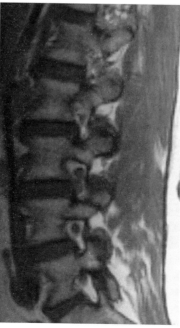

Fig. 4.56 a–c   Lateral intra- and extraforaminal disk herniation on the right side at the level of L3/L4:

a T2-weighted parasagittal image (TSE; TR = 3635ms, TE = 120 ms): The intraforaminal disk herniation compresses the L3 root. The signal intensity of the herniated disk is clearly higher than that of the parent disk.

b T1-weighted parasagittal image (TSE; TR = 800 ms, TE = 12 ms): The disk herniation is well recognizable due to the loss of signal in the intraforaminal fat. Broad area of contact with the L3 nerve root.

Fig. 4.**56 c** ▷

a

b

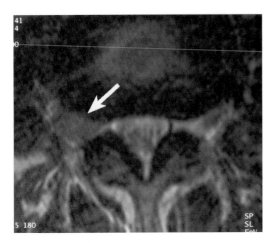

Fig. 4.**56 c** T2-weighted transverse section: Intra- and extraforaminal disk herniation on the right with high signal intensity in comparison with the parent disk (arrow) (TSE; TR = 4465ms, TE = 120 ms).

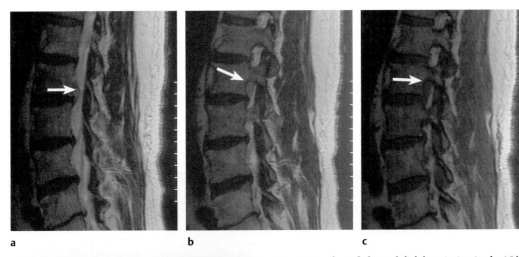

a

b

c

d

Fig. 4.**57 a–d Left-lateral disk herniation in the L2/L3 segment that has migrated cranially:**

a T2-weighted parasagittal image (TSE; TR = 3635ms, TE = 120 ms): The subligamentous disk herniation has migrated far cranially. It displays higher signal intensity than the parent disk.

b Slice 3 mm further lateral to **a**: The intraforaminal component is only poorly defined on this image.

c T1-weighted image in the same slice position as **b** (TSE; TR = 800, TE = 12 ms): The intraforaminal disk herniation is better recognizable on this sequence due to the signal loss of the fatty tissue.

d T2-weighted transverse section: High signal intensity of the herniated disk. Slight compression of the dural sac.

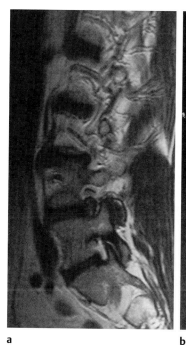
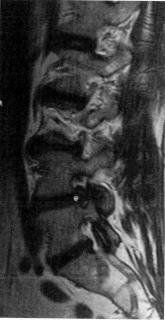

a　　　　　　　　b

Fig. 4.**58 a, b　Intraforaminal disk herniation at the level of L4/L5 on the right:**

a T2-weighted image (TSE; TR = 3635ms, TE = 120 ms): The intraforaminal disk herniation at the level L4/L5 extends in a cranial direction as far as the L4 root, although the root itself is not compressed.

b Image 3 mm lateral to **a**: The compression of the L4 root is recognizable on this slice, appearing flattened and elevated.

Intradural Disk Herniation

Intradural disk herniation is rare. Only 0.13 % of herniations extend in an intradural direction, whereby a differentiation is made between a subdural and subarachnoid location (Wasserstrom *et al.*, 1993). It is assumed that adhesions between the posterior longitudinal ligament and the dura prevent an epidural location of the disk herniation and instead result in an intradural prolapse. Intradural herniations may however be confused with intradural tumors on MRI due to their lack of any displacing character in relation to the dural sac, but the absence of contrast enhancement in the prolapse plus the residual continuity with the parent disk will, in individual cases, allow the correct diagnosis. This continuity is not always present which makes the distinction even more difficult.

Intradural disk herniations should always be considered:

- when the signal behavior and, especially, the contrast pattern of intradural structures do not unequivocally match those of a tumor,
- when, at the same time, the clinical symptoms of the patients have presented acutely,
- when there is continuity with the disk of origin, together with concomitant degenerative damage.

Limbus-Like Herniation

The so-called limbus-like herniation is a special form of disk alteration that is primarily found in younger patients. It is a disk herniation in which the dorsal ring apophysis has been separated from the vertebral body by a shearing force. In this case the apophysis looks dislocated while the bony contour has a rounded appearance in the region of the posterior margin and its junction with the end plate. The disk herniation lies adjacent to this rounded bony contour and displaces the detached fragment into the subligamentous space. The apophyseal fragment can also come to rest above the prolapse. Limbus-like herniations can also often present at a ventral location where, however, they are of no clinical significance.

Limbus-like herniations occur primarily in the upper lumbar spine at the level of L1/L2 and

L2/L3. The cause is assumed to lie in the fact that, due to the close relationship between Sharpey's fibers of the intervertebral disk and the apophysis of the vertebral body, the bone gives way to the disk herniation at the margin of the apophyseal ring, rather than Sharpey's fibers tearing away from the apophysis, thus causing the herniation to occur through the bone. This strong connection between Sharpey's fibers and apophysis is most notably found in adolescents in whom the bony stability between apophysis and vertebral body is still insufficient. This explains why the limbus-like herniation primarily occurs in the younger age groups and less often in older patients (Jinkins *et al.*, 1989).

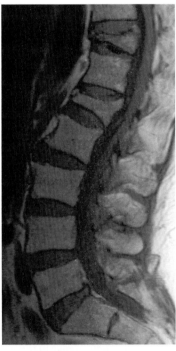

Fig. 4.**59** **Marked anterior disk herniation in the L2/L3 segment with discrete end plate indentation in the ventral part of L3.** T1-weighted sagittal image (TSE; TR = 800 ms, TE = 12 ms): Clear protrusion of the anterior longitudinal ligament. In addition, evidence of old fractures of the vertebral bodies T11 and L1. A distinct convex bulge of the posterior marginal strip of T11 is noticeable. The T11/12 disk demonstrates reduction in signal consistent with calcification. The posterior marginal strip of L1 is also reduced in height and altered in its contour.

Anterior Disk Herniation

Anterior disk herniation virtually always occurs at a subligamentous location due to the very strong anterior longitudinal ligament that is solidly attached to the bone and the annulus fibrosus. It can, however, assume considerable dimensions. The herniations can extend subligamentously along the vertebral-body margin in cranial and caudal directions. Anterior disk herniations result in extensive reactive marginal osteophytes, which can appear as a complete syndesmophytic bridge. The anterior disk herniation is typically and especially frequently found at L3/L4 and L4/L5, as opposed to the posterior herniation, which primarily occurs at L4/L5 and L5/S1 (Fig. 4.**59**).

The reason why anterior disk herniations are mainly found further cranially is because here the main load-bearing region within the spine lies more to the front. Conversely, due to the lordosis of the lumbar spine the main load-bearing region in the distal levels of the lumbar spine lies more dorsally. This favors the occurrence of dorsal disk herniations in these distal segments. The combination of anterior, lateral and posterior herniations, so-called *multidirectional disk herniations*, is also a not infrequent finding. They too are primarily found at L3/L4 and L4/L5.

Pathogenetically, a special weakness of the disks is considered to be present (Jinkins *et al.*, 1989). The clinical relevance of anterior disk herniations is disputed. It is usually assumed that they do not cause any symptoms. It is therefore not obligatory to include them in an MRI examination report, although their conspicuous syndesmophyte formations do draw attention on radiographic survey views. Pathophysiological studies are available, however, which prove that pain can radiate from an anterior disk herniation.

Spondylolisthesis

Incidence and Distribution

Spondylolisthesis secondary to spondylolysis is a relatively common finding in the region of the lumbar spine. According to estimates, approximately 7 % of the population is affected. Spondylolysis occurs primarily at the level L5/S1, with changes in the proximal sections of the lumbar spine appearing with decreasing frequency.

Pathogenesis

Anterior spondylolisthesis is the most common structural fault occurring as a result of a (mostly bilateral) spondylolysis or due to a subluxed position of the facet joints.

Spondylolysis usually occurs during childhood or adolescence, less frequently during adulthood. Apart from a familial disposition, various forms of damage to the interarticular portion are found which display the characteristics of a stress fracture. They arise from increased, extreme, and long-standing load bearing on the spine, especially loading in hyperextension and rotation. Pathological loading of proximal and distal segments after spinal fusion surgery can result in an acquired spondylolysis that primarily affects adults (Harris and Wiley, 1963). A further cause under discussion is an inflammatory reaction in the form of an osteochondritis or ostitis. Direct trauma should be considered a rare cause.

Degenerative anterior spondylolisthesis without the presence of lysis of the interarticular portion occurs as a result of disk degeneration and loss of disk height, which leads to instability in the small vertebral joints.

Clinical Presentation

Patients with anterior spondylolisthesis usually present clinically with low back pain and also, not infrequently, with radicular symptoms. The radicular complaints arise mainly from a stenosis of the intervertebral foramen at the level of the affected segment. The forward translation of one of the vertebra results in a concurrent compression of the corresponding infraforaminal portion of the nerve root, either from degenerative alterations at the facet joints or, alternatively, from the

development of hypertrophic connective tissue or the formation of cartilaginous tissue along the zone of lysis.

The clinical presentation of the patient does not therefore allow any differentiation between a spondylolisthesis that has developed secondary to spondylolysis and one due to a degenerative process.

Diagnostics

MRI

MRI evidence of spondylolysis is best provided on sagittal sections, with PD- or T1-weighted sequences being the most suited (Grenier *et al.*, 1989). Supplementary T1-weighted FLASH sequences with fat saturation or, if necessary, images using a STIR sequence can improve the diagnostic reliability by providing high contrast between bony structures and the bony cleft. The defect is oriented perpendicular to the pars interarticularis on sagittal sections (Figs. 4.**60** and 4.**61**).

Midsagittal slices allow a differentiation between anterior spondylolisthesis secondary to facet degeneration and anterior spondylolisthesis due to spondylolysis. In the case of a genuine spondylolysis, the row of spinous processes is stepped above the misalignment between the vertebral bodies, while a degenerative spondylolisthesis displays the step at the same level. This is because, in the case of a genuine spondylolysis, the distance between spinous process and posterior vertebral-body margin is increased in comparison with normal findings, i.e. the spinal process of this vertebra does not slip forward with the vertebral body, whereas the next higher vertebral body demonstrates forward displacement together with the spinous process. In the case of a degenerative anterior spondylolisthesis, the spinal process of the vertebra that has slipped forward is included in the anterior translation, so the step in the alignment of the spinal processes appears between the ventrally displaced vertebral body and the one distal to it (Fig. 4.**62**).

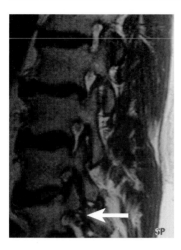

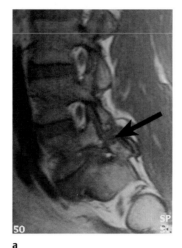

a

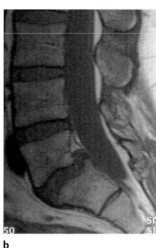

b

Fig. 4.**60 Spondylolisthesis L5 with no noteworthy anterior translation.** T2-weighted parasagittal section (TSE; TR = 3400 ms, TE = 120 ms): The vertical lysis is well shown in the interarticular portion. The bony cleft is filled with connective tissue. At the same time there is a clear protrusion of the L4/L5 disk and hypertrophy at the L5 facet joint with a corresponding narrowing of the intervertebral foramen.

Fig. 4.**61 a, b Interruption of the interarticular portion at the level of L5:**

a T1-weighted parasagittal section (TSE; TR = 800 ms, TE = 12 ms): Mild anterior translation of L5 over S1 (Grade I according to Meyerding). The intervertebral foramen L5/S1 is completely occluded by fibrous and osseous structures.

b Midsagittal section: Evidence of frank anterior slippage of L5 over S1. Mild disk herniation, occurring typically in an epidural location and in a cranial direction.

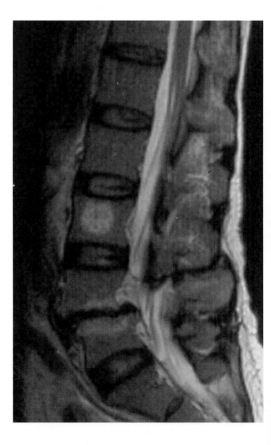

Fig. 4.**62 Spondylolysis L4 with obvious forward slippage of L4 over L5.** Concomitant erosive destruction of the inferior and superior end plates of L4 and L5, respectively. Deterioration of the disk, clear fatty-marrow degeneration. The dorsal step in the row of spinous processes is typical for spondylolisthesis secondary to genuine spondylolysis. Whereas the dorsal alignment of the posterior vertebral margins shows a step at the L4/L5 junction, the step in the row of spinal processes is at the L3/L4 level.

Degenerative Changes of the Thoracic Spine

Incidence and Distribution

Thoracic herniations are rare. According to the literature, only 4% of all disk herniations are found in the thoracic region (Ryan *et al.*, 1988; Alvarez *et al.*, 1988). However, the introduction of MRI has led to an increase in the detection of thoracic disk herniations.

Some 75% of these disk herniations affect the distal third of the thoracic spine, with the levels T10/11 and T11/12 being the most frequently affected (Ryan *et al.*, 1988). The proximal levels are less often involved because the kyphosis of the thoracic spine, which is most pronounced at the level T6 to T8, causes the point of stress concentration of these segments to lie more anteriorly. Therefore the anterior parts of the disk become more prone to degeneration. On the other hand, the consequence for the distal part of the thoracic spine is that there is a dorsal malalignment of the spinal axis at the junction between kyphosis and lordosis and a correspondingly increased loading of the dorsal parts of the intervertebral disks (Alvarez *et al.*, 1988; Parisel *et al.*, 1989).

Due to the kyphosis of the thoracic spine, the spinal cord lies far anteriorly within the spinal canal and in part even overlies the posterior contours of the vertebral bodies. This causes yet smaller disk herniations to come into direct contact with the spinal cord and elicit signs and symptoms. This is still more intensified by the fact that the spinal canal is relatively narrow in the thoracic region and there is therefore little room for the spinal cord to move out of the way.

Clinical Presentation

The primary clinical feature is myelopathy associated with the most varied and sometimes discrete symptoms. Combinations of radiculopathy and myelopathy are possible, although asymptomatic presentations are no rarity. It may be assumed that these asymptomatic disk herniations predominate, with up to two-thirds of all diagnosed herniations falling into this category (Ryan *et al.*, 1988; Alvarez *et al.*, 1988; Williams *et al.*, 1989).

Diagnostics

MRI

With optimal implementation, the diagnostic reliability of an MRI examination is comparable to that of CT myelography. It has a higher detection rate than conventional myelography, with CT myelography and MRI each achieving equally high detection rates without false-negative findings. MRI is therefore the method of choice for suspected thoracic disk herniation. If, however, a herniated disk cannot be confirmed using this technique, e.g. because of manifest motion artifacts, then the examiner will have to resort to CT myelography.

The signal patterns of disk herniations vary. Some disk herniations appear very dark on all sequences without calcifications necessarily being present in these cases—a finding that can be readily differentiated by CT (Ross *et al.*, 1987). The majority of disk herniations appear isointense with the corresponding disk. Using T2 weighting, the signal intensity of the herniated disk is lower than that of CSF, making a distinction possible between the disk herniation and the hyperintense subarachnoid space. The co-affected disks not infrequently demonstrate no reduction in signal in the area of the nucleus pulposus, so that signs of disk degeneration need not be apparent on MRI.

The proportion of calcified disk herniations is higher than in other regions of the spine. The cause of these calcifications is not clear. These calcified disk herniations are partly to be viewed in conjunction with calcifications of the nucleus pulposus of the corresponding disk. Calcified disk herniations are also detected, however, without the nucleus of the corresponding disk itself being affected. Apart from that, an association with the occurrence of Scheuermann's disease is currently under discussion. There is an increased incidence of thoracic disk herniations in association with Scheuermann's disease (Roosen *et al.*, 1987; Ryan *et al.*, 1988).

The diagnostic reliability of an MRI examination of a thoracic disk herniation can be limited by CSF-flow artifacts, particularly on T2-weighted images, as well as by artifacts resulting from the heart or major vessels. In this respect, T2-

weighted TSE images most notably display CSF-flow artifacts, while T2-weighted GRE images mainly demonstrate flow artifacts from the major vessels and heart. However, the latter can usually be readily suppressed by flow compensation. In addition, the appearance of overlapping in the field of examination due to flow artifacts can be avoided by switching the phase-encoding gradient to the craniocaudal direction. However, in some cases, this direction of switching can obscure a disk herniation because the resultant chemical shift artifacts of the bone marrow in the AP direction render delineation of the herniated disk impossible. In this respect, sagittal images of the spine should be obtained by switching the frequency-encoding gradient in the craniocaudal direction and the phase-encoding gradient in the AP direction (Enzmann *et al.*, 1987). Susceptibility and motion artifacts can also render detection of disk herniations difficult on T2-weighted sagittal images due to the increased sensitivity of these sequences to artifacts. The long repetition and echo times of T2-weighted SE images make them prone to motion artifacts. GRE sequences are not only particularly sensitive to motion and flow artifacts but also to susceptibility artifacts (Figs. **4.63–4.67**).

The diagnostic reliability of MRI is sufficient only if transverse sections are obtained in addition to T1- and T2-weighted images (Ross *et al.*,

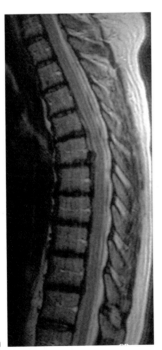 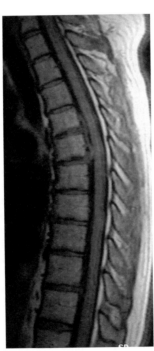

a

b

Fig. 4.**63 a–c Large thoracic disk herniations at T6/T7 and T10/T11:**

a T2-weighted sagittal image (TSE; TR = 3700 ms, TE = 120 ms): The large disk herniation at T6/T7 has migrated slightly cranially. It displays low signal intensity. The small disk herniation at T10/T11 also demonstrates low signal intensity corresponding to the disk. Marked respiratory artifacts.

b T1-weighted sagittal section (TSE; TR = 800 ms, TE = 12 ms): Both herniations are well defined. Clear CSF-flow artifacts in the region of T5 and T6. The sagittal slices were obtained by switching the phase-encoding gradient in the AP direction. As a result, there is a corresponding chemical-shift artifact of moderate degree visible in the craniocaudal direction of projection. The posterior vertebral-body margin is therefore sharply defined along the entire thoracic spine.

1987). These three sequences complement one another. In individual cases disk herniations are only seen on axial images and not on sagittal slices and, conversely, some herniations are only visible on sagittal and not on axial sections (Fig. 4.**68**).

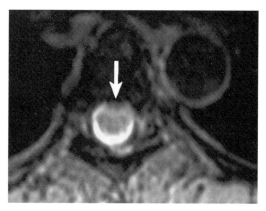

Fig. 4.**63 c** Transverse section using T2 weighting (FLASH; TR = 700 ms, TE = 15 ms, flip angle α = 20°): The medial disk herniation is well delineated. It demonstrates mild compression of the myelon.

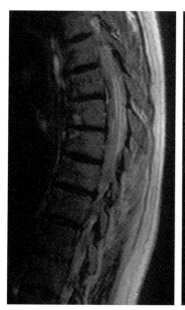

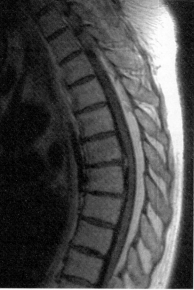

a

b

Fig. 4.**64 a–c** **Thoracic disk herniation at the T6/T7 level:**

a T2-weighted sagittal section (TSE; TR = 3900 ms, TE = 120 ms): Evaluation of the vertebral body margins is not possible due to flow artifacts. The disk herniation is therefore not delineated.

b T1-weighted sagittal section (TSE; TR = 800 ms, TE = 12 ms): The disk herniation is well defined. There is a surrounding signal enhancement due to the decelerated CSF flow.

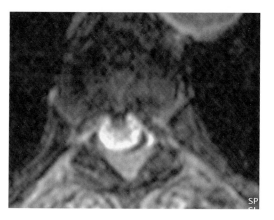

c Transverse section (FLASH; TR = 703 ms, TE = 15 ms, flip angle α = 20°): The disk herniation appears particularly well accentuated on this image. Note the small rounded structure with a clear compression of the myelon.

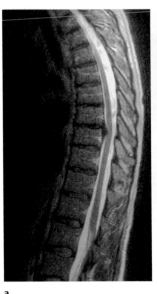
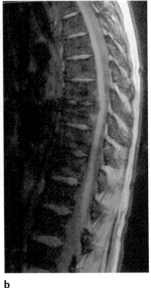

a

b

Fig. 4.65 a, b Unmistakable disk herniation in the middle region of the thoracic spine:

a T2-weighted sagittal section (TSE; TR = 5310 ms, TE = 112 ms): The disk herniation has migrated caudally and displays low signal intensity. Note the conspicuous compression. Mild CSF-flow artifacts, otherwise only few motion artifacts.

b GRE sequence (FLASH; TR = 465 ms, TE = 11 ms, flip angle α = 90°): The disk herniation is not recognizable on this image due to marked pulsation artifacts from the heart and vessels.

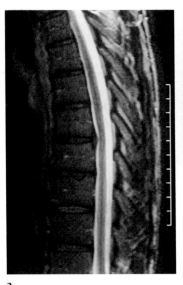
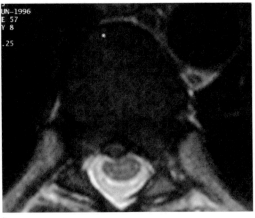

b

a

Fig. 4.66 a, b Subligamentous disk herniation in the T8/T9 region:

a T2-weighted sagittal section (TSE; TR = 5310 ms, TE = 112 ms): The disk herniation has migrated caudally and also slightly cranially, displaying an identical signal intensity to that of the parent disk. There is only a flat bulging dorsally.

b Transverse section using T2 weighting (TSE; TR = 5000 ms, TE = 120 ms): Here, there is a better presentation of the spinal cord compression. The disk herniation exhibits low signal intensity.

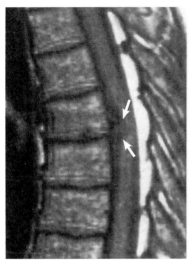
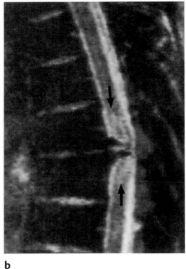

Fig. 4.**67 a, b** **Calcified disk herniation at T6/T7:**

a T1-weighted image (SE; TR = 685 ms, TE = 20 ms) showing disk herniation compromising the spinal cord (arrows).

b GRE sequence (FFE; TR = 600 ms, TE = 20 ms, flip angle α = 10°): The presentation of the disk herniation is all too obvious due to susceptibility artifacts (arrows). Slightly irregular signal losses are to be found. In addition, edema of the spinal cord can also be seen. The disk displays frank loss of height.

a   b

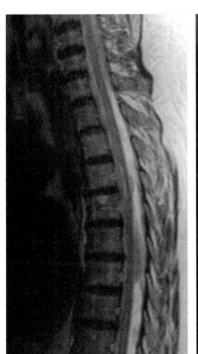
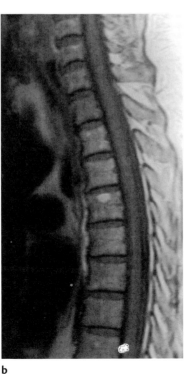

Fig. 4.**68 a–e** **69-year-old female patient with syringomyelia in the T3/T4 region with a herniation of the T5/T6 disk:**

a T2-weighted sagittal image with the phase switched in the AP direction (TSE; TR = 5300 ms, TE = 120 ms): The spinal canal is poorly assessable due to CSF flow and motion artifacts. Neither the syrinx nor the disk herniation is clearly definable.

b Image using T1 weighting (TSE; TR = 800 ms, TE = 12 ms): The described alterations are not clearly definable on this image either.

Fig. 4.**68 c–e** ▷

a   b

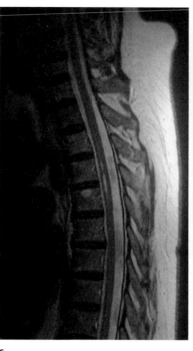
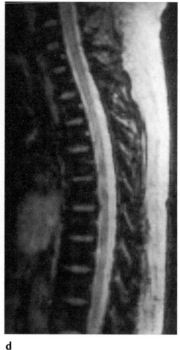

c

d

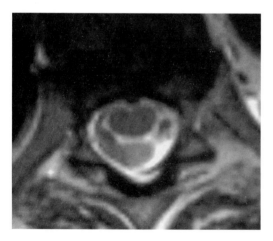

Fig. 4.**68 c–e**

c T2-weighted section after switching the phase in the craniocaudal direction (TSE; TR = 3390 ms, TE = 120 ms): The syrinx is now depicted free of artifacts. The spinal canal is on the whole clearly more readily evaluable. There is sharp delineation of the spinal cord. However, the disk herniation at the level of T5/T6 cannot be seen on this image either; only a slight bulge of the disk is visible.

d T2-weighted image using a GRE technique (two-dimensional FLASH; TR = 663 ms, TE = 22 ms, flip angle α = 35°): The image quality is heavily impaired by flow artifacts, so neither syrinx nor disk herniation is detectable.

e Transverse image using T2 weighting (TSE; TR = 5820 ms, TE = 120 ms): Only on the transverse T2-weighted slice orientation is there clear evidence of the small medial disk herniation causing a slight indentation of the spinal cord.

Degenerative Changes of the Cervical Spine

Diagnostics

MRI

MRI has acquired considerable significance for detecting degenerative changes of the cervical spine. With a suitable sequence selection, bulgings, herniations and bony changes can be readily displayed. MRI is superior to cervical myelography (Nakstadt *et al.*, 1989) and achieves the same detection rate as CT myelography, in some studies even surpassing it (Brown *et al.*, 1988; Neuhold *et al.*, 1991; Breidahl *et al.*, 1991; Youssem *et al.*, 1992). Recent studies have reported a sensitivity and specificity of up to 91 % (Youssem *et al.*, 1992). MRI is better suited for examining the entire spine than CT myelography, allowing additional depiction in the transverse and sagittal slice orientation without difficulty.

Unlike the thoracic and lumbar region, disk degeneration of the cervical spine is not so much recognizable from signal loss of the central parts than, above all, from the loss of disk height. Loss of disk height is always regarded as a sign of degeneration. The differentiation between annulus and nucleus is somewhat less easy than in the lumbar region because the annulus often only appears as a very thin structure. The attachment to the posterior longitudinal ligament is very firm.

The differentiation between protrusion and disk herniation is difficult, although also of less relevance, than it is in the region of the lumbar spine. Generally speaking, circumferential disk displacements tend to be interpreted as protrusions and the tongue-shaped ones, on the other hand, as disk herniations. Furthermore, unequivocal distinction between a sub- and an extraligamentous disk herniation is not possible. Here the rule is that the flat, mild herniations tend to have a subligamentous location, while the large, tongue-shaped or circumscribed massive herniations and more likely to be extraligamentous (Isu *et al.*, 1986). Massive herniations are seen less here than in the lumbar spine and are usually not associated with a corresponding loss of disk height. If protrusions or herniated disks have existed for a long time, there is always a reactive bony alteration of the end plates with corresponding reactive spondylotic bony bridging. This combination of a disk herniation with a retrospondylophytic bony reaction can lead to frank spinal stenosis and result in a severe compression of the myelon. The loss of disk height gives rise to uncovertebral joint arthrosis, the uncinate processes widen and become short and thick, which is associated with stenosis of the intervertebral foramina. Cases of severe polysegmental degenerative alterations of the intervertebral disks can result in long-segment spinal stenoses with a corresponding compression of the spinal cord and narrowing of the intervertebral foramina (Figs. 4.**69**–4.**74**).

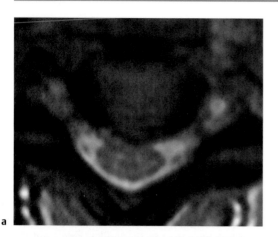

a

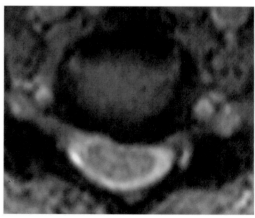

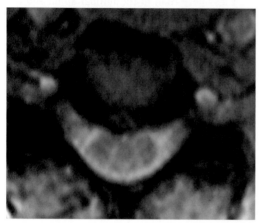

c

Fig. 4.**69 a–c Flat protrusion of the C3/C4 intervertebral disk with reactive bony bridging:**

a Transverse section at the level of the disk (two-dimensional FLASH; TR = 608 ms, TE = 15 ms, flip angle α = 20°): Flat, somewhat medially accentuated protrusion of the disk is recognizable here, stopping just short of the spinal cord. The ventral reserve space appears exhausted. The intervertebral foramina appear patent.

b Mid-laterally accentuated protrusion on the left, bridged by bone (two-dimensional FLASH; TR = 608 ms, TE = 15 ms, flip angle α = 20°): The protrusion reaches the spinal cord.

c Small medial tongue-shaped disk protrusion (two-dimensional FLASH; TR = 608 ms, TE = 15 ms, flip angle α = 20°).

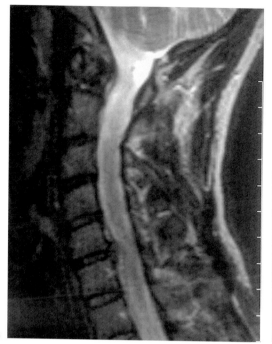

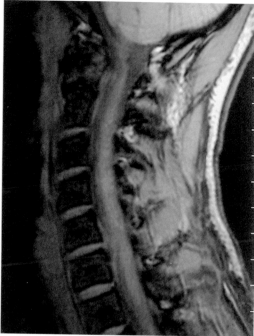

a

b

Fig. 4.70 a–c Large right mid-lateral disk herniation at the C5/C6 segment:

a T2-weighted sagittal image (TSE; TR = 4600 ms, TE = 112 ms): The disk herniation causes a displacement of the myelon. The dura appears slightly pushed aside. Note that the disk itself demonstrates no signal change in comparison with the other disks. At most, there is only a slight loss in height.

b T1-weighted image (two-dimensional FLASH; TR = 403 ms, TE = 11 ms, flip angle α = 90°): The disk is recognizable on this image as a space-occupying structure, although poorly defined relative to the spinal cord. There is a better presentation of the marked congestion of the epidural venous plexus, both proximal and caudal to the disk protrusion, than on the T2-weighted image.

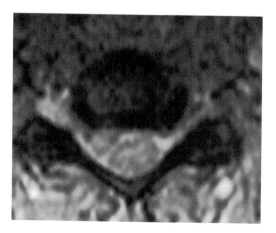

c T2-weighted transverse image: The tongue-shaped disk herniation situated to the right is easily recognizable, resulting in compression of the C5 root on the right side. The herniation reaches the spinal cord. The intervertebral foramen appears patent.

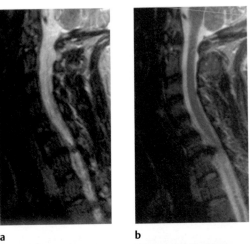

a

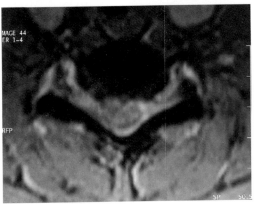

b

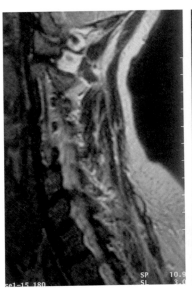

a

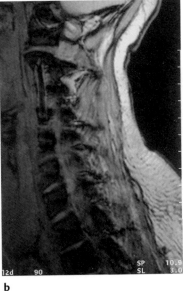

b

Fig. 4.71 a–c Right-lateral and intraforaminal disk herniation at the C6/C7 segment:

a T2-weighted parasagittal image (TSE; TR = 5300 ms, TE = 120 ms): The circumscribed disk herniation is well delineated laterally on the right.

b Slice 3 mm medial to **a**. Large disk herniation compromising the spinal cord can also be seen on this slice.

c Transverse section at the level of the foramina (two-dimensional FLASH; TR = 703 ms, TE = 15 ms, flip angle α = 20°): The disk herniation appears relatively ill defined against the myelon. It extends broadly into the intervertebral foramen on the right.

Fig. 4.72 a–c Left intraforaminal disk herniation at the C6/C7 segment:

a T2-weighted image (TSE; TR = 4600 ms, TE = 112 ms): The disk herniation extending broadly in an infraforaminal direction can hardly be seen on this image.

b T1-weighted image (two-dimensional FLASH; TR = 403 ms, TE = 11 ms, flip angle α = 90°): The disk herniation is much more readily recognizable on this image than with T2 weighting, displaying a spherical configuration and being displaced far caudally.

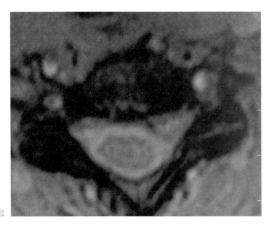

Fig. 4.**72c** Transverse section at the level of the foramina (two-dimensional FLASH; TR = 608 ms, TE = 15 ms, flip angle α = 20°): The disk herniation projects broadly in an infraforaminal direction and is easily distinguishable due to the displacement of the dura. It does not reach the spinal cord.

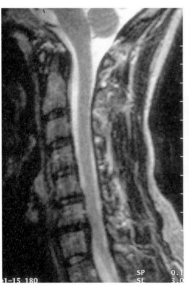

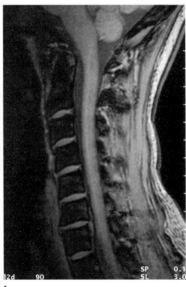

a

b

Fig. 4.**73a–c Subligamentous disk herniation originating from the C6/C7 disk:**
a T2-weighted sagittal section (TSE; TR = 4700 ms, TE = 112 ms): The C6/C7 disk demonstrates a slight signal reduction relative to the adjacent disks. The disk herniation extends far caudally down the posterior margin of C7.
b T1-weighted image (two-dimensional FLASH; TR = 403 ms, TE = 11 ms, flip angle α = 90°): The disk herniation is well demarcated due to the identical signal in comparison with the C6/C7 disk.

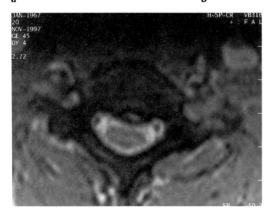

c T2-weighted image caudal to the C6/C7 disk (two-dimensional FLASH; TR = 703 ms, TE = 15 ms, flip angle α = 20°): The disk herniation displays a high signal intensity. The ligamentous structures appear dorsally displaced.

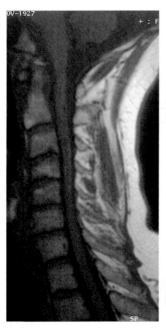
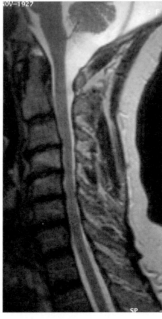

a b

Fig. 4.**74 a–e** **Bony spinal stenosis at the C3–C6 segment:**

a T1-weighted sagittal image (SE; TR = 800 ms, TE = 12 ms): Marked disk degeneration at C3/C4 and C4/C5 with a considerable subchondral reaction and a broad retrospondylosis. Anterior disk herniation C3/C4 and C4/C5.

b Sagittal image using T2 weighting (TSE; TR = 4800 ms, TE = 130 ms): The long-segment bony stenosis in the C3–C7 region is well depicted. The spinal cord appears compressed and atrophic. The vertebral bodies demonstrate clear bone-marrow changes, primarily in the form of a fatty-marrow reaction.

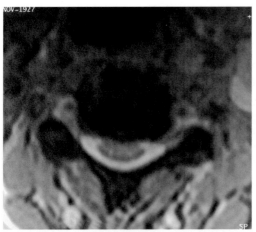
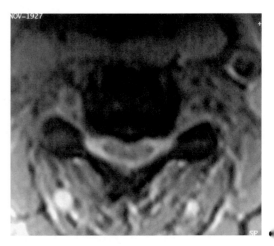

c d

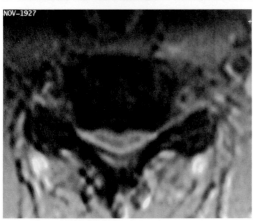

e

c–e Transverse images through the level of the disks C3/C4 (**c**), C4/C5 (**d**), and C5/C6 (**e**): The images each show a combined bony and diskal stenosis of the spinal canal, in part with a clear flattening and reduction in volume of the spinal cord consistent with the atrophy. In addition there is a bilateral stenosis of the intervertebral foramina recognizable at C5/C6 secondary to an uncovertebral joint arthrosis.

The compression of the spinal cord can lead to intramedullary signal enhancement. This signal enhancement is the expression of a reactive edema or gliosis. Long-lasting compressions can result in a circumscribed necrosis of the spinal cord. The origin of these alterations may be considered to lie in chronic ischemia caused by the disturbed circulation on the part of both the arterial and the venous limb. The formation of edema can be long-segment in appearance, or even round to oval. Should a contrast agent be administered, most cases will reveal a barrier disturbance with a corresponding clear signal enhancement resulting from the accumulation of contrast. Patients with signal enhancement of the myelon will in the majority of cases not enjoy any clinical improvement after surgery in comparison with patients without this finding. The cause is considered to lie in irreversible damage to the spinal cord. Fujiwara *et al.* (1989) found that the results

of surgery could be expected to be poor if the transverse area of the myelon was less than 30 mm².

Severe atrophy of the myelon is not infrequently considered to be a long-term sequel of this spinal-cord compression (Figs. 4.**75**–4.**78**).

The posterior displacement of disk material together with the reactive bony changes at the vertebral end plates can result in marked congestion of the epidural venous plexus. This congestion of the venous pathways can be recognized particularly well both above and below the affected segment, especially in the parasagittal, more laterally aligned sections. Should a contrast agent be administered, there will be a clear signal enhancement within these veins, primarily in the lateral parts up to and including the foramina. In some cases this facilitates the differentiation between disk herniation and venous congestion, particularly intraforaminally.

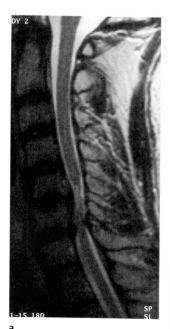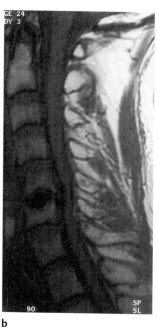

a   b

Fig. 4.**75 a, b Severe spinal stenosis especially in the C5–C7 region.** Postoperative sections after Cloward's procedure with insertion of a Palacos plug at C5/C6. Myelon atrophy and reactive gliosis at the level C5/C6:
a T2-weighted image (TSE; TR = 4600 ms, TE = 112 ms): High-degree spinal stenosis in the area of segment C5–C7. This is primarily due to the bony changes particularly in the region of the corresponding end plates C5/C6. In addition there is evidence of a C6/C7 disk herniation and a mild hypertrophy of the ligamentum flavum in the C6/C7 region. The spinal cord appears clearly atrophic. There is a pin-like signal enhancement at the C5/C6 level.
b T1-weighted image (SE; TR = 351 ms, TE = 12 ms): The Palacos plug can be seen easily on this image. Furthermore, the atrophy of the spinal cord is also shown well. The intramedullary signal enhancement on T2 weighting is associated with a reduction in signal on this image.

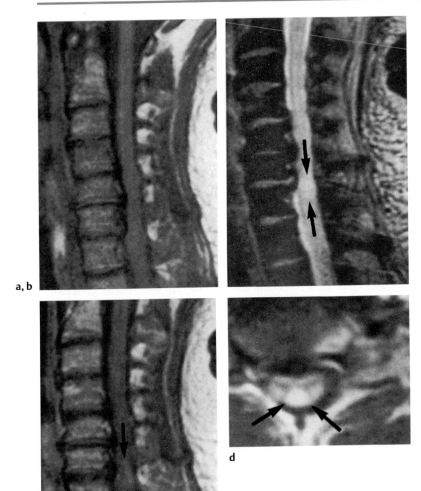

a, b

c

d

Fig. 4.**76 a–d   Old disk herniations in the regions C4/C5, C5/C6 and C6/C7 with marked retrospondylosis:**

a T1-weighted sagittal section (SE; TR = 650 ms, TE = 25 ms): Obvious compression of the spinal cord by the bony changes.

b T2-weighted GRE sequence: Finding of a long-segment compression of the spinal cord with evidence of myelon edema at the level C6/C7 (arrows).

c Contrast application: Finding consistent with a barrier breakdown at this level (arrow).

d On the transverse section there is a circumscribed, almost round, mid-dorsal enhancement with contrast (arrows).

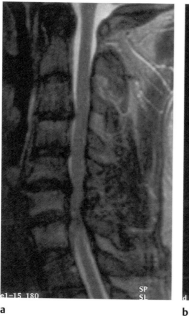

a

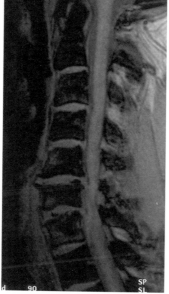

b

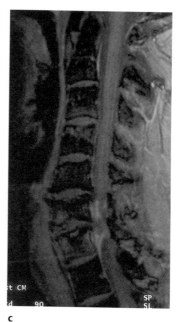

c

Fig. 4.**77 a–f** **Sequestered disk herniation at C6/C7.** Advantageous effect of contrast application for better delineation of the herniated disk:

a T2-weighted image of the spinal canal (TSE; TR = 5300 ms, TE = 112 ms): The disk herniation at the level C6/C7 is not clearly defined. Long-segment spinal stenosis secondary to marked disk degeneration in the region of C3–C7. Somewhat more marked disk protrusion and retrospondylosis at C5/C6.

b T1-weighted sagittal image (two-dimensional FLASH; TR = 403 ms, TE = 11 ms, flip angle α = 90°): The severe osteochondrotic changes, particularly at C5/C6 and C6/C7, are quite well defined on this image. The disk herniation, however, is not recognizable.

c Image after contrast application: The disk herniation is now well defined. In addition, the congestion along the course of the epidural venous plexus is easily discernible proximally and distally.

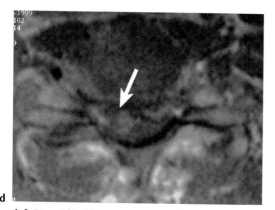

d

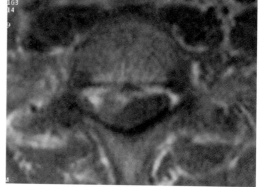

e

d–f *T1-weighted transverse images after contrast application at the level of C6/C7:*

d This figure shows the large sequestered disk herniation mid-laterally on the right with compression of the spinal cord (arrow).

e Slice 4 mm caudal to **d**: The disk herniation is partially transected on this section, next to it there is strong enhancement along the course of the epidural venous plexus.

Fig. 4.**77 f** ▷

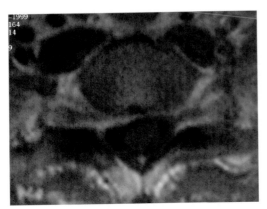

Fig. 4.**77 f**   Slice 4 mm caudal to **e**: The foramina C7/T1 are imaged on this slice. Easily identifiable enhancement in the infraforaminal area and right mid-laterally in the epidural regions. The nerve-root ganglia are well defined.

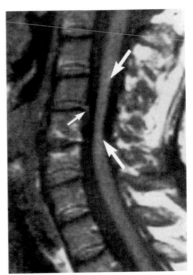

Fig. 4.**78   Postoperative image after Cloward's procedure for disk herniation at the level C5/C6.** C4/C5 disk herniation. The spinal cord demonstrates clear atrophy along the course of C4–C5/6 (SE; TR = 650 ms, TE = 25 ms).

Acquired Spinal Canal Stenosis

In collaboration with W. Weber, H. Henkes and D. Kühne

Definition

Stenosis of the spinal canal results in compression or narrowing of the dural sac or myelon. The neural structures are compromised in the spinal canal, in the lateral recess and in the intervertebral foramen. The disorder is congenital or acquired, or there is a combination of a primarily preformed narrow spinal canal with alterations of a mostly degenerative nature occurring later.

Etiology and Pathogenesis

Congenital causes of spinal canal stenosis include:

- idiopathic form with short pedicles of the vertebral arches,
- disorders encompassing disturbances of skeletal growth:

  - achondroplasia,
  - mucopolysaccharidosis,
  - multiple hereditary exostoses,
  - Down's syndrome,
  - progressive scoliosis,
  - congenital disturbances of vitamin D metabolism.

The *acquired causes* are of traumatic, postoperative (scar formation and instability), neoplastic, inflammatory (spondylodiskitis, epidural abscess, Paget's disease), metabolic-hormonal (acromegaly, epidural lipomatosis) or degenerative origin, with the latter predominating quantitatively (Remonda *et al.*, 1966; Jinkins, 1999) (Table 4.**1**).

In a population of 158 patients treated surgically for stenosis of the spinal canal, the cause was degenerative in 70 %, congenital in 16 %, and in 14 % of the cases the cause was a combination of both (Lemaire *et al.*, 1995). The degenerative changes involve not only the bony and ligamentous structures surrounding the dural sac but also the intervertebral disks. This can be explained by the fact that the bony spinal changes usually occur only after the development of disk degeneration with a corresponding protrusion or disk herniation. Since disk degeneration is usually also associated with loss of interspace height, this in turn promotes the development of spondylarthrotic changes, even to the extent of subluxation of the small vertebral joints, which consequently leads to hypertrophy of the ligamenta flava. From a pathogenetic viewpoint, therefore, the cause of spinal stenosis is disk degeneration together with the sequelae of protrusion or prolapse, loss of disk height and potential structural fault within a segment.

In detail, the following degenerative findings can be detected with the aid of imaging techniques, especially MRI and CT:

- intervertebral osteochondrosis (degeneration of the nucleus pulposus and the end plates),
- spondylosis deformans (degeneration of the annulus fibrosus with the formation of spondylophytes),

as well as the resultant disk displacements:
- spondylarthrosis (degeneration of the joint facets with the formation of bony extensions),
- degeneration and hypertrophy of the ligamenta flava,
- spondylolisthesis (spondylolysis or degeneration of the joint facets),
- intraspinal synovial cysts in association with spondylarthrosis.

Incidence

Degenerative changes of the lumbar spine increase with age and in 70-year-olds are detectable in 100 % of cases. Consequently, the majority of patients with stenosis of the spinal canal are in their middle and later lives, although degenerative changes of the spine can become symptomatic in the form of stenosis of the spinal canal as early as the fourth or fifth decade of life in the case of constitutionally narrow spinal canal.

Table 4.1   Acquired forms of spinal stenosis

Osseous:
- retrospondylosis
- facet joint hypertrophy
- spondylolisthesis
- Paget's disease
- rachitis
- post-traumatic

Ligamentous:
- hypertrophy of the ligamenta flava
- calcification and ossification of the ligaments (posterior longitudinal ligament, ligamentum flavum)
- DISH (diffuse idiopathic skeletal hyperostosis)
- gout
- oxalosis
- hyperparathyroidism and secondary hyperparathyroidism
- metabolic-hormonal
- lipomatosis
- acromegaly

Postoperative/post-inflammatory
neoplastic

Clinical Presentation

The lumbar segments L4/L5 and L5/S1 are most frequently affected. The patients present with:

- low back pain (87 %),
- radicular pain (82 %),
- neurogenic claudication (58 %).

A neurologic deficit manifests itself in 37 % of cases (Lemaire et al.1995).

Amundsen *et al.* (1995) report the following frequency distributions for the individual symptoms:

- low back pain (95 %),
- neurogenic claudication (91 %),
- leg pain (82 %),
- weakness in the legs (33 %),
- bladder or bowel disturbances (12 %).

Radicular symptoms were bilateral in 42 % of cases and unilateral in 58 % of cases. The L5 roots were affected in 91 % of cases, the S1 roots in 63 % of cases, the L1–L4 roots in 28 % of cases, and the S2–S5 roots in 5 % of cases. In 47 % of cases two levels were affected, in 35 % of cases one level, in 17 % of cases three levels, and in 1 % of cases four levels.

Vascular and neurogenic forms of spinal claudication can be difficult to differentiate on clinical grounds. Classically, the symptoms of neurogenic spinal claudication consist of diffuse pain in both legs associated with numbness and weakness. The complaints are bilateral and of longer duration. Symptoms are exacerbated by walking and standing upright and alleviated by flexion of the spine. Facultatively, radicular pain, paresthesias and sexual dysfunction can also occur (Jinkins, 1999).

Rare differential diagnoses include degenerative disorders of the hips, knees and pelvic ring, neurological diseases such as diabetic neuropathy and amyotrophic lateral sclerosis, demyelinating diseases, as well as cervical myelopathy. And finally, a retroperitoneal tumor can also be the cause of the symptoms (Hilibrand and Rand, 1999).

Both radicular and myelopathic symptoms, as well as their combinations, can occur in cervical forms of spinal stenosis. The radicular symptoms can be associated with paresthesias, numbness and muscular weakness, initially unilaterally. Numbness and weakness is observed in both legs in cervical myelopathy, with disturbances of depth perception also occurring.

Parameters and Morphology

The normal form of the lumbar spinal canal is a transverse oval, i.e. the transverse diameter (interpeduncular distance) is larger than the sagittal diameter. Although there are interindividual differences regarding the normal width of the spinal canal, depending on height, weight and age (Karantanas *et al.*, 1998), the following dimensions can be regarded as points of reference (Ciric *et al.*, 1980; Lackner *et al.*, 1982; Dorwart *et al.*, 1983).

- interpeduncular distance at least 16 mm,
- sagittal diameter at least 11.5 mm,
- width of the lateral recess at least 3 mm,
- maximum thickness of the ligamenta flava 4–5 mm.

These dimensions are the absolute values of the bony spinal canal alone without reference to the width of the dural sac and dural sac stenoses not resulting from bony changes, such as a disk herniation (Helms and Vogler, 1983).

Two measuring techniques in particular have proven themselves for determining bony stenosis of the cervical canal:

- Measurement of the sagittal diameter of the cervical canal and the vertebral body and calculation of their ratio (Torg *et al.*, 1986; Pavlov *et al.*, 1987):

$$\frac{\text{sagittal diameter of the cervical canal}}{\text{sagittal diameter of the vertebral body}}$$

- A technique that determines the absolute diameter of the spinal canal. These measured values have been derived exclusively with the aid of conventional radiographs.

The disadvantage of this method, which is based upon absolute values, lies in the fact that these values are subject to the magnification factor with which the x-rays were obtained. This factor, however, is not always known. If one considers that measuring differences from 20–30 % can occur due to the magnification factor, then this shows how uncertain this method is.

Torg's ratio method, on the other hand, has found widespread use in the literature. It was originally based on the results compiled from top athletes with and without clinical complaints in the region of the cervical spine. The average value determined by Torg in asymptomatic athletes was 0.94 ± 0.125 (examination of 3314 cervical segments). According to Castro et al., (1997), findings with a Torg ratio of 0.8 were not clinically conspicuous. However, according to reports in the literature, symptoms were frequently found with ratios of 0.70 and lower. The most advanced cervical stenosis was most frequently measured at the C7 segment.

The mean values calculated using the absolute method are summarized in Table 4.2.

Table 4.2 Mean values according to the absolute method

	Males	Females
Mean value (C3–C6)	19 mm ± 0.19	17 mm ± 0.14
Range of variation	14–23.5 mm	15–20 mm

Studies comparing these parameters with those obtained from conventional radiography as well as from CT and MRI (Herzog *et al.*, 1991) revealed only a slight correlation between these three examination methods. Although the correlation coefficient comparing plain radiographs with CT amounted to 0.82, which may be regarded as a good score, the correlation coefficient between CT and MRI was only 0.64. This results from the difficulties of imaging bony structures by MRI.

The deformation of the spinal canal and the subsequent constriction of the dural sac are more important than these parameters for practical purposes. This constriction can extend even to the complete compression of the dural sac, as can be demonstrated by myelography and postmyelo- graphic CT. The concave-shaped or the erect-shaped form resulting from broadening of the bony and ligamentous structures is characteristic of degenerative lumbar stenosis of the spinal canal. This form can be demonstrated on axial sections of the affected spinal segment. The epidural fat in the spinal canal is no longer visible and is an indication of the clinical significance of the stenosis (Helms and Vogler, 1983).

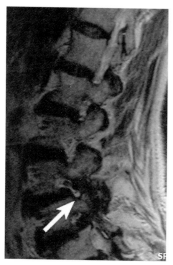 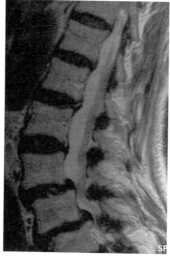 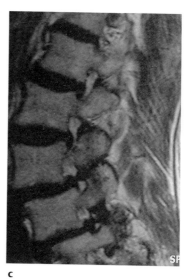

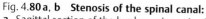
a   b   c

Fig. 4.79 a–c Marked, degenerative spinal stenosis in the distal lumbar spine:

a T2-weighted parasagittal section through the foramina (TSE; TR = 3700 ms, TE = 120 ms): There are obvious stenoses in the intervertebral foramina at L3/L4 and L4/L5 of diskal and bony origin. A disk protrusion is one cause, particularly obvious at L3/L4, with the other being facet hypertrophy of the superior articular surface of L4, which is causing narrowing of the foramen from a dorsal direction (arrow).

b Slice displaced a few millimeters further in a midsagittal direction: Marked stenosis, above all in the region of L4, secondary to considerable hypertrophy of the ligamenta flava with concomitant mild retrospondylophytic reaction and disk protrusion.

c Parasagittal slice through the foramina of the contralateral side: Here too, stenosis of the foramina L3/L4, L4/L5 and L5/S1 is identifiable.

Fig. 4.80 a, b Stenosis of the spinal canal: ▷

a Sagittal section of the lumbar spine using T1 weighting (TSE; TR = 800 ms, TE = 12 ms): Combined bony, diskal and ligamentous stenosis at the sections L2–L5. The spinal canal clearly appears narrowed. There is, in part, an increased fatty deposition visible in the dorsal sections.

Fig. 4.80 b s. p. 234

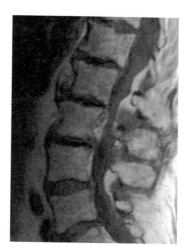

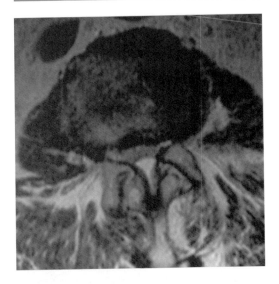

Special attention should be paid to any obliteration in the cervical canal of the subarachnoid space ventrally and dorsally and to a possible compression of the myelon, which can be further intensified by folds in the ligamenta flava.

Fig. 4.80 b T2-weighted transverse section (TSE; TR = 5640 ms, TE = 120 ms): The spinal canal displays an almost trifoliate, triangular narrowing, resulting primarily from hypertrophy of the facet joints. The dural sac clearly appears flattened. The epidural space is filled with fatty tissue dorsally, resulting in a mild convex bulge of the dural margin. The individual nerve roots are not delineated.

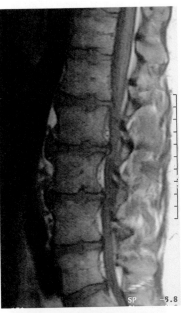
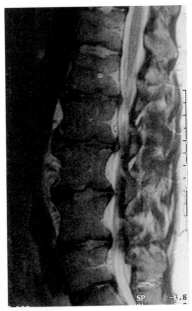
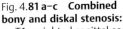

a

b

Fig. 4.81 a–c Combined bony and diskal stenosis:

a T1-weighted sagittal section (TSE; TR = 800 ms, TE = 12 ms): Long-segment stenosis of the lumbar spine in the region L2–S1. Disk protrusions with reactive bony changes of the vertebral end plates. Evidence of multiple Schmorl's nodes.

b T2-weighted image (TSE; TR = 3700 ms, TE = 120 ms): The image clearly demonstrates compression of the dural sac. The individual nerve roots are clustered together and not definable. The signal inside the spinal canal is reduced as a result of the altered CSF flow, yet distal to the stenosis in the region L5/S1 it is increased because in this segment CSF flow is reduced.

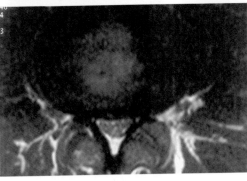

c Transverse image through the level C3/C4 (TSE; TR = 5400 ms, TE = 120 ms): Frank narrowing of the spinal canal. The nerve roots completely fill the dural sac.

Diagnostics

X-ray Diagnostics

For most patients imaging diagnostics for back pain will begin with conventional survey views of the spine in two planes. If this does not assist diagnosis and the patient's symptoms persist despite conservative treatment, then modern sectional imaging is employed for further diagnostics. If the conventional views reveal no pathological finding and the patient complains of insufferable pain or a newly occurring neurological deficit is found, then MRI or CT or both should be used immediately for further diagnostics. Watching and waiting are not indicated when an infection or neoplasia is the cause for the complaints, or with newly occurring symptoms after surgery.

MRI and CT

Initially, *MRI* is the diagnostically most reliable method for differentiating between congenital, neoplastic and degenerative causes of spinal canal stenosis and associated pathological findings.

MRI allows assessment of the bone marrow, the ligaments, the myelon with the cauda equina, and the nerve roots. Due to the pathological blood-nerve barrier, the latter will demonstrate enhancement after intravenous application of a paramagnetic contrast material when compression secondary to spinal canal stenosis is present (Jinkins, 1999).

The form and width of the spinal canal is also adequately displayed, even though *plain CT* provides more precise results in the assessment of bony changes (Figs. 4.**79**–4.**85**).

Myelography with subsequent myelo-CT is diagnostically very reliable, especially for spinal canal stenosis whether with or without possible multi-level involvement, which is not infrequent. The inflow of contrast agent into the dural sac can first be assessed as a dynamic process by using fluoroscopy. If there is a cut-off in the contrast column, the neurosurgeon will gain most valid information about the disk segment where the maximum of stenosis is located (Jinkins, 1999) (Fig. 4.**86**).

Furthermore, a *postmyelographic CT* can assess the form and width of the dural sac very well. This procedure allows a precise differentiation between bony and soft tissue-related compressions

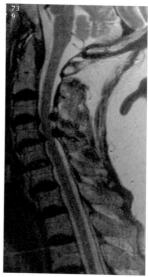

Fig. 4.**82 Combined ligamentous, diskal, and bony stenosis at the segmental region of C3–C5.** T2-weighted sagittal section (TSE; TR = 3640 ms, TE = 120 ms): Noticeable is the considerable hypertrophy of the ligamenta flava contributing to a conspicuous compression of the spinal cord from a dorsal direction, in addition to the compression by the disks. There is also an identifiable structural fault with mild anterior listhesis of C4 over C5.

of the dural sac and offers advantages over MRI in the presence of severely scoliotic spines.

MR myelography is also being increasingly used to assess the dural sac. Basically two techniques can be employed:

- *three-dimensional TSE myelography* with corresponding three-dimensional postprocessing with the aid of MIP (maximum intensity projection).
- *single-shot T2 sequences* using high-volume scanning with which an image can be acquired within seconds are much less time-consuming. Here, several projections can be obtained in a short time and postprocessing of the images is not necessary (Demaerel *et al.*, 1997).

Other working groups prefer strongly *T2*-weighted three-dimensional GRE sequences* for MR-myelography and obtain results comparable to those of conventional myelography (Ramsbacher *et al.*, 1997) (Fig. 4.**87**).

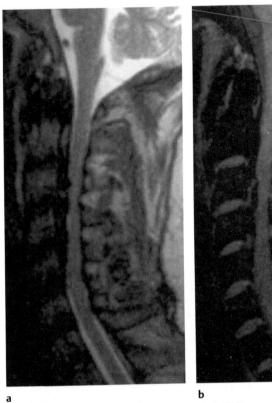

a

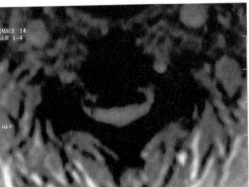

b

c

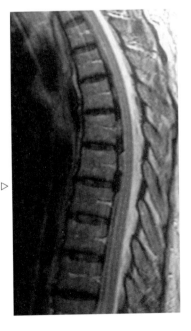

Fig. 4.**83 a–c** **Extensive calcification of the posterior longitudinal ligament in the cervical spine:**
a T2-weighted sagittal section (TSE; TR = 4600 ms, TE = 112 ms): Long-segment calcification of the posterior longitudinal ligament primarily in the region C2–C5. High-grade narrowing of the spinal canal with compression of the myelon.
b T1-weighted sagittal section (GRE sequence; TR = 403 ms, TE = 11 ms, flip angle α = 90°): The calcification along the length of the longitudinal ligament is also well shown on this image.
c Transverse section (GRE sequence): The use of a GRE sequence results in an overemphasis of the calcification of the longitudinal ligament in the presence of scleroderma. The hypertrophy is particularly clear due to the susceptibility artifacts.

Fig. 4.**84** **Long-segment calcification of the posterior longitudinal ligament in the region of the thoracic spine with clear compression of the spinal cord.** The T2-weighted sagittal image (TSE; TR = 5300 ms, TE = 120 ms) shows the calcification in the proximal and middle region of the thoracic spine, appearing as a rather irregularly formed contour along the length of the calcified posterior longitudinal ligament. The kyphosis of the thoracic spine brings the spinal cord to lie directly over this calcification, thus causing compression of the myelon.

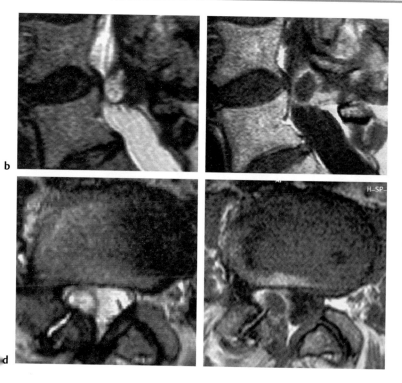

Fig. 4.**85 a–d** Synovial cyst at L3/L4 on the right side secondary to facet degeneration:

a T2-weighted sagittal section with compressive intraspinal cyst.

b T1-weighted sagittal section after contrast application: Peripheral enhancement.

c, d Corresponding transverse sections: T2-weighted (**c**) and T1-weighted after contrast administration (**d**).

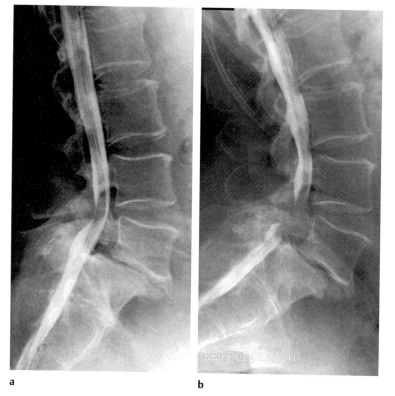

Fig. 4.**86 a, b** Functional myelography in a patient with spondylolisthesis:

a Flexion: Narrowing of the spinal canal from a dorsal direction at the level L4/L5.

b Extension: Interruption of the contrast column at L5.

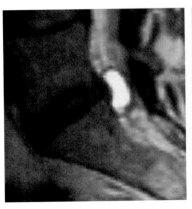
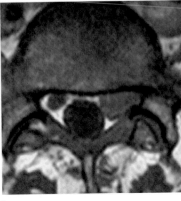

a   **b**

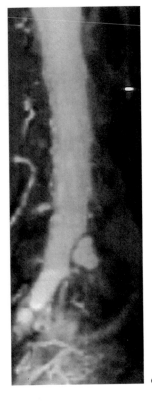

c

Fig. 4.**87 a–c Juxta-articular cyst at L5/S1:**
a T2-weighted sagittal section: Depiction of the signal-intense cyst.
b T1-weighted transverse section: Cyst outlined on the left in the lateral recess.
c MR-myelography: Cyst and CSF space appear signal-intense.

Since CSF serves as an endogenic contrast medium, segments distal to any obstruction of the contrast column that intrathecal contrast medium is unable to reach when using conventional myelography become assessable with MR-myelography (Freund *et al.*, 1997). Pilot studies examining *MR-myelography with intrathecal application of gadolinium* have already been conducted (Zeng *et al.*, 1999).

Because of the lack of space in the coil, functional studies of the lumbar spine are performed in the supine or prone position in order to simulate extension and flexion. Other approaches try to simulate functional states of the lumbar spine during MRI and CT by axial loading, similar to functional myelographic studies of the lumbar spine taken while standing (Willén *et al.*, 1997).

MRI Findings after Lumbar Disk Surgery

The indication for postoperative MRI examination is if no adequate resolution of symptoms has been achieved after surgery or when pain reappears after a symptom-free interval. These symptoms are covered by the term "failed back surgery syndrome" (FBSS) and can be of the most varied origins.

Recurrent herniation is regarded as the cause in only about 5–10 % of these cases. In the remaining cases the symptomatic picture is elicited by scar changes or segmental instability. Whereas patients with recurrent herniation can often undergo successful revision surgery, this is not the case in patients with scar changes of the epidural space.

MRI allows a differentiation to be made between recurrent herniation and scar tissue, provided the examination is performed using contrast material. MRI can also assist in verifying or excluding other causes of symptoms occurring after surgery, such as postoperative spondylodiskitis or bony spinal stenosis, especially of the lateral recess and the foramina.

Postoperative Course

The histological picture undergoes considerable changes, particularly within the first 6 months after surgery. Seroma formation is found during the early days, sometimes accompanied by a hematoma, which can take on a considerable space-occupying character. This can result in deformation of the dural sac and displacement of the nerve roots, not dissimilar to the preoperative effect of the herniated disk. This effect is usually most conspicuous in the early days after surgery and may lead to misinterpretation of the MRI findings.

The formation of granulation tissue in association with marked vascularization is encountered at a very early stage. This tissue, which develops during the first weeks and months, leads to an increasing retraction of the scar tissue in the surrounding structures so that the initial compression of the dural sac then turns into scarry retraction, usually posterolaterally. The nerve root can be included in this scar tissue and also appears displaced in some cases (Annertz *et al.*, 1995). Ac-

cording to experimental studies by Nguyen *et al.* (1993), scar tissue demonstrates various degrees of density and organization. Apart from regions with a high density and a high degree of organization of the fibrous tissue, there are also areas that consist of more loosely organized collagen and protein-containing extracellular material. The consequence is that not only are there regions with varying degrees of vascularization, including zones with a large amount of vascular ingrowth, but also sections with only slight vascularization. In contrast with old scar tissue, newly developed scar tissue usually displays a higher degree of inhomogeneity with zones of only poorly organized tissue structure. This is of importance when using a contrast agent during MRI studies.

MRI Findings

■ Sequences

First of all non-contrast MRI should be performed using standard sequences and obtaining sagittal and transverse sections.

After contrast application, the use of a fat-saturated T1-weighted sequence with a transverse slice orientation is recommended because fat saturation can further improve diagnostic reliability (Georgy *et al.*, 1995). Although differentiation of scar from herniated disk with the use of a contrast medium is already 96 % accurate without fat saturation (Ross *et al.*, 1990), the addition of fat saturation clearly increases contrast and thus improves reliability even further. The distinction between recurrent disk herniation or residual disk herniation and scar tissue becomes clear and the extent of the scar-tissue structures can be better assessed. In addition, visualization of further areas of enhancement, such as the intervertebral disk space and dorsal structures of the disk, nerve roots, ganglia and facet joints, can be improved with regard to their contrast behavior (Georgy *et al.*, 1995).

The examination should be rounded off with a sagittal sequence using T1-weighting without fat saturation.

■ Signal Behavior after Surgery

The seroma, which appears during the first weeks after surgery, displays intermediate signal intensity on T1-weighted images, similar to that of disk tissue. During the first few days after the operation, this signal can appear somewhat inhomogeneous due to hemorrhage. A largely homogeneous signal enhancement is found on the T2-weighted image. Surgery will render the posterior margin of the disk less definable. This is explained by the fact that the annulus and the posterior longitudinal ligament are partially removed during the operation to facilitate access to the disk space. The dark posterior margin of annulus and ligament is therefore lacking, the granulation tissue that forms after surgery directly overlies the disk and also encroaches in part upon the disk space.

Once scar tissue formation is complete in the following months, its signal behavior does not change on plain images. The scar tissue structures display intermediate signal intensity on the T1-weighted image and intermediate to high signal intensity on the T2-weighted image. Years after surgery, scar tissue can appear isointense or hypointense on the T2-weighted image in comparison with the nucleus of the disk.

The surgical defect in the posterior margin of the disk becomes less visible and is sometimes even closed completely. This is the reason why the annulus can appear intact on these images (Hochhauser *et al.*, 1988). The distinction between recurrence and scar formation on plain images can also be rendered impossible in this phase (Figs. **4.88–4.93**).

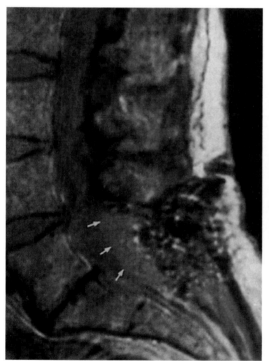

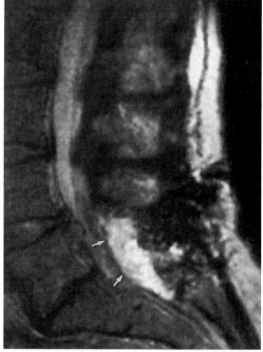

a

Fig. 4.88 a, b Postoperative images 14 days after left-sided disk surgery on L5/S1:

a Laminectomy L5. Numerous small metal artifacts dorsally in the soft tissues and in the region of the laminectomy. Dorsal epidural seroma with an intermediate signal intensity, which is somewhat en-

hanced in comparison with the dura (arrows) (SE; TR = 2100 ms, TE = 20 ms).

b T2-weighted image (SE; TR = 2100 ms, TE = 80 ms): Signal enhancement of the tissue structures after surgery (arrows).

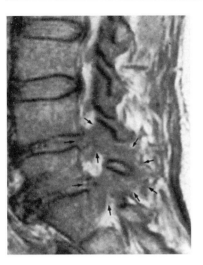

◁ Fig. 4.**89** **Postoperative images following left-sided disk surgery on L4/L5 and L5/S1.** The image demonstrates interruption of the darkly outlined posterior margin of the disk at both levels and in its stead a wide attachment of the dorsal aspect of the disks to the scar tissue which also fills out the epidural fat, resulting in a corresponding reduction in signal in the epidural space. The scar tissue even extends far paravertebrally. The dark boundary of the posterior margins of disks L2/L3 and L3/L4 results from a summation of annulus fibrosis, Sharpey's fibers, and posterior longitudinal ligament (arrows).

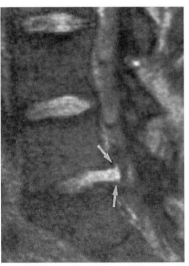

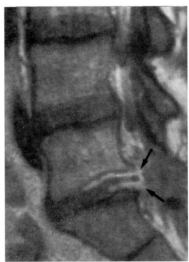

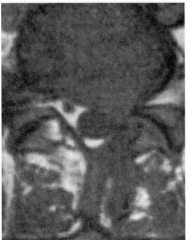

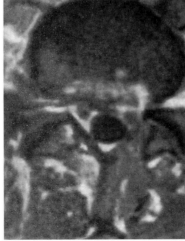

Fig. 4.**90 a–d** **Postoperative images following left-sided disk surgery at L5/S1 several months previously:**

a T2-weighted parasagittal image (SE; TR = 2100 ms, TE = 80 ms): Marked formation of granulation tissue reaching intraspinally and merging into the disk space. The tissue displays a very high signal intensity (arrows).

b Sagittal image (SE; TR = 550 ms, TE = 20 ms): After contrast application, evidence of a strong accumulation of granulation tissue with the contrast enhancement extending far intradiskally along the cartilaginous end plate (arrows).

c Transverse section through the level L5/S1 (SE; TR = 550 ms, TE = 20 ms): Here the scar tissue is insufficiently outlined against both the dural sac and the disk. The S1 root on the left appears obscured.

d After contrast application, conspicuous enhancement of the scar tissue with wide involvement of the intradiskal components. Dural sac and nerve root are now well defined. A recurrent herniation can be ruled out.

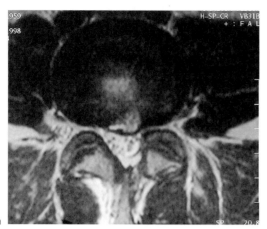

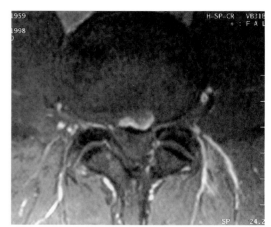

a

Fig. 4.91 a, b Postoperative images after disk surgery:
a T2-weighted transverse image a few months after surgery on the L3/L4 disk (TSE; TR = 4900 ms, TE = 120 ms): The interruption in the bony margin of the lamina is visible on the left side of this image, as is the postoperative defect in the ligamenta flava on

the left. The granulation tissue in the posterior fiber ring of the disk shows a mild compression of the dural sac. It displays high signal intensity. In the posterior margin of the disk there is a wide interruption in the course of the annulus.
b After contrast application there is a strong marginal enhancement along the granulation tissue.

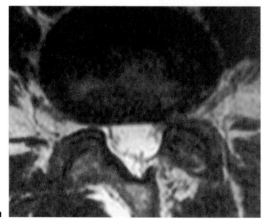

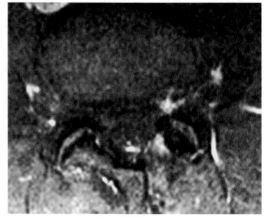

a

Fig. 4.92 a, b Postoperative images after disk surgery several years previously at the level L4/L5:
a T2-weighted transverse image (TSE; TR = 4500 ms, TE = 120 ms): Evidence of the bone defect in the lamina on the left. There is no clear surgery-related finding, either epidurally or in the region of the posterior margin of the intervertebral disk.

b Image after contrast application: Subtle contrast enhancement in the dorsal epidural space on the left at the level of the bony window and in the region of the posterior disk margin on the left side consistent with low-grade formation of granulation tissue.

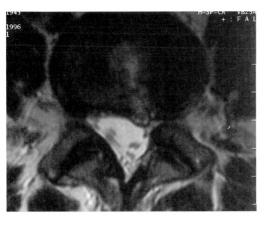

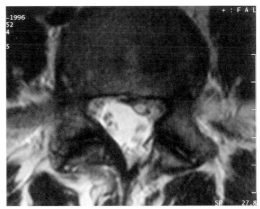

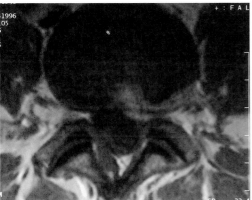

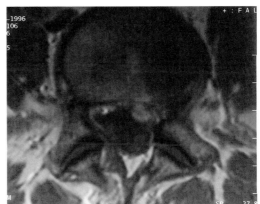

Fig. 4.93 a–d 6 years after left-sided surgery of disk L4/L5:

a T2-weighted transverse image through the level L4/L5: Tongue-shaped contour alteration at the dorsal disk margin left-midlaterally. Mild signal enhancement in this section with additional enhancement running linearly deep into the disk.

b T2-weighted transverse image 4 mm caudal to **a**: Questionable herniation toward the recess on the left, encroaching on nerve root L5.

c T1-weighted transverse image after contrast application through an identical level to **a**: Conspicuous wide contrast enhancement with inclusion of the annulus, consistent with scar tissue formation. The left intraforaminal disk margin is also enhanced with contrast agent.

d Image at an identical level to **b**: Contrast enhancement on the left at the level of the recess and linearly in the disk space: Granulation-tissue formation, no recurrent herniation.

■ Administration of Contrast Medium

After contrast application in the first few days after surgery, there is only a marginal signal enhancement corresponding to a fringe of granulation tissue growing into the postoperative seroma from its border. The anterior components of the epidural space facing the disk can be spared from contrast uptake, making differentiation between disk herniation and seroma difficult or impossible (Fig. 4.**94**).

During the subsequent weeks and months after surgery there is a largely homogeneous enhancement of the scar tissue after contrast application,

with inhomogeneities possibly appearing, depending on the stage of scar maturity and the density of the vascular structures. The contrast enhancement effect is the result of the flow of the contrast agent into the extra-cellular space. The following three preconditions are necessary for this effect:

- capillary supply of the region,
- large interstitial extracellular space,
- loose junctions between the endothelial cells as a prerequisite for contrast flow, which is dependent upon the molecular structure of the contrast agent administered.

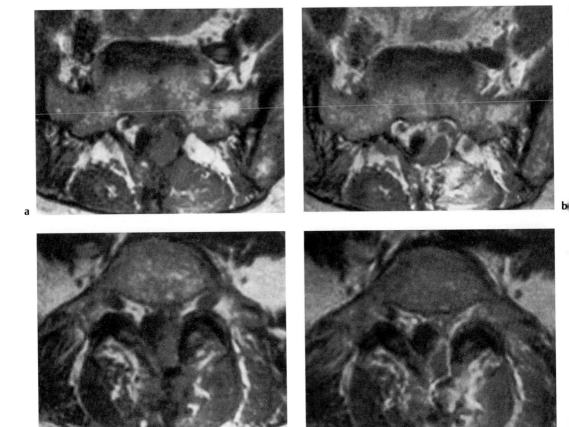

Fig. 4.**94 a–d   Seroma formation 14 days after left-sided surgery of disk L5/S1:**

a T1-weighted plain image (SE; TR = 750 ms, TE = 25 ms): The image shows a structure with a space-occupying effect to the left of the dural sac with intermediate signal intensity.

b Marginal circumferential enhancement after contrast application. The central areas of the tissue, which has formed after surgery, do not enhance with contrast.

c Slice at the level of the foramina L5 (SE; TR = 950 ms, TE = 25 ms): Here too, the left-epidural tissue that has formed after surgery gives a space-occupying impression.

d After contrast application the image again shows marginal enhancement.

Contrast enhancement is considerably stronger in the scar than in the herniated disk, amounting to an average of 120–150 % in the scar tissue as opposed to an almost lack of contrast uptake by the recurrent herniation. This allows differentiation between recurrent or residual herniation and scar tissue in a high percentage of cases (Figs. 4.**95**–4.**102**).

It is, however, important to know that enhancement of scar tissue reaches its peak during the first 15 minutes after the injection and declines afterward. The herniated disk can display a very delayed and slow contrast uptake, causing delayed images 30–45 minutes after contrast administration to produce a false-positive effect. The herniated disk then demonstrates the same or a higher contrast enhancement in comparison with scar tissue (Fig. 4.**103**) (Ross *et al.,* 1989, Hamm *et al.,* 1993).

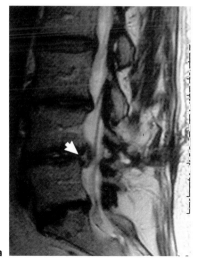

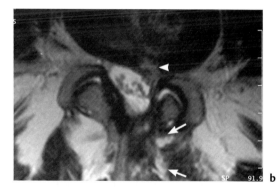

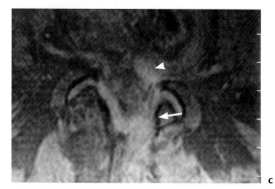

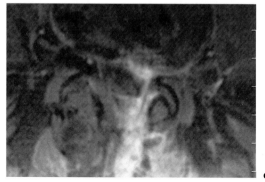

Fig. 4.**95 a–d** **Postoperative images 3 months after disk surgery at the segment L4/L5:**

a T2-weighted sagittal image (TSE; TR = 4000 ms, TE = 120 ms): The image clearly shows dorsal scar tissue, which corresponds to the surgical approach to the spinal canal. Brighter zones are recognizable in some sections, more likely as an expression of fluid retention. Dorsal to the disk there is relatively bright epidural tissue with a somewhat space-occupying effect and a marginal reduction in signal (arrow).

b T2-weighted image in transverse slice orientation (TSE; TR = 4800 ms, TE = 120 ms): The image shows to the left of the spinous process the relatively strong inhomogeneous granulation tissue, which is not yet completely interspersed with scar tissue. The interruption in the region of the ligamentum flavum is also filled with scar tissue. Access to the disk via a left-epidural approach can be seen as a signal-intense interruption along the course of the annulus fibrosus (arrows).

c T1-weighted plain image (SE with fat saturation; TR = 1040 ms, TE = 14 ms): Relatively substantial granulation tissue making a wide appearance along the spinous process and reaching epidurally into the diskal structures (arrows).

d Image after contrast application: There is a homogeneous, strong enhancement of the granulation tissue with the enhanced structures also extending to the opening in the disk area along the course of the annulus fibrosus.

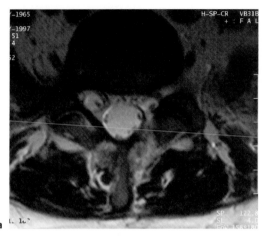

a

Fig. 4.**96 a–e Images 2 years after disk surgery at the level L5/S1:**

a T2-weighted transverse image (TSE; TR = 4500 ms, TE = 120 ms): The interruption of the lamina can be recognized easily on this slice orientation, as can the interruption of contour along the ligamentum flavum on the left side. There is no particular scar formation.

b T2-weighted sagittal image (TSE; TR = 3635 ms, TE = 120 ms): Interruption along the lamina at L5/S1. Relatively signal-intensive tissue is visible with individual discrete streaks of compact components, for the most part representing newly formed fatty tissue. High signal intensity within the dorsal disk elements with the annulus not demarcated. Signs of instability with corresponding hypervascularization in the caudal marginal area of L5.

c T1-weighted sagittal plain image (TSE; TR = 800 ms, TE = 12 ms): Contour defect in the posterior marginal region of the spinal canal at the level of L5/S1 with the tissue defect filled with fibrolipid tissue.

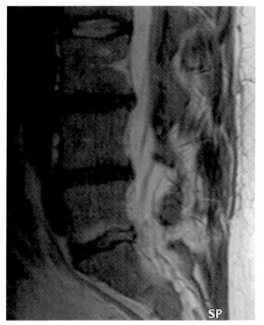

b

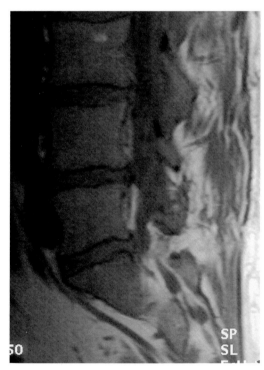

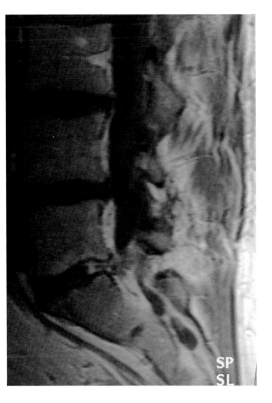

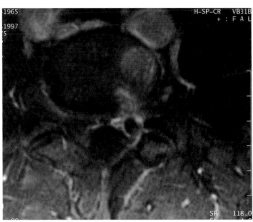

Fig. 4.**96 d–e**

d Image after contrast application: There is enhancement particularly around the posterior disk margin indicating the surgical defect at the annulus, which is filled with granulation tissue.

e Transverse image with fat saturation after contrast application (SE; TR = 540 ms, TE = 20 ms): The epidural contrast enhancement is easily identifiable on the left of this image, particularly the signal enhancement around the S1 root consistent with the envelopment of S1 by scar tissue. In addition, the section shows signal enhancement along the annulus fibrosus and the deeper disk components on the left side, reflecting the curettage that has been performed here.

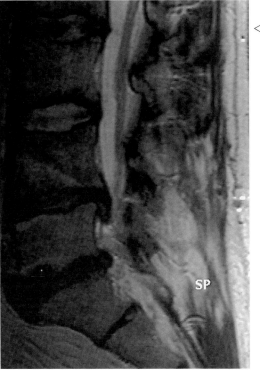

Fig. 4.**97 a–g Images 4 years after disk surgery at the level L4/L5:**

◁ **a** T2-weighted sagittal image (TSE; TR = 5000 ms, TE = 120 ms): An epidural tissue structure is visible at L4/L5, dorsal to the posterior margin of the vertebral body, which is not defined relative to the caudally extruded disk herniation. Note the relatively high signal intensity of this tissue. The dorsal surgical approach to the spinal canal is recognizable by the interruption in the course of the ligamentum flavum. The space is filled with a fibrous structure.

Fig. 4.**97 b–g** ▷

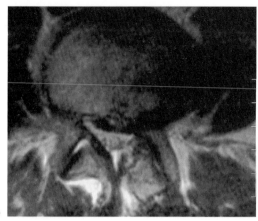
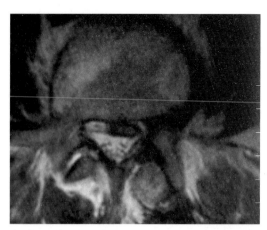

b

Fig. 4.**97 b**, **c** T2-weighted transverse images (TSE; TR = 5000 ms, TE = 120 ms): The images show tissue expanding in a caudal direction, noticeable in the sagittal slice orientation. There is marked compression of the dural sac. The slice of **c** lies 4 mm caudal to **b** and represents the posterior margin of L5. Note the clear signal enhancement in the vertebral joint on the right.

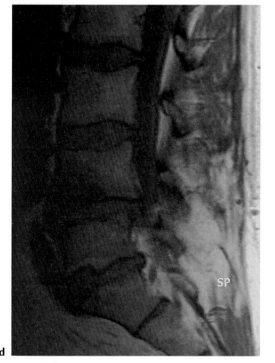
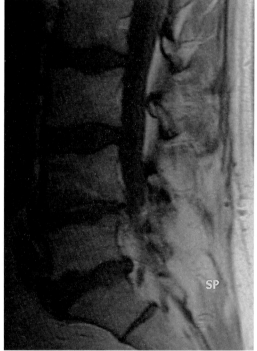

d

Fig. 4.**97 d, e**

d T1-weighted sagittal image (TSE; TR = 800 ms, TE = 12 ms): Marked scar formation at the level of L4/L5 involving both the dorsal surgical approach to the intervertebral disk and the epidural space. Conspicuous reduction in signal, particularly in the anterior part of L4.

e T1-weighted sagittal section after contrast application: Note the teardrop-shaped tissue projecting in a caudal direction and showing contrast enhancement.

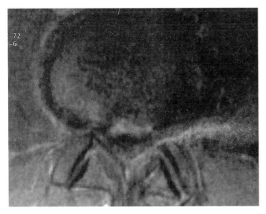

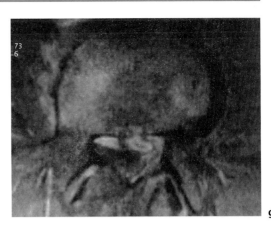

g

Fig. 4.97 f, g

f Transverse section with fat saturation after contrast application. This image is at the corresponding level to **b**: Clear contrast enhancement dorsally in the region of the granulation tissue so that the structures in **b**, resembling a possible disk herniation with a space-occupying effect, appear merely as granulation tissue.

g T1-weighted transverse image with fat saturation after contrast application: The image corresponds to the slice of **c**. Strong contrast enhancement is visible in the granulation tissue dorsally along the posterior margin of L5 on the left side. Recurrent herniation in this region is therefore ruled out.

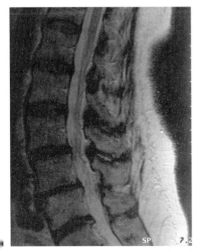

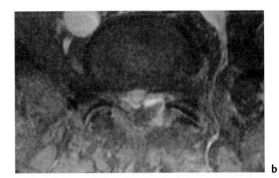

b

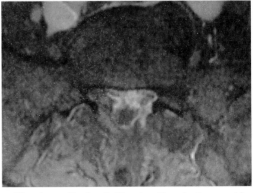

c

Fig. 4.98 a–c Images 18 years after left-sided disk surgery at the level L5/S1:

a T2-weighted sagittal image (TSE; TR = 3400 ms, TE = 120 ms): Even after the long interval between surgery and MRI examination, the granulation tissue appears signal intense in the region of the dorsal disk margin at the level L5/S1 and assumes a pseudo space-occupying character.

b, c *Transverse images with fat saturation after contrast application:*

b There is also strong contrast enhancement consistent with granulation tissue, especially in the dorsal sections of the disk. The S1 root on the right displays enhancement.

c Slice 4 mm distal to **b**: Here too there is strong epidural contrast enhancement consistent with the conspicuous formation of granulation tissue. No evidence of recurrent herniation.

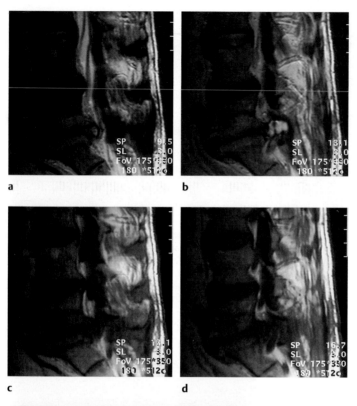

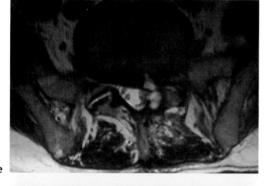

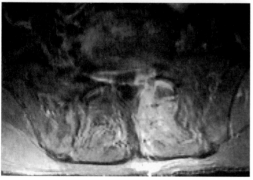

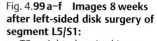

Fig. 4.**99 a–f Images 8 weeks after left-sided disk surgery of segment L5/S1:**

a T2-weighted sagittal image (TSE; TR = 4000 ms, TE = 120 ms): Very high signal intensity in the epidural granulation tissue at the level L5/S1 extending as far as the disk space. Otherwise, marked osteochondrosis as well as evidence of an anterior disk herniation, which appears bridged by osteophytes.

b Image 4 mm lateral to **a**: Marked fluid accumulation at the level of the surgical access to L5/S1 along the ligamentum flavum.

c T1-weighted image in the same slice position as **a**: Homogeneous signal in the operative region rendering differentiation between disk, granulation tissue, and ligamentous structures impossible.

d Corresponding image to **b**: Here too there is a uniform homogeneous tissue of intermediate signal intensity. Differentiation of the dorsal epidural fluid accumulation at the level of the lamina is not possible.

e T2-weighted transverse image (TSE; TR = 4850 ms, TE = 120 ms): The epidural surgical approach is easily identifiable from the signal enhancement of the highly vascularized granulation tissue. There is a wedge-shaped dorsal defect in the disk margin. A conspicuous disk protrusion is still present to the right of this defect.

f T1-weighted image with fat saturation after contrast application: Very strong homogeneous enhancement of the entire granulation tissue. The disk protrusion remains spared as a hypointense structure.

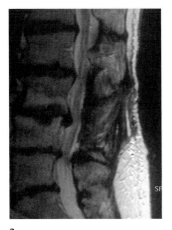

a

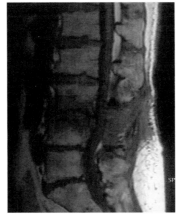

b

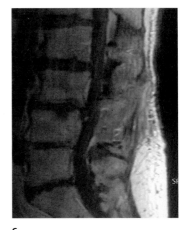

c

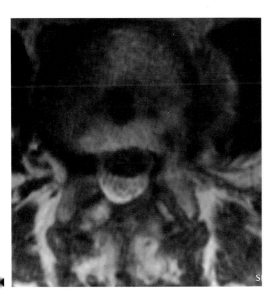

Fig. 4.100 a–e Images after disk surgery and extensive laminectomy at L3/L4 for spinal canal stenosis.
Evidence of recurrent herniation at the L3/L4 segment:

a T2-weighted sagittal section (TSE; TR = 3640 ms, TE = 120 ms): Postoperative laminectomy with the surgical defect filled with scar tissue. The L3/L4 disk displays a clear signal reduction. A Schmorl's node is present in the superior end plate of L4. Osteochondrotic bony changes. Large recurrent herniation with considerable compression of the dural sac displaying no signal.

b T1-weighted sagittal image: Extensive dorsal epidural scar tissue.

c Image after contrast application: Diffuse enhancement of the scar tissue in the dorsal sections. The disk herniation remains spared from contrast enhancement.

d T2-weighted transverse section with evidence of recurrent medial herniation.

Fig. 4.**100 e** ▷

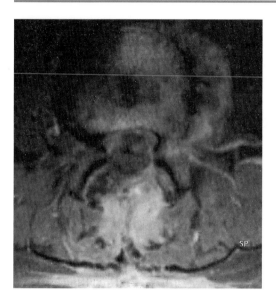

Fig. 4.**100 e** T1-weighted image with fat saturation after contrast application: The disk herniation remains spared from contrast enhancement. Most extensive paravertebral contrast enhancement, particularly on the left side, consistent with a mild concomitant inflammatory reaction (arrow). The recurrent disk herniation has been surgically removed.

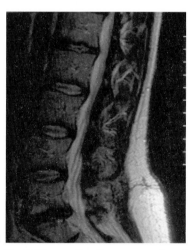

a

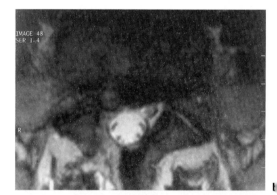

b

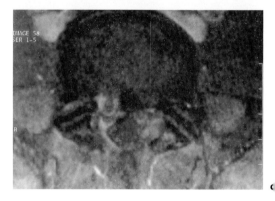

c

Fig. 4.**101 a–c Small recurrent herniation on the right side at the level L5/S1. Images after disk surgery 2 years previously:**

a T2-weighted sagittal section (TSE; TR = 5300 ms, TE = 120 ms): The L5/S1 disk displays clear reduction in height, signal loss and a relatively strong epidural tissue dorsally. No clear differentiation is possible between recurrence and scar tissue.

b Transverse section using T2 weighting (TSE; TR = 4500 ms, TE = 120 ms): Well recognizable laminectomy window on the right with epidural surgical access towards the right. There is a mild signal enhancement along the posterior margin of the disk.

c Corresponding section to **b** after contrast application (SE with fat saturation; TR = 540 ms, TE = 20 ms): The image shows marginal contrast enhancement along the scar tissue. This applies to the posterior margin of the disk with sparing of a recurrent herniation. This disk herniation is the cause of the compression of the S1 root on the right. The S1 nerve root is also enveloped by scar tissue, which has a marginal appearance.

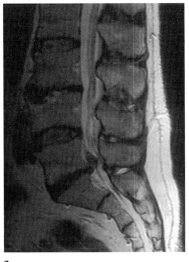
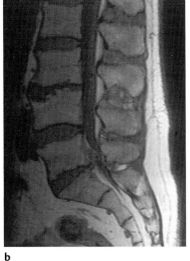

a b

Fig. 4.**102 a–c** **Recurrent herniation L5/S1.** Images after disk surgery 6 years previously:
a T2-weighted sagittal image (TSE; TR = 3400 ms, TE = 120 ms): Osteochondrosis in segment L5/S1, marked concomitant signal reduction in the disk. Recurrent herniation luxated in a cranial direction.
b T1-weighted plain sagittal image (TSE; TR = 800 ms, TE = 12 ms): The recurrent herniated disk is only poorly defined against the dural sac.

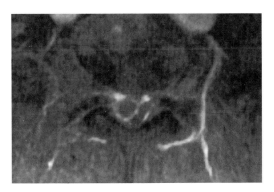

c Transverse image with fat saturation after contrast application (SE; TR = 540 ms, TE = 120 ms): The recurrent herniation displays a marginal contrast reaction. There is no contrast enhancement recognizable within the herniated disk.

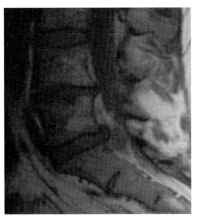
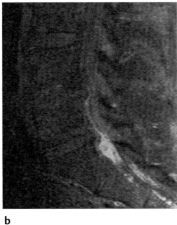

a b

Fig. 4.**103 a–d** **L5/S1 disk herniation:**
a Parasagittal section using T1 weighting (TSE; TR = 800 ms, TE = 17 ms) with evidence of a herniated disk lying in the epidural fat at the level L5/S1.
b Sagittal image obtained 1 hour after contrast application (with fat saturation): Strong enhancement within the disk tissue.

Fig. 4.**103 c** and **d** ▷

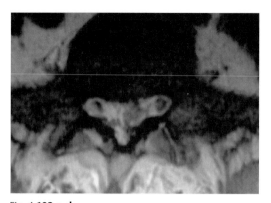

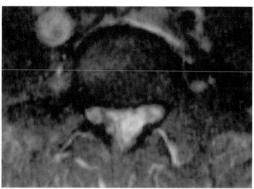

Fig. 4.**103 c, d**
c T2-weighted transverse section (TSE; TR = 5400 ms, TE = 120 ms): Left midlateral disk herniation.

d Transverse section corresponding to Fig. **c** obtained 1 hour after contrast application (SE with fat saturation; TR = 690 ms, TE = 20 ms): Strong, very homogeneous enhancement of the herniated disk. Note the strong contrast enhancement particularly in the vertebral joint on the left.

■ Dosage

It has been shown that signal enhancement can be significantly heightened by increasing the dose of contrast medium to 0.2 or 0.3 mmol, thus improving the diagnostic reliability of the examination (Nguyen *et al.*, 1993). This statement only applies, however, for examinations without the use of fat-saturation sequences after contrast application. No scientific studies to date have examined whether the use of fat saturation will also achieve the same good effect with the lower dose of 0.1 mmol/kg body weight as with the higher dose.

■ Contrast Medium Enhancement in Relation to Scar Age

Contrary to initial opinions (Steiner, 1989), later studies have shown that contrast enhancement declines with the age of the scar (Hamm *et al.*, 1993). This is linked to the fact that the degree of scar-tissue vascularization decreases during the process of ageing. This can result in scars no longer displaying any appreciable contrast reaction after some years.

■ Further Effects of Contrast Administration

There are numerous other effects of contrast application described in the literature (Georgy *et al.*, 1995):

- enhancement of the nerve roots,
- enhancement of the spinal ganglia,
- enhancement of the facet joints.

Enhancement of the nerve roots. Enhancement of the nerve roots applies to both the intradural components and those lying within the nerve sleeve. This reaction in the form of a neuritis or arachnoiditis can have various causes. On the one hand it has been proposed that, depending on the contrast medium used, myelography can cause arachnoiditis when performed before surgery (as it often is). While alternatively, this finding is often encountered secondary to irritation of the nerve root by the herniated disk. And last but not least, it is argued that there is a connection with the operation itself in the form of pressure-related damage. It is not clear which significance is to be attached to this reaction (Fig. 4.**104**).

Enhancement of the spinal ganglia. It is also not possible to assess contrast enhancement of the spinal ganglia unequivocally with respect to its clinical relevance. Enhancement of the spinal ganglia is also observed in patients who have not been operated on. This can be most impressively demonstrated by additional fat saturation (Fig. 4.**105**).

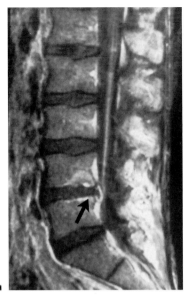

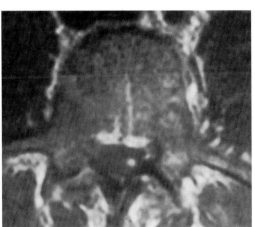

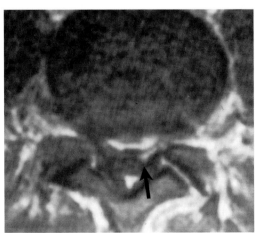

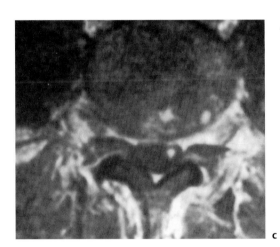

Fig. 4.104 a–d   Severe neuritis of the L5 root on the left side secondary to APLD (automated percutaneous lumbar diskectomy) 4 days previously:

a Sagittal section of the spine after contrast application: There is slight contrast uptake with a corresponding signal enhancement along the end plates in the segmental region L4/L5 (arrow). Furthermore, there are signs of a contrast reaction in the annulus. Note the marked signal enhancement along the L5 root consistent with a severe neuritis.

Fig. 4.104 b–d   Transverse images, each 4 mm caudal to the course of the L5 root on the left: An isolated, strong contrast enhancement of the root can be traced on these images as far as the intervertebral foramen. The exit point of the nerve root at the level of the foramen is conspicuous in **d**. Here the horizontal course is directed to the left (arrow). Conspicuous contrast enhancement of the epidural venous complex consistent with damage and granulation tissue formation in the region of the annulus fibrosus. In addition there is also contrast enhancement of the left facet joint.

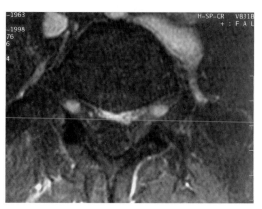

Fig. 4.**105** **T1-weighted transverse image with fat saturation after contrast application** (SE; TR = 540 ms, TE = 20 ms): Strong enhancement both along the course of the epidural venous plexus and bilaterally in the L5 root ganglion on the right and left.

Enhancement of the facet joints. Enhancement of facet joints is sometimes observed even years after disk surgery. The relevance of this is unclear, and whether this effect is related to the operation is just as uncertain because it is also seen in non-operated patients with spondylarthrosis (Figs. 4.**103** and 4.**104**, 4.**106**–4.**108**).

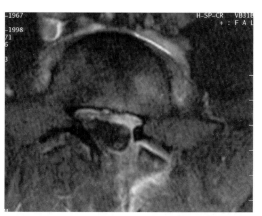

Fig. 4.**106** **Image after left-sided disk surgery of L4/L5.** The images display strong enhancement of the epidural scar tissue and a unilateral enhancement of the vertebral joint on the left side (SE with fat saturation: TR = 540 ms, TE = 20 ms).

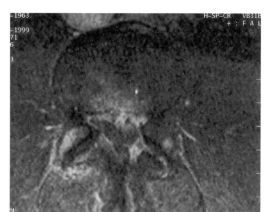

Fig. 4.**107** **Image after disk surgery via a left-sided approach.** Transverse image after contrast application: In particular, there is enhancement of the periarticular soft tissues on the right at the level of the vertebral joint L3/L4 with additional hyperemia of the bone along the facets on the right side. There is a discrete intra-articular contrast enhancement on the left. Enhancement is also present along the ligamentum flavum with extensive epidural enhancement involving the intradiskal components.

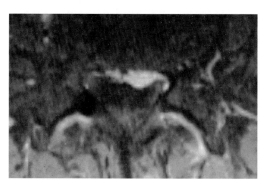

Fig. 4.**108** **Strong bilateral intra-articular enhancement at the level L4/L5.** Marked, slightly asymmetric contrast enhancement of the epidural venous plexus (SE with fat saturation: TR = 690 ms, TE = 20 ms).

■ Limitations

MRI for the purpose of clarifying an FBSS after disk surgery has its limitations. These arise, on the one hand, from the behavior of the contrast medium already described, and, on the other, from differential-diagnostic problems.

Very small recurrent herniations can escape detection due to a partial volume effect because an apparent false-positive contrast enhancement of this tissue appears on the contrast-assisted image. This applies to fragments of 3 mm and less. Spondylophytes can also give rise to misinterpretation, particularly when fat saturation is used, because they can be mistaken for a recurrent or residual herniation. These limitations should be taken into account when interpreting findings and eliminated where necessary by adjusting the examination techniques.

Pseudomeningocele

A rare complication after spinal surgery is the development of a pseudomeningocele. A tear in the dura is a prerequisite for this. If this injury is insufficiently repaired, there will be an accumulation of CSF, which is either enveloped by the arachnoid membrane or a fibrous capsule. The finding can be recognized on MRI from the CSF signal intensity in the sac (cele) (Figs. 4.**109** and 4.**110**).

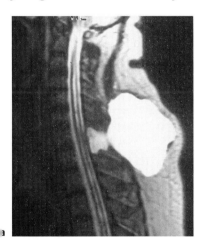

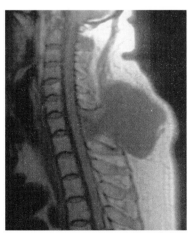

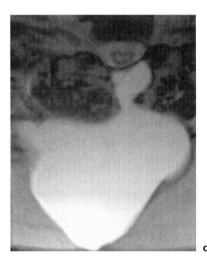

Fig. 4.**109 a–c Large pseudomeningocele following surgery of the cervical spine with insertion of a syringosubarachnoid shunt for syringomyelia involving the entire length of the spinal cord:**
a T2-weighted sagittal image (TSE; TR = 5400 ms, TE = 120 ms): Evidence of an extensive pseudomeningocele at the level C6/C7, which is well defined by the high signal intensity of the fluid. There is a laminar defect at the level C7.
b T1-weighted sagittal image: The fluid is isointense with CSF and is easily seen on this image. The accumulation of CSF produces a dorsal bulge of the skin.
c Transverse section using T2 weighting (TSE; TR = 5600 ms, TE = 120 ms): Evidence of a wide area of contact between the pseudomeningocele and the dura.

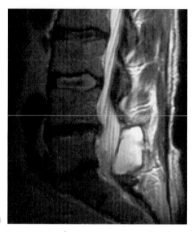

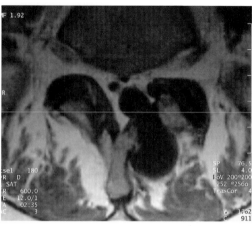

Fig. 4.**110 a, b   Postoperative lumbar pseudomeningocele at the level L5/S1 after disk surgery:**
a T2-weighted sagittal section (TSE; TR = 4000 ms,
TE = 90 ms): Evidence of a large dorsal pseudomeningocele at the level L5.

b T1-weighted transverse section (TSE; TR = 600 ms,
TE = 12 ms): The meningocele extends dorsally along
the bony defect on the left at the level of the lamina.
Delineation from the dural sac is not possible.

Spinal Fusion

Spinal fusion is primarily performed when disk
surgery has not resulted in relief of symptoms.

MRI can assist in providing information on the
stability of the fused segment (Fig. 4.**111**).

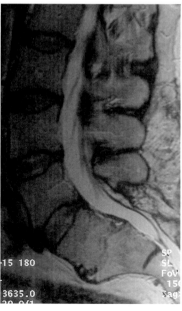

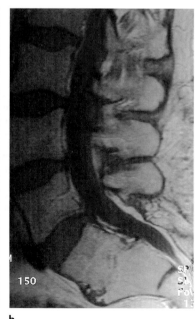

Fig. 4.**111 a, b   Postoperative image after spinal fusion in the L5/S1 segmen-
tal region after previously
failed disk surgery:**
a T2-weighted sagittal
  section: Solid bony fu-
  sion in the segmental
  region L5/S1.
b T1-weighted sagittal
  section: Here too, there
  are no signs of instability in the L5/S1 segmental region.

a

b

MRI Findings after Cervical Disk Surgery

Whereas compressive effects of the disk material secondary to a protrusion or a prolapse primarily elicit clinical symptoms of the lumbar spine, disk herniation of the cervical spine only plays a minor role as a cause of radiculopathy or myelopathy in comparison with cervical spondylosis. This means that, apart from removal of the disk material, it is above all the bony changes that must be surgically addressed. Only about 60–70 % of patients treated have little or no symptoms after surgery, while from 10–15 % deteriorate. There are various reasons for this:

- Inadequate decompression (which refers to the degree of decompression on the one hand and to the affected segment on the other). This is seen on MRI by a persisting deformation of the spinal cord, recognizable along with the offending compressive structure and a corresponding obliteration of the subarachnoid space. If several stenosing segments are present, a mistake in segment selection will be made if only one element is decompressed. In more pronounced cases, a diffuse stenosis of the spinal canal is present, in which case a

segmental operation would not be not indicated (Fig. 4.**112**).

- Spinal cord atrophy secondary to a long-standing compression despite an otherwise adequate decompression (Fig. 4.**78**). Atrophy of the spinal cord is defined as a narrowing of the spinal cord, although sometimes it is merely a change in form without any apparent residual compression. Measurement techniques will confirm atrophy if the cross-sectional diameter is less than 50 mm. It is the result of long-standing compression with irreversible damage to the spinal cord.

- Malacia of the spinal cord, which is defined as an area of persisting signal enhancement in the spinal cord on T2-weighted images. The individual case will reveal a barrier disturbance at this level with corresponding contrast enhancement. Spinal cord malacia is also the result of a long-standing compression of the spinal cord. The finding can develop into a cyst or syrinx.

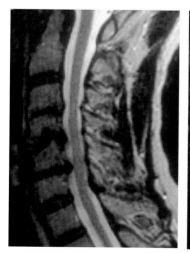 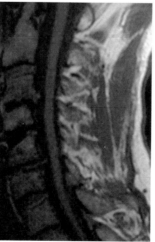

a b

Fig. 4.**112 a–e Postoperative image after Cloward's procedure in the segmental regions C3/C4 and C4/C5.** Inadequate decompression in both segments. Spinal cord atrophy at the level C3/C4 and evidence of mild spinal cord malacia at this level. Additional disk herniation in the C5/C6 segment:

a T2-weighted sagittal image (TSE; TR = 4600 ms, TE = 112 ms): Conspicuous retrospondylosis at C3/C4 and C5/C6. Narrowing of the spinal cord at the level C3/C4. Mild intramedullary signal enhancement consistent with spinal cord malacia. Disk herniation C5/C6 causing malacia of the spinal cord.

b T1-weighted transverse section (SE; TR = 351ms, TE = 12 ms): Clearly recognizable retrospondylosis at C3/C4 and C4/C5. Disk herniation C5/C6.

Fig. 4.**112 c–e** ▷

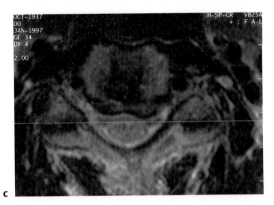

c

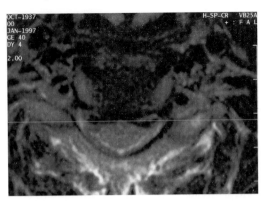

d

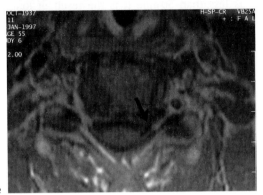

e

Fig. 4.112 c–e

c Transverse section using T2 weighting at the level C3/C4 (TSE; TR = 4320 ms, TE = 120 ms): Easily identifiable bilaterally accentuated retrospondylosis, mild bilateral narrowing of the foramina. Speckled intramedullary signal enhancements.

d Transverse section using T2 weighting at the level C5/C6 (TSE; TR = 4320 ms, TE = 120 ms): Clear bilaterally accentuated disk herniation.

e Transverse image after contrast application (SE; TR = 640 ms, TE = 15 ms): Depiction in this segment of a wide bilateral disk herniation, slightly accentuated on the left. Additional narrowing of the left intervertebral foramen (arrow).

- Development of a recurrent disk herniation after successful fusion of the segment. Fusion of the segment as part of the operation inevitably results in hypermobility of the proximal and distal segments. This finding not infrequently leads to disk herniation in one of the sections adjacent to the fused segment (Fig. 4.**113**).
- Occurrence of spondylosis deformans in an adjoining segment. This finding can also occur in association with increased loading of an adjacent segment proximal and distal to an operated section and, in addition to uncovertebral joint arthrosis and the subsequent impingement of the nerve roots in the foramina, can result in the corresponding development of myelopathy and radiculopathy.

The signal intensity of the adjacent vertebral bodies is inconsistent after surgical fusion. Both reduction in signal on T1-weighted images and signal enhancement on T2-weighted images can occur as an indication of the formation of edema, as well as signal enhancements on the T1-weighted image with an isointense signal on the T2 image as an expression of fatty-marrow degeneration. Not least, sclerosing changes are also known and are associated with a corresponding reduction in signal on T1 and T2 weighting. On T1 and T2 weighting, a signal can appear in the vertebral bodies that is isointense with the adjacent vertebral sections. If a bone dowel is present, then decreased signal intensity is usually found on T1 and T2 weighting.

MR images obtained after cervical disk surgery often display metal-induced artifacts, either as a result of metal abrasion or from inserted metal interposition bodies or, in the case of vertical fusions, from inserted screw material. This should be borne in mind when selecting the sequences, with SE sequences as a rule being preferable to GRE sequences.

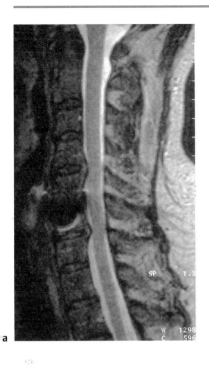

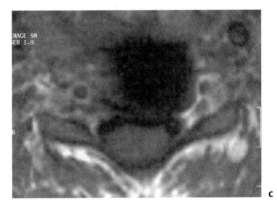

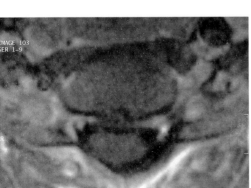

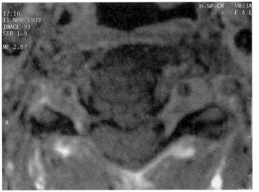

Fig. 4.**113 a–d** Postoperative image after disk surgery in the segment C5/C6 with insertion of a titanium interbody spacer. This female patient was initially asymptomatic after surgery. She redeveloped symptoms after some years, originating from herniations in the adjacent proximal and distal segments:

a T2-weighted sagittal image (TSE; TR = 5300 ms, TE = 112 ms): Signal loss in the region C5/C6 due to the titanium implant. Evidence of a fresh disk herniation at the levels C4/C5 and C6/C7.

b Transverse image at the level C4/C5 after contrast application (SE; TR = 420 ms, TE = 14 ms): Easily recognizable medial compressive disk herniation. The intervertebral foramina appear patent.

c Transverse image at the level C5/C6 after contrast application: Normal appearance of the spinal cord with inconspicuous depiction of the foramina. Signal loss at the level of the vertebral body due to the implanted titanium material.

d Transverse image at the level C6/C7 after contrast application: Here too, the medially accentuated disk herniation is well recognizable. The foramina have an inconspicuous appearance.

Summary

- *Degenerative processes* of the diskovertebral and synovial joints as well as the ligamentous system are all included under the term "degenerative disorders of the spine."
- The intervertebral disk is subject to an ageing process, which can be demonstrated on MRI by using T2-weighted sequences. Consequently, a distinction can be made among four types:
  - Type I (neonatal disk),
  - Type II (child and juvenile disk),
  - Type III (younger adult disk),
  - Type IV (older adult disk).
- With increasing age the signal intensity of the nucleus pulposus on T2-weighted SE sequences diminishes. In the older adult, T2-weighted images no longer allow differentiation between annulus and nucleus.
- The signal intensity of the vertebral body on T1-weighted SE sequences is also subject to physiological alterations. Whereas the signal intensity of the vertebral body of the juvenile and young adult appears lower than that of the intervertebral disk, the opposite is seen in the older adult due to the formation of fatty marrow. This can be regarded as a differential-diagnostic sign if diffuse infiltrations of the bone marrow are present.
- Tears of the annulus fibrosus are recognizable by MRI on strongly T2-weighted images. Four *types of annular tears* are distinguished:
  - concentric tear (disruption of the short longitudinal connecting fibers between the annular lamellae),
  - transverse tear (frequently found in the outermost Sharpey's fibers),
  - radial tear (fissures in the annulus with connections to the nucleus),
  - complete tear (broad disruption of the annulus).
- Mucoid material with additional ingrowth of fibrovascular tissue is found in the cracks of the tears. The tears can become the cause of pain.
- The vertebral bodies are particularly subject to a *process of ageing and remodeling* in the region of the inferior and superior end plates, which can be diagnosed by MRI on T1- and T2-weighted SE sequences. Three types are distinguished:
  - Type I: T1-weighted reduction in signal, T2-weighted signal enhancement,
  - Type II: T1-weighted signal enhancement, T2-weighted signal enhancement,
  - Type III: T1-weighted reduction in signal, T2-weighted reduction in signal.
- Type I corresponds to the formation of edema and fibrovascular tissue, type II to fatty-marrow transformation, type III to sclerosis. Types I and III are often associated with back pain.
- Disk herniations are classified into the *protrusion*, in which the annulus fibers are still largely intact, and the *prolapse* in which the annulus is disrupted. The protrusion is subdivided into the circumscribed form and the bulging form. The prolapse is classified into those of subligamentous and extraligamentous location, while the sequester is no longer attached to the parent disk.
- *Special forms* of disk herniations include the lateral (intra- and extraforaminal), intradural, and anterior forms, as well as the limbus-type herniation in which a shear fracture is found at the posterior margin of the vertebral body.
- *Spondylolisthesis* is often combined with a dorsal disk herniation that has migrated cranially. An intraforaminal stenosis can occur as a result of the spondylolysis.
- The examination technique comprises T1- and T2-weighted images, which should be obtained in transverse and sagittal slice orientation. Whereas GRE sequences are important for imaging the cervical spine, the best results for the lumbar spine are obtained with conventional SE and TSE sequences.
- The main clinical symptoms of patients with degenerative disorders of the spine and disk herniations are lumbalgia and radicular pain, sometimes accompanied by paresthesia. Myelopathy can occur in the region of the cervical spine. Patients with spinal canal stenosis can present a special type of clinical symptoms, which manifest themselves in the form of *spinal claudication*.

Summary

- *Thoracic disk herniations* are often small, but nevertheless elicit clinical symptoms due to their close contact with the spinal cord. Their demonstration demands special requirements from the examination technique because flow, motion and chemical shift artifacts can make imaging difficult.
- Soft and hard disk herniations often occur in combination in the region of the *cervical spine*. MRI can differentiate them with the combined use of SE and GRE sequences.
- Apart from using various measurement options to detect spinal stenosis, *typical image findings* should be looked for:
  - the characteristic concave-shaped or the erect-shaped form in the lumbar region,
  - the obliteration of the subarachnoid space and compression of the myelon in the cervical region.
- As a rule, images after lumbar disk surgery should be obtained with and without contrast application because differentiation between scar tissue and recurrent herniation is only possible after contrast administration. Supplementary fat saturation can prove useful. Care should be taken to obtain thin slices, and the *examination* should be performed *in two planes*.

- Scar tissue already enhances with contrast a few weeks after surgery, whereas a herniated disk does not. However, this is only valid within a time window of about 20 minutes.
- Further effects after surgery are found in the nerve roots, the ganglia, and the facet joints. These inflammatory changes can be made visible by administering a contrast agent.
- The inserted fusion implant material often restricts studies after cervical disk surgery. GRE sequences should be avoided. Signs of incorporation of the inserted material or instability should be looked for.
- Furthermore, the following alterations are often seen:
  - spinal cord atrophy,
  - malacia of the myelon,
  - disk herniation at another level,
  - retrospondylosis.

References

Aguila, L. A., D. W. Piraino, M. T. Modic, A. W. Dudley, P. M. Duchesneau, M. A. Weinstein: The intranuclear cleft of the intervertebral disk: magnetic resonance imaging. Radiology 155 (1985) 155–158

Allgayer, B., A. Frank, D. Daller, H. v. Einsiedel, A. Trappe: Die Magnetresonanztomographie (MRT) in der Diagnostik des Failed Back Surgery Syndroms (FBSS). Fortschr. Röntgenstr. 158 (1993) 160–165

Alvarez, O., C. T. Roque, M. Pampati: Multilevel thoracic disk herniations: CT and MR studies. J. Comput. assist. Tomogr. 12 (1988) 649–652

Amundsen, T., H. Weber, F. Lileas et al.: Lumbar spinal stenosis: clinical and radiologic features. Spine 20 (1995) 1178

Anand, A. K., B. C. P. Lee: Plain and metrizamide CT of lumbar disk disease: comparison with myelography. Amer. J. Neuroradiol. 3 (1982) 567–571

Anda, S., J. Stovring, M. Ro: CT of extraforaminal disc herniation with associated vacuum phenomenon. Neuroradiology 30 (1988) 76–77

Annertz, M., B. Jönsson, B. Strömqvist, S. Holtas: Serial MRI in the early postoperative period after lumbar discectomy. Neuroradiology 37 (1995) 177–182

Awwad, E. E., D. S. Martin, K. R. Smith jr.: The nuclear trail sign in thoracic herniated disks. Amer. J. Neuroradiol. 13 (1992) 137–143

Barakos, J. A., P. G. D'Amour, W. P. Dillon, T. H. Newton: Trigeminal sensory neuropathy caused by cervical disk herniation. Amer. J. Neuroradiol. 11 (1990) 609

Bauduin, E., P. Flandory, A. Jodaitis, A. Stevenaert: Foraminal herniation of a thoracic calcified nucleus pulposus. Neuroradiology 31 (1989) 287–288

Beyer, H. K., G. Oppel, R. Blümm, D. Uhlenbrock: Die MRT bei der Diagnostik der lumbalen Discushernie. Röntgenpraxis 41 (1988) 37–42

Boden, S. D., D. O. Davis, T. S. Dina, N. J. Patronas, S. W. Wiesel: Abnormal magnetic-resonance scans of the lumbar spine in asymptomatic subjects. J. Bone Jt Surg. 72 (1990a) 403–408

Boden, S. D., P. R. McCowin, D. O. Davis, T. S. Dina, A. S. Mark, S. Wiesel: Abnormal magnetic-resonance scans of the cervical spine in asymptomatic subjects. J. Bone Jt Surg. 72 (1990b) 1178–1184

Boden, S. D., D. O. Davis, T. S. Dina, C. P. Parker, S. O'Malley, J. L. Sunner, S. W. Wiesel: Contrast-enhanced MR imaging performed after successful lumbar disk surgery: prospective study. Radiology 182 (1992) 59–64

Bolender, N.-F., N. S. R. Schönström, D. M. Spengler: Role of computed tomography and myelography in the diagnosis of central spinal stenosis. J. Bone Jt Surg. 67 (1985) 240–246

Bonneville, J. F., M. Runge, F. Cattin, P. Potelon, Y.-S. Tang: Extraforaminal lumbar disc herniations: CT demonstration of Sharpey's fibers avulsion. Neuroradiology 31 (1989) 71–74

Braitinger, S., H. Heller, R. Petsch, B. Kunkel, H. W. Dörnemann, P. Stass: MRT der operierten Lendenwirbelsäule. Fortschr. Röntgenstr. 147 (1987) 185–191

Braun, J.-P., A. Tournade: Le canal de conjugaison cervical. J. Neuroradiol. 6 (1979) 327–334

Braun, I. F., J. P. Lin, A. E. George, I. I. Kricheff, J. C. Hoffman: Pitfalls in the computed tomographic evaluation of the lumbar spine in disc cisease. Neuroradiology 26 (1984) 15–20

Breidahl, W. H., V. Low, M. S. Khangure: Imaging the cervical spine: a comparison of MR with myelography and CT myelography. Aust. Radiol. 35 (1991) 306–314

Breton, G.: Is that a bulging disk, a small herniation or a moderate protrusion? Canad. Ass. Radiol. J. 42 (1991) 318

Brown, B. M., R. H. Schartz, E. Frank, N. K. Blank: Preoperative evaluation of cervical radiculopathy and myelopathy by surface-coil MR imaging. Radiology 151 (1988) 1205–1212

Bundschuh, C. V., M. T. Modic, J. S. Ross, T. J. Masaryk, H. Bohlman: Epidural fibrosis and recurrent disk herniation in the lumbar spine: MR imaging assessment. Amer. J. Roentgenol. 150 (1988) 923–932

Capesius, P., F. Smaltino, M. Kaiser, S. Meoli, A. Gambardella: Computed tomography of the cervical spinal canal. J. neurosurg. Sci. 25 (1981) 265–270

Castillo, M., J. A. Malko, J. C. Hoffman: The bright intervertebral disk: An indirect sign of abnormal spinal bone marrow on T_1-weighted MR images. Amer. J. Neuroradiol. 11 (1990) 23–26

Castro, F. P., J. Ricciardi, M. E. Brunet, M. T. Busch, Th. S. Whitecloud III: Stingers, the Torg ratio, and the cervical spine. Amer. J. Sports. Med. 25 (1997) 603–608

Chafetz, N., C. E. Cann, J. M. Morris, L. S. Steinbach, H. I. Goldberg: Pseudarthrosis following lumbar fusion: Detection by direct coronal CT scanning. Radiology 162 (1987) 803–805

Ciric, I., M. A. Mikhael, J. A. Tarkington, N. A. Vick: The lateral recess syndrome. A variant of spinal stenosis. J. Neurosurg. 53 (1980) 433–443

Claussen, C., Th. Grumme, J. Treisch, B. Lochner, E. Kazner: Die Diagnostik des lumbalen Bandscheibenvorfalls. Fortschr. Röntgenstr. 136 (1982) 1–8

Demaerel, P., H. Bosmans, G. Wilms et al.: Rapid lumbar spine MR myelography using rapid acquisition with relaxation enhancement. Amer. J. Roentgenol. 168 (1997) 277

Dietemann, J. L., J. F. Bonneville, M. Runge, M. Y. Jeung, A. Weintraub, A. Wackenheim: Computed tomography of lumbar apophyseal joint lipoma: report of three cases. Neuroradiology 31 (1989) 60–62

Dihlmann, W.: Computertomographie des lumbalen Diskusprolaps und der Vertebralkanalstenose. Z. Rheumatol. 43 (1984) 153–159

Dihlmann, W.: Lumbaler Reprolaps oder Narbengewebe? Fortschr. Röntgenstr. 146 (1987) 330–334

Dorwart, R. H., J. B. Vogler, C. A. Helms: Spinal stenosis. Radiol. Clin. N. Amer. 21 (1983) 301–325

Edelman, R. R., G. M. Shoukimas, D. D. Stark, K. R. Davis, P. F. J. New, S. Saini: High-resolution surface-coil imaging of lumbar disk disease. Amer. J. Roentgenol. 144 (1985) 1123–1129

Enomoto, H., N. Kuwayama, T. Katsumata, T. Doi: Ossification of the ligamentum flavum. Neuroradiology 30 (1988) 571–573

Enzmann, D. R., C. Griffin, J. B. Rubin: Potential false-negative MR images of the thoracic spine in disk disease with switching of phase- and frequency-encoding gradients. Radiology 165 (1987) 635–637

Enzmann, D. R., J. B. Rubin: Cervical spine: MR imaging with a partial flip angle, gradient-refocused pulse sequence. Part. I. General considerations and disk disease. Radiology 166 (1988a) 467–472

Enzmann, D. R., J. B. Rubin: Cervical spine: MR imaging with a partial flip angle, gradient-refocused pulse sequence. Part II. Spinal cord disease. Radiology 166 (1988b) 473–478

Enzmann, D. R., J. B. Rubin: Short TR, variable flip angle, gradient echo scans of the cervical spine: comparison of 2DFT and 3DFT techniques. Neuroradiology 31 (1989) 213–216

Firooznia, H., V. Benjamin, I. I. Kricheff, M. Rafii, C. Golimbu: CT of lumbar spine disk herniation: Correlation with surgical findings. Amer. J. Roentgenol. 142 (1984) 587–592

Fitt, G. J., J. M. Stevens: Postoperative arachnoiditis diagnosed by high resolution fast spin-echo MRI of the lumbar spine. Neuroradiology 37 (1959) 139–145

Fletcher, G., V. M. Haughton, K.-C. Ho, S. Yu: Age-related changes in the cervical facet joints: Studies with cryomicrotomy, MR. and CT. Amr. J. Neuroradiol. 11 (1990) 27–30

Francavilla, T. L., A. Powers, T. Dina, H. V. Rizzoli: MR imaging of thoracic disk herniations. J. Comput. assist. Tomogr. 11 (1987) 1062–1065

Freund, M., A. Hutzelmann, C. Steffens et al.: MR-Myelographie bei Spinalkanalstenosen. Fortschr. Röntgenstr. 167 (1997) 474

Fujiwara, F., K. Yonenobu, S. Ebara, K. Jamashita, K. Ono: The prognosis of surgery for cervical compression myelopathy (An analysis of the factors involved). J. Bone Jt Surg. 71-B (1989) 393–398

Galanski, M., A. Weidner, H. Vogelsang: Der enge lumbale Spinalkanal. Röntgen-Bl. 35 (1982) 450–458

Gallucci, M., A. Bozzao, B. Orlandi, R. Manetta, G. Brughitta, L. Lupattelli: Does postcontrast MR enhancement in lumbar disk herniation have prognostic value? J. Comput. assist. Tomogr. 19 (1995) 34–38

Gentry, L. R., C. M. Strother, P. A. Turski, M. J. Javid, J. F. Sackett: Chymopapain chemonucleolysis: Correlation of diagnostic radiographic factors and clinical outcome. Amr. J. Roentgenol. 145 (1985) 351–360

Georgy, B. A., J. R. Hesselink, M. S. Middleton: Fat-suppression contrast-enhanced MRI in the failed back surgery syndrome: a prospective study. Neuroradiology 37 (1995) 51–57

Grenier, N., H. Y. Kressel, M. L. Schiebler, R. I. Grossman, M. K. Dalinka: Normal and degenerative posterior spinal structures: MR imaging. Radiology 165 (1987a) 517–525

Grenier, N., R. I. Grossman, M. L. Schiebler, B. A. Yeager, H. I. Goldberg, H. Y. Kressel: Degenerative lumbar disk disease: Pitfalls and usefulness of MR imaging in detection of vacuum phenomenon. Radiology 164 (1987b) 861–865

Grenier, N., H. Y. Kressel, M. L. Schiebler, R. I. Grossman: Isthmic spondylolysis of the lumbar spine: MR imaging at 1.5 T. Radiology 170 (1989a) 489–493

Grenier, N., J. F. Greselle, J. M. Vital, P. Kien, D. Baulny, J. B. Broussin et al.: Normal and disrupted lumbar longitudinal ligaments. Correlative MR and anatomic study. Radiology 171 (1989b) 197–205

Grenier, N., J.-F. Greselle, C. Douws, J.-M. Vital, J. Senegas, J. Broussin, J.-M. Caille: MR imaging of foraminal and extraforaminal lumbar disk herniations. J. Comput. assist. Tomogr. 14 (1990) 243–249

Geum-Ju Hwang, J.-S. Suh, J.-B. Na, H.-M. Lee, N.-H. Kim: Contrast enhancement pattern and frequency of previously unoperated lumbar discs on MRI. J. magn. Reson. Imag. 7 (1997) 575–578

Hackenbroch, M. H., B. Waldecker, K. H. Prömper: Der lumbale Bandscheibenvorfall – Korrelation computertomographischer und myelographischer Befunde mit Operationsbefunden. Röntgen-Bl. 36 (1983) 50–55

Hamm, B., B. Häring, H. Traupe, M. Mayer: Diagnostischer Stellenwert der kontrastmittelunterstützten MR-Tomographie in der Diagnostik des Postdiskektomie-Syndroms. Fortschr. Röntgenstr. 159 (1993) 269–277

Hammer, B., H. Böhm-Jurkovic, D. zur Nedden, E. Valencak, I. Moshenipour: Der Wert der frühen postoperativen CT-Untersuchung nach lumbaler Bandscheibenoperation. Fortschr. Röntgenstr. 145 (1986) 586–590

Harris, R. J., J. J. Wiley: Acquired spondylosis as a sequel to spine fusion. J. Bone Jt Surg.45-A (1963) 1159–1170

Hartjes, H. K. Roosen, W. Grote, A. Buch, A. Brenner, K. Ruhnau et al.: Cerivcal disk syndromes: Value of metrizamide myelography and diskography. Amer. J. Neuroradiol. 4 (1983) 644–645

Haughton, V. M., O. P. Eldevik, B. Magnaes, P. Amundsen: A prospective comparison of computed tomography and myelography in the diagnosis of herniated lumbar disks. Radiology 142 (1982) 103–110

Healy, J. F., B. B. Healy, W. H. M. Wong, E. M. Olson: Cervical and lumbar MRI in asymptomatic older male lifelong athletes: frequency of degenerative findings. J. Comput. assist. Tomogr. 20 (1996) 107–112

Hedberg, M. C., B. P. Drayer, R. A. Flom, J. A. Hodak, C. R. Bird: Gradient echo (GRASS) MR imaging in cervical radiculopathy. Radiology 150 (1988) 683–689

Heller, H., R. Petsch, Th. Auberger, K. Decker: MRT der Wirbelsäule. Fortschr. Röntgenstr. 142 (1985) 419–426

Helms, C. A., J. B. Vogler: Spinal stenosis and degenerative lesions. In Newton, T. H., D. G. Potts: Modern Neuroradiology, Vol. 1: Computed Tomography of the Spine and Spinal Cord. Clavadel, San Anselmo 1983 (pp. 251 ff.)

Hering, K. G., G. Stetter, K. Meydam: Der enge Lumbalkanal – Vorteile der Computertomographie gegenüber Nativdiagnostik und Myelogramm. Radiol. Prax. 4 (1985) 107–115

Herzog, R. J., J. J. Wiens, M. F. Dillingham, M. J. Sontag: Normal cervical spine morphometry and cervical spinal stenosis in asymptomatic professional football players. Plain film radiography, multiplanar computed tomography, and magnetic resonance imaging. Spine 16 (1991) 178–186

Hilibrand, A. S., N. Rand: Degenerative lumbar stenosis: diagnosis and management. J. Amer. Acad. orthop. Surg. 7 (1999) 239

Ho, P. S. P., S. Yu, L. A. Sether, M. Wagner, K.-C. Ho, V. M. Haughton: Ligamentum flavum: appearance on sagittal and coronal MR images. Radiology 168 (1988a) 469–472

Ho, P. S. P., S. Yu, L. A. Sether, M. Wagner, K.-C. Ho, V. M. Haughton: Progressive and regressive changes in the nucleus pulposus. Part I. The neonate. Radiology 169 (1988b) 87–91

Hochhauser, L., St. A. Kieffer, E. D. Cacayorin, G. R. Petro, W. F. Teller: Recurrent postdiskectomy low back pain: MR surgical correlation. Amer. J. Roentgenol. 151 (1988) 755–760

Hofmann, W., M. Grobovschek, H. Rahim: Spinale Computertomographie lumbosakral/lumbosakrale Funktionsmyelographie. Fortschr. Röntgenstr. 145 (1986) 392–396

Holtas, S., C.-H. Nordström, E.-M. Larsson, H. Pettersson: MR imaging of intradural disk herniation. J. Comput. assist. Tomogr. 11 (1987) 353–356

Hueftle, M. G., M. T. Modic, J. S. Ross, T. J. Masaryk, J. R. Carter, R. G. Wilber et al.: Lumbar spine: postoperative MR imaging with Gd-DTPA. Radiology 167 (1988) 817–824

Hwang, G.-J., J.-S. Suh, J.-B. Na, H.-M. Lee, N.-H. Kim: Contrast enhancement pattern and frequency of previously unoperated lumbar discs on MRI. J. magn. Reson. Imag. 7 (1997) 575–578

Ishida, Y., K. Suzuki, K. Ohmori: Dynamics of the spinal cord: an analysis of functional myelography by CT scan. Neuroradiology 30 (1988) 538–544

Isu, T., I. Y. Iwasaki, K. Miyasaka, H. Abe, K. Tashiro, T. Ito: A reappraisal of the diagnosis in cervical disc disease: the posterior longitudinal ligament perforated or not. Neuroradiology 28 (1986) 215–220

Jend, H.-H., K. Helmke, M. Heller, D. Kühne: Die Computertomographie bei Fehlbildungen, entzündlichen und degenerativen Veränderungen der Wirbelsäule. Fortschr. Röntgenstr. 137 (1982) 523–529

Jensen, M. E., C. W. Hayes, G. G. DeBlois, F. J. Laine: Hemispherical spondylosclerosis: MR appearance. J. Comput. assist. Tomogr. 13 (1989) 540–542

Jinkins, J. R.: MR evaluation of stenosis involving the neural foramina, lateral recess and central canal of the lumbosacral spine. MRI Clin. N. Amer. 7 (1999) 493

Jinkins, J. R., A. G. Osborn, D. Garrett., S. Hunt, J. L. Story: Spinal nerve enhancement with Gd-DTPA: MR correlation with the postoperative lumbosacral spine. Amer. J. Neuroradiol. 14 (1993) 383–394

Jinkins, J. R., A. R. Whitemore, W. G. Bradley: The anatomic basis of vertebrogenic pain and the autonomic syndrome associated with lumbar disk extrusion. Amer. J. Neuroradiol. 10 (1989) 219–231

Jinkins, J. R.: MR of enhancing nerve roots in the unoperated lumbosacral spine. Amer. J. Neuroradiol. 14 (1993) 193–202

Junges, R., H. Zwicker: Die Wertigkeit der CT-Untersuchung bei Bandscheibenvorfällen. Fortschr. Röntgenstr. 136 (1982) 166–170

Kaiser, M. C., P. Capesius, A. Roilgen, G. Sandt, D. Poos, G. Gratia: Epidural venous stasis in spinal stenosis. Neuroradiology 26 (1984) 435–438

Kaisser, P., W. Gördes, R. Reither, H.-J. Heller: Erfahrungen mit der Diskolyse – Korrelation von klinischen und radiologischen Befunden. Orthop. Prax. 12 (1985) 944–949

Karantanas, A. H., A. H. Zibis, Papaliaga et al.: Dimensions of the lumbar spinal canal: variations and correlations with somatometric parameters using CT. Europ. Radiol. 8 (1998) 1581

Karnaze, M., H. Gado, K. Sartor, F. J. Hodges: Comparison of MR and CT myelography in imaging the cervical and thoracic spine. Amer. J. Roentgenol. 150 (1988) 397–405

Klumair, J., K. Fochem: Zur Problematik der Wirbellochmessung in der Computertomographie. Radiologe 20 (1980) 203–204

Kornberg, M., G. R. Rechtine: Quantitative assessment of the fifth lumbar spinal canal by computed tomography in symptomatic L4–L5 disc disease. Spine 10 (1985) 328–330

Lackner, K., S. Schroeder: Computertomographie der Lendenwirbelsäule. Fortschr. Röntgenstr. 133 (1980) 124–131

Lackner, K., S. Schroeder, O. Köster: Quantitative Auswertung, Indikationen und Wertigkeit der Computertomographie der Lendenwirbelsäule. Fortschr. Röntgenstr. 137 (1982) 309–315

Landman, J. A., J. C. Hoffman, I. F. Braun, D. L. Barrow: Value of computed tomographic myelography in the recognition of cervical herniated disk. Amer. J. Neuroradiol. 5 (1984) 391–394

Lane, J. I., K. K. Koeller, J. D. L. Atkinson: MR imaging of the lumbar spine: enhancement of the radicular veins. Amer. J. Roentgenol. 166 (1996) 181–185

Lane, J., K. Koeller, J. Atkinson: Contrast-enhanced radicular veins on MR of the lumbar spine in an asymptomatic study group. Amer. J. Neuroradiol. 16 (1995) 269–273

Lane, J., K. Koeller, J. Atkinson: Enhanced lumbar nerve roots in the unoperated spine: radiculitis or radicular veins? Amer. J. Neuroradiol. 15 (1994) 1317–1325

Lang, Ph., H. K. Genant, N. Chafetz, P. Steiger, D. Stoller: Magnetresonanztomographie bei der Beurteilung funktioneller Stabilität posterolateraler lumbaler Spondylodesen. Fortschr. Röntgenstr. 147 (1987) 420–426

LeBlanc, A. D., E. Schonfeld, V. S. Schneider, H. J. Evans, K. H. Taber: The spine: changes in T_2 relaxation times from disuse. Radiology 169 (1988) 105–107

Lee, B. C. P., E. Kazam, A. D. Newman: Computed tomography of the spine and spinal cord. Radiology 128 /1987) 95–102

Lemaire, J. J., J. L. Sautreaux, J. Chabannes et al.: Lumbar canal stenosis. Retrospective study of 158 operated cases. Neurochirurgia 41 (1995) 89

Li Wang, Z., S. Yu, L. A. Sether, V. M. Haugthon: Incidence of unfused ossicles in the lumbar facet joints: CT, MR and cryomicrotomy study. J. Comput. assist. Tomogr. 13 (1989) 594–597

Lochner, B., Th. Grumme, C. Claussen: Computertomographische Diagnostik einer Pseudomeningozele nach lumbaler Bandscheibenoperation. Fortschr. Röntgenstr. 137 (1972) 224–225

Lochner, B., A. Halbsguth, H.-W. Pia, P.-A. Fischer: Die spinale MRT. Nervenarzt 56 (1985) 174–185

Lorenz, R.: Indikation und Aussagekraft radiologischer Meßmethoden bei Wirbelsäulenerkrankungen. Röntgen-Bl. 34 (1981) 192–197

Maravilla, K. R., P. Lesh, J. C. Weinreb, D. K. Selby, V. Mooney: Magnetic resonance imaging of the lumbar spine with CT correlation. Amer. J. Neuroradiol. 6 (1985) 237–245

Masaryk, T. J., J. S. Ross, M. T. Modic, F. Boumphrey, H. Bohlman, G. Wilber: High-resolution MR imaging of sequestered lumbar intervertebral disks. Amer. J. Roentgenol. 150 (1988) 1155–1162

Meyer, J. D., R. E. Latchaw, H. M. Ropolo, K. Ghoshhajra, Z. L. Deeb: Computed tomography and myelography of the postoperative lumbar spine. Amer. J. Neuroradiol. 3 (1982) 223–228

Milette, P. C., D. Melanson, P. R. Pupuis et al.: A simplified terminology for abnormalities of the lumbar disc. Canad. Ass. Radiol. J. 42 (1991) 319–325

Milette, P. C., S. Fontaine, L. Lepanto, R. Déry, G. Breton: Clinical impact of contrast-enhanced MR imaging reports in patients with previous lumbar disk surgery. Amer. J. Roentgenol. 167 (1996) 217–223

Modic, M. T., T. Masaryk, F. Boumphrey, M. Goormastic, G. Bell: Lumbar herniated disk disease and canal stenosis: prospective evaluation by surface coil MR, CT, and myelography. Amer. J. Neuroradiol. 7 (1986) 709–717

Modic, M. T., T. J. Masaryk, J. S. Ross, J. R. Carter: Imaging of degenerative disk disease. Radiology 168 (1988) 177–186

Modic, M. T., J. S. Ross, T. J. Masaryk: Magnetic Resonance Imaging of the Spine. Year Book, Chicago 1989

Müller, H. A., W. Sachsenheimer, G. van Kaick: Die Wertigkeit der CT bei der präoperativen Diagnostik von Bandscheibenvorfällen. Fortschr. Röntgenstr. 135 (1981) 353–540

Murayama, S., Y. Numaguchi, A. E. Robinson: The diagnosis of herniated intervertebral disks with MR imaging: a comparison of gradient-refocused-echo and spin-echo pulse sequences. Amer. J. Neuroradiol. 11 (1990) 17–22

Nakstad, P. H., J. K. Hald, S. J. Bakke, I. O. Skalpe, J. Wiberg: MRI in cervical disk herniation. Neuroradiology 31 (1989) 382–385

Neuhold, H., M. Stiskal, Ch. Platzer, G. Pernecky, M. Brainin: Combined use of spin-echo and gradient-echo MR imaging in cervical disk disease. Neuroradiology 33 (1991) 422–426

Nguyen, C. M., K.-C. Ho, S. Yu, V. M. Haughton, J. A. Strandt: An experimental model to study contrast enhancement in MR imaging of the intervertebral disk. Amer. J. Neuroradiol. 10 (1989) 811–814

Nguyen, C. M., V. M. Haughton, K.-C. Ho: Effect of repeated injections of chymopapain in the epidural space. Radiology 174 (1990) 417–419

Nguyen, C. M., V. M. Haughton, K.-C. Ho, H. S. An: MR contrast enhancement: an experimental study in postlaminectomy epidural fibrosis. Amer. J. Neuroradiol. 14 (1993) 997–1002

Nicolas, V., Th. Krahe, W. Dewes, R. Venbrocks, A. Steudel, Th. Harder: MR-Tomographie zur Therapiekontrolle nach Chemonukleolyse. Fortschr. Röntgenstr. 147 (1987) 537–542

Norman, D., C. M. Mills, M. Brant-Zawadzki, A. Yeates, L. E. Crooks, L. Kaufman: Magnetic resonance imaging of the spinal cord and canal: potentials and limitations. Amer. J. Roentgenol. 141 (1983) 1147–1152

Nowicki, B. H., V. M. Haughton, Shiweiyu, S. A. Howard: Radial tears of the intervertebral disc. Int. J. Neuroradiol. 3 (1997) 270–284

Oppel, U., H. K. Beyer, H. Fett, A. Hedtmann: Magnetresonanztomographische Untersuchungen mit Kontrastmitteln beim Postdiskotomie-Syndrom. Orthopäde 18 (1989) 41–52

Osborn, A. G., R. S. Hood, R. G. Sherry, W. R. K. Smoker, H. R. Harnsberger: CT/MR Spectrum of far lateral and anterior lumbosacral disk herniations. Amer. J. Neuroradiol. 9 (1988) 775–778

Parizel, P. M., G. Rodesch, D. Baleriaux, D. Zegers de Beyl, J. D'Haens, J. Noterman et al.: Gd-DTPA-enhanced MR in thoracic disc herniations. Neuroradiology 31 (1989) 75–79

Paulsen, R. D., G. A. Call, F. R. Murtagh: Prevalence and percutaneous drainage of cysts of the sacral nerve root sheath (Tarlov-cysts). Amer. J. Neuroradiol. 15 (1994) 293–297

Pavlov, H., J. St. Torg, B. Robie, C. Jahre: Cervical spinal stenosis: Determination with vertebral body ratio method. Radiology 164 (1987) 771–775

Postacchini, F., G. Pezzeri, A. Montanaro, G. Natali: Computerised tomography in lumbar stenosis. J. Bone Jt Surg. 62-B (1980) 78–82

Ramsbacher, J., A. M. Schilling, K. J. Wolf et al.: Magnetic resonance myelography (MRM) as a spinal examination technique. Acta neurochir. 139 (1997) 1080

Remonda, L., A. Lukes, G. Schroth: Die spinale Stenose: Stand der bildgebenden Diagnostik und Therapie. Schweiz. med. Wschr. 126 (1996) 220

Resnick, D., G. Niwayama: Intervertebral disc herniations: cartilaginous (Schmorl's) nodes. Radiology 126 (1978) 57–65

Resnick, D., G. Niwayama: Diagnosis of Bone and Joint Disorders, 2nd ed. Saunders, Philadelphia 1988

Roosen, N., U. Dietrich, N. Nicola, G. Irlich, D. Gahlen, W. Stork: MR imaging of calcified herniated thoracic disk. J. Comput. assist. Tomogr. 11 (1987) 733–735

Ropper, A. H., D. C. Poskanzer: The prognosis of acute and subacute transverse myelopathy based on early signs and symptoms. Ann. Neurol. 4 (1978) 51–59

Rosenthal, D. I., J. A. Scott, H. J. Mankin, G. L. Wismer, T. J. Brady: Sacrococcygeal Chordoma: magnetic resonance imaging and computed tomography. Amer. J. Roentgenol. 145 (1985) 143–147

Ross, J. S., N. Perez-Reyes, T. J. Masaryk, H. Bohlman, M. T. Modic: Thoracic disk herniation: MR imaging. Radiology 165 (1987a) 511–515

Ross, J. S., T. J. Masaryk, M. T. Modic, H. Bohlman, R. Delamater, G. Wilber: Lumbar spine: Postoperative assessment with surface-coil MR imaging. Radiology 164 (1987b) 851–860

Ross, J. S., T. J. Masaryk, M. T. Modic: Postoperative cervical spine: MR assessment. J. Comput. assist. Tomogr. 11 (1987c) 955–962

Ross, J. S., R. Delamarter, M. G. Hueftle, T. J. Masaryk, M. Aikawa, J. Carter et al.: Gadolinium-DTPA-enhanced MR imaging of the postoperative lumbar spine: Time course and mechanism of enhancement. Amer. J. Roentgenol. 152 (1989) 825–834

Ross, J. S., M. T. Modic, T. J. Masaryk, J. Carter, R. E. Marcus, H. Bohlman: Assessment of extradural degenerative disease with Gd-DTPA-enhanced MR imaging: correlation with surgical and pathologic findings. Amer. J. Roentgenol. 154 (1990a) 151–157

Ross, J. S., M. T. Modic, T. J. Masaryk: Tears of the anulus fibrosus: Assessment with Gd-DTPA-enhanced MR imaging. Amer. J. Roentgenol. 154 (1990b) 159–162

Ross, J. S., T. M. Masaryk, M. Schrader, A. Gentili, H. Bohlman, M. T. Modic: MR imaging of the postoperative lumbar spine: assessment with gadopentetate dimeglumine. Amer. J. Neuroradiol. 11 (1990c) 771 – 776

Rothfus, W. E., A. L. Goldberg, Z. L. Deeb, R. H. Daffner: MR recognition of posterior lumbar vertebral ring fracture. J. Comput. assist. Tomogr. 14 (1990) 790–794

Ryan, R. W., J. F. Lally, Z. Kozic: Asymptomatic calcified herniated thoracic disks: CT recognition. Amer. J. Neuroradiol. 9 (1988) 363–366

Sartor, K.: Spinale Computertomographie. Radiologe 20 (1980) 485–493

Sartor, K., S. Richert: Computertomographie des zervikalen Spinalkanals nach intrathekalem Enhancement: Zervikale CT-Myelographie. Fortschr. Röntgenstr. 130 (1979) 261–269

Schipper, J., J. W. P. F. Kardaun, R. Braakman, K. J. van Dongen, G. Blaauw: Lumbar disk herniation: Diagnosis with CT or myelography? Radiology 165 (1987) 227–231

Schreiber, A., N. Walker: Enger lumbaler Spinalkanal und seine klinische Bedeutung. Orthop. Prax. 4 (1985) 270–275

Schulze-Röbbecke, R., S. Schroeder, K. J. Münzenberg, K. Lackner: Die Form- und Größenbestimmung des lumbalen Spinalkanals mit Hilfe von röntgenologischen Kriterien der Lendenwirbelsäule. Orthop. Prax. 4 (1985) 276–282

Sether, L. A., C. Nguyen, S. Yu, V. M. Haughton, K.-C. Ho, D. S. Biller et al.: Canine intervertebral disks: Correlation of anatomy and MR imaging. Radiology 175 (1990) 207–211

Silverman, C. S., L. Lenchik, P. M. Shimkin, K. L. Lipow: The value of MR in differentiating subligamentous from supraligamentous lumbar disk herniations. Amer. J. Neuroradiol. 16 (1995) 571–579

Sobel, D. F., J. Zyroff, R. P. Thorne: Diskogenic vertebral sclerosis: MR imaging. J. Comput. assist. Tomogr. 11 (1987) 855–858

Sotiropoulos, S., N. I. Chafetz, P. Lang, M. Winkler, J. M. Morris, P. R. Weinstein et al.: Differentiation between postoperative scar and recurrent disk herniation: prospective comparison of MR, CT, and contrast-enhanced CT. Amer. J. Neuroradiol. 10 (1989) 639–643

Stanley, J. H., S. I. Schabel, G. D. Frey, G. D. Hungerford: Quantitative analysis of the cervical spinal canal by computed tomography. Neuroradiology 28 (1986) 139–143

Steiner, G., H. K. Beyer, D. Uhlenbrock, B. Lehmann, E. Dickmann, U. Oppel: Analyse des NMR-Signals auf biologische Information in der Diagnostik der Wirbelsäule. Fortschr. Röntgenstr. 145 (1986) 189–192

Steiner, H.: MR-Tomographie nach lumbalen Bandscheibenoperationen: differentialdiagnostische Möglichkeiten durch Gd-DTPA. Fortschr. Röntgenstr. 151 (1989) 179–185

Steiner, H., J. Lammer, H. Schreyer, G. Papaefthymiou, G. H. Schneider: Computertomographische und myelographische Befunde nach lumbalen Bandscheibenoperationen. Fortschr. Röntgenstr. 146 (1987) 697–704

Stevens, J. M., D. M. O'Driscoll, Y. L. Yu, B. E. Kendall, S. Anathapavan: Some dynamic factors in compressive deformity of the cervical spinal cord. Neuroradiology 29 (1987) 136–142

Stoeter, P., I. Schneider, R. Bergleiter, U. Ebeling: Diagnostischer Wert der computertomographischen Untersuchung der Lumbalsakralregion bei Patienten mit Lumboischialgien. Fortschr. Röntgenstr. 136 (1982) 515–524

Swartz, J. D.: Letter form the guest editor: protrusion, extrusion, confusion! Semin. Ultrasound 14 (1993) 383–384

Takahashi, M., Y. Sakamoto, M. Miyawaki, H. Bussaka: Increased MR signal intensity secondary to chronic cervical cord compression. Neuroradiology 29 (1987) 550–556

Teresi, L. M., R. B. Lufkin, M. A. Reicher, B. J. Moffit, F. V. Vinuela, G. M. Wilson et al.: Asymptomatic degenerative disk disease and spondylosis of the cervical spine: MR imaging. Radiology 164 (1987) 83–88

Torg, J., H. Pavlov, S. Genuario et al.: Neuropraxia of the cervical spinal cord with transient quadriplegia. J. Bone Jt Surg. 68-A (1986) 1354–1370

Torricelli, P., V. Spina, C. Martinelli: CT diagnosis of lumbosacral conjoined nerve roots. Neuroradiology 29 (1987) 374–379

Toyone, T., K. Takabashi, H. Kitahara et al.: Vertebral bone-marrow changes in degenerative lumbar disc disease: an MRI study of 74 Patients with low back pain. J. Bone Jt Surg. 76-B (1994) 757–764

Tsuji, H., T. Tamaki, T. Itoh, H. Yamada, T. Motoe, S. Tatezaki, T. Noguchi, H. Takano: Redundant nerve roots in patients with degenerative lumbar spinal stenosis. Spine 10 (1985) 72–82

Tsuruda, J. S., D. Norman, W. Dillon, T. H. Newton, D. G. Mills: Three-dimensional gradient-recalled MR imaging as a screening tool for the diagnosis of cervical radiculopathy. Amer. J. Roentgenol. 154 (1990) 375–383

Tyrrell, P. N., V. N. Cassar-Pullicino, I. W. McCall: Gadolinium-DTPA enhancement of symptomatic nerve roots in MRI of the lumbar spine. Europ. Radiol. 8 (1998) 116–122

Ullrich, C. G., E. F. Binet, M. G. Sanecki, S. A. Kieffer: Quantitative assessment of the lumbar spinal canal by computed tomography. Radiology 134 (1980) 137–143

Ulmer, J. L., A. D. Elster, V. P. Mathews, A. M. Allen: Lumbar spondylosis: reactive marrow changes seen in adjacent pedicles on MR images. Amer. J. Roentgenol. 164 (1995) 429–433

VanDyke, C., J. S. Ross, J. Tkach, T. J. Masaryk, M. T. Modic: Gradient-echo-MR imaging of the cervical spine: Evaluation of extradural disease. Amer. J. Roentgenol. 153 (1989) 393–398

Verbiest, H.: Stenosis of the bony lumbar vertebral canal. In Wackenheim, A., E. Babin: The Narrow Lumbar Canal. Springer, Berlin 1980

Wackenheim, A., D. Vallier, E. Babin: Die konstitutionelle Stenose des Lumbalkanals. Radiologe 20 (1980) 470–477

Wasserstrom, R., A. C. Mamourian, J. F. Black, R. A. W. Lehman: Intradural lumbar disk fragment with ring enhancement on MR. Amer. J. Neuroradiol. 14 (1993) 401–404

Watanabe, A. T., G. P. Teitelbaum, R. B. Lufkin, J. S. Tsuruda, J. R. Jinkins, W. G. Bradley: Gradient-Echo MR imaging of the lumbar spine: Comparison with Spin-Echo Technique. J. Comput. assist. Tomogr. 14 (1990) 410–414

Weinreb, J. C., L. B. Wolbarsht, J. M. Cohen, C. E. L. Brown, K. R. Maravilla: Prevalence of lumbosacral intervertebral disk abnormalities on MR images in pregnant and asymptomatic nonpregnant women. Radiology 170 (1989) 125–128

Willén, J., B. Danielson, A. Gaulitz et al.: Dynamic effects on lumbar spinal canal. Axial loaded CT-myelography and MRI in patients with sciatica and/or neurogenic claudication. Spine 22 (1997) 2968

Williams, M. P., G. R. Cherryman, J. E. Husband: Significance of thoracic disc herniation demonstrated by MR imaging. J. Comput. assist. Tomogr. 13 (1989) 211–214

Wilmink, J. T., L. Penning, M. van den Burg: Role of stenosis of spinal canal in L4 – L5 nerve root compression assessed by flexion-extension myelography. Neuroradiology 26 (1984) 173–181

Wimmer, B., H. Friedburg, J. Hennig, G. W. Kaufmann: Möglichkeiten der diagnostischen Bildgebung durch MRT. Radiologe 26 (1986) 137–143

Yousem, D. M., S. W. Atlas, D. B. Hackney: Cervical spine disk herniation: comparison of CT and 3 D FT gradient echo MR scans. J. Comput. assist. Tomogr. 16 (1992) 345–351

Yu, S., V. M. Haughton, P. S. P. Ho, L. A. Sether, M. Wagner, K.-C. Ho: Progressive and regressive changes in the nucleus pulposus. Part II. The adult. Radiology 169 (1980) 93–97

Yu, Y. L., G. H. du Boulay, J. M. Stevens, B. E. Kendall: Computed tomography in cervical spondylotic myelopathy and radiculopathy: visualisation of structures, myelographic comparison, cord measurements and clinical utility. Neuroradiology 28 (1986) 221–236

Yu, S., L. A. Sether, P. S. P. Ho, M. Wagner, V. M. Haughton: Tears of the anulus fibrosus: Correlation between MR and pathologic findings in cadavers. Amer. J. Neuroradiol. 9 (1988a) 367–370

Yu, S., V. M. Haughton, L. A. Sether, M. Wagner: Anulus fibrosus in bulging intervertebral disks. Radiology 169 (1988b) 761–763

Yu, S., V. M. Haughton, L. A. Sether, K.-C. Ho, M. Wagner: Criteria for classifying normal and degenerated lumbar intervertebral disks. Radiology 170 (1989) 523–526

Yussen, P. S., J. D. Swartz: The acute lumbar disc herniation: imaging diagnosis. Sem. Ultrasound, CT MRI 14 (1993) 389–398

Zaunbauer, W., S. Däpp, M. Haertel: Anatomische Normalmaße im zervikalen Computertogramm. Radiologe 25 (1985) 521–524

Zeng, Q., L. Xiong, J. R. Jinkins et al.: Intrathecal Gadolinium-enhanced MR-myelography and cisternography. Amer. J. Roentgenol. 173 (1999) 1109

Zur Nedden, D., R. Putz: Anatomie und Computertomographie des lumbalen Wirbelkanals. Röntgenpraxis 38 (1985) 153–157

5 Tumors of the Spine and Spinal Canal

D. Uhlenbrock and V. Kunze

Contents

Tumors of the Spine

V. Kunze

Bone Tumors

A large number of histologically different, benign and malignant bone tumors are found in the skeletal system. These tumors differ in their radiological appearance as well as in age and site of predilection. Patients usually present with only unspecific symptoms, which are often misinterpreted as "rheumatic" or "degenerative." There are only a few exceptions to this rule, such as cases of osteoid osteoma with its typical nocturnal pain, which responds well to acetylsalicylic acid.

Compared with other sites, the spine and sacrum are only rarely affected by primary bone tumors. Thus, only a total of 7 % of benign and 15 % of malignant bone tumors are found at these locations.

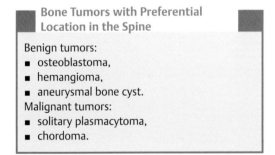

Bone Tumors with Preferential Location in the Spine

Benign tumors:
- osteoblastoma,
- hemangioma,
- aneurysmal bone cyst.

Malignant tumors:
- solitary plasmacytoma,
- chordoma.

Other tumor entities are also observed in the spine, but these have a predominantly extra-axial location (Resnick *et al.*, 1988).

Generally speaking, bone tumors also display changes in signal intensity on MRI similar to those of other lesions, e.g. inflammatory reactions. They therefore usually exhibit low signal intensity on T1-weighted images, while T2-weighted images will show marked signal enhancement. Due to the normally high proportion of fatty marrow in the spine, T1-weighted sequences, T2-weighted fat sat sequences or T2-weighted GRE sequences, for example, should be selected for intra-osseous delineation. T2-weighted sequences or contrast-enhanced T1-weighted sequences, on the other hand, exhibit a high extraosseous contrast (Aisen *et al.*, 1986; Bohndorf *et al.*, 1986; Weigert *et al.*, 1987; Hesnick and Niwayama, 1988).

Inflammatory changes also display a similar signal pattern at MRI. In contrast to these, however, bone tumors are usually confined to a single vertebral body. The intervertebral disks are normally not involved unless there is extensive destruction of the vertebral body. In the presence of inflammation, on the other hand, more often than not an involvement of two adjacent vertebrae is usually seen, together with their common intervertebral disk (Dihlmann, 1987; Reiser *et al.*, 1990).

■ Osteoblastoma

Incidence

The age of predilection for benign osteoblastomas is the second or third decade of life during which period about 70 % of all cases occur. Males are more often affected than females by a ratio of 2:1.

Clinical Presentation

Pain is a typical symptom associated with osteoblastomas, although it is generally only of a mild degree. Afflictions of the spine can be associated with scoliosis, muscular tension and neurological manifestations, including paresthesias and weakness.

Location

The thoracic and lumbar segments are the areas of the spine primarily affected, although involvement of the vertebral body itself is less typical. Pedicle and lamina are often involved and the spinous and transverse processes slightly less often. *Intracortical osteoblastomas* are surrounded by a marked sclerotic zone, not unlike osteoid osteomas but with the nidus of osteoblastomas being larger. *Intratrabecular osteoblastomas* show no surrounding zone of osteosclerosis because the periosteum does not become stimulated to produce a local sclerotic reaction. Unlike osteoblastomas of the long tubular bones, vertebral osteoblastomas have a tendency for epidural expansion and invasion of paravertebral tissue with infiltration of the adjacent vertebral bodies.

Histology

The nidus of the osteoblastoma contains a well-vascularized fibrous stroma that produces osteoid and primitive bone. Histologically there is no clear distinction from an osteoid osteoma, but the osteoblastoma is defined as such once the nidus has reached a certain size. Complete surgical removal of the tumor generally results in healing.

Diagnostics

Conventional Radiograph

On conventional radiographs osteoblastomas appear as sharply circumscribed, expansive, osteolytic lesions with partial or extensive calcification or ossification, occurring, in particular, in the posterior bony elements of the thoracic or lumbar spine. Sometimes a nidus similar to an osteoid osteoma is recognizable; sometimes it appears as a large osteolysis similar to an aneurysmal bone cyst. Scoliosis is often found, although less frequently than with osteoid osteomas (Aisen *et al.*, 1986; Resnick *et al.*, 1988; Krahe *et al.*, 1989).

MRI (Fig. 5.**1**)

The T1-weighted MR image shows a hypointense or isointense lesion relative to muscle. Depending on the degree of bony sclerosis or calcification, there is a signal-free, or almost signal-free, marginal zone around the central tumor. After contrast application, a marked increase in signal intensity of the central tumor component is seen. Whereas good delineation from bone marrow, though poor differentiation in the presence of paravertebral expansion, can be obtained on the plain T1-weighted image, the application of contrast will allow a useful separation from the surrounding soft tissue while the contrast decreases relative to bone marrow. The tumor displays high signal intensity on the T2-weighted image and on T2-weighted fat sat (fat saturated) sequences. Considerable variations may be encountered, however, depending on the degree of sclerosis of the lesion.

■ Hemangioma

Incidence and Location

It may be assumed that after appropriate histopathological processing about 10 % of all spines will reveal hemangiomas. They are located mainly in the region of the thoracic spine where they are to be found in the vertebral bodies. They are less frequently encountered extending into, or primarily located in, the posterior bony elements of the vertebrae.

Clinical Presentation

Hemangiomas are often discovered as incidental findings during examinations performed for other reasons. Only rarely do they elicit clinical symptoms, such as soft-tissue swelling or pain, which are then sometimes secondary to pathological fractures. In rare cases symptoms arise as a result of compression of the myelon due to expansion into the epidural space, as a result of epidural hemorrhage or compression fractures.

Histology

Hemangiomas of the spine usually reach a maximum of about 1 cm in diameter. Cavernous and capillary hemangiomas are the most frequently found.

Cavernous hemangiomas have large, thin-walled vessels, which are delimited by narrow rows of endothelial cells and filled with blood. *Capillary hemangiomas* are characterized by similar, but smaller, vessels and narrower lumina. Whereas cavernous hemangiomas are predominantly situated in the skull and the rest of the skeletal system, capillary hemangiomas are found preferentially in the spine. The bony trabeculae in the vicinity of the lesion become absorbed while the remainder thicken in compensation. Reactive bony regenerations are also observed. Apart from the blood-filled vessels, histology reveals fatty components within the tumor.

Diagnostics

Conventional Radiograph

Hemangiomas of the spine demonstrate a characteristic pathognomonic appearance on conventional radiographs. A vertical trabecular striation

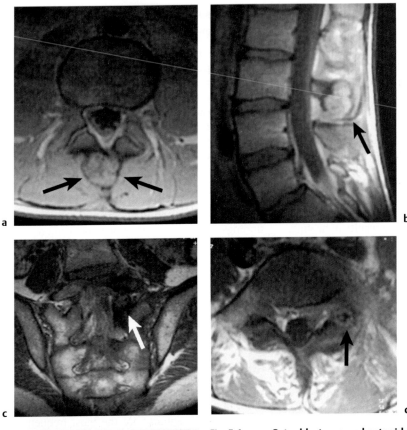

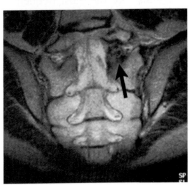

Fig. 5.1 a–e Osteoblastoma and osteoid osteoma (Images courtesy of Dr. Dörfler, University Clinic, Münster, Germany):
a T1-weighted transverse image with depiction of a bullous widening of the spinous process (arrows).
b T1-weighted sagittal section after contrast application: No appreciable enhancement of the tumor detectable (arrow).
c T1-weighted coronal section with depiction on the left of an osteoid osteoma of the articular process. The nidus displays intermediate signal intensity; the marginal sclerosis appears dark (arrow).
d T1-weighted transverse section: The nidus reveals a delicate bright margin (arrow).
e T2-weighted coronal section. No signal enhancement of the nidus. The marginal sclerosis also remains dark (arrow).

of the vertebral bodies is found, together with a marked reduction in density between the individual trabeculae (Resnick *et al.*, 1988; Krahe *et al.*, 1989).

MRI

The lesion also has a characteristic appearance on MRI. Markedly high signal intensity is already observed on the plain T1-weighted image so that the lesion clearly "lights up" within the surrounding hemopoetic bone marrow. The high signal intensity of hemangiomas can be explained by the relatively high proportion of fat present in these lesions (Fig. 5.**2**).

Hemangiomas can exhibit a signal intensity that is exactly equal to that of bone marrow on fat saturated sequences (Fig. 5.**3**).

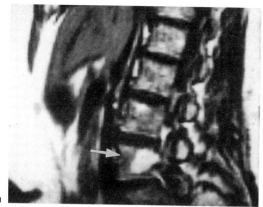

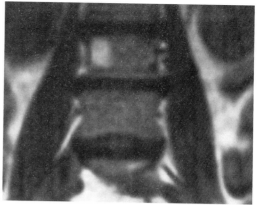

Fig. 5.**2a, b** **Hemangioma of the L3 vertebral body:**
a T1-weighted sagittal image (SE; TR = 600 ms, TE = 20 ms): Evidence of a hyperintense lesion in the L3 vertebral body (arrow) with extension into the right pedicle.

b T1-weighted coronal image (SE; TR = 550 ms, TE = 20 ms): Evidence also of the hyperintense, right-sided hemangioma.

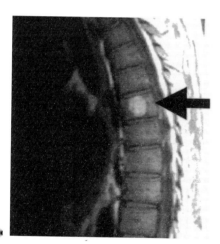

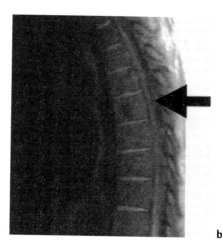

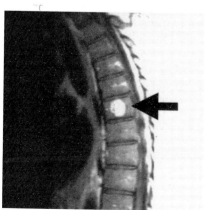

Fig. 5.**3 a–c** **Hemangioma of the T7 vertebral body:**
a T1-weighted sagittal image: Hyperintense lesion in the T7 vertebral body (arrow), characteristic of a hemangioma.
b T1-weighted image with frequency-selective fat suppression: The hemangioma in the T7 vertebral body is no longer depicted due to suppression of the fat signal (arrow).
c T1-weighted image after contrast application: Slight contrast enhancement of the hemangioma (arrow).

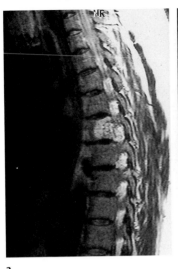
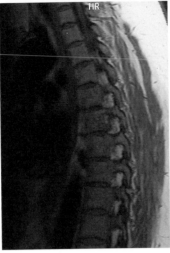
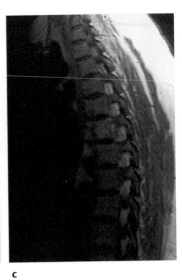

a b c

Fig. 5.**4 a–c Hemangioma of the T5 vertebral body:**
a T2-weighted sagittal image (TSE; TR = 5300 ms, TE = 120 ms): High, slightly inhomogeneous, signal intensity of the vertebral body hemangioma.
b T1-weighted sagittal image (SE; TR = 800 ms, TE = 12 ms): Only slight signal intensity, therefore poor delineation against the other structures of the vertebral body. At most, individual small punctate signal enhancements are recognizable.
c T1-weighted image after contrast application: Slight signal enhancement in the region of the hemangioma.

Rare cases will demonstrate extension into the paraspinal tissue. The lesion also displays high signal intensity on T2-weighted sequences (Fig. 5.**4**).

Hemorrhages, e.g. into the epidural space, appear with varying degrees of signal intensity, depending on their age. The administration of contrast is not necessary with this form of tumor entity. The appearance of focal fatty deposits in the bone marrow is the most important differential-diagnostic criterion on MRI (Ross *et al.*, 1987; Wiegert *et al.*, 1987; Fruehwald *et al.*, 1988).

■ **Aneurysmal Bone Cyst**

Incidence

The aneurysmal bone cyst is primarily found during the first to third decades of life. About 80 % of aneurysmal bone cysts affect patients under 20 years of age.

Clinical Presentation

Various symptoms are presented, depending on location. Apart from local tenderness and swelling, involvement of the spine is associated with neurological deficits. Pathological fractures can cause severe acute pain.

Pathogenesis

Pathogenetically, trauma appears to play an important role in the development of some aneurysmal bone cysts. Local alterations of hemodynamics secondary to venous occlusions or arteriovenous fistulae are held responsible for the development of aneurysmal bone cysts. In addition, they are often found in association with other benign or malignant bone tumors. A large number of aneurysmal bone cysts, however, are considered to be idiopathic. Up to 30 % of cases occur in the spine (Kransdorf, 1995). Here, the aneurysmal bone cyst is primarily located in the posterior bony elements such as the vertebral arches, the transverse and spinous processes, less often in the vertebral bodies. The aneurysmal bone cyst is observed in decreasing order in the thoracic, lumbar, cervical spine and the sacrum.

Histology

The aneurysmal bone cyst is an expansive lesion with thin-walled, blood-filled cystic cavities. Histopathological processing of the material reveals either a large solitary cystic cavity or, more commonly, multiple cysts of sizes ranging between a few millimeters and a few centimeters. The cysts are separated from each other by thin fibrous septations. The cavernous blood-filled cysts do not comprise real vascular cavities, but are bordered by fibroblasts and multinuclear osteoclast-like giant cells. Typical components of vessel walls are not encountered in aneurysmal bone cysts. The fibrous septations can also contain osteoid and lamellar bone, multinuclear giant cells, histiocytes and hemosiderin deposits. The cysts themselves may be filled with fresh blood, while fibrinous clots are less commonly found. Even though the aneurysmal bone cyst is primarily a benign lesion with no tendency to metastasize, local expansive growth with penetration into the soft tissues is possible so that the aim of surgery must be complete removal to prevent recurrence.

Diagnostics

Conventional Radiograph

The aneurysmal bone cyst of the spine appears on conventional radiographs as an osteolytic and expansive lesion involving either the posterior elements of the bony spine or both the posterior elements and the vertebral body itself. A major finding will reveal involvement of adjacent vertebrae, expansion into the spinal canal, the ribs, or the paraspinal soft tissue.

CT

In some cases CT demonstrates a fluid–fluid level within the lesion, especially if the patient has remained motionless in the exposure position for more than 10 minutes (Resnick *et al.*, 1988; Krahe *et al.*, 1989).

MRI

Aneurysmal bone cysts have a characteristic appearance on MRI (Figs. 5.**5** and 5.**6**).

An intralesional structure is found within the cyst that is not usually identified in bone lesions of other origins, such as osteolytic metastases. The lesion itself is characterized by an inhomogeneous signal intensity surrounded by a low-signal rim.

In some cases a fluid–fluid level is identifiable within the cyst that is also detectable on CT. Fluid–fluid levels within a lesion, however, are not proof of an aneurysmal bone cyst. They are also observed in solitary bone cysts, bone metastases, osteosarcomas, fibrosarcomas and cavernous hemangiomas. In these cases, the fluid–fluid levels represent blood in the cysts, hemorrhage in the tumor, or telangiectatic components of an osteosarcoma (Sone, 1992). The lesion will demonstrate varying degrees of signal intensity, depending on the age of the hemorrhage within the cyst. Relatively low signal intensity is therefore observed on T1-weighted images in cases of fresh hemorrhage. After only a few days this signal intensity changes to higher signal intensities on the T1-weighted image due to erythrocyte and hemoglobin degradation. Acute hemorrhages are displayed with relatively low signal intensity on T2-weighted images. Hemorrhages of various ages can appear within the individual cystic spaces so that inhomogeneous signal intensity is sometimes observed. After intravenous application of Gd-DTPA, marginal enhancement of signal intensity is revealed, while the central components demonstrate no signal increase at all (Beltran *et al.*, 1986; Bohndorf *et al.*, 1986; Weigert *et al.*, 1987; Resnick and Niwayama, 1988).

Because aneurysmal bone cysts occur relatively frequently secondary to other primary bone tumors, an underlying primary disease should also be considered despite this typical form of appearance. Precursor lesions are found in about one-third of cases:

- common:
  - giant cell tumor (most common),
  - osteoblastoma,
  - angioma,
  - chondroblastoma,

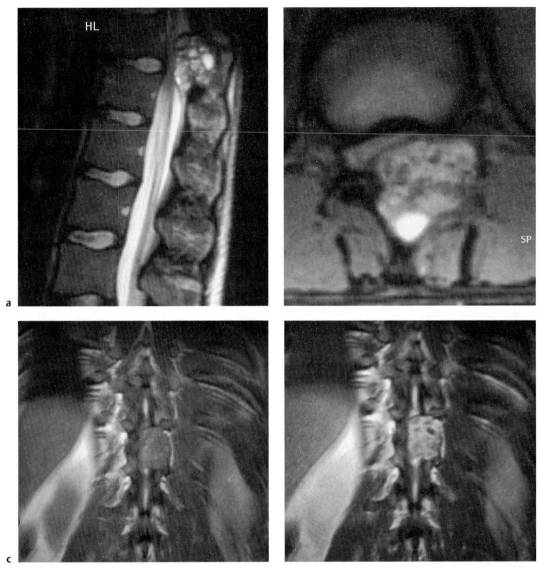

Fig. 5.5 a–d Aneurysmal bone cyst in the region of the vertebral arch of T11 with high-grade stenosis of the spinal canal and the left neuroforamen:

a T2-weighted sagittal section (TSE; TR = 5000 ms, TE = 112 ms): Evidence of a bone tumor originating from the vertebral arch of T11 displaying marked septation. The fluid within the cyst exhibits high signal intensity.

b T2-weighted GRE sequence (TR = 282 ms, TE = 8 ms, flip angle α = 20°): Somewhat mottled inhomogeneous signal intensity of the bone tumor. Predomi-

nantly homogeneous signal. The destruction of the vertebral arch on the left side with involvement of the vertebral joint and the spinous process is clearly seen.

c T1-weighted plain coronal section (TSE; TR = 644 ms, TE = 12 ms): Somewhat mottled inhomogeneous signal intensity, in part with punctate signal enhancements.

d Identical section after contrast application: Relatively clear contrast enhancement of the bone cyst. A homogeneous signal pattern remains.

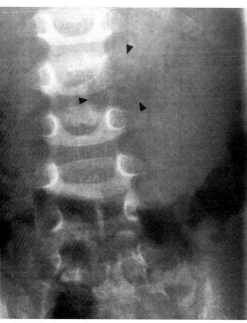

Fig. 5.**6 a–d** **Aneurysmal bone cyst on the left side at L2/L3:**

a Radiograph of the lumbar spine: Depiction of an osteolytic enlargement of the transverse process of L2, a left-sided loss of contour of the L2 vertebral body and destruction of the pedicle. Arrows indicate the full extent of the cyst.

b CT of the bone cyst: The plain (upper) and contrast-enhanced (lower) images show the enlargement and destruction of the bone. There is also a fluid level as an indication of hemorrhage (left, upper and lower).

c T1-weighted sagittal image (SE; TR = 1600 ms, TE = 120 ms): Reduction in signal of the cellular blood components (arrow) relative to the remaining cystic fluid (from Jansen, J., B. Terwey, B. Rama, E. Markakis: MRI diagnosis of aneurysmal bone cyst. *Neurosurg. Rev.* 1990; **13**(2): 161–6)

d Transverse MRI slice (SE; TR = 1600 ms, TE = 30 ms): Signal intense tumor with expansion far into the muscles of the back. The fluid level here (arrow) is also appreciable.

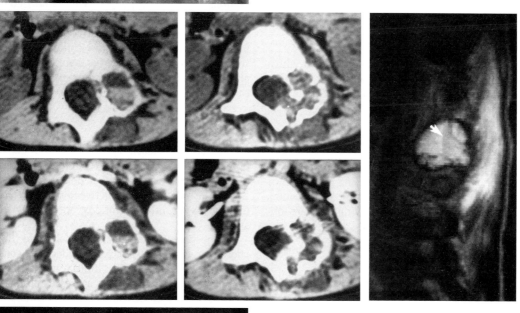

c

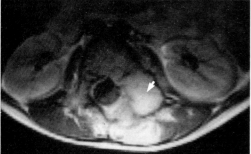

- less common:
  - fibrous dysplasia,
  - non-ossifying fibroma,
  - chondromyxoid fibroma,
  - solitary bone cyst,
  - fibrous histiocytoma,
  - eosinophilic granuloma,
  - osteosarcoma (Kransdorf, 1995).

The occurrence of an additional aneurysmal bone cyst in the stage of development should be included among the differential-diagnostic considerations when an expansive cystic structure with progressive growth is detected in the presence of a known primary lesion (Resnick *et al.*, 1988). Fluid–fluid levels, both on the CT and the MRI scan, are an important indication of the presence of an aneurysmal bone cyst; different signal intensities relative to the age of the hemorrhages and evidence of intralesional structures on the MRI scan also make the diagnosis of an aneurysmal bone cyst likely.

■ Chordoma

Incidence

Chordomas are found in all age groups but with a predilection for older ages from about 50 years onwards. Men are more often affected than women by a ratio of 2:1.

Clinical Presentation

Initially only few and unspecific symptoms are usually presented. With increasing expansion of the tumor and depending on its location, however, various signs and symptoms are observed, including:

- gastrointestinal symptoms where there is involvement of the rectum,
- urological symptoms in cases of bladder involvement,
- neurological symptoms where the nerve roots or the myelon are affected.

Rectal palpation can identify sacral chordomas as fixed presacral space-occupying lesions.

Location

Chordomas are tumors arising from remnants of the embryonic notochord. These remnants can be found in the bones of the skull. In accordance with the tissue of origin, there is a particular predominance of chordomas in the cranial parts of the spine (approximately 30 %), at the clivus and at the occipitocervical junction. More than 50 % of chordomas are located in the caudal parts of the axial skeleton (sacrum, coccyx). Tumors of cranial origin predominate in the younger age groups. Spinal chordomas are usually located in the vertebral bodies, although a multifocal involvement is uncommon. Extraosseous involvement or the involvement of extra-axial bones is very rare. Chordomas relatively often exhibit a large extraosseous extension. The chordoma is the commonest aggressive retrorectal tumor.

Histology

The macroscopic appearance of chordomas is that of a *lobular pattern* of growth. The actual appearance depends on the degree of chondroid and mucinous material. Hemorrhage and cystic formations can also be present. The extraosseous component is usually contained within a pseudocapsule. Intracellular and extracellular mucin predominates histologically in chordomas. The solid tumor components consist mainly of cells of an epithelioid character, reminiscent of adenocarcinomas.

Growth

Chordomas can reach enormous sizes. Chordomas with a size of over 30 cm are sometimes found in the sacrococcygeal region. The typical size in this region reaches between 5 and 20 cm. Chordomas of other locations are somewhat smaller.

By the time the diagnosis is established, the chordoma has usually already undergone considerable expansion and is infiltrating the surrounding structures due to its aggressive form of growth. If complete resection of these tumors is not achieved then local recurrence is a regular feature. In about 30 % of cases hematogenous metastases are found (lung, liver, skeleton, soft tissue and other parenchymatous organs), especially with chordomas of the spine, less often with those of the skull.

Diagnostics

Conventional Radiograph

Chordomas manifest themselves radiologically as osteolysis with and without calcifications and cortical erosions. An irregular destruction of the bone is found in the sacrum, along with presacral fibrous elements. Loss of vertebral height is seen in the spine. Sometimes infiltration of the adjacent vertebral bodies by continuous growth is also found, accompanied by infiltration of the intervertebral space (Resnick *et al.*, 1988; Krahe *et al.*, 1989).

MRI

Like most other bone tumors, chordomas also appear on MRI as a hypointense formation on T1-weighted images. Calcifications, which occur in the paraosseous elements in up to 30% of cases, cannot usually be directly depicted on MRI and are much more clearly seen on CT. Intravertebral expansion is clearly seen on T1-weighted sequences and even on fat-suppressed T2-weighted images. Exclusion or proof of infiltration of the rectum is also possible with T1-weighted images. The detection of a continuous layer of fat separating the rectum from the presacral space-occupying lesion militates in favor of infiltration of the rectum (Fig. 5.**7**).

The paraosseous component can otherwise be displayed with more contrast on T2-weighted images. The tumor clearly enhances relative to the surrounding soft tissue. After injection of contrast, chordomas also demonstrate a marked increase in signal intensity, although sometimes this may be only slight, (Fig. 5.**8**) (Sarrazin, 1996).

Intraspinal expansion of the chordoma is particularly well displayed on contrast-enhanced T1-weighted images because in this case the hyperintense tumor contrasts with the hypointense CSF (Rosenthal *et al.*, 1985; Sze *et al.*, 1988).

MRI is indicated for preoperative planning for surgery of chordomas. Sagittal or coronal sections allow an overview of the intraosseous expansion. MRI is also outstandingly suited for assessing soft-tissue infiltrations. It is not always possible, however, to decide whether organ infiltration is actually present with tumors that have already reached the bowels.

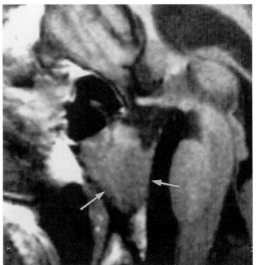

a

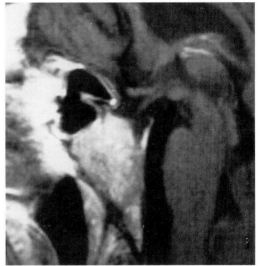

b

Fig. 5.**7 a**, **b**   **Chordoma**
a T1-weighted sagittal image (SE; TR = 550 ms, TE = 15 ms): Hypointense space-occupying lesion of the clivus, which has almost completely replaced the normal bone marrow (arrows).
b T1-weighted sagittal image (SE; TR = 550 ms, TE = 15 ms) after intravenous administration of 0.1 mmol/kg body weight Gd-DTPA: Clear increase in signal intensity in comparison with the plain scan. Decreased contrast relative to fatty marrow, yet better delineation against CSF. The signal pattern does not allow a differential diagnosis to be made.

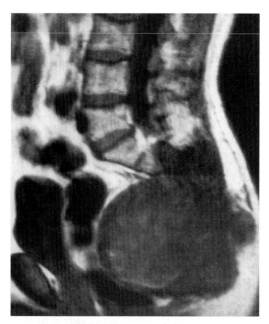

Fig. 5.8 Chordoma of the sacrococcygeal region. The large tumor has resulted in extensive destruction of the bone and has grown far forward into the presacral region. The rectum is displaced anteriorly by the tumor. A dividing layer of fat is still detectable (SE; TR = 500 ms, TE = 20 ms).

■ Plasmacytoma

Incidence

According to the 1972 WHO classification of bone tumors, plasmacytomas rank among the primary bone tumors. If plasmacytomas are regarded as primary malignant bone tumors, then, with an incidence of about 50%, they are by far the most common malignoma. Middle-aged and older patients, between 45 and 65 years, are usually affected. There is a slight sex predisposition in favor of males by a ratio of 3:2. Individual bones can be affected, although involvement of larger skeletal elements is more frequently encountered.

Clinical Presentation

The following clinical complaints are foremost in the presence of a plasmacytoma:

- exhaustion,
- weight loss,
- recurrent infections.

Laboratory examinations reveal:

- greatly elevated blood sedimentation rate (BSR),
- anemia,
- alterations in serum proteins.

The production of monoclonal immunoglobulins is found in the majority of cases. The occurrence of bone pain can be regarded as a clinical indication of bone involvement. Proliferations of plasma cells with a plasma fraction of over 10% and various degrees of differentiation are found in the bone marrow. Osteolytic bone destruction and spontaneous fractures can also be the first sign of the disease.

Therapy

Treatment for plasmacytoma is oriented on laboratory and radiological findings. The Salmon and Durie staging system has established itself as one of the most popular classification schemes (Table 5.1).

This classic staging system does not take MRI findings into account, but confines itself more to staging on the basis of conventional survey radiographs. Asymptomatic patients in stage I do not usually require treatment.

It has emerged in some more recent studies that positive MRI findings, i.e. evidence of bone marrow infiltration, have a positive prognostic reliability in patients with stage I as regards the possibility of proceeding to more aggressive stages (Vande Berg, 1997; Weber, 1997). The mon-

Table 5.1 Staging system for plasmacytoma according to Salmon and Durie

Stage I	all of the following criteria fulfilled: • Hb > 100 g/l • serum calcium value normal • IgG value < 5 g/dl • IgA value < 3 g/dl • Bence-Jones proteinuria < 4 g/24 h • a maximum of one solitary skeletal osteolysis
Stage II	one of the following criteria fulfilled: • Hb < 85 g/l • calcium > 12 mg/dl • IgG value > 7 g/dl • IgA value > 5 g/dl • Bence-Jones proteinuria > 12 g/24 h • extensive lytic bone lesions
A	normal renal function
B	disturbed renal function

oclonal gammopathies should also be regarded in this light. These do not as yet represent a disease requiring treatment, but they do have the tendency in about 19% of patients of developing into a hematological neoplastic disease within 10 years. Laboratory findings are remarkable with these gammopathies, although there are no clinical or radiological alterations. However, MRI does also reveal bone marrow changes in some of these patients, usually in the form of a focal or variegated pattern of involvement. If bone marrow infiltration is diagnosed on MRI in these patients, then the probability of a disease that requires treatment being present is significantly higher in comparison with a population with gammopathies yet without MRI findings. According to various studies, all patients requiring therapy had demonstrated MRI alterations one to several years beforehand (Vande Berg, 1997).

Diagnostics

Skeletal Scintigraphy

Skeletal scintigraphy has a significantly low sensitivity for detecting plasmacytoma. This must be due to the fact that the prevalent feature of plasmacytoma is osteoclast activity with resorption of adjacent bone trabeculae. The radiograph of the spine correspondingly reveals coarse-meshed osteoporosis with and without circumscribed osteolysis. The osteolyses usually display clear margins. Despite MRI evidence of focal involvement of the vertebral bodies, less than one half of cases demonstrate a correlative finding on the survey radiograph (Baur, 1996).

These skeletal changes principally involve the vertebral bodies and, only later on in the course of the disease, the posterior vertebral elements, reflecting the general tendency for plasmacytomas to involve mainly those parts of the skeleton containing red bone marrow. In addition mottled, moth-eaten, destructive bone patterns are also observed. Multiple compressed vertebrae secondary to pathological fractures are not infrequently seen. A typical sight is the collapsed vertebra associated with a fish vertebra deformity, similar to that found in osteoporosis. Large paravertebral soft-tissue tumors are also no rarity (Freyschmidt, 1980; Resnick and Niwayama, 1988; Resnick *et al.*, 1988).

MRI

MRI is the method best suited for detecting bone marrow infiltration. A differentiation is made between various forms of involvement:

Focal marrow involvement. Here, tumor nodules consisting entirely of myeloma cells are found in the bone marrow. On MRI they appear as focal, signal-reduced lesions with a signal intensity lower than, or similar to, that of muscle. An in-

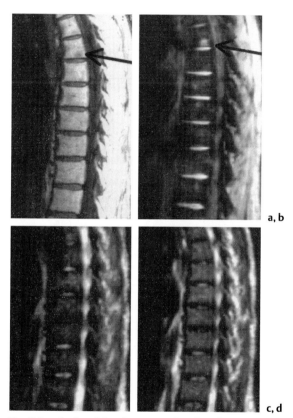

a, b

c, d

Fig. **5.9 a–d   Focal involvement of T6 by plasmacytoma:**
a   T1-weighted image: A circumscribed hypointense lesion that is highly suspect of a focal involvement by plasmacytoma (arrow) is displayed near the inferior end plate of T6.
b   Opposed-phase image: The lesion, which was depicted hypointense on the T1-weighted image, now appears hyperintense (arrow). No evidence of any further lesions.
c, d   STIR and T2-weighted images: The lesion demonstrated in **a** and **b** is no longer apparent.

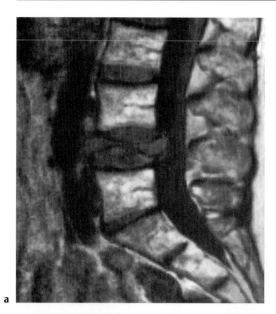

a

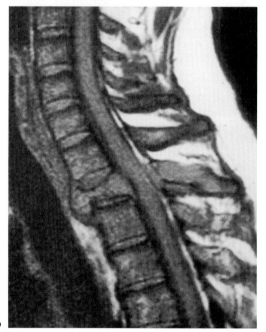

b

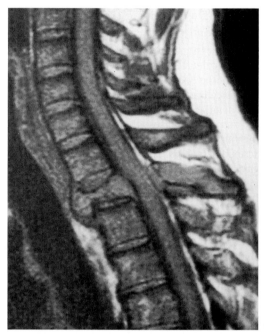

crease in homogeneous signal intensity is observed after contrast application. Individual cases have been reported of primary hyperintense lesions on T1-weighted images. This has been explained by the possible presence of hemorrhage (Moulopoulos, 1992). Both T1- and T2-weighted image sequences are required to display tumor involvement in its entirety because focal lesions are sometimes detectable only on T1- or T2-weighted sequences (Figs. 5.**9** and 5.**10**) (Libshitz, 1992).

The most sensitive sequences are

- T1-weighting: SE, opposed-phase GRE,
- T2-weighting: STIR.

Fig. 5.**10 a–c Localized involvement of the spine by plasmacytoma:**

a T1-weighted image (SE; TR = 550 ms, TE = 20 ms): Involvement of L4, which is clearly reduced in height. The tumor does not exceed the bony contours on this image.

b,c T1- and T2-weighted images of a plasmacytoma: Isointense signal of the tumor on the T1-weighted image (SE; TR = 650 ms, TE = 25 ms), clear signal enhancement on the T2-weighted image (FFE; TR = 600 ms, TE = 20 ms, flip angle α = 10°), and collapse of the vertebral body.

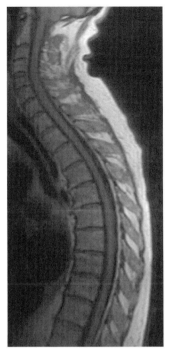

Fig. 5.**11 Variegated form of infiltration by plasmacytoma.** T1-weighted sagittal image (SE; TR = 800 ms, TE = 12 ms): The images display focal variegated reductions of signal in the bone marrow.

Variegated (salt and pepper) pattern of marrow involvement. The smallest of innumerable hypointense lesions are found dispersed in the normal marrow on T1-weighted images, displaying an increase in signal intensity after contrast application (Fig. 5.**11**).

Diffuse pattern of marrow involvement. The diffuse pattern of involvement is the complete replacement of normal bone marrow throughout the entire spine with an increase in signal intensity after contrast application (Moulopoulos, 1994). Unlike the focal pattern of involvement, this form of infiltration correlates highly significantly with the results of iliac crest biopsy (Fig. 5.**12**) (Baur, 1996).

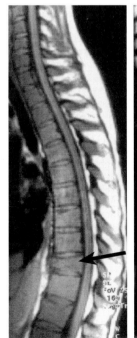

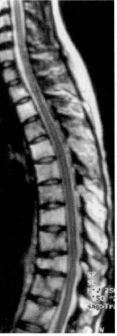

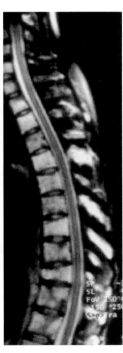

Fig. 5.**12 a–h Diffuse involvement by plasmacytoma before (a–e) and after (f–h) therapy:**

a T1-weighted image: Homogeneous signal reduction in all vertebrae. The intervertebral disks and the adjacent muscles display the same, or lower, signal intensity relative to the bone marrow of the vertebral bodies. Compression fracture of T10 (arrow).

b, c TSE T2-weighted image without (**b**) and with (**c**) frequency-selected fat suppression: The bone marrow of the vertebral bodies appears hyperintense due to homogeneous involvement by the plasmacytoma.
Fig. 5.**12 d–h** ▷

a   b   c

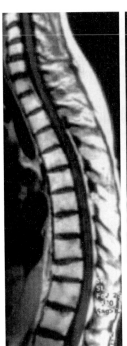

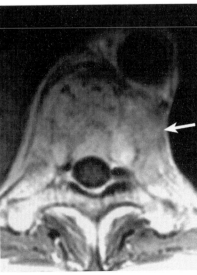

e

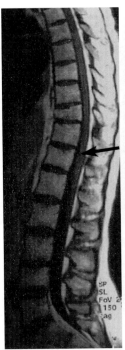

Fig. 5.**12 d, e** T1-weighted image after intravenous application of contrast medium: Massive contrast uptake in all (affected) vertebral bodies. The vertebral bodies now appear clearly brighter than the intervertebral disks. In the transverse image through T10 a paravertebral soft-tissue component is displayed (arrow). Penetration into the spinal canal is not evident.

d

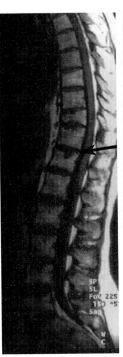

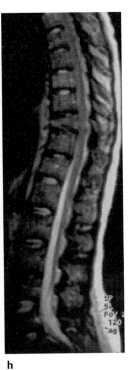

Fig. 5.**12**
f, g T1-weighted images before (**f**) and after (**g**) intravenous application of contrast medium: Signal intensities have returned to normal with the exception of a small focal lesion with contrast enhancement near the superior end plate of T12 (arrow). The bone marrow appears slightly inhomogeneous.

h T2-weighted image: There is merely the slightest hint of the focal lesion in T12. Otherwise the signal intensities have returned to normal.

f

g

h

Mixed (focal and diffuse) pattern of marrow involvement. The mixed pattern of involvement comprises (Figs. 5.**13** and 5.**14**) (Baur, 1996):

- diffuse infiltrations,
- focal involvement.

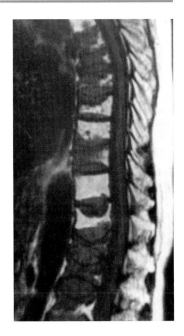

Fig. 5.**13** **Mixed pattern of involvement by plasma-** ▷ **cytoma.** On the T1-weighted image (SE; TR = 650 ms, TE = 25 ms) the non-involved vertebral bodies are depicted bright (fatty marrow), the involved vertebral bodies dark. The vertebral bodies with infiltration of the marrow in part display marked collapse. The plain radiograph was unable to distinguish between osteoporosis and plasmacytoma.

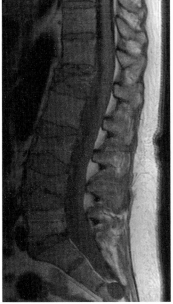
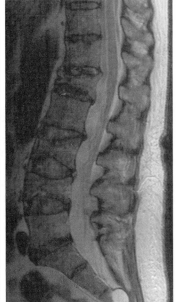
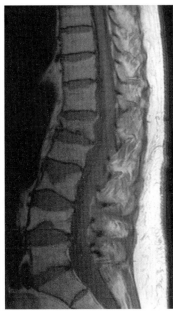

a   b   c

Fig. 5.**14 a–c** **Mixed pattern of involvement by plasmacytoma.** 60-year-old female patient:
a T1-weighted image (SE; TR = 800 ms, TE = 12 ms): Very extensive involvement of the spine with partly diffuse, partly mottled, reduction in signal.
b T2-weighted image (TSE; TR = 4000 ms, TE = 120 ms): Slightly mottled signal intensity in the vertebral bodies, in part somewhat signal enhanced. On the whole, assessment of bone involvement is markedly poorer.

c Finding after therapy (TSE; TR = 800 ms, TE = 12 ms): Marked signal enhancement of the entire bone marrow as an indication of tumor regression. There is a corresponding increased amount of fatty marrow. The vertebral bodies now display a hyperintense signal relative to the disks. Numerous indentations of the vertebrae, primarily involving L1, L3 and L4.

Diffuse bone marrow infiltration, in which tumor cells and normal hematopoietic cells lie close together, is particularly difficult to diagnose using conventional radiography because only a depletion of bone calcium is seen, possibly combined with wispy trabecular thinning. These cases may also be difficult to diagnose on MRI because vertebrae with normal signal intensity may be not be available for comparison. Assessment of the signal intensity of the bone marrow should be made by comparison with that of surrounding structures, especially the intervertebral disk or muscle. In older patients the signal intensity of the bone marrow on T1-weighted images is slightly higher than that of the disk. If this difference is not present, then diffuse involvement of the bone marrow must be taken into consideration. In the case of diffuse bone marrow infiltration, a marked increase in signal intensity by over 40 % will be found after contrast application. In healthy individuals this contrast enhancement is age-related. With increasing age (plasmacytoma is a disease of older age), a significant decrease in contrast enhancement is found. A diffuse reduction in signal intensity is also observed, however, in benign stimulation of bone-marrow cells, e.g. by inflammation or anemia (Bauer, 1996, 1997). These criteria are equally valid for cases of diffuse metastatic invasion of the bone marrow (Dooms *et al.*, 1985; Porter *et al.*, 1986; Kaplan *et al.*, 1987; McKinstry *et al.*, 1987; Uhlenbrock *et al.*, 1988; Josten *et al.*, 1991).

Differential Diagnosis

An established radiological or MRI method for distinguishing an osteoporotic collapse fracture from a fracture secondary to plasmacytoma or other such tumor is not as yet available (Fig. 5.**15**). At the moment, diffusion-weighted images, which have permitted a good differentiation in initial studies, are under discussion. Further results remain to be seen (Baur 1998).

Purely morphological points of reference for benign and malignant fractures are listed in Table 5.**2**.

According to these criteria the majority of compression fractures appear as benign fractures, even in plasmacytoma patients, yet these patients will still demonstrate plasmacytoma cells in their vertebral bodies. A plasmacytoma, therefore, cannot be ruled out even in fractures that appear

Table 5.2   MRI criteria for differentiating benign from malignant fractures (according to Lecouvet)
Benign: ● normal signal intensity on all sequences (chronic fracture)   ● band of low signal intensity adjacent to the inferior or superior end plate (acute fracture)   ● normal bone marrow signal intensity in the other vertebral bodies   ● homogeneous signal intensity after contrast application   ● bulging protrusion dorsally
Malignant: ● diffuse signal reduction on T1-weighted images (Fig. 5.**15**)   ● high or inhomogeneous signal intensity on T2-weighted images   ● round or irregular focal lesions of the bone marrow   ● involvement of pedicles   ● epidural soft-tissue mass (Fig. 5.**16**)   ● high or inhomogeneous contrast enhancement   ● convex posterior margin

benign on MRI. The more pronounced the bone marrow infiltration detected on MRI (diffuse involvement or a large number of foci), the sooner should the occurrence of compression fractures be anticipated (Lecouvet, 1997).

Therapy Monitoring

The monitoring of therapy has become an important indication for MRI. Histologically, edematous hypocellular tissue is found immediately after radio- and chemotherapy. The deposition of structural fat starts during the second week as a prerequisite for bone marrow regeneration. The replacement of red marrow commences in the periphery of the vertebral bodies. From 3–15 weeks after therapy, increased amounts of fat are found in the bone marrow as compared with a healthy reference population. At this point the differential diagnosis between regenerating bone marrow and residual malignant cells is difficult on T1-weighted images.

On T2-weighted images residual foci of malignant cells appear hyperintense, although necroses and inflammatory changes also demonstrate a similar signal pattern so that here too an unequivocal classification of the lesion is still not possible. However, after contrast application far more than 50 % of the changes still recognizable in

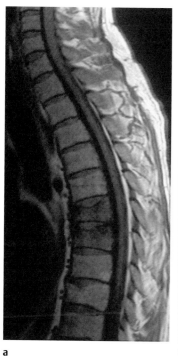

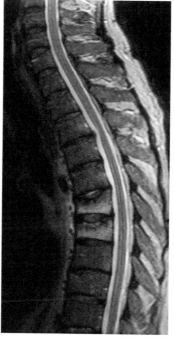

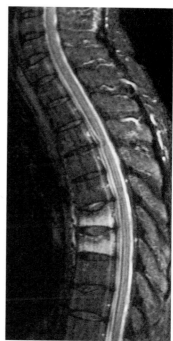

a

b

c

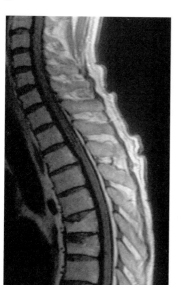

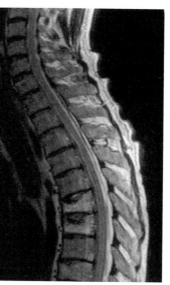

Fig. 5.15 a–e Compression fractures at T6 and T7. There was no known tumor involvement in this patient:

a T1-weighted sequence (SE; TR = 800 ms, TE = 12 ms): Complete reduction in signal of the two thoracic vertebrae is seen.

b T2-weighted SE sequence (SE; TR = 5310 ms, TE = 112 ms): On the whole, complete signal enhancement of the vertebral bodies T6 and T7 with end plate disruption.

c STIR sequence: Here too, there is clear homogeneous signal enhancement of the thoracic vertebrae 6 and 7.

d Follow-up image 5 months later. T1-weighted image (SE; TR = 800 ms, TE = 12 ms): Normalization of the bone-marrow signal.

d

e

e TSE (TR = 3635 ms, TE = 120 ms): Using T2 weighting, a mild signal enhancement of the thoracic vertebrae is still recognizable. This shows that the diffuse signal reduction on the T1-weighted image is not always the decisive factor in differentiating between a malignant and benign fracture. Further criteria must be taken into account for this differential diagnosis; in some cases only the clinical course will allow a final decision.

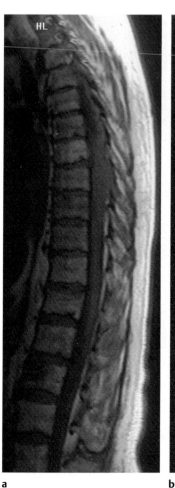

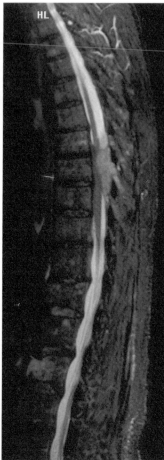

a   b

Fig. 5.16 a–c Plasmacytoma with extensive epidural soft-tissue component:

a T1-weighted image (SE; TR = 800 ms, TE = 12 ms): Mottled inhomogeneous reduction in signal in the vertebral bodies with evidence of an epidural space-occupying lesion in the region of T7–T9.

b The images obtained with T2 weighting (STIR) show the epidural tumor component with a clearly better delineation against the spinal cord and CSF in comparison with the T1-weighted images.

c T2-weighted image (TSE; TR = 3995 ms, TE = 120 ms): The tumor arises from the appendant structures of the vertebrae and encroaches far into the spinal canal.

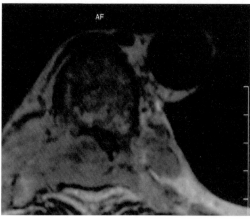

c

patients with a complete response to therapy display neither increased signal intensity nor a marginal enhancement. If a marginal enhancement is seen, then it is explained as representing peripheral processes of repair. A lack of, or only marginal, contrast enhancement is an MRI indicator for a treated inactive tumor. However, persistent homogeneous contrast enhancement is also found in fresh compression fractures or after radiotherapy. In individual cases enhancement is still observed even years later. These enhancements therefore pose a difficult differential-diagnostic problem because they do not necessarily indicate the presence of residual tumor (Moulopoulos, 1994).

In the case of a diffuse or variegated pattern of involvement, the bone marrow of responders usually reverts back to a normal appearance on MRI. With the focal pattern, however, residual abnormalities remain, possibly due also to local destruction of bone and the resulting fibrotic changes (Fig. 5.**12**).

■ Eosinophilic Granuloma

Incidence and Clinical Presentation

Eosinophilic granuloma is a common tumor of childhood, which involves the spine. Pain, local swelling, as well as fever and leukocytosis are typical observations. Eosinophilia is an occasional finding.

Histology

Histologically, eosinophilic granuloma is included among the diseases of Langerhans' cell histiocytosis (previously known as histiocytosis X), together with Hand–Schüller–Christian syndrome and Letterer–Siwe disease. These three entities are characterized by:

● histiocytes,
● eosinophilic granulocytes,
● other inflammatory cells.

Pigment, hemosiderin and fat are formed in the cells by phagocytosis.

Occurrence

The majority of cases present with a solitary lesion, multiple involvement is less common. The appearance of eosinophilic granulomas varies, depending on location. Whereas a sharply demarcated osteolysis is observed in long tubular bones, destruction of the vertebra can ultimately result in almost complete collapse (vertebra plana). In less marked cases, formation of a bullous lytic lesion of the vertebral body and the posterior bony elements is seen. Involvement of adjacent vertebrae is also possible; the disk interspace, however, maintains its normal height. The thoracic and upper lumbar spine are most commonly involved (Resnick *et al.*, 1988).

Diagnostics

MRI

The picture found on MRI is uncharacteristic and shows a hypointense formation on the T1-weighted image with a marked increase in signal intensity after intravenous contrast application. Eosinophilic granulomas show on the T2-weighted image with increased signal intensity, as do the majority of the other tumors. Paraspinal hemorrhages are recognizable by their characteristic signal intensity, which is related to the age of the hemorrhage. T1-weighted sagittal images are particularly suited for detecting involvement of adjacent vertebrae. A reduction in the height of the vertebral body is also well recognizable (Fig. 5.**17**). Transverse images are well suited for displaying paraspinal involvement of the soft tissues (Bohndorf *et al.*, 1986).

■ Other Bone Tumors

Apart from the bone tumors hitherto mentioned, which have a predilection for the spine, the majority of the remaining benign and malignant bone tumors can also present with vertebral manifestations, albeit less commonly. Usually these tumors also display low signal intensity on T1-weighted images and high signal intensity on T2-weighted images. Differential diagnostic information cannot be deduced from MRI, with just a few exceptions. Thus, some tumors or tumorlike lesions such as *giant-cell tumors, telangiectatic osteosarcomas* and *hemophilic pseudotumors*, as well as *aneurysmal bone cysts* can exhibit characteristic signal intensities due to acute or subacute hemorrhages or chronic hemosiderin deposits. In these cases high signal intensities can be found on the T1-weighted image and decreased signal intensities on the T2-weighted image and above all on T2-weighted GRE sequences (Davis, 1992; Aoki, 1996).

High signal intensity on the T1-weighted image with little reduction on the T2-weighted image can be observed with *lipomas* and *liposarcomas*. Intraosseous lipomas are an uncommon finding, however, despite the high content of fat in bone marrow. *Cystic tumors* with high protein content can also demonstrate high signal intensity on T1-weighted images. Low signal intensity, both on the T1-weighted and also on the T2-weighted image, is demonstrated by tumors with a high proportion of collagenous fibrous tissue or

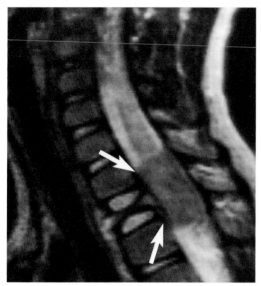

a

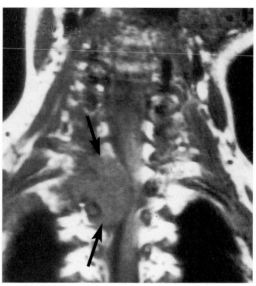

b

Fig. 5.**17 a, b** **Eosinophilic granuloma of T3:**
a T2-weighted image (SE; TR = 2100 ms, TE = 80 ms): Typical finding of a vertebra plana with an intraspinal tumor extension (arrows).

b Coronal section (SE; TR = 500 ms, TE = 120 ms): Better assessment of the compression of the myelon by the intraspinal tumor component (arrow).

with widespread ossifications or calcifications. These include, for example, *fibrous dysplasia* and *fibroblastic osteosarcoma* (Fig. 5.**18**).

A similar pattern is recognizable in the sclerotic zone of *osteoid osteomas*, with both the nidus and the surrounding edema appearing hyperintense. The MRI presentation of the osteoid osteoma, however, is not always typical (Fig. 5.**1**). It is possible, therefore, that in some cases, instead of the nidus, only an ill-defined increase in signal intensity on the T2-weighted image is all that is demonstrated (Hachem, 1997). A variation is also seen in *chondroid tumors*, which display intermediate signal intensity on the T1-weighted image and a greatly increased signal intensity on the T2-weighted image (Fig. 5.**19**).

The differentiation between malignant and benign tumors is only possible to a certain degree with the aid of MRI. There are some indications, however, which are strongly suggestive of benign or malignant tumors.

Benign tumors usually have a homogeneous appearance with:

- displacement of the surrounding structures,
- only slight perifocal edema,
- formation of a pseudocapsule,
- sharp demarcation,
- a slight or delayed increase in signal intensity after intravenous application of Gd-DTPA.

A perifocal zone of edema (reactive zone) is strongly suggestive of a malignant tumor. An intravenous bolus injection of Gd-DTPA using a dynamic scanning technique will produce a rapid and marked increase in signal strength. For this purpose, rapid (GRE) sequences are acquired at short intervals before and during Gd-DTPA administration, without pausing between images. The signal intensity time course of important structures can be assessed by performing region of interest (ROI) analysis. This technique can also be employed for monitoring therapy (Freyschmidt, 1980; Ramsey and Zacharias, 1985; Aisen *et al.*, 1986; Bohndorf *et al.*, 1986; Reiser *et al.*, 1987; Weigert *et al.*, 1987; Resnick *et al.*, 1988; Sze *et al.*, 1988c; Krahe *et al.*, 1989).

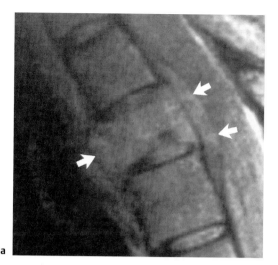

a

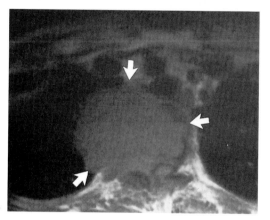

b

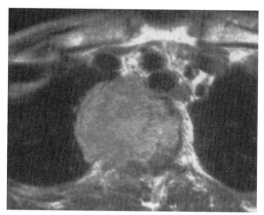

c

Fig. 5.18 a–c Fibroblastic osteosarcoma of T4:

a T2-weighted sagittal section (SE; TR = 1600 ms, TE = 60 ms): The tumor extends beyond the vertebral contours and displays a signal intensity isointense with the other vertebral bodies (arrows).

b T1-weighted transverse section: Extensive mediastinal and right thoracic space-occupying tumor is evident (arrows).

c Only slight enhancement is identifiable after contrast application.

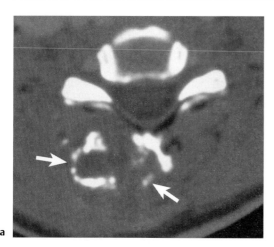

a

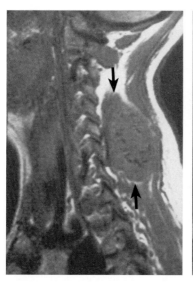

b

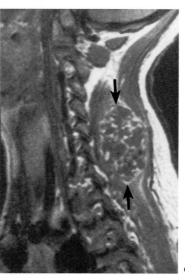

c

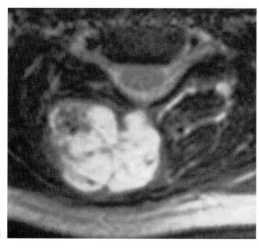

d

Fig. 5.**19 a–d Ecchondroma developing from the spinous process of C6:**

a CT of the tumor region with mottled, flaky tumor calcifications and large dorsal space-occupying lesion (arrows).

b MRI sagittal section (SE; TR = 650 ms, TE = 25 ms): The calcifications are recognizable as a discrete reduction in signal. The extent of the tumor is more readily assessable (arrows).

c Mottled enhancement after contrast application (arrows).

d T2-weighted image: Marked signal enhancement with mottled signal voids.

Metastases to the Vertebrae and the Epidural Space

The most common malignant changes of bone are caused by metastases, with about one-quarter of all malignant tumors showing evidence of skeletal metastases at autopsy. There is a predilection for metastases to involve those parts of the apparatus of locomotion and support that have a higher proportion of red bone marrow. The vast majority of skeletal metastases (about two-thirds) are found in the spine and sacrum. Hematogenous metastatic spread is the commonest form, while lymphogenous spread or tumor invasion by continuous spread is by far less common.

Incidence

Not all tumors metastasize equally often to the skeletal system. In decreasing order of frequency, skeletal metastases are found in the following disorders:

- mammary carcinoma,
- prostatic carcinoma,
- bronchial carcinoma,
- renal carcinoma,
- carcinoma of the uterus,
- thyroid carcinoma,
- gastric carcinoma,
- colonic carcinoma, among others.

Clinical Presentation

The clinical appearance of spinal metastases is nonuniform. In some cases no clinical symptoms are presented despite considerable tumor expansion, while in other cases fractures, vertebral collapse and epidural expansion of tumor components result in compression of the myelon. The presenting clinical symptoms in these cases include:

- pain,
- muscular weakness,
- disturbances of sensation,
- bowel and bladder dysfunction.

Diagnostics

Conventional Radiograph

Metastases are only recognizable on conventional images when more than 40% of the cancellous bone of the vertebral body involved has been destroyed by metastasis (Fig. 5.**20**).

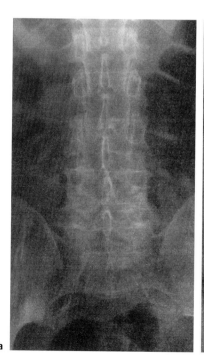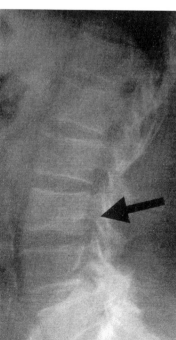

Fig. 5.**20 a–d** **Metastases from prostatic carcinoma.** Patient with incipient symptoms of transverse spinal lesion and marked pain of the lumbar spine:

a Conventional radiograph in two planes: Disruption of the inferior end plate of L3 (arrow) without there being any indication of osteolysis or osteoblastic metastasis. The fracture was classified as old.

a

Fig. 5.**20 b–d** ▷

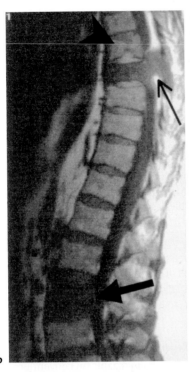

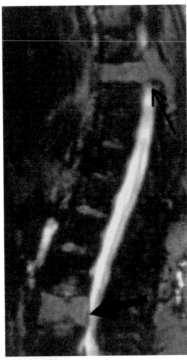

b

c

Fig. 5.**20 b, c** T1-weighted (**b**) and T2-weighted (**c**) fat sat sequence: Complete metastatic infiltration of L3. Posterior cortex is convex toward the spinal canal (large arrow). Besides that, metastatic involvement of T8 with reduction in height and involvement of the pedicles and spinous process. The sagittal images already give the impression of penetration into the spinal canal (small arrow). Schmorl's node in T7 as a secondary finding (arrowhead)

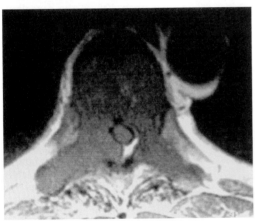

d T1-weighted transverse section after intravenous contrast application: Penetration into the spinal canal on the right with displacement of the dural sac.

Depending on whether an osteoblastic or osteolytic type of metastatic disease is present, osteolysis of the vertebral bodies, in particular, or homogeneous or inhomogeneous sclerosis is observed on conventional radiographs. Myelography will clearly demonstrate epidural spread, including craniocaudal expansion. In most cases, the height of the intervertebral disk remains unaffected, even when two adjacent vertebral bodies demonstrate metastatic involvement. This finding is an important differential-diagnostic criterion over inflammatory changes (Resnick and Niwayama, 1988). Disk involvement, however, has also been reported in individual cases in the presence of metastatic disease (Gupta, 1996).

MRI

MRI allows very sensitive and specific portrayal of metastases of the vertebral bodies. The first exploratory examination sequence is the T1-weighted sagittal image (Fig. 5.**21**).

In older age, when the majority of metastases are found, the hematopoietic marrow of the spine is largely replaced by fatty marrow, so that at this age normal bone marrow appears hyperintense on T1-weighted sequences. This imaging technique displays the metastases as hypointense circumscribed circular lesions or as hypointense formations involving the entire, or almost the entire, vertebral body (Fig. 5.**22**).

It is also usually possible to distinguish metastases from degenerative changes of the spine, which are seen in particular in the marginal areas (lateral, anterior or posterior) of the vertebral bodies as hypointense zones. It is more difficult to recognize diffuse bone-marrow carcinosis because an almost homogeneous reduction in signal intensity of the bone marrow is seen which then appears more hypointense than the disk tissue (Figs. 5.**23** and 5.**24**).

A very high percentage of these metastases appear as hyperintense lesions on T2*-weighted GRE sequences, whereas a much smaller percentage display an increase in signal intensity on T2-weighted SE sequences (Sardanelli, 1997). The use of T2-weighted fat-saturated sequences, however, clearly increases the detection rate for these lesions, even though fat-saturated sequences are associated with a deterioration of the signal-to-noise ratio (Mehta, 1995; Pozzi-Mucelli, 1997). According to Layer *et al.* (1988), opposed-phased GRE studies are even higher in contrast than SE and GRE sequences when assessing vertebral metastases.

The application of contrast material results in a lower detection rate for metastases on SE sequences because the signal is brought into line with that of vertebral fat. There is, however, a useful indication for the application of contrast material in the assessment of intraspinal tumor masses and for a more precise classification of the lesions, especially in pretreated patients (Table 5.**3**).

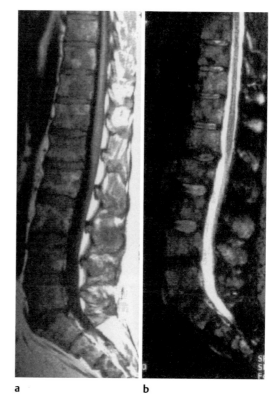

a   b

Fig. 5.**22** **Metastasis of a bronchial carcinoma.** T1-▷ weighted coronal image (SE; TR = 600 ms, TE = 15 ms): The metastases in the spine and pelvis are delineated from the hyperintense bone marrow as circumscribed hypointense circular lesions (arrow heads).

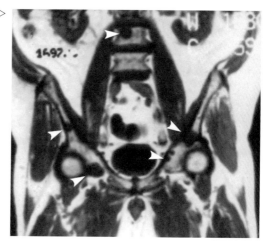

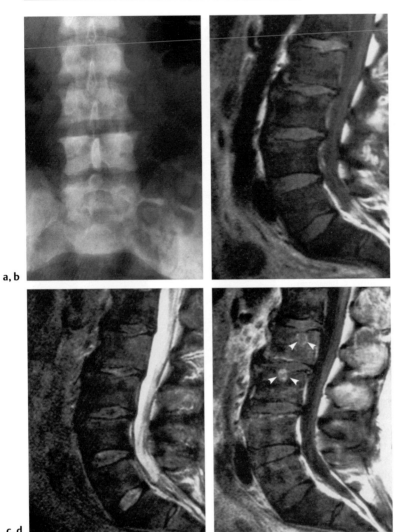

a, b

c, d

Fig. 5.23 a–d Diffuse bony metastases secondary to prostatic cancer.

a Survey radiograph of the lumbar spine: Diffuse sclerosis of all imaged vertebrae due to osteoblastic metastases.

b T1-weighted sagittal image (SE; TR = 650 ms, TE = 25 ms): The bone-marrow signal of all imaged vertebrae is decreased. The intervertebral disks are displayed with higher signal intensity than the bone marrow.

c 2-weighted sagittal image (SE; TR = 2100 ms, TE = 80 ms): Here there is no circumscribed increase in signal intensity. The bone marrow is diffusely hypointense in all the vertebral bodies.

d 1-weighted image (SE; TR = 650 ms, TE = 25 ms) after intravenous application of 0.1 mmol/kg body weight Gd-DTPA: In comparison with the image without contrast, there is a partly circumscribed increase in signal intensity in the vertebral bodies. The difference of signal intensity between bone marrow and disks is smaller. There is an additional circumscribed focal contrast enhancement of L2 and L3 (arrow heads).

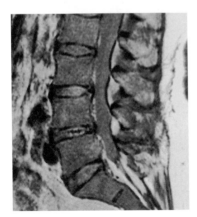

◁ Fig. 5.**24 use bony metastases secondary to mammary carcinoma** (SE; TR = 600 ms, TE = 15 ms). The posterior vertebral margin of L5 is destroyed. There is a homogeneous reduction in signal intensity of all vertebral bodies, making the disks appear hyperintense to the spine.

In comparison with the detection of vertebral metastases, MRI is less sensitive in detecting involvement of the pedicles, transverse and spinous processes (Fig. 5.**25**) (Kosuda, 1996).

The majority of metastases are found in the thoracic and lumbar spine, while the cervical spine is less commonly affected. Because the dens can also display an inhomogeneous signal intensity, even in normal patients, differential-diagnostic problems may possibly arise in equivocal cases of minor involvement of the dens; they are, however, only seen in rare cases. During staging, coronal images through the pelvis and the proximal femur should be obtained, in addition to images of the spine.

Fractures of the sacrum are particularly associated with gynecological tumors that have undergone radiotherapy in the region of the pelvis. Here the differential diagnosis is between a pure fracture and metastatic involvement. Band-like lesions with low signal intensity on both T1- and T2-weighted images constitute the typical appearance of a fracture, while high signal intensity on the T2-weighted image is seen in cases of metastases (Nakahara, 1995). However, the differential diagnosis cannot always be established clearly because fractures can also demonstrate an increase in signal intensity, after contrast application, and sometimes ill-defined peripheral margins (Mammone, 1995). According to Stäbler (1995), a large number of insufficiency fractures display a vacuum phenomenon on CT imaging.

During the routine follow-up of carcinoma patients, skeletal bone scanning certainly remains the method of choice for asymptomatic patients. Patients with local symptoms, however, can be monitored reasonably well by using a combination of conventional radiography and MRI. It should be borne in mind that over one-third of radiographic changes in carcinoma patients are due to benign causes such a degenerative alterations, sequelae of irradiation and osteoporosis (Sze *et al.*, 1988c; Josten *et al.*, 1991; Soderlund, 1996). MRI is sometimes more sensitive than a conventional bone scan, especially for the staging of small-cell bronchial carcinoma. This applies particularly for the histological pattern of intertrabecular involvement without significant osteolysis or osteosclerosis. The prognostic reliability of this, however, has not yet been clarified (Link, 1995; Hochstenbag, 1996; Yamaguchi, 1996; Sauvage, 1996). Not all metastases display a typical

signal behavior. In cases of hemorrhage or partial hemorrhage, hyperintense regions can be seen on the T1-weighted image, while osteoblastic metastases, especially from prostatic and mammary carcinomas, can also appear hypointense or have an inhomogeneous signal intensity on the T2-weighted image (Fig. 5.**26**) (Feydy, 1995).

Differential Diagnosis

The differential diagnosis of inflammatory changes of the spine can be established without a shadow of a doubt in the majority of cases because focal metastatic lesions clearly differ with regard to decrease in signal intensity near the end plates and involvement of the intervertebral disk. The disk remains uninvolved in normal cases of metastatic disease (Table 5.**4**).

Table 5.3 Suitable sequences for examining the spine in the presence of metastases

Basic sequence:
- T1-weighted SE sequence
- T2-weighted TSE sequence with fat saturation
- T2*-weighted GRE sequences
- Opposed-phased GRE sequences

Contrast application:
- for larger intraspinal tumor components
- for purposes of differential diagnosis
- for monitoring response to therapy

Table 5.4 Differential diagnosis of vertebral metastasis versus spondylodiskitis

	Metastasis	**Spondylodiskitis**
Disk	not involved	increased signal intensity on T2-weighted images
Inferior and superior end plate	partially destroyed, otherwise well defined	not defined on T1-weighted images
Vertebral arches	often involved	often uninvolved
Paravertebral soft tissues	asymmetrically involved	circumferentially involved

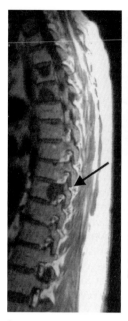

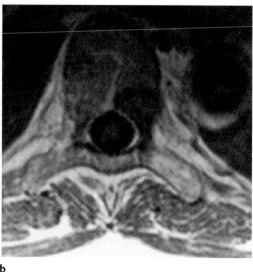

Fig. 5.**25 a, b** **Non-small cell bronchial carcinoma; multiple metastases to the vertebral bodies:**
a T1-weighted SE sequence: Several metastases to the vertebral bodies. Involvement of the vertebral arch of T8 (arrow).
b T1-weighted transverse SE sequence after intravenous contrast application: No penetration into the spinal canal, nor is the transverse process affected. The hypointense metastasis is recognizable left dorsally in the vertebral body and in the pedicle.

a

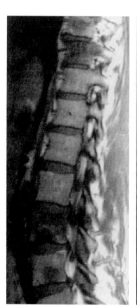

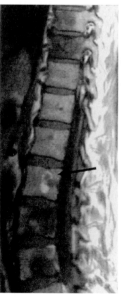

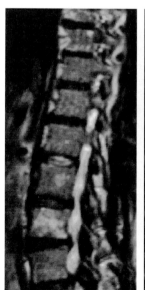

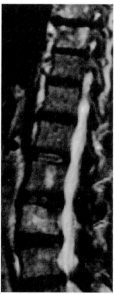

a

b

Fig. 5.**26 a, b** **Mammary carcinoma.** Multiple focal metastases appearing hypointense on the T1-weighted image and hyperintense on the T2-weighted image. Hyperintense formation in L1 (arrow). In the upper components there is only a hyperintense ring with central hypodensity. Here there is the possibility of a partially hemorrhaged metastasis:
a T1-weighted SE sequence.
b T2-weighted TSE sequence.

Tumors of the Spinal Canal

D. Uhlenbrock

Epidural, Non-metastatic Space-Occupying Lesions

■ Spinal Epidural Lipomatosis

Spinal epidural lipomatosis is a disease that is associated with an increase in fatty tissue and usually involves only a few segments. Individual cases may show a diffuse increase of fatty tissue in the spinal canal. The distal lumbar spine as well as the middle and distal sections of the thoracic spine are predominantly affected. Epidural lipomatosis is only rarely encountered in the cervical spine. Involvement of the distal sections of the lumbar spine can extend as far as the sacral canal.

Pathogenesis

The disorder is most commonly seen in association with the following factors:

- excessive alimentary obesity,
- usually long-standing steroid therapy.

In both cases there is an increased production of epidural fat, becoming so pronounced over the years that it leads to compression of the dural sac or myelon. Compression in the region of the thoracic spine primarily occurs from a dorsal direction, while in the region of the lumbar spine the compression usually involves ventral as well as dorsal and lateral elements.

Clinical Presentation

Paresthesias occur in addition to radicular pain, resembling a disk herniation in presentation. Weakness of the extremities is also found, similar to spinal claudication secondary to spinal stenosis.

Diagnostics

Conventional Radiograph

Marked cases of spinal epidural lipomatosis already display changes on conventional radiographs. Thinning of the pedicles and lamina as well as widening of the spinal canal as an indication of increased spinal pressure are found. Myelography reveals an epidural structure constricting the dural sac, usually over several segments.

CT

The diagnosis is easily established on CT because epidural fat is well differentiated by its typical density values. Anterior displacement of the myelon is found in the thoracic spine due to the particularly marked increase of posterior fatty-tissue components, associated in part with compression and flattening of the spinal cord (Buthiau *et al.*, 1988; Maehara *et al.*, 1988: Gero and Chynn, 1989).

MRI

MRI readily displays the increased epidural fat on T1-weighted images by means of its characteristic signal pattern. Dorsal, and sometimes ventral, compression of the dural sac is well recognizable on sagittal images, particularly in the distal sections of the lumbar and the sacral spine. Extradurally, the nerve roots are completely invested by fat (Figs. 5.**27**, 5.**28** and 5.**29**). The "Y" configuration of the dural sac is a characteristic appearance and is the result of compression (Fig. 5.**30**).

On T2-weighted images the lipomatosis also reveals a typical signal intensity that is equivalent to that of fat. In addition, secondary alterations of the myelon, such as compression-related myelon edema, are also detectable from the signal enhancement of the spinal cord (Gero and Chynn, 1989).

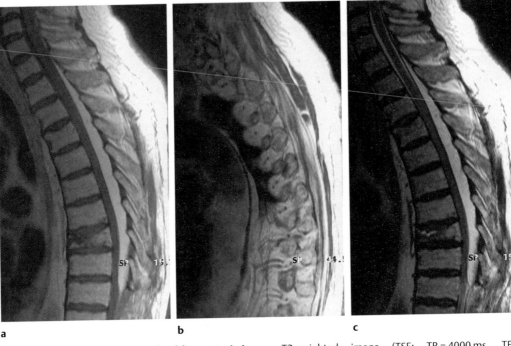

a   b   c

Fig. 5.**27 a–c** **Long-segment epidural lipomatosis in the region of the thoracic spine:**

a T1-weighted image (TSE; TR = 520 ms, TE = 12 ms): There is an epidural lipomatosis with dorsal compression in the region of the thoracic spine. The spinal cord appears clearly flattened. The subarachnoid space is no longer delineated, in contrast to the region of the cervical spine where dark CSF is still well displayed.

b Paramedian section (TSE; TR = 520 ms, TE = 12 ms): The nerve roots in the foramina are completely embedded in fat.

c T2-weighted image (TSE; TR = 4000 ms, TE = 120 ms): The CSF appears bright on this sequence and is well delineated in the cervical region. A CSF signal is no longer recognizable in the area of the cervical spine due to compression of the dural sac. A laminectomy of the T10 and T11 sections was initially performed in this patient, yet without any tendency toward improvement. An additional polysegmental laminectomy over the entire region of the thoracic spine was then undertaken which resulted in an overall improvement of the clinical symptoms.

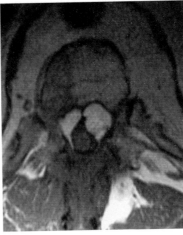

Fig. 5.**28 a, b** **Image after polysegmental laminectomy secondary to epidural lipomatosis:**

a Sagittal section (TSE; TR = 790 ms, TE = 17 ms): Residual islands of lipomatous tissue at the levels T12 and L4–L5. Otherwise, signs of an extensive laminectomy in the proximal region of the lumbar spine.

b Transverse section (SE; TR = 630 ms, TE = 15 ms): Widespread epidural lipomatosis with deformation of the dural sac is still recognizable.

a   b

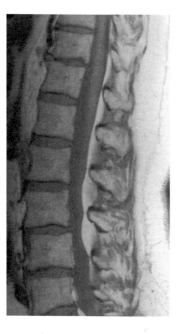

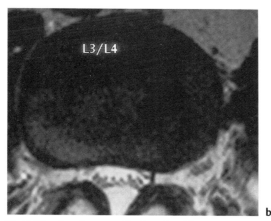

Fig. 5.29 a, b **Circumscribed epidural lipomatosis in the region of the lumbar spine:**
a Sagittal section (TSE; TR = 800 ms, TE = 12 ms): Compression of the dural sac by a dorsal epidural lipomatosis at the level of L3/L4.
b Transverse section through this level (TSE; TR = 6060 ms, TE = 120 ms): Marked compression of the dural sac by the dorsal fatty depositions.

Fig. 5.30 a–c **Spinal epidural lipomatosis:**
a T2-weighted sagittal image (SE; TR = 1800 ms, TE = 90 ms): Narrowing of the spinal canal in the lumbar spine.
b, c T1-weighted paraxial images (SE; TR = 550 ms, TE = 15 ms): Increased deposition of hyperintense fat with compression of the dural sac. The nerve roots are completely invested by extradural fat.

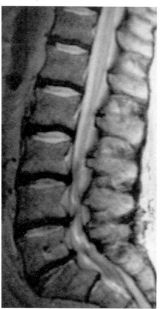

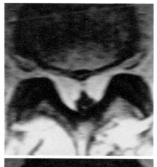

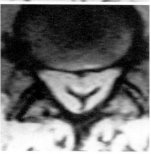

Therapy

If the cause of the disease cannot be directly influenced therapeutically (e.g. change of medication or nutritional habits), laminectomy is regarded as the method of choice. The symptoms usually improve rapidly as a result (Maehara *et al.*, 1988; Buthiau *et al.*, 1988; Gero and Chynn, 1989).

■ Intraspinal Synovial Cyst

The intraspinal synovial cyst is an uncommon finding. It represents a cystic space-occupying lesion that is usually found in the lumbar spine, less commonly in the cervical spine. The thoracic spine is only involved in individual cases. The cyst has contact with the facet joint from where it spreads in a dorsolateral direction. It compresses the spinal cord or the dural sac to varying degrees, depending on its size. Sometimes very small cysts of only a few millimeters are found, however, which are of little clinical relevance.

Pathogenesis

There is some controversy concerning the pathogenesis of the synovial cyst. The cause is assumed to be leakage of joint fluid secondary to rupture of the joint capsule. The joint fluid in turn becomes encapsulated secondarily. Another theory assumes a herniation of the synovial membrane that subsequently expands relative to the amount of intra-articular fluid. Furthermore, the possibility cannot be excluded that it is in fact a bursa that has come into contact with the facet joint via small communication channels and gains its space-occupying character from the leakage of fluid. Synovial cysts are commonly found in association with degenerative changes of the small vertebral joints. Furthermore, the cysts are often seen in patients with rheumatoid arthritis. An association with spinal trauma is also under discussion (Dihlmann, 1987; Jackson *et al.*, 1989).

Clinical Presentation

The clinical presentation of the patients depends on the site of the synovial cyst. If it is a finding in the region of the lumbar spine, nerve root compression can occur accompanied by corresponding radicular symptoms. Back pain has also been reported. Pathological proprioceptive reflexes, sensory disturbances or muscular atrophy can develop. The rare occurrence of a cyst in the region of the cervical spine can also result in compression of the spinal cord with symptoms typical of myelopathy.

Diagnostics

Myelography
At myelography, the synovial cyst appears as an extradural dorsolateral space-occupying lesion. Myelography allows no further differentiation.

CT
The cyst is easily recognizable on CT by its density values, which parallel those of fluid. Assigning the cyst to the facet joint can pose problems in individual cases, however, especially with large cysts that also extend far ventrally. The cyst wall usually appears as a thick capsular margin and is sometimes calcified. In some cases the cyst is also filled with gas, giving the cystic contents density values equivalent to those of air (Hemminghytt *et al.*, 1982; Spencer *et al.*, 1983; Schulz *et al.*, 1984; Resnick *et al.*, 1988; Silbergleit *et al.*, 1990).

MRI
MRI does not offer any significant advantages over CT in the diagnosis of synovial cysts. The posterolateral location and contact with the facet joint are suggestive of a synovial cyst. A further sign is its frequent location dorsal to the ligamentum flavum, while in other cases the synovial cyst is indistinguishable from the ligamentum flavum. On T1-weighted images, the cyst reveals signal intensity similar to that of CSF. The cyst can, however, demonstrate a higher signal intensity if it is rich in protein. If the cyst is filled with blood, then the signal intensity is also higher than that of CSF. Marked reductions in signal intensity of the cyst wall can be signs of calcification. Depending on the extent of these calcifications, differential diagnostic problems may arise on MRI. This is also the case with gas-filled cysts because these gas inclusions appear signal free on MRI and are therefore difficult to distinguish from bone (Jackson *et al.*, 1989; Silbergleit *et al.*, 1990). Signal intensity is high on T2-weighted images and can also differ from that of CSF, depending on the composition of the cystic content. (Figs. 5.**31** and 5.**32**).

Evidence of gas in the cyst should be regarded as a pathognomonic sign and therefore allows a differential diagnosis.

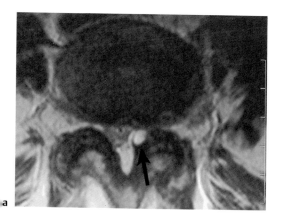

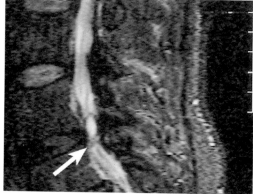

Fig. 5.**31 a–c** **Small synovial cyst at the level L4/L5 on the left side:**

a T2-weighted image (TSE; TR = 4465 ms, TE = 120 ms): The cyst, measuring only a few millimeters, is located epidurally on the left and has resulted in mild compression of the dural sac (arrow).

b T2-weighted sagittal sequence (STIR): The cyst is well delineated and displays a relatively thick capsular structure, which appears hypointense (arrow).

c T1-weighted sequence after contrast application (SE; TR = 420 ms, TE = 14 ms): There is marginal contrast enhancement while the cystic contents remain hypointense (arrow).

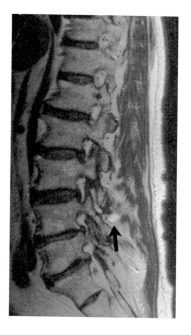

◁ Fig. 5.**32** **Small synovial cyst extending dorsally and extraspinally at the level L3/L4.** T2-weighted sagittal image (TSE; TR = 3695 ms, TE = 120 ms): The cyst displays high signal intensity and has contact with the facet joint (arrow).

Intradural Tumors

Incidence

Intraspinal tumors are seen considerably less often than brain tumors. The ratio is about 1:6. Depending on their relation to the spinal cord and it meninges, a distinction is made between:

- intradural extramedullary tumors,
- intramedullary tumors.

From 40–50 % of all spinal tumors are intradural-extradural in location. The ratio of intradural-extramedullary to intramedullary and extradural tumors is about 3 : 1 : 2 or 50 % : 17 % : 33 %. The figures vary from author to author, depending on whether metastases are included and how broadly the term "extradural" is defined. The differences in the figures result from whether they are derived from autopsy populations of institutes of pathology or from neurosurgical departments. Tumors that were proven to have been clinically silent, or to which no clinical significance was attached, are not infrequently found at autopsy. This applies particularly to small neurinomas of the cauda equina as well as to meningiomas. On the other hand, figures from a neurosurgical patient population are influenced by the urgency of the operation and operability. A distinction should also be made between figures from adult patient populations and those of children.

> **Commonest tumors with intradural extramedullary growth**
>
> - neurinoma,
> - meningioma.
>
> Commonest intramedullary tumors:
> - astrocytoma,
> - ependymoma.
>
> Extradural tumors:
> Extradural tumors are mostly metastases.

Location

About 19 % of all spinal tumors are of cervical location; almost 50 % are thoracic. About 31 % of all tumors are of lumbosacral origin. The most common tumor in the cervical region is the meningioma, followed a great way behind by neurinomas, astrocytomas, ependymomas and hemangioblastomas. Neurinomas, astrocytomas, ependymomas and hemangioblastomas are mainly seen in the thoracic region. Hemangioblastomas are more commonly found at a thoracic location than cervical, the same applies to ependymomas.

The most common conus and cauda tumor is the myxopapillary ependymoma. Meningiomas are rarely seen in this region. This also applies to the lumbar area where neurinomas frequently occur. Furthermore, malformation tumors are often seen in this region (Kernohan and Sayre, 1952).

Metastases should be distinguished from primary intradural tumors. A distinction is made between the following forms:

- metastasizing CNS tumors,
- tumors arising from outside the CNS with intraspinal dissemination.

Intraspinal metastases of brain tumors are seen above all in children and comprise mainly medulloblastomas, primitive neuroectodermal tumors (PNET) and ependymomas. In adults they are usually glioblastomas and tumors of the pineal gland (Figs. 5.**33**–5.**35**).

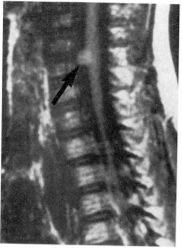

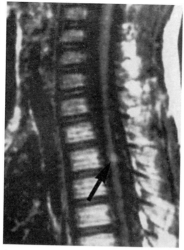

a

b

Fig. 5.**33** **Metastases from a medulloblastoma.** The images after contrast application show two lesions at the level of C6/C7 and T4, which only slightly enhance with contrast and demonstrate a higher signal intensity relative to the spinal cord. They partially overlie the spinal cord and also reveal intramedullary invasion (SE; TR = 780 ms, TE = 25 ms).

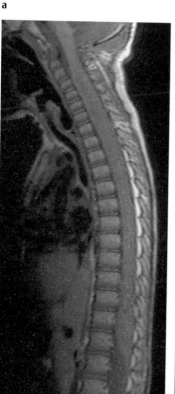

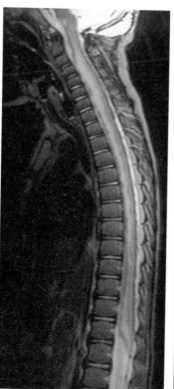

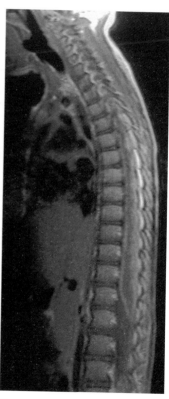

a

b

c

Fig. 5.**34 a–d** **Diffuse leptomeningeal metastatic disease after surgery for medulloblastoma:**

a T1-weighted image (SE; TR = 800 ms, TE = 12 ms): Operative defect in the posterior cranial fossa. Marked enlargement of the entire spinal cord in the spinal canal with concomitant reduction in signal intensity.

b T2-weighted image (TSE; TR = 5300 ms, TE = 120 ms): Marked enlargement of the spinal cord with

considerable signal enhancement, particularly in the proximal section.

c Image of the spinal canal (SE; TR = 800 ms, TE = 12 ms) after contrast application with evidence of a marked, irregularly delineated, relatively strong leptomeningeal metastatic disease.

Fig. 5.**34 d** ▷

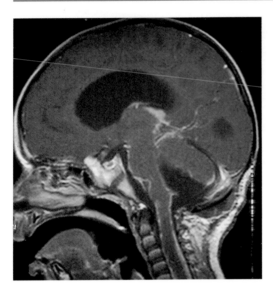

Fig. 5.**34d** T1-weighted image after contrast application; sagittal section in the region of the craniocervical junction after contrast application (SE; TR = 722 ms, TE = 17 ms): Marked signal enhancement along the spinal cord. Hypointense presentation of the myelon. Considerable tumor dissemination also present in the region of the CSF pathways.

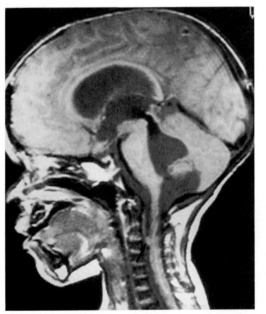

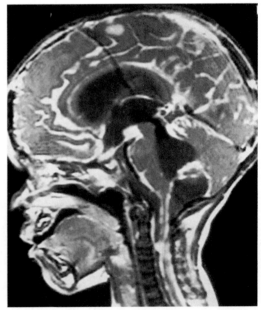

a

Fig. 5.**35a–c Diffuse metastatic spread into all the CSF spaces (primary tumor: extraneural sarcoma):**
a T1-weighted plain image (SE; TR = 650 ms, TE = 25 ms) with indications of faulty circulation of CSF (large ballooned internal CSF spaces) secondary

to a reduced CSF absorption capacity. Nodular structure anterior to the spinal cord at C3 (arrow).
b Diffuse enhancement along the CSF spaces after contrast application. The nodule also displays a homogeneous contrast enhancement.

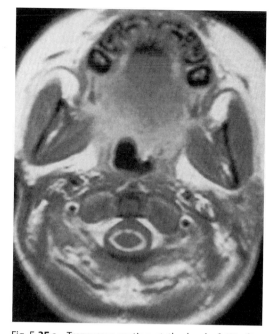

Fig. 5.**35 c** Transverse section at the level of C2 after contrast application: Marginal contrast enhancement around the spinal cord along the pia mater.

Oligodendrogliomas and astrocytomas rarely metastasize into the spinal canal. In individual cases, metastatic spread by a choroid plexus papilloma is also observed in children.

Among those tumors located outside the CNS, intraspinal metastatic spread is above all seen in mammary and bronchial carcinoma as well as in malignant melanoma (Figs. 5.**36** and 5.**37**).

Leptomeningeal metastases are most frequently found in the lumbosacral region (Fig. 5.**38**).

This predilection for lumbosacral spread may be explained by gravity causing the tumor cells to descend within the spinal canal until they become lodged at a lumbosacral site in the region of the conus and cauda. In cases of leptomeningeal dissemination in the cervical and thoracic region, the finding is more common in a dorsal than a ventral location. This may be a consequence of the direction of CSF flow, which proceeds in a caudal direction dorsally and in cranial direction ventrally.

Intramedullary metastases are relatively uncommon, being found most often with bronchial carcinoma, secondly with mammary carcinoma, and otherwise with melanoma and lymphoma, rarely in cases of colonic tumor and hypernephroma. It is assumed that intramedullary metastases are spread via a hematogenous route, although a direct route via nerve roots is also under discussion. This is conceivable for bronchial carcinomas. Intramedullary metastases are predominantly found in the thoracic region (Fig. 5.**39**).

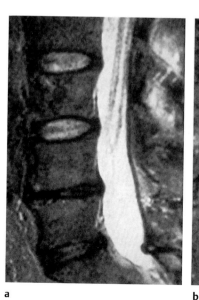

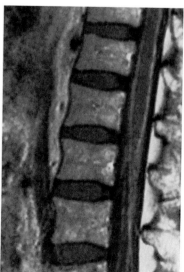

a   b

Fig. 5.**36 a, b** **Leptomeningeal metastatic spread of a mammary carcinoma** (confirmed by CSF cytology):
a T2-weighted image (SE; TR = 2100 ms, TE = 80 ms): Evidence of short and thickened nerve roots.
b T1-weighted image (SE; TR = 720 ms, TE = 20 ms): Diffuse enhancement along the spinal cord and cauda equina after contrast application without formation of nodules.

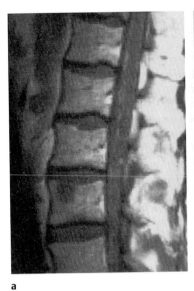

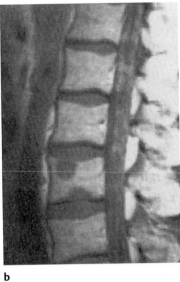

a

b

Fig. 5.**37 Bronchial carcinoma with intraspinal metastatic invasion.** These images obtained after contrast application show a diffuse enhancement along the spinal cord and cauda equina with numerous small nodular structures.

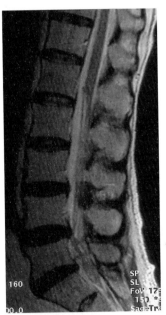

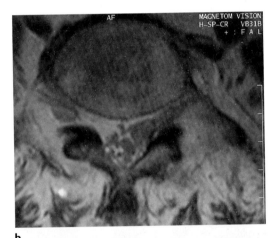

b

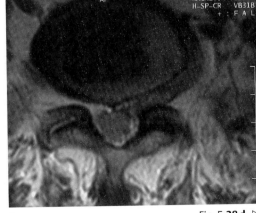

a

Fig. 5.**38 a–d Lumbosacral metastatic spread of a known bronchial carcinoma:**
a T2-weighted sequence (TSE; TR = 5000 ms, TE = 120 ms): Intradural tumor components recognizable in the L5/S1 region with irregular contouring and subsequent lack of delineation of some of the neural structures.
b, c T2-weighted transverse images (TSE; TR = 4465 ms, TE = 120 ms): Conglomeration within the spinal canal with the nodular tumors partially overlying the individual nerves.

c

Fig. 5.**38 d** ▷

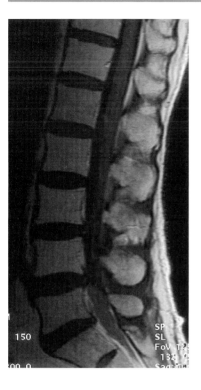

Fig. 5.**38 d** After contrast application (SE; TR = 800 ms, TE = 12 ms): Only very low-grade enhancement along the cauda. Small tumor nodule ventrally showing contrast enhancement at the level of L1.

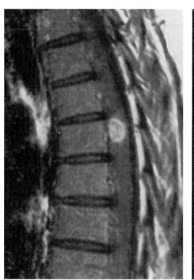

a

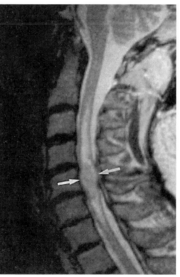

b

Fig. 5.**39 a, b** **Intramedullary metastases:**

a Metastasis of a renal carcinoma at the level of T8 enhancing strongly with contrast. The spinal cord is not particularly enlarged (SE; TR = 680 ms, TE = 25 ms).

b Metastasis of a bronchial carcinoma (arrows). T2-weighted image (SE; TR = 2200 ms, TE = 90 ms): Enlargement of the spinal cord and extensive edema proximally and distally.

Tumor cyst and syringomyelia. Tumors of the spinal canal are often associated with syringomyelia. This applies particularly to intramedullary tumors. According to the literature, the occurrence rate for syringomyelia in association with an intramedullary tumor lies between 30 and 50%; above all, cervical tumors frequently present with syringomyelia (Barnett and Rewcastle, 1973). Syringomyelia rarely develops on the basis of extramedullary tumor growth. In the majority of cases the syrinx develops in the immediate vicinity of the tumor, less frequently is it a part of the tumor or arises within the tumor. In this case it is referred to as an intratumoral cyst, as distinct from syringomyelia. If the syrinx begins to develop in the vicinity of the tumor, it can be delineated from the tumor by a narrow zone of gliosis. In these cases the syrinx does not contain malignant cells at its rostral and caudal ends. Cysts that lie within the tumor usually contain tumor cells at their proximal or caudal margins. Intratumoral cysts can develop exclusively in one direction or in both tumor directions.

As regards the pathogenesis of the syrinx, it is assumed that tumor-related faulty circulation of CSF secondary to the space-occupying lesion in the spinal canal leads to an intraspinal increase in pressure, which is associated with drainage of CSF into the spinal cord via small fissures and gaps. The ensuing myelomalacia then develops further into a syringomyelia. The high occurrence rate of cervical syringomyelias is due to the fact that the cervical cord is particularly subject to the effects of traction and pressure because of the greater mobility of the cervical spine, which can more easily lead to myelomalacia.

Intratumoral cysts develop as a result of tumor degeneration and necrosis, with the cysts in this case being lined by tumor tissue. Active secretion by the tumor can also result in the formation of a cyst (Barnett and Rewcastle, 1973).

Intratumoral cysts often contain a xanthochromic fluid with evidence of elevated protein levels, producing signal intensities on MRI that differ from those of CSF and more resemble those of the tumor. The typical case will reveal a more pronounced T1 shortening relative to CSF and, when using a moderately long echo time (70–120 ms), a signal enhancement on the T2-weighted image, which appears stronger than that of CSF. Depending on the composition of the fluid in the intratumoral cyst, its separation on

MRI from the tumor can be rendered more difficult or impossible. Strong reductions in signal intensity are seen on T2-weighted images after hemorrhage as a result of hemosiderin deposits. Reactive cysts in the form of a syrinx, on the other hand, tend to contain a fluid that is isointense with CSF. They are smooth and have regular circumscribed margins, while intratumoral cysts are more often irregular and associated with a variable width and discontinuous expansion (Goy *et al.*, 1986; Williams *et al.*, 1987; Schubeus *et al.*, 1989). The syrinx can reveal pulsation artifacts on the T2-weighted (non-flow-compensated) image. Intratumoral cysts on the other hand usually have no connection with CSF.

Finally, these criteria allow no certain conclusion as to whether the lesion is a reactive or tumor cyst. The administration of contrast material can facilitate this differentiation because tumor cysts demonstrate contrast enhancement of their walls, while reactive cysts do not. The administration of contrast has therefore proven itself worthwhile for purposes of differentiation (Figs. 5.**40**–5.**42**) (Slasky *et al.*, 1987; Fenzl *et al.*, 1988; Kahn *et al.*, 1989; Schubeus *et al.*, 1989).

Clinical Presentation

The clinical presentation of intraspinal tumors can extend over years. With intradural extramedullary tumor location, the symptoms not infrequently begin with radicular pain. It is typical for the pain to be made worse by coughing, sneezing and straining. Further tumor growth will give rise to additional spinal cord symptoms, which are determined by the positional relationship of the tumor to the spinal cord.

Asymmetric cord compression by the extramedullary tumor not infrequently gives rise to Brown-Séquard syndrome. Intramedullary tumors tend to exhibit bilateral sensory loss with interference of dissociated sensation at the level of the lesion. Depending on the extent of the tumor, spastic paresis (symptoms of pyramidal tract lesion) or flaccid paresis (symptoms of anterior horn lesion) may appear. Bladder and rectal disturbances are typical for both cases, although they are seen slightly more often with intramedullary tumor location.

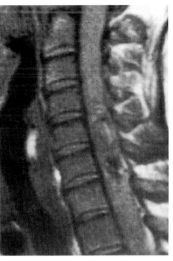
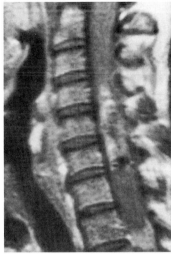
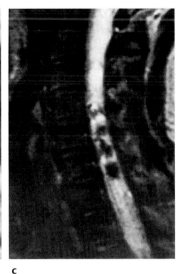

a   b   c

Fig. 5.**40 a–c** **Ependymoma.** 41-year-old female patient:

a T1-weighted image (SE; TR = 650 ms, TE = 25 ms): Intramedullary tumor from C4 to C7. Reduction of signal intensity evident in the distal tumor region.

b Mottled inhomogeneous enhancement after contrast application (SE; TR = 650 ms, TE = 25 ms): Central tumor components remain spared of contrast enhancement.

c T2-weighted image with multiple zones of marked signal reduction (SE; TR = 2100 ms, TE = 80 ms): Histological examination of this tumor, which extended from C4 to C7 revealed multiple cysts with residual hemorrhage.

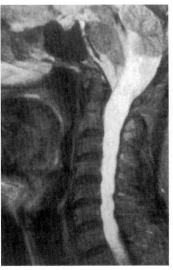
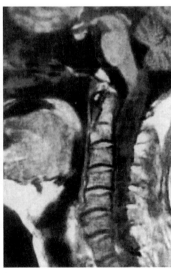
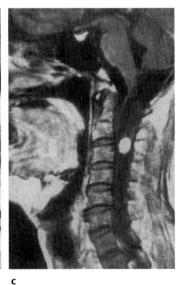

a   b   c

Fig. 5.**41 a–c** **Hemangioblastoma.** Reactive cystic formation proximal and distal to the tumor. 7-year-old female patient:

a T2-weighted image (SE; TR = 1600 ms, TE = 90 ms): Diffuse signal enhancement in the spinal cord and the medulla oblongata.

b T1-weighted image (FLASH; TR = 315 ms, TE = 14 ms, flip angle α = 90°): Intramedullary cavitation with enhanced CSF signal pattern. No evidence of a tumor.

c After contrast application (FLASH; TR = 315 ms, TE = 14 ms, flip angle α = 90°): Evidence of a tumor nodule at the level of C3. Reactive cyst proximal and distal to the nodule.

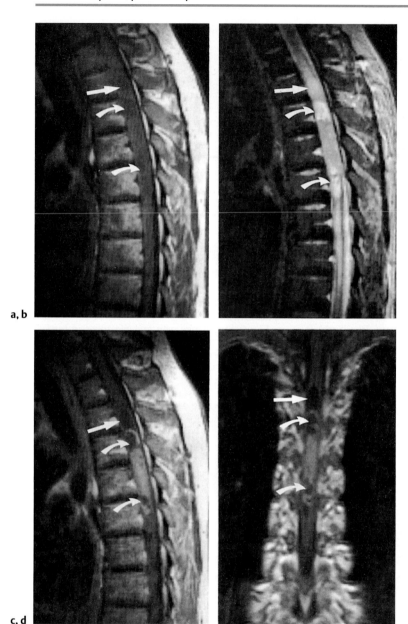

a, b

c, d

Fig. 5.**42 a–d Astrocytoma grade II.** Multiple cystic structures. 47-year-old patient:

a T1-weighted sagittal section (SE; TR = 500 ms, TE = 15 ms): Enlargement of the spinal cord from T4 to T9. Tumor necrosis marked by curved arrows, the proximal reactive cyst by a straight arrow. The image does not, however, allow a distinction between the two.

b T2-weighted image (SE; TR = 2500 ms, TE = 90 ms): This image does not allow any differentiation between the cystic structures either. Marked edema of the myelon proximal and distal to the tumor.

c After contrast application: Enhancement of the tumor. The proximal reactive cyst remains spared of contrast enhancement.

d Finding after contrast application in coronal section.

Differential Diagnosis

In the presence of an intramedullary process, a whole series of disorders must be included among the differential-diagnostic options. *Encephalomyelitis disseminata* with an intramedullary lesion can mimic an intramedullary tumor just as a *myelitis* of other origin can. Both cases can demonstrate expansion of the spinal cord. Other alterations such as *irradiation-induced myelopathy* can produce a picture similar to that of a tumor. Contrast administration is often of help because intramedullary tumors of the spinal cord nearly always demonstrate a more or less strong, albeit sometimes inhomogeneous, enhancement. Individual cases of myelitis will indeed also show a barrier disturbance, but it is usually less pronounced and is therefore associated with only slight signal enhancement after contrast application (Fenzl *et al.*, 1988).

Table 5.5 summarizes some of the differential diagnoses.

Leptomeningeal metastatic disease must be differentiated from arachnoiditis. In each case MRI can give an identical image. This applies especially for diffuse forms of leptomeningeal carcinomatosis without nodular formations. If nodular changes are present, however, the diagnosis of metastatic disease can be made with relative certainty.

■ Intradural Extramedullary Tumors

Neurinoma

The commonest intradural extramedullary tumor is the neurinoma. Synonymous terms are:

- neurilemoma,
- schwannoma.

A distinction should also be made from the neurofibroma.

The tumor is derived from Schwann cells of the dorsal nerve roots or the cauda equina.

Incidence

It is difficult to provide exact frequency figures because neurinomas can in some cases remain clinically silent and are only seen at autopsy. It is assumed that about 16–30% of all intraspinal tumors are attributed to neurinomas.

The frequency peak is during the fourth to fifth decade of life; however, the tumors are seen in all ages, although very rarely in children and infants (Nittmer, 1976).

Location

The tumors most commonly occur in the thoracic and lumbar regions. Apart from the intradural extramedullary site, the tumor is also seen, albeit

Table 5.5 Differential diagnosis of intramedullary tumor

	Intramedullary tumor	Encephalomyelitis disseminata	Transverse myelitis	Arteriovenous fistula
Configuration of the spinal cord	enlargement typical	mild enlargement (rare)	slight enlargement	slight enlargement possible
Signal T1-weighted	(in)homogeneous signal reduction, sometimes cysts and syrinx	normal findings	slight signal reduction possible	normal findings
Signal T2-weighted, transverse	(in)homogeneous signal enhancement, cross section of the cord completely filled	eccentric signal enhancement, in the white matter	central signal enhancement with central sparing (central dot sign); sharp peripheral margin	signal enhancement in white and gray matter, thick veins with intradural course
Pattern of contrast enhancement	in part, mottled enhancement, strong pattern	contrast enhancement within the lesion possible during acute episode	marginal enhancement	slight contrast enhancement possible
Tumor extent	several segments, pan-medullary	1 segment per lesion, several lesions	several segments, poor prognosis with 10 and more segments	several segments

rarely, at intramedullary or exclusively extramedullary sites. The tumors are commonly thoracic and lumbar in location and adapt their growth to the surrounding structures. A quite typical direction of growth is from intradural to extradural via the intervertebral foramen, which usually may already demonstrate marked widening on plain radiographs as a result of pressure atrophy and bone erosion.

Intramedullary neurinomas may be pinhead in size. Larger space-occupying intramedullary tumors are a rarity. Neurinomas do not usually envelop the nerve roots, but rather tend to enlarge them in a fusiform fashion or displace them. Neurinomas which grow along the cauda equina often do not cause any symptoms at all due to the lack of any compressive effect along the nerve roots and are therefore not infrequently seen at MRI as an incidental finding.

Clinical Presentation

Neurinomas present clinically with pain and paresthesia in the form of radiculopathy. These symptoms can exist for years without the diagnosis of a tumor being made. Neurinomas located along the cauda equina are not infrequently clinically silent because signs of compression are often lacking, despite displacement of the cauda.

Histology

Histologically, two types of neurinomas are differentiated:

- Antoni type A,
- Antoni type B.

Antoni type B is based on regressive changes of the tumors cells with interstitial mucus production and loosening of the tissue structure, while these features are lacking in Antoni type A.

Spinal neurinomas tend to form cysts more frequently than do intracranial neurinomas. The cysts can sometimes reach a considerable size.

Diagnostics

MRI

The signal pattern of neurinomas depends on the macromorphological appearance of the tumor. Homogeneous solid tumors show an isointense or slightly hypointense signal on the T1-weighted sequence relative to the spinal cord. Rarely is there a clear reduction in signal intensity, although in cases of marked cystic formation the corresponding predominant signal may be isointense with CSF. On T2-weighted images, neurinomas are usually clearly hyperintense. The signal pattern can appear homogeneous or even inhomogeneous, depending on the degree of regressive changes. Regions with reduction in signal intensity may be apparent on T2-weighted images, representing areas of increased collagen formation and tightly packed Schwann cells. The tumors usually demonstrate a homogeneous and strong contrast enhancement, although cystic areas do remain demarcated as voids. Parts with a dense fibrous matrix also reveal a very strong contrast enhancement effect (Figs. 5.**43**–5.**49**).

MRI provides no evidence to allow a differentiation between Antoni A and Antoni B histological types, neither with regard to signal pattern on native images nor after contrast application (Demachi *et al.*, 1990).

The differentiation of malignant forms is difficult because malignant schwannomas are more prone to infiltrate with an irregular margin. Also these tumors are usually particularly large.

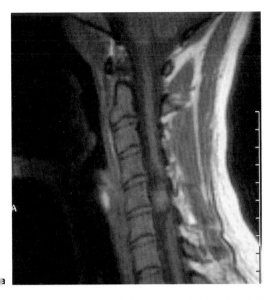

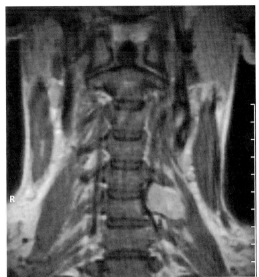

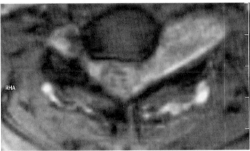

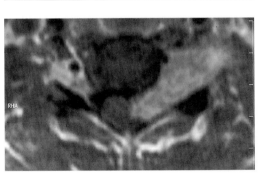

Fig. 5.**43 a–d Hourglass neurinoma at the level of C5.** 27-year-old female patient:

a T1-weighted image (TSE; TR = 693 ms, TE = 12 ms): The tumor demonstrates a signal intensity that is hyperintense to the spinal cord. It shows marked displacement.

b T2-weighted image (FLASH; TR = 688 ms, TE = 22 ms, flip angle α = 25°): Slightly increased signal intensity of the entire tumor, which is growing extradurally from an intraspinal location. Marked enlargement of the intervertebral foramen.

c After contrast application (TSE; TR = 640 ms, TE = 12 ms): There is a homogeneous, and on the whole moderate, enhancement.

d The coronal image reveals displacement of the vertebral artery by the tumor on the left side.

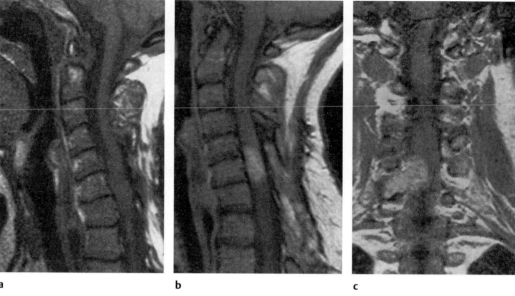

a b c

Fig. 5.**44 a–c Hourglass neurinoma at C6.** 64-year-old patient:

a T1-weighted image (SE; TR = 560 ms, TE = 17 ms): Largely isointense space-occupying extramedullary lesion at the level of C6, anterior to the spinal cord.

b After contrast application there is uniform enhancement of the tumor.

c The coronal section demonstrates the extraspinal growth of the tumor via the right intervertebral foramen.

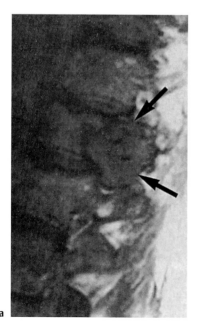

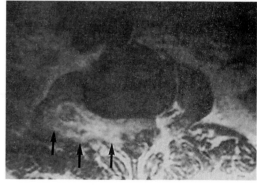

Fig. 5.**45 a, b Hourglass neurinoma at the level of T11.** 65-year-old female patient:

a T1-weighted parasagittal image (SE; TR = 560 ms, TE = 30 ms): The tumor demonstrates expansion into the right intervertebral foramen with extensive bone erosion (arrows).

b Transverse section after contrast application: Significant extraspinal extension with tumor growth into the psoas muscle on the right (arrows).

a b

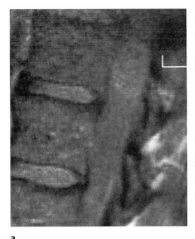

a

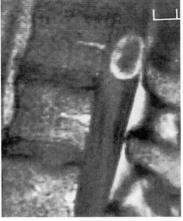

b

Fig. 5.**46 a, b** **Cellular schwannoma at the level of T12.** 26-year-old patient.
a PD-weighted image (SE; TR = 2100 ms, TE = 20 ms): The tumor appears slightly hyperintense to the spinal cord.
b Marginal enhancement after contrast application.

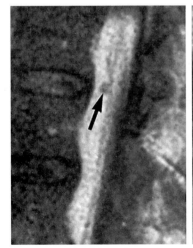

a

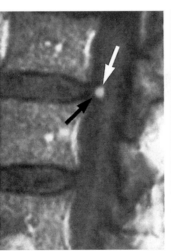

b

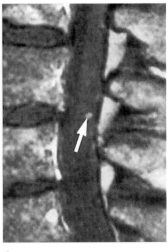

c

Fig. 5.**47 a–c** **Neurinomas at the levels T12/L1 and L3/L4.** 54-year-old female patient:
a T2-weighted image (SE; TR = 2100 ms, TE = 80 ms): Low signal intensity of the neurinoma (arrow).

b T1-weighted image (SE; TR = 785 ms, TE = 25 ms): After contrast application evidence of a tumor measuring only a few millimeters with homogeneous signal enhancement (arrows).
c After contrast application: A further small tumor at the level of L3/L4 (arrow).

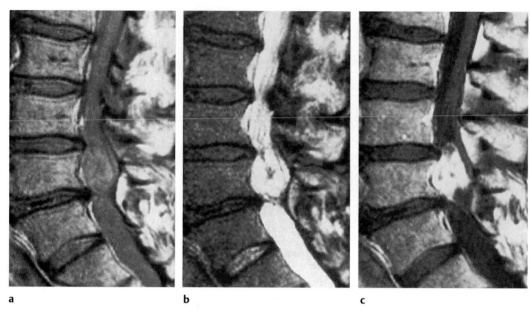

a   b   c

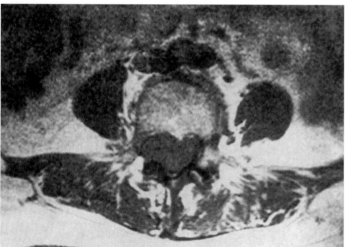

d

Fig. 5.48 a–d　Neurinoma at L4.
67-year-old female patient:
a PD-weighted image (SE;
　TR = 2100 ms, TE = 20 ms): En-
　largement of the spinal canal
　by a space-occupying tumor at
　L4, which is slightly hyperin-
　tense to CSF.
b T2-weighted image (SE;
　TR = 2100 ms, TE = 80 ms):
　High and slightly inhomo-
　geneous signal intensity of the
　tumor.
c After contrast application: Still
　somewhat inhomogeneous,
　yet strong signal enhance-
　ment.
d Transverse image (SE;
　TR = 650 ms, TE = 25 ms): Evi-
　dence of bone erosion along
　the intervertebral foramen on
　the right.

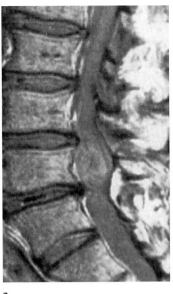
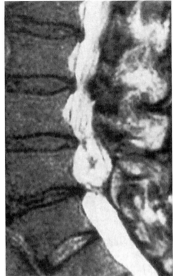
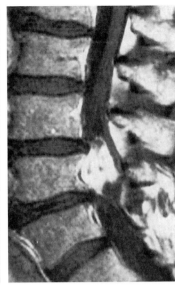

a   b   c

Fig. 5.**49 a–d** **Neurinoma at the level T12/L1:**
a T1-weighted image (TSE; TR = 800 ms, TE = 12 ms): Depiction of the intraspinal portion of the tumor. The tumor appears slightly hyperintense to CSF.
b T2-weighted image (TSE; TR = 3635 ms, TE = 120 ms): Slightly inhomogeneous signal intensity of the tumor. The cauda equina is spread out with a corresponding displacement of the nerves in an anterior and posterior direction.
c After contrast application (TSE; TR = 800 ms, TE = 12 ms): Homogeneous enhancement.
d Coronal image after contrast application: The intra- and extraspinal portions of the tumor are well recognizable.

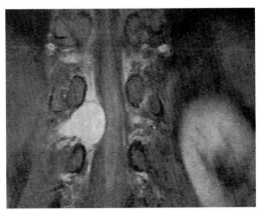

d

Neurofibroma

Neurofibromas are primarily seen in association with von Recklinghausen's neurofibromatosis. They are usually prone to multiple occurrences, although singular occurrence does not militate against the association with von Recklinghausen's disease. The tumors are found in all areas of the spinal canal. With von Recklinghausen's disease they can be associated with bony changes and anterior or lateral meningoceles, dural ectasia with vertebral scalloping, enlargement of the spinal canal, and bony dysplasias of the long tubular bones and skull base. Neurofibromas can also produce extensive erosions of the bone secondary to pressure atrophy. Small neurofibromas associated with von Recklinghausen's disease can occur with an intramedullary location.

Histology

Neurofibromas have an architecture similar to that of neurinomas, yet differ on account of their significant amount of fibrous tissue. In contrast to neurinomas, however, they do envelop the nerve roots.

Location

The tumors frequently appear intra- and extradural in location, at the same time. Small neurofibromas associated with von Recklinghausen's disease can occur with an intramedullary location.

With the occurrence of a plexiform lesion, considerable parts of the tumor can be found extraspinal-paraspinally, resulting in mediastinal tumor masses, which appear as mediastinal widening, even on plain radiographs.

Diagnostics

MRI

On T1-weighted images, neurofibromas display a signal intensity that is similar to, or higher than, that of muscle. This slightly greater signal intensity with a relative shortening of T1 due to interaction of large mucopolysaccharide molecules is ascribed to the presence of tissue water (Burk *et al.*, 1987).

There is a clear signal enhancement on T2-weighted images, not infrequently with additional well-circumscribed central regions of reduced signal intensity as a possible expression of the fibrous components of the tumor. Contrast application reveals a variably strong enhancement (Fig. 5.**50**).

Meningioma

Incidence

The meningioma is the second most common intradural extramedullary tumor. It has a predilection for advanced age; the age-specific prevalence rate increases with age. Nevertheless, children and adolescents can also become affected by meningiomas. Among adults, females are clearly more commonly affected: according to some data, up to 85 % of all intraspinal meningiomas are seen in women (Jänisch *et al.*, 1988). This clear predilection for the female sex does not, however, apply to children and adolescents. It is assumed that hormone receptors in the tumor tissue are responsible for this predilection of intraspinal meningiomas for women.

Location

Spinal meningiomas are preferentially found in the thoracic region, secondly in the cervical region and only rarely in the lumbar area. The ratio is about 80 % : 16 % : 4 %.

The regions C3/C4 are most commonly involved in the cervical area, with the exception of the foramen magnum. The tumors are generally more posterolateral than anterior in location. In the cervical region the anterior site is, however, not atypical.

Tumor Expansion

In the vast majority of cases, tumors are intradural extramedullary in location and displace the spinal cord. An exclusively extradural or combined intradural-extradural growth is the exception. A higher percentage of extradural meningiomas are associated with malignancy. In cases of a combined intradural-extradural growth, the tumor is located along the spinal nerve roots inside and outside the intervertebral foramen, thus exhibiting an hourglass configuration. The meningioma of the foramen magnum is a unique variety. It is the most common tumor in this region. Not only can it expand far caudally, but it

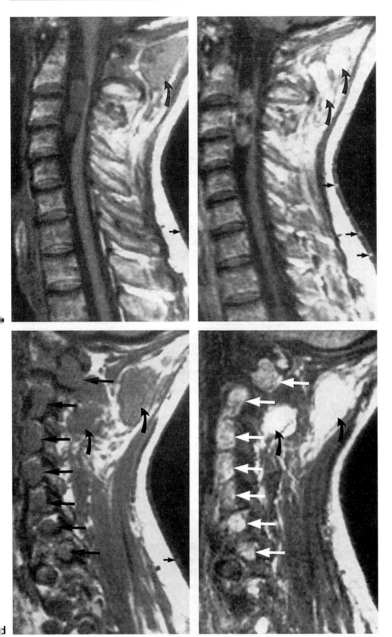

Fig. 5.**50 a–d   Von Reckling-hausen's neurofibromatosis.**
43-year-old female patient:
a T1-weighted sagittal image (SE; TR = 650 ms, TE = 25 ms): Two neurofibromas anteriorly in the spinal canal, demarcated at the level C2–C4. Marked compression of the spinal cord. Large nodule in the nuchal region (curved arrow) and small cutaneous nodules (small arrow).
b After contrast application: Slight enhancement of the intraspinal nodules, clear enhancement in the nuchal region and in the intracutaneous nodules.
c Parasagittal image (SE; TR = 650 ms, TE = 25 ms): Multiple nodules along the intervertebral foramina.
d T2-weighted image (SE; TR = 2100 ms, TE = 80 ms): In part, marked signal enhancement of the nodules.

can also display a considerable space-occupying effect in the posterior cranial fossa. Apart from the nodular tumor formation, a plaque-like type of growth in the spinal canal is very rarely encountered, unlike the intracranial type of meningioma.

The tumors can be multiple in occurrence and appear both intracranially and intraspinally. Bony defects and erosions can develop at the vertebrae secondary to pressure. New bone formations in the form of reactive hyperostosis are typically found more in the region of the calvaria.

Histology

The tumors arise from the arachnoid cap cells, taking their origin from persisting arachnoid cell remnants in the spinal canal. They do not originate from the dura, to which they nevertheless often reveal firm fixation as a result of dural infiltration. The tumors can also arise from the dentate ligaments, the nerve roots or from the spinal cord itself.

Histologically meningiomas are classified into different subtypes:

- The commonest type is the syncytial meningioma, which is ranked by the WHO as grade I (benign) (synonym: meningothelial or endothelial meningioma).
- Further subtypes:
  - fibroblastic meningioma (WHO grade I),
  - transitional meningioma (WHO grade I),
  - psammomatous meningioma (WHO grade I),
  - angiomatous meningioma (WHO grade I),
  - hemangioblastic meningioma (WHO grade I),
  - hemangiopericytic meningioma (WHO grade II),
  - papillary meningioma (WHO grade II to III),
  - anaplastic meningioma (WHO grade III).

The hemangioblastic meningioma does not arise from arachnoid cap cells. It develops from the capillary walls and exhibits a similar histological architecture to that of the cerebellar hemangioblastoma.

The hemangiopericytic meningioma develops from pericytes and demonstrates a higher degree of malignancy, for which reason it has a tendency to recur.

About 70 % of meningiomas reveal calcifications in the spinal canal, which are sometimes very extensive (Zimmerman and Bilaniuk, 1988).

Diagnostics

MRI

Meningiomas appear on MRI as extramedullary space-occupying tumors, often only monosegmental, whose contrast pattern on plain images differs only slightly from that of the spinal cord (Takemoto *et al.*, 1988). This applies in particular to T1-weighted images. Apart from a signal intensity that is isointense with the spinal cord, T2-weighted images can also demonstrate clearly higher signal intensity. In the presence of marked calcification of the tumor (e.g. with the psammomatous form), the signal intensity on T2-weighted images can also appear distinctly lower than that of the spinal cord.

The application of contrast improves delineation from the other tissue structures of the spinal canal, although a very strong enhancement is not always to be seen. Contrast enhancement can be low in individual cases. A calcified tumor will not infrequently demonstrate a mottled inhomogeneous contrast reaction. It is helpful to analyze exactly the meninges of the spinal cord after contrast application. The discovery of contrast enhancement in the contiguous meninges is not infrequent and is an indication of the tumor in relation to other differential diagnostic options (Figs. 5.51–5.59).

Tumors with an exclusively extradural pattern of expansion are not diagnostically distinguishable from other types of tumor, especially from neurinomas. An indication of extradural location of the tumor is when the dura is distinguishable as a thin black line between tumor and spinal cord. This is proof of location and is nearly always present.

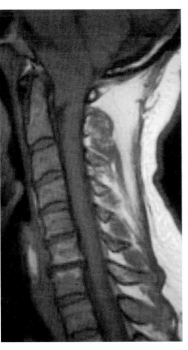

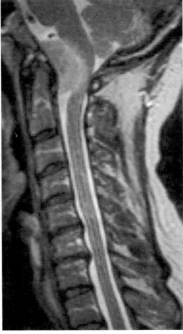

a

b

Fig. 5.**51 a, b Meningioma in the region of the foramen magnum:**
a T1-weighted sagittal image (TSE; TR = 693 ms, TE = 12 ms): The tumor demonstrates a signal intensity identical to that of the brain stem and spinal cord. There is a marked space-occupying effect stretching far rostrally along the clivus.
b T2-weighted sagittal image (TSE; TR = 5000 ms, TE = 112 ms): On this image there is a homogeneous signal intensity in the meningioma, which appears slightly enhanced relative to the spinal cord.

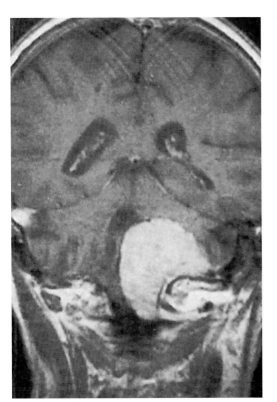

Fig. 5.**52 Large meningioma of the posterior cranial fossa with expansion into the cervical canal:** Coronal section after contrast application (SE; TR = 612 ms, TE = 20 ms): The tumor reveals a marked space-occupying effect with corresponding displacement of the cerebellar structures.

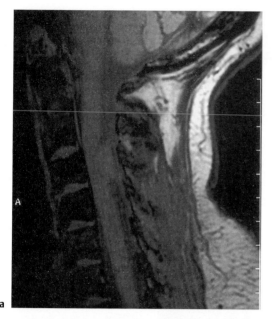

a

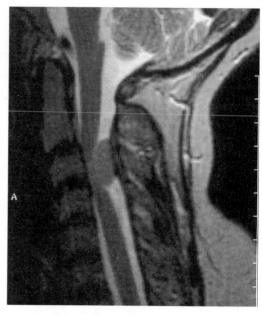

b

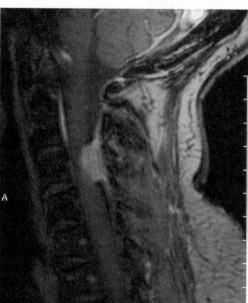

c

Fig. 5.**53 a–c Cervical meningioma at the level of C3.** 62-year-old patient:

a Sagittal section (FLASH; TR = 403 ms, TE = 11 ms, flip angle α = 90°): The tumor is encroaching on the spinal canal dorsally, demonstrating a signal intensity that corresponds to that of the spinal cord. Marked myelon compression.

b T2-weighted image (TSE; TR = 4602 ms, TE = 112 ms): The tumor reveals a slightly increased signal intensity relative to the spinal cord.

c After contrast application (FLASH; TR = 403 ms, TE = 11 ms, flip angle α = 90°): Here there is a homogeneous signal enhancement of the tumor. A concomitant reaction in the dura is clearly recognizable, appearing thickened proximally and caudally and revealing a correspondingly increased contrast enhancement.

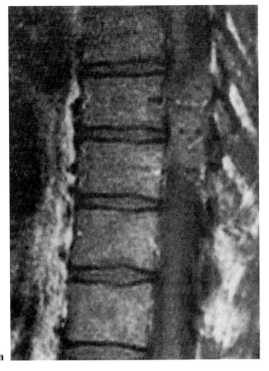

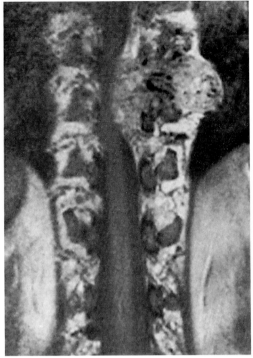

b

△
Fig. 5.**54 a, b** **Hemangioblastic meningioma with in-tradural/extradural direction of growth.** 53-year-old patient:
a T1-weighted sagittal section (SE; TR = 550 ms, TE = 25 ms): Image of the slightly hyperintense tumor showing small punctiform signal losses (vascular structures).
b Coronal section after contrast application: The space-occupying effect of the tumor is well recognizable, as is the hourglass pattern of growth. Slight enhancement with somewhat inhomogeneous contrast filling.

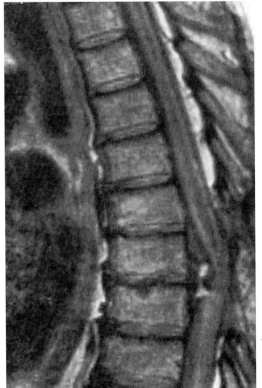

◁ Fig. 5.**55** **Calcifying psammomatous thoracic me-ningioma at the level T7/T8.** Marked compression of the spinal cord, proximal to which there is a syringomy-elia (SE; TR = 680 ms, TE = 20 ms). 52-year-old patient.

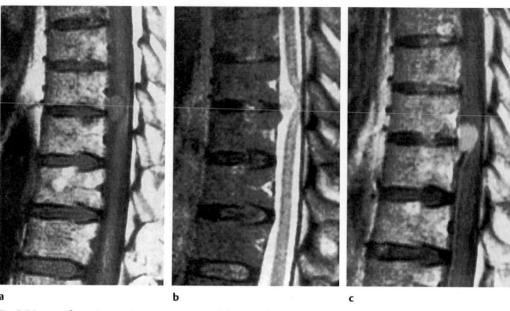

a   b   c

Fig. 5.**56 a–c Thoracic meningioma.** 68-year-old patient:

a T1-weighted image (SE; TR = 780 ms, TE = 25 ms): Isointense signal in the tumor relative to the spinal cord.

b T2-weighted image (SE; TR = 2100 ms, TE = 80 ms): The tumor appears clearly hyperintense.

c After contrast application: Strong enhancement of the tumor with concomitant involvement of the pia mater.

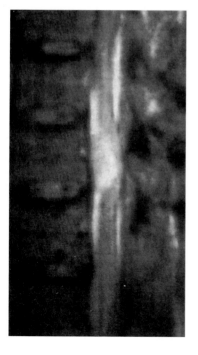

◁ Fig. 5.**57 Meningioma at the level T9.** T2-weighted image with clear signal enhancement of the tumor (SE; TR = 2100 ms, TE = 80 ms). 52-year-old patient.

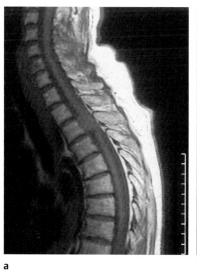
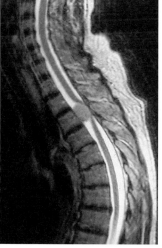
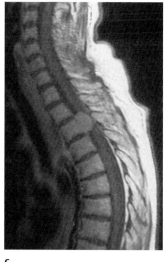

a b c

Fig. 5.**58 a–c Meningioma at the level T3.** The tumor is invading the spinal canal anteriorly, resulting in a marked compression of the spinal cord:

a T1-weighted sagittal image (TSE; TR = 800 ms, TE = 12 ms): The tumor is isointense with, and is growing anterior to, the spinal cord leading to massive displacement.

b T2-weighted sagittal image (TSE; TR = 5310 ms, TE = 112 ms): The tumor displays a slightly increased signal intensity relative to the spinal cord.

c After contrast application (TSE; TR = 800 ms, TE = 12 ms): Strong enhancement.

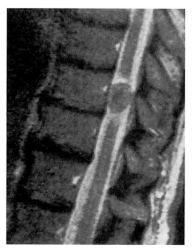
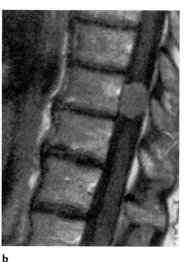

a b

Fig. 5.**59 a, b Thoracic meningioma.** 62-year-old female patient:

a T2-weighted image (SE; TR = 2100 ms, TE = 80 ms): Tumor isointense with the spinal cord.

b T1-weighted image after contrast application: Only moderate enhancement so that the tumor appears slightly hyperintense to the spinal cord (the plain image demonstrated an isointense signal; not shown).

Primary Melanoma

Primary melanomas are seen either as nodules or, in cases of diffuse spread, as leptomeningeal melanoblastosis. Macroscopically they appear as brown-black spots or in the form of a diffuse blackening of the leptomeninges, which is also associated with thickening. The tumors can also invade the spinal cord. The patients also usually present with large cutaneous pigmented nevi, although a form without skin affections is also known.

Primary Meningeal Sarcoma of the CNS

Primary meningeal sarcomas of the CNS are tumors that arise from undifferentiated leptomeningeal cells of the meninges of the brain and spinal cord, from the stromal plexus, the blood vessels and dystopic mesenchymal tissue. These sarcomas can have a nodular presentation or appear diffuse in the form of sarcomatosis. The diagnosis should only be made if a primary extracranial sarcoma has been ruled out.

The primary meningeal sarcoma has a predilection for children, adolescents and young adults. From 0.7–1.3 % of all intracranial tumors in children are primary meningeal sarcomas. It is a very aggressively growing tumor with a poor prognosis. The one-year survival rate after tumor resection is around 50 %.

The nodular form presents on MRI as a circumscribed tumor that is not sharply demarcated. It has contact with the leptomeninges, not infrequently allows visualization of cystic elements and demonstrates clear enhancement after contrast application. Differential diagnostic considerations include astrocytoma, neuroblastoma, lymphoma and PNET.

Diffuse sarcomatous infiltration exhibits tumor involvement of the leptomeninges, which becomes particularly conspicuous from enhancement after contrast application. The differential diagnosis includes other forms of leptomeningeal metastatic disease, meningitis, Sturge-Weber syndrome, and leptomeningeal melanosis (Pfluger *et al.*, 1997).

Paraganglioma

Paragangliomas belong to the group of neuroendocrine tumors (NET), a term which has largely replaced the name "apudoma." Neuroendocrine tumors consist of cells that display neural characteristics and have a potential endocrine function. Furthermore, the cells have peptide-containing secretory granula and are present, for example, in the adenohypophysis, the thyroid gland (medullary carcinoma), the islet cells of the pancreas (insulinoma), in the gastrointestinal tract (carcinoid), in the tracheobronchial tree (carcinoid), in the adrenal marrow, in the skin (Merkel cell tumor), in the lung (small-cell carcinoma) and in the chemoreceptor system (paraganglioma, especially the glomus jugulare tumor and the carotid body tumor). Paragangliomas are rarely found in the CNS where they are then seen primarily in the region of the pineal body, the petrous bone, the sella and in the spinal canal. The cell structures in the spinal canal from which the tumor arises have not yet been identified.

The tumors occur principally during middle age, with men being slightly more often affected than women. This tumor originates most commonly from the filum terminale, less often from the caudal nerve roots.

Usually a long period of clinical complaints with back pain and sciatica-like symptoms precedes before the tumor diagnosis is made.

The tumor has a tendency to recur if total resection is not possible.

Diagnostics

MRI

The tumor is usually isointense with the spinal cord on T1-weighted images. On T2-weighted images the tumor can also appear isointense relative to the spinal cord, although inhomogeneous signal intensities have been reported, with signal enhancements seen particularly in the region of the proximal and caudal tumor margin. The tumor usually demonstrates strong contrast enhancement. It is well vascularized and not infrequently intraspinal serpiginous vascular structures are recognizable flowing towards the tumor from a proximal direction. This is a very characteristic sign of the tumor and demonstrates the hypervascularized character of paragangliomas. The hypervascularized structure of the tumor can be visualized on MRI as a flow-void phenomenon in the form of punctiform zones of signal loss. In extreme cases, therefore, a mottled image can appear on T2-weighted images (a "salt and pepper" pattern).

The distinction from a neurinoma or an ependymoma is not always possible.

Myxopapillary Ependymoma

Incidence

The myxopapillary ependymoma is a well-vascularized tumor growing almost exclusively in the region of the thoracolumbar junction and arising from the filum terminale or the conus medullaris. About 40–60 % of all tumors of the spinal cord are ependymomas, of which almost 50 % originate in the region of the cauda equina. Up to 80 % of ependymomas in this region are assigned to the myxopapillary type.

Histology and Tumor Expansion

Histologically the myxopapillary ependymoma is a tumor rich in fibrous connective tissue, with a mucinous degeneration of the stroma and a mucoid secretion of the tumor cells. The tumor is rarely extradural in location.

Although the majority of the tumors extend over only 1–2 segments in the thoracolumbar region, an expansion over up to 10 segments can also be observed. In addition, individual cases exhibit multifocal tumors.

The tumor can lead to an enlargement of the spinal canal with corresponding bony erosion. Rarely does it extend into the intervertebral foramina (Fig. 5.**60**).

Diagnostics

MRI

In the majority of cases the tumor appears isointense with the spinal cord on T1 weighting, less frequently hypointense, and in exceptional cases hyperintense. The tumor practically always appears hyperintense on T2-weighted sequences. A strong characteristic enhancement is found after contrast application, although it can be inhomogeneous if smaller intratumoral cysts are present.

Contrast application delineates the extent of the tumor better. In individual cases it is the only way to detect the presence of cysts (Fig. 5.**61**).

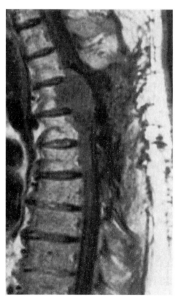 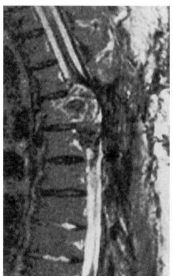 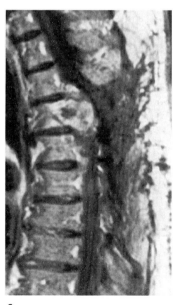

a b c

Fig. 5.**60 a–c** **Myxopapillary ependymoma (grade 1) with destruction of T6. Image after biopsy:**
a T1-weighted image (SE; TR = 770 ms, TE = 17 ms): Evidence of an intra- and extramedullary tumor isointense with the spinal cord and invading the bone anteriorly.

b T2-weighted image (SE; TR = 2100 ms, TE = 80 ms): The tumor demonstrates a slightly inhomogeneous signal intensity. Note the clear decrease in signal of those portions of the spinal cord that are adjacent proximally and distally. Hemosiderin deposits?

c After contrast application: Clear, yet inhomogeneous, tumor enhancement.

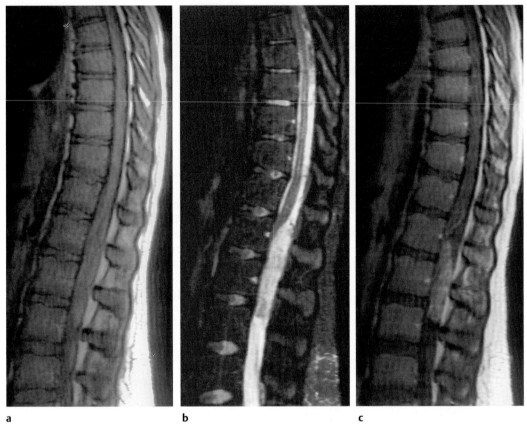

a   b   c

Fig. 5.**61 a–c Myxopapillary ependymoma in the region of the thoracolumbar junction:**

a T1-weighted sagittal section (TSE; TR = 800 ms, TE = 12 ms): Isointense tumor at the level of the conus and along the cauda with poor delineation relative to the spinal cord. Tumor extent is approximately from L1–L3.

b T2-weighted sagittal section (TSE; TR = 5300 ms, TE = 120 ms): Relatively homogeneous high signal intensity of the tumor, clear anterior displacement of the cauda and parts of the spinal cord.

c After contrast application (TSE; TR = 800 ms, TE = 12 ms): Here there is clear tumor enhancement, in part also involving the pia along the caudal parts of the spinal cord.

Subependymoma of the Filum Terminale

Subependymomas constitute a histological sub-entity of ependymomas and are characterized by a dense fibrillar and loose cellular stroma with corresponding ependymal cells. Proliferating fibrillar subependymal astrocytes dominate the histological picture. The cells can exhibit rosette forms, perivascular pseudo rosettes or clumps of polygonal cells with no particular alignment. The cell of origin of subependymomas is not exactly known.

The tumors can develop in the entire spinal canal. At the level of the filum terminale they are extramedullary in location, otherwise they are intramedullary.

One case study reports a hyperintense signal both on T1-weighted and T2-weighted SE sequences. A striking feature was that there was no significant signal enhancement on the contrast-assisted images. This is in accordance with the fact that the tumor is usually very avascular. It can have an appearance similar to that of a neurinoma or meningioma as regards its macro-morphological structure, so that these two tumors should be primarily included in any differential-diagnostic considerations (Roeder *et al.*, 1994).

Leptomeningeal Metastases

Pathogenesis and Clinical Presentation

Leptomeningeal metastases can develop both from intracranial tumors and systemic extracranial tumors (p. 304 *et seq.*).

Leptomeningeal metastatic disease often remains asymptomatic for a long time. Apart from that, very unspecific symptoms are also seen:

- headache,
- back pain,
- cranial nerve symptoms where there is involvement of the craniocervical junction.

Signs and symptoms arising from involvement of the spinal nerve roots are typical and sometimes take on a radicular form.

Diagnostics

MRI

The diagnosis may escape detection on plain images if there are no nodular changes seen along the leptomeninges. Nodular tumor metastases are, however, frequently well visualized both on T1- and on T2-weighted images. The highest detection rate for leptomeningeal metastatic disease is achieved by administering contrast medium, which demonstrates both nodular formations and also, in particular, any diffuse infiltration of the leptomeninges in the form of a sometimes quite distinct enhancement. Severe cases can result in enhancement of the entire dural sac, sometimes with involvement the nerve roots when marked tumor infiltration is present (Figs. 5.**62**–5.**65**).

The detection rate of MRI for leptomeningeal metastatic disease can be considered as low. It is assumed that no more than 10–15 % of all cases with metastatic spread are in fact detectable by MRI.

In individual cases the procedure is inferior to myelography, especially with small nodular structures. But as a rule, myelography, including CT myelography, is the poorer technique and MRI scanning is therefore the method of choice.

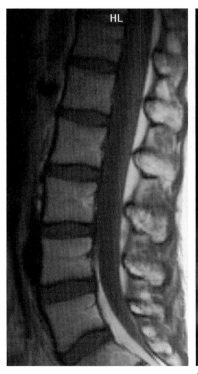 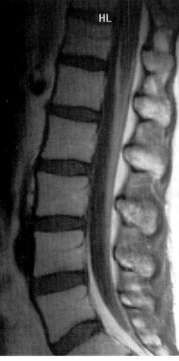

Fig. 5.**62 a–d** **Metastatic mammary carcinoma.** 25-year-old female patient:

a T1-weighted sagittal section (TSE; TR = 600 ms, TE = 12 ms): This image shows nothing obvious.

b Image after contrast application: Diffuse strong enhancement along the conus medullaris and the cauda equina with a uniform thickening of the leptomeningeal structures in the form of diffuse leptomeningeal metastatic disease.

Fig. 5.**62 c** and **d** ▷

a   b

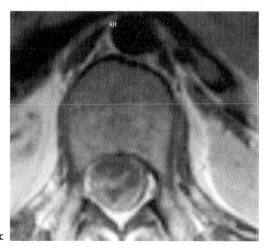

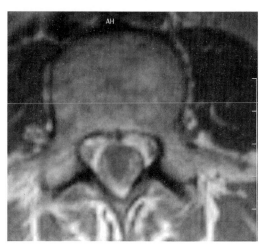

c

Fig. 5.62 c, d

c Transverse section immediately distal to the conus after contrast application: Irregular enhancement along the clumped nerve roots, which are in contact with each other.

d Transverse section after contrast application: The nerve roots course in a dorsolateral direction. They are attached to the dura and adherent to each other, producing a U-shaped configuration along the course of the nerve roots.

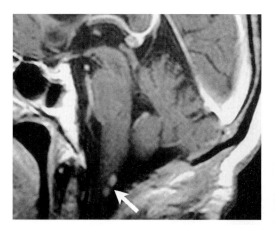

Fig. 5.**63 Two metastases overlying the cervical cord in a case of known carcinoma of the breast.** Sagittal section after contrast application; arrow (SE; TR = 722 ms, TE = 17 ms).

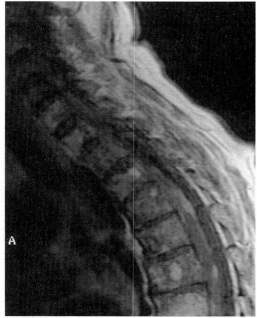

A

Fig. 5.**64 Diffuse osseous and intraspinal metastatic disease in a case of known bronchial carcinoma.** Image after contrast application (TSE; TR = 800 ms, TE = 12 ms): The image shows a mottled structure of the vertebral bodies with marked decreases in signal intensity. There are macronodular deposits along the spinal cord that display signal enhancement relative to the myelon.

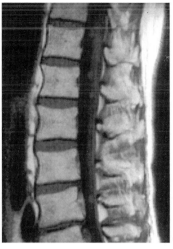 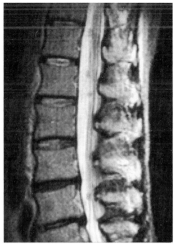 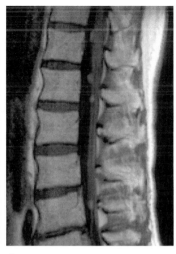

a
b
c

Fig. 5.**65 a–c Metastatic bronchial carcinoma.** 57-year-old patient:
a Sagittal section using T1 weighting (TSE; TR = 587 ms, TE = 12 ms): Multiple nodular structures along the conus medullaris and the cauda equina.

b T2-weighted image (TSE; TR = 5000 ms, TE = 112 ms): The small nodules are well delineated along the course of the cauda. They show a signal intensity that is isointense with the spinal cord.
c Image after contrast application: The small nodules reveal a relatively clear contrast enhancement.

Acquired Arachnoid cysts

Etiology and Pathogenesis

Acquired arachnoid cysts often develop after surgery on the spinal canal. Other causes include trauma, possibly in association with intraspinal hemorrhage, inflammation, spontaneous hemorrhage or (penetrating) injuries. The cysts are found with varying degrees of expansion and at differing locations, depending on the various etiological factors responsible for their development.

Diagnostics

MRI

They are recognizable on MRI both by their compressive effect on the spinal cord and by their enhanced CSF signal intensities. Difficulties arise if the cystic contents are not isointense with CSF, but are instead richer in protein or are xanthochromic. In such cases their signal pattern differs much from that of CSF. Separation from the spinal cord can sometimes be difficult. This is particularly the case when the spinal cord has undergone change in the form of myelomalacia secondary to compression, resulting in a marked in-tramedullary signal enhancement on T2-weighted images. Syringomyelias can also develop. Cavitations can expand after surgical drainage (the so-called balancing effect; Andrews *et al.*, 1988).

MRI is the imaging technique of choice and is often superior to CT myelography (Figs. 5.**66** and 5.**67**) (Sklar *et al.*, 1989).

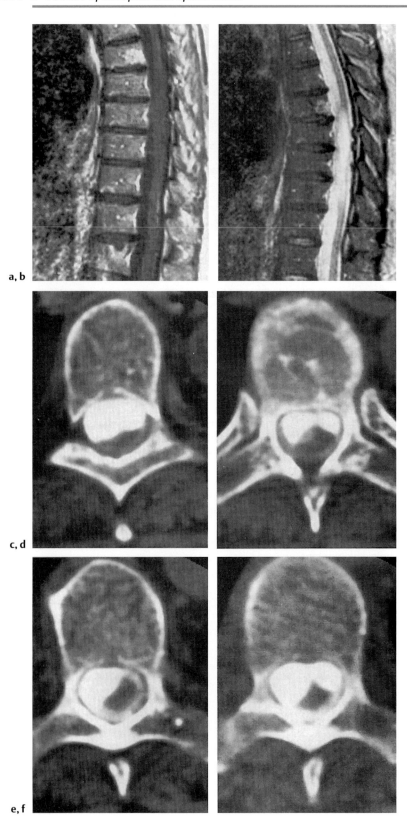

a, b

c, d

e, f

Fig. 5.**66 a–f Arachnoid cysts at the level T6–T10 after surgery for cervical hemangioblastoma.** Finding verified at surgery:

a T1-weighted image after contrast application (TSE; TR = 550 ms, TE = 25 ms): The arachnoid cysts display an increased signal intensity on the T1-weighted image and are not separated from the spinal cord.

b T2-weighted image (SE; TR = 2100 ms, TE = 80 ms): There is a hyperintense space-occupying lesion with a corresponding compression of the spinal cord.

c–f CT myelography at the level of the vertebrae T7 (**c**), T8 (**d**), T9 (**e**), and T10 (**f**). Six hours after intrathecal contrast application the images demonstrate small contrast concentrations within the arachnoid cysts, compression of the spinal cord, and partial elimination of the contrast medium from the subarachnoid space.

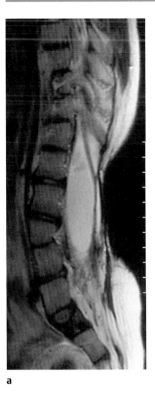

a

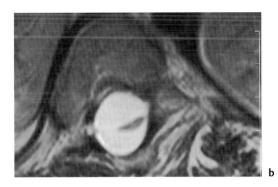

b

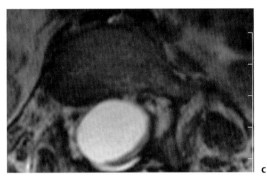

c

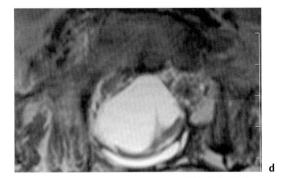

d

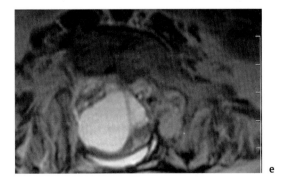

e

Fig. 5.**67 a–e** **Extensive arachnoid cysts in the lumbar region after surgery for myelomeningocele.** 9-year-old patient:

a T2-weighted sagittal image (TSE; TR = 3635 ms, TE = 120 ms): Clear enlargement of the spinal canal secondary to the underlying disease. Marked scarring at the operative site involving the attenuated and elongated myelon. Dysplasia of the distal lumbar vertebrae and the first sacral vertebra.

b–e Transverse sections obtained from cranial to caudal which show the dorsal displacement of the spinal cord originating from the arachnoid cyst (**c, d** and **e**). Cord-like scar formation stretching from posterior to anterior and radiating here into the dura (**d** and **e**).

■ **Intramedullary Tumors**

Astrocytoma

Incidence

About 10–25 % of all tumors of the spinal canal are gliomas, of which about one half are astrocytomas. The tumor is particularly common in children; it constitutes the largest proportion of intramedullary tumors in infancy. Altogether the frequency peak lies in the third to fourth decade of life.

Location and Grading

The tumor is most commonly seen in the thoracic cord, with the second most common location being the cervical cord; rarely are astrocytomas found at a lumbar location. The astrocytoma extends over on average of about six segments. Some tumors involve the entire spinal cord and are known as *panmedullary* astrocytomas.

Apart from the peg-like, diffusely infiltrating form of growth, which is associated with a sometimes only mild expansion of the spinal cord, an expansile, displacing manner of growth is also reported. These tumors are well delineated from the spinal cord and can sometimes be removed *in toto* at surgery (intradural extramedullary growth).

The commonest tumors are the grade I or grade II types.

Diagnostics

MRI

At MRI the tumors are predominantly slightly hypointense on T1-weighted images. On T2-weighted images they display a clear signal enhancement, which is mainly of homogeneous signal intensity. Inhomogeneities can however occur secondary to hemorrhage and necrosis with subsequent cystic formations. Differentiation between tumor and edema can prove difficult on plain images, as can the distinction between a reactive cyst or syrinx and tumor necrosis. The administration of contrast, however, will render this possible. Tumor cysts display marginal enhancement with contrast, while reactive cysts do not. The application of contrast is therefore useful to visualize better the full extent of the tumor and usually produces an inhomogeneous enhancement. These tumors nearly always take up contrast material, unlike intracranial astrocytomas (Figs. 5.**68**–5.**70**).

Surgical removal is the therapy of choice, usually followed up by radiotherapy. Histological grading is of crucial prognostic relevance. Patients with a higher-grade astrocytoma usually experience rapid deterioration, not least due to tumor dissemination into the CSF.

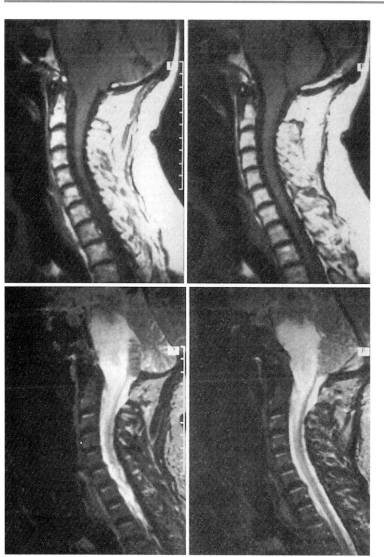

Fig. 5.68 a–d   Long-segment astrocytoma with intracranial and cervical location:

a, b T1-weighted image (SE; TR = 500 ms, TE = 15 ms): Diffuse expansion of the pons, medulla oblongata, and upper cervical cord. No difference in signal intensity relative to the non-involved parts of the brain.

c, d T2-weighted image (SE; TR = 2500 ms, TE = 90 ms): Diffuse and homogeneous signal enhancement of the tumor.

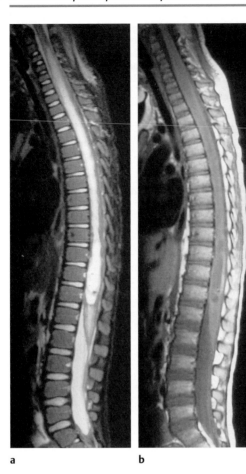

a   b

Fig. 5.**69 a, b** **Long-segment astrocytoma.** 5-year-old boy:
a T1-weighted sagittal image (STIR): Tumor extending from C4 to L1 with in part clear enlargement of the spinal cord. High signal intensity in the entire portion of the affected myelon.
b T1-weighted image (TSE; TR = 642 ms, TE = 12 ms): Enlargement of the spinal cord with a marked intramedullary decrease in signal intensity.

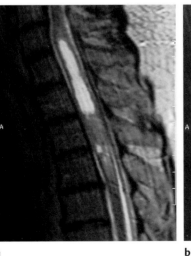

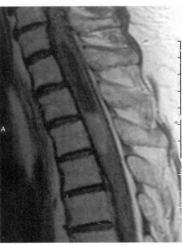

a   b

Fig. 5.**70 a, b** **Astrocytoma.** 64-year-old patient:
a T2-weighted sagittal image (TSE; TR = 5310 ms, TE = 112 ms): Clear enlargement of the spinal cord at the level of C7–T4 with inhomogeneous mottled, in part very high, signal intensity.
b After contrast application a viable, contrast-enhancing portion of the tumor becomes apparent caudally with a reactive cyst proximal to it.

Ependymoma

Incidence

The ependymoma is the commonest intramedullary tumor in adulthood. The age peak lies in the fourth decade, although ependymomas are also seen in infancy and at high age.

Location

The tumor is particularly common in the thoracic cord, less often in the cervical cord. Tumors occurring at the dorsolumbar junction are principally extramedullary in location. They are usually of the myxopapillary type.

Apart from the ependymoma, a rare intramedullary tumor is the subependymoma, which is also found at an extramedullary location along the filum terminale (p. 330).

Growth

The tumors mainly grow in a peg-like fashion, sometimes extending over the entire spinal cord. Spindle-shaped and nodular forms of growth are also known. They are usually situated in a central location. Cystic formations are seen in up to 50 %

of cases. Calcifications are rare with spinal ependymomas, unlike their intracranial counterparts.

Diagnostics

MRI

On the T1-weighted plain image the tumor displays hypointensive or isointensive signal intensity relative to the spinal cord, while a clear signal enhancement is seen on T2-weighted images. Regions of hemorrhage can differ considerably with respect to their signal pattern. Hemosiderin deposits are not infrequently found, particularly in the region of the proximal and caudal marginal contours of the tumor. Enhancement is always seen after contrast application, appearing very strong in some cases. It can appear homogeneous, although it is usually displayed as irregular and mottled.

The distinction between ependymoma and astrocytoma is difficult. The view of Scotti *et al.* (1987) that the contrast pattern contributes towards differentiation has basically not been confirmed. However, the contrast enhancement of ependymomas does usually appear stronger and more homogeneous than that of astrocytomas.

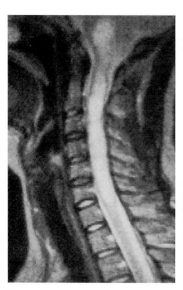 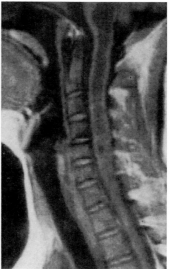 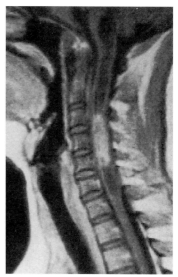

a   b   c

Fig. 5.**71 a–c Ependymoma.** 28-year-old female patient:
a T2-weighted image (SE; TR = 1600 ms, TE = 90 ms): Signal-intense expansion of the medulla oblongata and the cervical cord as far as C6/C7.
b Plain T1-weighted image (FLASH; TR = 315 ms, TE = 14 ms, flip angle α = 90°): Syringomyelia extend-

ing from the medulla oblongata to C6, revealing inhomogeneities suggestive of tumor between C3 and C5.
c After contrast application, solid portions of the tumor between C3 and C5, very strong and almost homogeneous contrast enhancement.

Ependymomas are recognizable by their more central location as compared with the more eccentrically growing astrocytomas. Moreover, an ependymoma is more likely in the presence of hemorrhage than an astrocytoma. And not least, tumors in the cervical region are more likely to be classified as an astrocytoma and those in the dorsolumbar region as an ependymoma (Figs. 5.**71**–5.**76**).

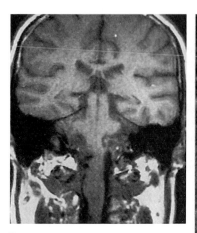

a

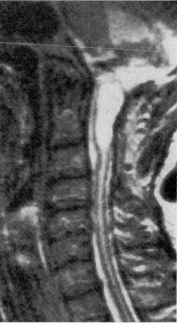

b

Fig. 5.**72 a, b** **Ependymoma at the level C2/C3.** Image obtained after partial removal of the tumor:
a T1-weighted coronal image (SE; TR = 550 ms, TE = 20 ms): Spindle-shaped portions of the tumor in the cervical canal, the signal of which appears slightly hypointense to the brain stem.
b T2-weighted image (SE; TR = 2100 ms, TE = 80 ms): Clear signal enhancement of the tumor, enlargement of the spinal cord, and peg-shaped expansion of the myelon edema caudally.

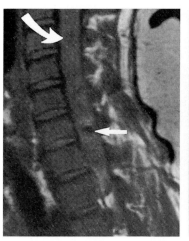

a

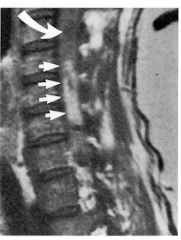

b

Fig. 5.**73 a,b** **Ependymoma in the cervical cord:**
a T1-weighted sagittal image (SE; TR = 650 ms, TE = 25 ms): Multiple nodular zones, in part with decreased signal intensity secondary to hemorrhage (arrows).
b After contrast application: Enhancement in the region of the tumor (arrows). The circumscribed myelomalacia of the cord at the level C3 can be regarded as reactive and not as tumor cavitation (curved arrow).

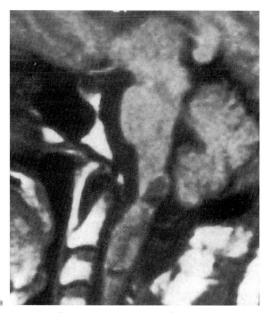

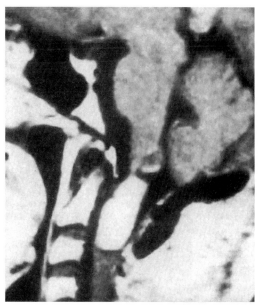

b

Fig. 5.**74 a, b   Ependymoma at C2/C3.**
a Plain image (SE; TR = 550 ms, TE = 20 ms): Enlargement of medulla oblongata and the upper cervical
cord by the tumor. In part, slightly decreased signal
intensity.

b Strong and homogeneous enhancement after contrast application

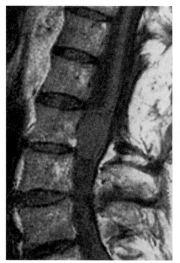

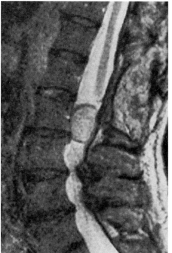

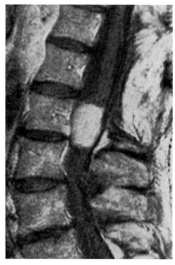

a   b   c

Fig. 5.**75 a–c   Recurrent ependymoma at L2.**
a T1-weighted   plain   image   (SE;   TR = 785 ms,
TE = 25 ms): The tumor shows a signal intensity that
parallels that of the spinal cord.

b T2-weighted image (SE; TR = 2100 ms, TE = 80 ms):
Low signal intensity. Hypointense pseudocapsular peripheral margin.
c Clear homogeneous signal enhancement after contrast application.

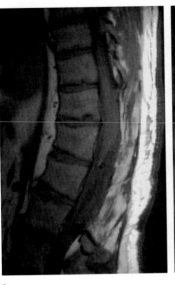
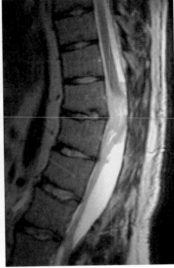
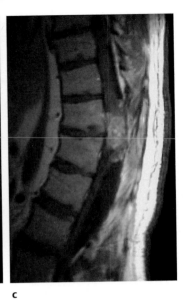

a   b   c

Fig. 5.**76 a–c** **Ependymoma in the conus region.** Recurrent tumor after previous surgery. 28-year-old
patient:
a T1-weighted image: Enlargement of the conus by a
tumor that is isointense with the spinal cord. Postlaminectomy image of the segments T12–L2.

b T2-weighted image: The tumor appears slightly signal-intense relative to the spinal cord.
c After contrast application: Strong, relatively homogeneous enhancement.

Primitive Neuroectodermal Tumor (PNET)

PNET is a collective term for tumors of the CNS
whose tumor matrix consists of undifferentiated
cells arising from the germinal matrix of the
primitive neural tube. They have the capability of
neuronal, glial or ependymal differentiation. Included here are:

- medulloblastoma of the cerebellum,
- pineoblastoma,
- neuroblastoma.

The terms "primary cerebral neuroblastoma,"
"undifferentiated small-cell tumor" and "blue
tumor" stem from the size and staining properties
of the tumor cells.

The common characteristic of these tumors is
their aggressive infiltrative growth with a strong
tendency to disseminate into the CSF. They are
very sensitive to radiation. A tumor manifestation
in the spinal canal is often to be regarded as secondary, although it can develop primarily from
the spinal cord. The tumors can be found in an intramedullary as well as a diffuse leptomeningeal
location particularly along the cauda equina. The
spinal canal should always be examined with
contrast medium for an exact assessment of the
extent of any intraspinal dissemination (Fig. 5.**77**).

Further Rare Intramedullary Tumors

Further rare intramedullary tumors worthy of
mention include, among others:

- gangliocytoma (Fig. 5.**78**),
- ganglioglioma (extremely rarely seen in extramedullary intradural locations),
- oligodendroglioma,
- glioblastoma.

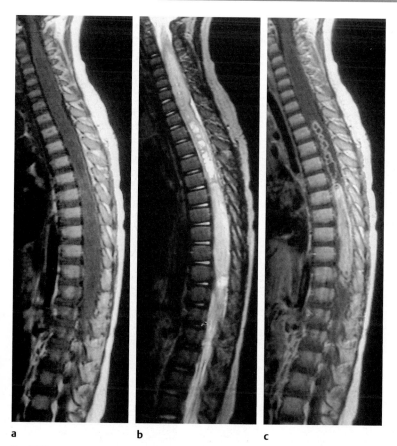

a   b   c

Fig. 5.**77 a–c Primitive neuroectodermal tumor (PNET) of the spinal cord.** 2-year-old girl:

a T1-weighted sagittal image (SE; TR = 405 ms, TE = 12 ms): Massive enlargement of the entire spinal cord along the course of the spinal canal with marked reduction in signal intensity. Cystic structures are in part separable, particularly in the mid-region of the thoracic spine.

b T2-weighted sagittal image (TSE; TR = 5310 ms, TE = 112 ms): The cystoid structures in the mid-region of the thoracic spine are more readily demonstrated on T2 weighting. Extensive, in part strong, signal enhancement of the myelon.

c Image after contrast application (SE; TR = 405 ms, TE = 12 ms): Strong contrast enhancement in the entire area of the tumor. The cystic structures are in part surrounded by a fringe of contrast medium, allowing the assumption of tumor cysts. The enlargement of the myelon recognizable in the region of the cervical spine is reactive and not secondary to tumor infiltration.

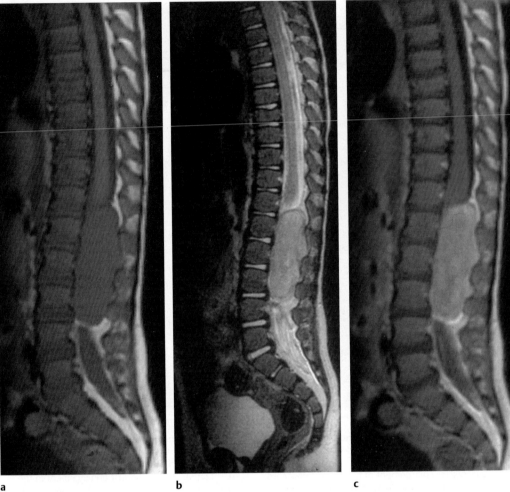

a   b   c

Fig. 5.**78 a–d Gangliocytoma.** The gangliocytoma originates from the distal part of the myelon and encroaches on the cauda equina. 16-year-old boy:

a T1-weighted sagittal image (SE; TR = 700 ms, TE = 19 ms): The tumor extends from T12 to the junction L3/L4. It demonstrates a homogeneous signal intensity that appears lower than that of the spinal cord. Note the marked distension of the spinal canal with corresponding erosion of the bone.

b T2-weighted image (TSE; TR = 3000 ms, TE = 108 ms): The tumor displays a largely homogeneous signal intensity that is slightly enhanced relative to the spinal cord.

c Image after contrast application: There is a strong, largely homogeneous contrast enhancement.

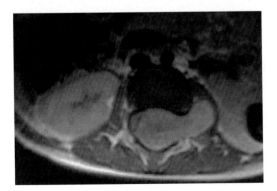

Fig. 5.**78 d** Transverse section after contrast application: The tumor extends further into the psoas muscle via the intervertebral foramen on the left side. The spinal canal appears distended secondary to tumor growth, as does the intervertebral foramen on the left.

Intramedullary Metastases

Intramedullary metastases are seen most commonly in the thoracic cord, especially in the caudal sections. The second most common area is the cervical region, with the lumbar region being most rarely affected. The metastases are usually small tumors confined to one segmental region.

Diagnostics

MRI

Intramedullary metastases are only rarely associated with the formation of cysts. The metastases are often hypointense on T1-weighted images and hyperintense on T2-weighted images. After contrast application there is usually a strong homogeneous enhancement. As with intracerebral metastases the size of the metastasis and the reactive perifocal edema are disproportionate. The perifocal edema is usually extensive and can be taken as an indication for an intramedullary metastasis. Intramedullary metastases rarely demonstrate hemorrhage with a subsequently different signal pattern (Fig. 5.**79**, see also Fig. 5.**39**).

Extradural, Intradural, Extramedullary, and Intramedullary Tumor manifestations

■ Primary Malignant Lymphoma, Secondary Lymphomatous Manifestation, Leukemic Infiltrate

Epidural Malignant Lymphoma

Incidence and Tumor Expansion

A primary epidural site is observed in approximately 2–6 % of all cases of malignant lymphoma. The tumor may have a circumscribed epidural location, although both intradural and extradural sites are also found that demonstrate a corresponding invasion of paravertebral structures via the intervertebral foramina. In individual cases the paravertebral part of the tumor may turn out to be larger than the intraspinal tumor mass.

The most commonly found tumors are those with intermediate-grade malignancy, followed by those with low-grade malignancy. They are rarely lymphomas with high-grade malignancy. Compression of the spinal cord is particularly typical

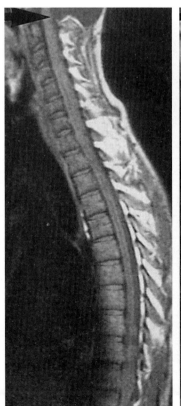
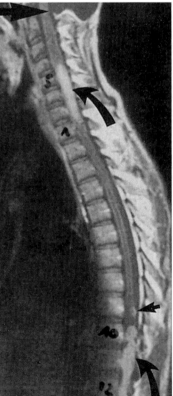

Fig. 5.**79 a, b** **Intramedullary metastases of a medulloblastoma:**
a T1-weighted plain image (SE; TR = 500 ms, TE = 15 ms): Enlargement of the cervical cord and the spinal cord at the level T10–T12 without any difference in signal intensity. Image obtained after surgery for medulloblastoma in the posterior cranial fossa (large straight arrow).
b After contrast application: Evidence of an intramedullary peg-shaped metastasis at the level C5–T1 and T10–T12 (curved arrows). Additional small nodule at T9 (small straight arrow). Edema-related enlargement of the upper cervical cord (large straight arrow).

a   b

of non-Hodgkin's lymphoma, less so of Hodgkin's lymphoma.

The tumors either originate from a vertebra and develop into the epidural space or, on the other hand, they may be encountered with no vertebral involvement at all. Some cases may be diagnosed in which vertebrae at other levels are also involved, in addition to the epidural invasion. Additional epidural compression, however, does not always develop from these vertebrae. The lymphomatous infiltration usually extends over 2–6 vertebral segments. It can be found both in a purely anterior as well as a posterior location, but the combined circumferential tumor infiltration is observed most commonly.

The thoracic space is the site of predilection, followed by the lumbar, cervical and lumbosacral spinal canal.

Diagnostics

MRI

Epidural lymphomas usually demonstrate an isointense signal intensity relative to the spinal cord on T1 weighting, a high signal intensity on PD weighting and an isointense signal, or even high signal, on T2 weighting. The majority of cases display homogeneous signal intensity. After contrast application there is usually a strong, less frequently a moderate, enhancement.

A differentiation between tumors with low-, moderate- or high-grade malignancy based on MRI appearance is not possible (Fig. 5.**80**).

Intramedullary Tumor Involvement

Incidence and Pathogenesis

Malignant lymphomas arising primarily in the spinal cord are rare. Primary malignant lymphomas of the CNS originate from pluripotent mesenchymal vascular cells and the leptomeninges of the brain or spinal cord. At first a dense accumulation of cell nests in the adventitia of the blood vessels develops, from where the tumor begins its diffuse perivascular spread; once adjacent vessels are involved, tumor cell nests merge to form larger areas, which can be nodular or long-segment.

This mechanism of development is the reason why primary malignant lymphomas assume a

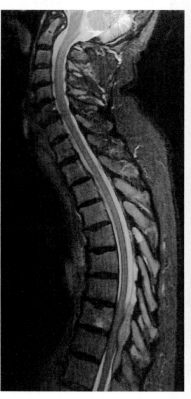

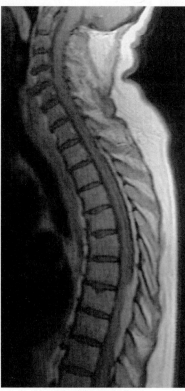

Fig. 5.**80 a, b Epidural lymphoma at the level T7–T10 with concomitant involvement of T8:**

a T2-weighted sagittal image (STIR): Space-occupying malignant lymphoma with epidural location and corresponding elevation of the dura dorsally. Somewhat higher signal intensity of the lymphoma relative to the spinal cord. Marked dorsal compression. Concomitant evidence of a mottled signal inhomogeneity with mild signal enhancements of T8.

b Sagittal section after contrast application (TSE; TR = 800 ms, TE = 12 ms): The tumor enhances homogeneously with contrast. The changes in T8 are not recognizable on this image.

a   b

non-tumor-like (non-space occupying) character and therefore, for a long time, are not, or only poorly, definable macroscopically. The lesions show a tendency to metastasize into the CSF spaces (Fig. 5.**81**).

There is considered to be an association between the occurrence of malignant lymphomas and immunosuppressive therapy. Malignant lymphomas are thus commonly seen in association with sustained drug therapy after renal transplantation; congenital or acquired immune defects also increase the incidence.

Intradural Extramedullary Tumor Dissemination

Incidence and Pathogenesis

Extramedullary tumor dissemination is found, on the one hand, in the presence of a primary cerebral malignant lymphoma, which not infrequently results in tumor metastasis to the spinal canal. On the other hand, CNS involvement can occur in the presence of a systemic lymphatic disease. The grade of malignancy of malignant lymphomas is, however, not the decisive factor for involvement of the CNS; even low-grade lymphomas metastasize into the CNS with a frequency from 15–83 % (mycosis fungoides), as do high-grade non-Hodgkin lymphomas where the figures vary from 23–47 %. The majority of cases display a subarachnoid spread with infiltration of the leptomeninges. The metastatic invasion can occur in the form of a diffuse dissemination along the leptomeninges that is sometimes associated with nodular tumor cell nests.

CNS involvement is not infrequently seen in leukosis among children, where the probability of CNS infiltration depends on the duration of the disease course. Concomitant involvement of the CNS is most common in acute lymphatic leukemia. In principle, involvement of the CNS can also occur in adults with leukemia, although it is considerably less frequent than in children. Here, too, it usually involves a diffuse infiltration of the leptomeninges and the entire subarachnoid space. Perivascular cell accumulations can predominate when the spinal cord is affected.

Diagnostics

MRI

According to studies comparing MRI with CSF cytology, the detection rate for leptomeningeal infiltration using MRI in patients with malignant lymphoma is regarded as low and amounts to under 10 % (Yousem *et al.*, 1990). This also applies for the use of contrast administration, although the detection rate can be clearly raised as compared with plain images.

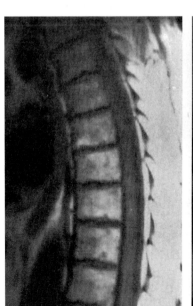
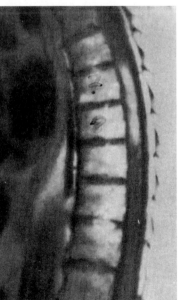

Fig. 5.**81 a, b** **Intramedullary malignant lymphoma T7/T8:**
a T1-weighted plain image (SE; TR = 320 ms, TE = 15 ms): No certain evidence of a pathological change.
b After contrast application strong intramedullary enhancement.

a   b

The overall low detection rate is explained by the tumors being frequently non-nodular. Only in the presence of larger cell accumulations is a strong enhancement usually to be expected after contrast application, which then confirms the finding (Fig. 5.**82**).

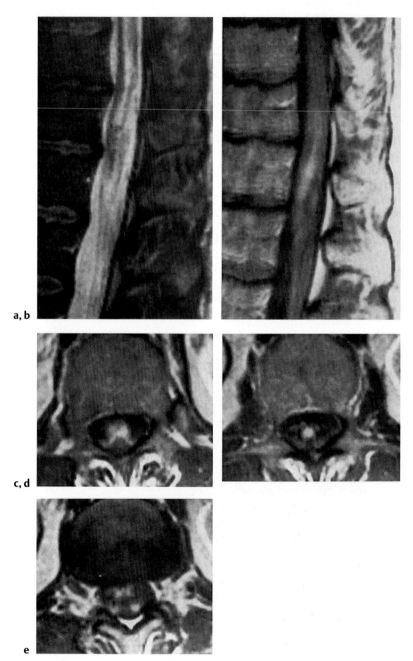

a, b

c, d

e

Fig. 5.**82 a–e Non-Hodgkin lymphoma (B-cell lymphoma with involvement of the CNS):**
a T2-weighted image (SE; TR = 2100 ms, TE = 80 ms): Streaky signal enhancement of the spinal cord at the level of the thoracolumbar junction.
b T1-weighted image after contrast application (SE; TR = 785 ms, TE = 25 ms): Signal enhancement in the region of the conus and the cauda equina.
c Transverse section after contrast application: Evidence of an intramedullary signal enhancement, which also extends in part to the nerve roots.
d Section further caudal to **c**.
e Section further caudal to **d**. Enhancement of the nerve roots of the cauda equina, concomitant thickening of the nerves is recognizable.

Summary

- The following bone tumors are found preferentially in the spine:
  - osteoblastoma,
  - hemangioma,
  - aneurysmal bone cyst,
  - chordoma,
  - plasmacytoma,
  - metastases.
- The *osteoblastoma* is a benign tumor that is usually seen in the vertebral appendages of the thoracic and lumbar spine. On MRI it appears as a hypo- or isointense structure on the T1-weighted image and on the T2-weighted image as a hyperintense tumor relative to muscle.
- *Hemangiomas* are discovered in about 10 % of all examinations. It is often an incidental finding. Complaints occur with expansive growth or pathological fractures. MRI reveals a relatively characteristic presentation with signal enhancement on the T1- and T2-weighted image.
- The *aneurysmal bone cyst* is an expansive lesion with thinned-walled, blood-filled cavities. There is inhomogeneous signal intensity on MRI, frequently associated with fluid–fluid levels caused by hemorrhage.
- The *chordoma* is preferentially found at the clivus and at the craniocervical junction, as well as caudally at the level of the sacrum or coccyx. An uncharacteristic signal pattern is found on MRI with a reduction in signal on the T1-weighted image and signal enhancement on the T2-weighted image.
- With an incidence of 50 %, the *plasmacytoma* is by far the commonest malignant bone tumor. MRI is the technique best suited for diagnosing involvement of the bone marrow. A distinction is made between a focal, variegated, diffuse and mixed pattern of involvement. The most sensitive sequences for detecting bone marrow infiltration are:
  - T1-weighted spin echo sequence,
  - opposed-phase GRE sequence,
  - STIR sequence.
- The eosinophilic granuloma is a common tumor of infancy. It displays a solitary lesion of the vertebral body that is associated with vertebral collapse (vertebra plana). The signal pattern on MRI is uncharacteristic.
- *Skeletal metastases* are a particularly common finding with mammary, prostatic and bronchial carcinomas. Whereas evidence of involvement of the vertebral body can be obtained successfully, diagnosing invasion of the pedicles and the transverse and spinous processes can pose problems. MRI should be run with the following sequences:
  - T1-weighted SE sequence,
  - opposed-phase GRE sequence,
  - STIR sequence.
- *Epidural lipomatosis* is counted among the most frequent epidural space-occupying lesions and can occur secondary to alimentary and hormonal factors. The increased adipose tissue is easily recognized on MRI from its characteristic signal pattern. Surgery to provide relief of symptoms may be indicated when appropriate signs and symptoms are present.
- *Intraspinal synovial cysts* are the result of spondylarthrotic alterations of the small vertebral joints. Their posterolateral location in contact with the vertebral joint is a characteristic feature. The signal intensity on MRI can differ from that of CSF.
- The commonest intradural extramedullary tumors are the *meningioma* and the *neurinoma*. The meningioma in particular is a tumor of the female sex; a hormone-stimulated form of growth is postulated. Meningiomas tend to be cervical in location, while neurinomas are found more often at thoracolumbar sites. Both types of tumor enhance strongly with contrast. Meningiomas are prone to form calcifications, neurinomas can develop large cysts. T1- and T2-weighted images do not usually allow a differentiation between the two tumors. Both tumors demonstrate on T1 weighting a pattern that is iso- or hypointense relative to the spinal cord and a moderate to strong signal enhancement on T2 weighting. A characteristic feature of the neurinoma worth noting is its hourglass type of growth.
- *Neurofibromas* are usually seen in association with von Recklinghausen's neurofibromatosis. The tumors show a multiple occurrence by preference. A combined intraspinal-extraspinal growth is common with considerable space-occupying effects resulting from multiple tumors. The plexiform neurofibroma, which has an extensive growth pattern and can result in widespread infiltrations, is a noteworthy type. The

Summary

signal intensity seen on the T1-weighted MR image is isointense with muscle or slightly hyper-intense, while there is a clear signal intensity enhancement on T2 weighting. A strong enhancement is observed after contrast application.

- *Paragangliomas* belong to the group of neuroendocrine tumors. They are slow-growing tumors whose characteristic is their marked hypervascularity. Not infrequently, vessels can be seen on MRI flowing toward the tumor from a proximal direction. Sometimes present within the tumor is a mottled image with small punctiform signal losses as a flow-void phenomenon, resulting in the so-called salt-and-pepper pattern on T2 weighting. A strong enhancement is seen after contrast application.

- A common tumor of the conus-cauda region is the *myxopapillary ependymoma*, which is extramedullary in location. The tumor usually extends over 1–2 segments only. It can lead to erosion of the vertebral body. The tumor is isointense on T1 weighting, rarely hypointense, and on the T2-weighted image nearly always hyperintense. A strong enhancement is typically seen after contrast application.

- The *subependymoma of the filum terminale* is a relatively avascular tumor found extramedullary in location at the level of the filum; otherwise it has an intramedullary site. It displays little contrast enhancement.

- *Leptomeningeal metastatic disease* can present in the diffuse, nodular or cluster form. The detection rate of MRI for metastatic spread is rather low, with only 10–15 % of all cases being discovered on MRI. The highest rate of detection is achieved after contrast application

- *Acquired arachnoid cysts* arise from surgery, trauma, hemorrhage and inflammation. They display a characteristic CSF signal and are recognizable by their space-occupying effect. However, their identification can be difficult on MRI, when either there is a variation in signal intensity or where there are myelon changes present.

- From 10–25 % of all intramedullary tumors are *gliomas*, of which about 50 % are *astrocytomas*. The tumor is particularly frequently seen in children. The highest frequency is found during the third and fourth decades. The thoracic cord is most commonly affected. The astrocytoma usually extends over six or more segments. A panmedullary form of growth can occur. A non-specific signal pattern is seen at MRI on T1- and T2-weighted plain images. After contrast application there is a strong, sometimes mottled, enhancement due to the possible presence of tumor necrosis. Reliable criteria for differentiating astrocytomas from other intramedullary tumors, especially ependymomas, are not available.

- *Ependymomas* are the commonest intramedullary tumors of adulthood. The tumor is most frequently of thoracic location, less often cervical. It displays a peg-like form of growth; sometimes a panmedullary expansion is present. Cystic formations are typical, while calcifications are rare. The signal pattern is uncharacteristic, both on T1- and T2-weighted images. Nor do contrast enhancement patterns allow any differential diagnostic conclusions.

- *PNETs* occur particularly in children. They exhibit a particularly aggressive form of growth with a tendency to disseminate into the CSF. The application of contrast is particularly important for demonstrating the total extent of the tumor.

- *Intramedullary metastases* occur less frequently than leptomeningeal metastases. They are preferentially seen in a thoracic location. As with cerebral metastases, intramedullary metastases have a tendency for extensive edema formation.

- *Malignant lymphomas* or *non-Hodgkin lymphomas* are not infrequently found in an extradural location. The tumor can arise in the vertebral bodies, but can also develop independent of the vertebrae. Lymphomatous infiltration usually extends over 2–6 vertebral segments.

- Malignant lymphomas are rarely found in the spinal cord. Their development is often associated with immunosuppressive therapy.

- Malignant lymphomas can present in the form of tumor dissemination into the subarachnoid space, with a malignant systemic disease or even a cerebral manifestation being the cause. Detection is often only possible after contrast application. On the whole, detection of tumor dissemination into the CSF is less likely by MRI than with lumbar puncture for CSF.

References

Aggarwal, S., J. H. N. Deck, W. Kucharczyk: Neuroendocrine tumor (paraganglioma) of the cauda equina: MR and pathologic findings. Amer. J. Neuroradiol. 14 (1993) 1003–1007

Aisen, A. M., W. Martel, E. M. Braunstein, K. I. McMillin, W. A. Phillips, T. F. Kling: MRT and CT evaluation of primary bone and soft-tissue tumors. Amer. J. Roentgenol. 146 (1986) 749–756

Andrews, B. T., P. R. Weinstein, M. L. Rosenblum, N. M. Barbaro: Intradural arachnoid cysts of the spinal canal associated with intramedullary cysts. J. Neurosurg. 68 (1988) 544–549

Aoki, J., H. Tanikawa, K. Ishii, G. S. Seo, O. Karakida, S. Sone et al.: MR findings indicative of hemosiderin in giant-cell tumor of bone: frequency, cause, and diagnostic significance. Amer. J. Roentgenol. 166, (1996) 145–148

Augustin, J. J. T., E. G. Martinench, F. C. Corretger, L. C. Salcines, A. D. Errando: Computed tomography of a post traumatic spinal arachnoid cyst. Neuroradiology 31 (1989) 354–355

Barloon, T. J. W., T. C. Yuh, C. J. C. Yang, D. H. Schultz: Spinal subarachnoid tumor seeding from intracranial metastasis: MR findings. J. Comput. assist. Tomogr. 11 (1987) 242–244

Barnett, M. J. M., N. B. Rewcastle: Syringomyelia and tumors of the nervous system. In Barnett, M. J. M., J. B. Foster, P. Hudgron: Syringomyelia. Saunders, Philadelphia 1973 (pp. 261 –301)

Baur, A., A. Stäbler, R. Bartl, R. Lamerz, M. Reiser: Infiltrationsmuster des Plasmozytoms in der Magnetresonanztomographie. Fortschr. Röntgenstr. 164 (1996) 457–463

Baur, A., A. Stäbler, R. Bartl, R. Lamerz, J. Scheidler, M. Reiser: MRI gadolinium enhancement of bone marrow: age-related changes in normals and in diffuse neoplastic infiltration. Skelet. Radiol. 26 (1997) 414–418

Baur, A., A. Stäbler, R. Brüning, R. Bartl, A. Krödel, M. Reiser et al.: Diffusion-weighted MR imaging of bone marrow: Differentiation of benign versus pathologic compression fractures. Radiology 207 (1998) 349–356

Beltran J., D. C. Simon, M. Levy, L. Herman, L. Weis, C. F. Mueller: Aneurysmal bone cysts: MR imaging at 1,5 T. Radiology 158 (1986) 689–690

Beres, J., P. Pech, Th. F. Berns, D. L. Daniels, A. L. Williams, V. M. Haughton: Spinal epidural lymphomas: CT features in seven patients. Amer. J. Neuroradiol. 7 (1986) 327–328

Berns, D. H., S. Blaser, J. S. Ross, Th. J. Masaryk, M. T. Modic: MR imaging with Gd-DTPA in leptomeningeal spread of lymphoma. J. Comput. assist. Tomogr. 12 (1988) 499–500

Blews, D. E., H. Wang, A. J. Kumar, P. A. Robb, P. C. Phillips, R. N. Bryan: Intradural spinal metastases in pediatric patients with primary intracranial neoplasms: Gd-DTPA enhanced MR vs CT myelography. J. Comput. assist. Tomogr. 14 (1990) 730–735

Bohndorf, K., M. Reiser, B. Lochner, W. Féaux de Lacroix, W. Steinbrich: Magnetic resonance imaging of primary tumours and tumour-like lesions of bone. Skelet. Radiol. 15 (1986) 511–517

Boncoeur-Martel, M.-P., A. Lesort, J.-J. Moreau et al.: MRI of paraganglioma of the filum terminale. J. Comput. assist. Tomogr. 20 (1996) 162–164

Boukobza, M. C. Mazel, E. Touboul: Primary vertebral and spinal epidural non-Hodgkin's lymphoma with spinal cord compression. Neuroradiology 38 (1996) 333–337

Breger, R. K., A. L. Williams, D. L. Daniels, L. F. Czervionke, L. P. Mark, V. M. Haughton et al.: Contrast enhancement in spinal MR imaging. Amer. J. Roentgenol. 153 (1989) 387–391

Britton, J., H. Marsh, B. Kendall, D. Kingsley: MRI and hydrocephalus in childhood. Neuroradiology 30 (1988) 310–314

Burk jr., D. L., J. A. Brunberg, E. Kanal, R. E. Latchaw, G. L. Wolf: Spinal and paraspinal neurofibromatosis: surface coil MR imaging at 1,5 T. Radiology 162 (1987) 797–801

Buthiau, D., J. C. Piette, M. N. Ducerveau, G. Robert, P. Godeau, F. Heitz: Steroid-induced spinal epidural lipomatosis: CT survey. J. Comput. assist. Tomogr. 12 (1988) 501–503

Bydder, G. M., J. Brown, H. P. Niendorf, I. R. Young: Enhancement of cervical intraspinal tumors in MR imaging with intravenous Gadolinium-DTPA. J. Comput. assist. Tomogr. 9 (1985) 847–851

Campbell, A. N., H. S. L. Chan, L. E. Becker, A. Daneman, T. S. Park, H. J. Hofman: Extracranial metastases in childhood primary intracranial tumors: a report of 21 cases and review of the literature. Cancer 53 (1984) 974–981

Campoy, F., P. Stiefel, E. Stiefel, J. M. Loizaga, J. Arduan, F. Campoy: Pilomatrix carcinoma: role played by MR imaging. Neuroradiology 31 (1989) 196–198

Chui, M. C., B. L. Bird, J. Rogers: Extracranial and extraspinal nerve sheath tumors: computed tomographic evaluation. Neuroradiol. 30 (1988) 47–53

Cohen, M. D., E. C. Klatte, R. Baehner, J. A. Smith, P. Martin-Simmerman, B. E. Carr et al.: Magnetic resonance imaging of bone marrow disease in children. Radiology 151 (1984) 715–718

Daffner, R. H., A. R. Lupetin, N. Dash, Z. L. Deeb, R. J. Sefczek, R. L. Schapiro: MRT in the detection of malignant infiltration of bone marrow. Amer. J. Roentgenol. 146 (1986) 353–358

Davies, A. M., R. M. Wellings: Imaging of bone tumors. Curr. Opin. Radiol. 4 (1992) 32–38

Demachi, H., T. Takashima, M. Kadoya, M. Suzuki, H. Konishi, K. Tomita et al.: MR imaging of spinal neurinomas with pathological correlation. J. Comput. assist. Tomogr. 14 (1990) 250–254

Dihlmann, W.: Gelenke, Wirbelverbindungen, 3. Aufl. Thieme, Stuttgart 1987

Dillon, W. P., D. Norman, T. H. Newton, K. Bolla, A. Mark: Intradural spinal cord lesions: Gd-DTPA-enhanced MR imaging. Radiology 170 (1989) 229–237

Dooms, G. C., M. R. Fisher, H. Hricak, M. Richardson, L. E. Crooks, H. K. Genant: Bone marrow imaging: Magnetic resonance studies related to age and sex. Radiology 155 (1985) 429–432

Enzmann, D. R., J. O'Donohue, J. B. Rubin, L. Shuer, P. Cogen, G. Silverberg: CSF pulsations within nonneoplastic spinal cord cysts. Amer. J. Roentgenol. 149 (1987) 149–157

Fenzl, G., S. H. Heywang, Th. Vogl: Die Kernspintomographie mit Gadolinium-DTPA in der Diagnostik spinaler Läsionen. Fortschr. Röntgenstr. 148 (1988) 415–418

Feydy, A., R. Carlier, C. Vallee, D. Mompoint, A. Chevallier, S. Engerand et al.: Imaging of osteosclerotic metastases. J. Radiol. 76 (1995) 561–572

Filling-Katz, M. R., P. L. Choyke, N. J. Patronas, M. B. Gorin, D. Barba, R. Chang et al.: Radiologic screening for von Hippel-Lindau disease: the role of Gd-DTPA enhanced MR imaging of the CNS. J. Comput. assist. Tomogr. 13 (1989) 743–755

Fontaine, S., D. Melanson, R. Cosgrove, G. Bertrand: Cavernous hemangiomas of the spinal cord: MR imaging. Radiology 166 (1988) 839–841

Fredericks, R. K., A. Elster, F. O. Walker: Gadolinium-enhanced MRT: a superior technique for the diagnosis of intraspinal metastases. Neurology 39 (1989) 734–736

Freyschmidt, J.: Knochenerkrankungen im Erwachsenenalter. Röntgenologische Diagnose und Differenzialdiagnose. Springer, Berlin 1980

Friedburg, H., M. Schumacher, J. Hennig: Pathologie des kraniozervikalen Übergangs in der magnetischen Resonanztomographie. Fortschr. Röntgenstr. 145 (1986) 315–320

Frocrain, L., R. Duvauferrier, J.-L. Husson, J. Noel, A. Ramee, Y. Pawlotsky: Recurrent postoperative sciatica: Evaluation with MR imaging and enhanced CT. Radiology 170 (1989) 531–533

Frühwald, F., St. Frühwald, P. Ch. Hajek, B. Schwaighofer, A. Neuhold, L. Wicke: Fokale Fetteinschlüsse im Knochenmark der Wirbelsäule – MR-Befunde. Fortschr. Röntgenstr. 148 (1988) 75–78

Gero, B. T., K. Y. Chynn: Symptomatic spinal epidural lipomatosis without exogenous steroid intake. Neuroradiology 31 (1989) 190–192

Goy, A. M. C., R. S. Pinto, B. N. Raghavendra, F. J. Epstein, I. I. Kricheff: Intramedullary spinal cord tumors: MR imaging, with emphasis on associated cysts. Radiology 161 (1986) 381–386

Gupta, R. K., P. Agarwal, H. Rastogi, S. Kumar, R. V. Phadke, N. Krishnani; Problems in distinguishing spinal tuberculosis from neoplasia on MRI. Neuroradiology 38 (1996) 97–104

Hachem, K., S. Haddad, N. Aoun, J. Tamraz, N. Attalah: MRI in the diagnosis of osteoid osteoma. J. Radiol. 78 (1997) 635–641

Hemminghytt, S., D. L. Daniels, A. L. Williams, V. M. Haughton: Intraspinal synovial cysts: natural history and diagnosis by CT. Radiology 145 (1982) 375–376

Hochstenbag, M. M., G. Snoep, N. A. Cobben, A. M. Schols, F. B. Thunnissen, E. F. Wouters et al.: Detection of bone marrow metastases in small lung cell cancer. Comparison of magnetic resonance imaging with standard methods. Europ. J. Cancer 32A (1996) 779–782

Jackson jr., D. E., S. W. Atlas, J. R. Mani, D. Dorman,: Intraspinal synovial cysts: MR imaging. Radiology 170 (1989) 527–530

Jänisch, W., D. Schreiber, H. Güthert: Neuropathologie. Tumoren des Nervensystems. Fischer, Stuttgart 1988

Josten, N., B. Sander, W. Schörner, A. Hackl, H. Henkes, P. Schubeus et al.: Kernspintomographische Screeninguntersuchungen des Knochenmarks mit Gradientenecho-Sequenzen. Fortschr. Röntgenstr. 154 (1991) 614–620

Kaffenberger, D. A., C. P. Shah, F. R. Murtagh, C. Wilson, M. L. Silbiger: MR imaging of spinal cord hemiangioblastoma associated with syringomyelia. J. Comput. assist. Tomogr. 12 (1988) 495–498

Kahn, Th., N. Roosen, G. Fürst, E. Lins, W. J. Bock, H.-G. Lenard et al.: MRT mit Gadolinium-DTPA bei spinalen intraduralen Raumforderungen. Fortschr. Röntgenstr. 151 (1989) 602–610

Kaplan, P. A., R. J. Asleson, L. W. Klassen, M. J. Duggan: Bone marrow patterns in aplastic anemia: Observations with 1,5-T MR imaging. Radiology 164 (1987) 441–444

Karnaze, M. G., M. H. Gado, K. J. Sartor, F. J. Hodges III: Comparison of MR and CT myelography in imaging the cervical and thoracic spine. Amer. J. Roentgenol. 150 (1988) 397–403

Katz, B. H., R. M. Quencer, R. S. Hinks: Comparison of gradient-recalled-echo and T_2-weighted spin-echo pulse sequences in intramedullary spinal lesions. Amer. J. Neuroradiol. 10 (1989) 815–822

Kernohan, J. W., G. P. Sayre: Tumors of the Central Nervous System. Armed Forces Institute of Pathology, Washington 1952

Kleihues, P., M. Kiessling, G. Wagner, F. Amelung: Tumoren des Nervensystems. Standardisierte Nomenklatur, biologisches Verhalten und klinisch-pathologische Definitionen. Springer, Berlin 1988

Kleinman, G. M., F. H. Hochberg, E. P. Richardson: Systemic metastases from medulloblastoma. Report of two cases and review of the literature. Cancer 48 (1981) 2296–2309

Kosuda, S., T. Kaji, H. Yokoyama, T. Yokokawa, M. Katayama, T. Iriye et al.: Does bone SPECT actually have lower sensitivity for detecting vertebral metastasis than MRI? J. nucl. Med. 37 (1996) 975–978

Krahe, Th., V. Nicolas, S. Ring, M. Warmuth-Meth, O. Köster: Diagnostische Aussagefähigkeit von Röntgenübersichtsaufnahme und Computertomographie bei Knochentumoren der Wirbelsäule. Fortschr. Röntgenstr. 150 (1989) 13–19

Kramer, E. D., S. Rafto, R. J. Pacher, R. A. Zimmermann: Comparison of myelography with CT follow-up versus Gadolinium MRI for subarachnoid metastatic disease in children. Neurology 41 (1991) 46–50

Kransdorf, M. J., D. E. Sweet, Aneurysmal bone cyst: concept, controversy, clinical presentation, and imaging. Amer. J. Roentgenol. 164 (1995) 573–580

Krol, G., G. Sze, M. Malkin, R. Walker: MR of cranial and spinal meningeal carcinomatosis: Comparison with CT and myelography. Amer. J. Roentgenol. 151 (1988) 583–588

Lanir, A., E. Aghai, J. S. Simon, R. G. L. Lee, M. E. Clouse: MR imaging in myelofibrosis. J. Comput. assist. Tomogr. 10 (1986) 634–636

Layer, G., T. Sommer, M. Busch, H. Schüller, H. H. Schild: Quantitative Evaluierung der Eignung von Magnetresonanzsequenzen zum Nachweis von Wirbelsäulenmetastasen solider Tumoren. Fortschr. Röntgenstr. 168 (1998) 20–26

Lecouvet, F. E., B. C. Vande Berg, B. E. Maldague, L. Michaux, E. Laterre, J.-L. Michaux et al.: Vertebral compression fractures in multiple myeloma. Part I. Distribution and appearance at MR imaging. Radiology 204 (1997a) 195–199

Lecouvet, F. E., J. Malghem, L. Michaux, J.-L. Michaux, F. Lehmann, B. E. Maldague et al.: Vertebral compression fractures in multiple myeloma. Part II. Assessment of fracture risk with MR imaging of spinal bone marrow. Radiology 204 (1997b) 201–205

Lewis, T. T., D. P. E. Kingsley: Magnetic resonance imaging of multiple spinal neurofibromata-neurofibromatosis. Neuroradiology 29 (1987) 562–564

Libshitz, H., S. R. Malthouse, D. Cunningham, A. D. Mac Vicar, J. E. Husband: Multiple myeloma: appearance at MR imaging. Radiology 182 (1992) 833–837

Link, T. M., J. Sciuk, H. Frundt, W. Konermann, O. Schober, P. E. Peters: Wirbelsäulenmetastasen. Wertigkeit diagnostischer Verfahren bei der Erstdiagnostik und im Verlauf. Radiologe 35, 1 (1995) 21–27

Maehara, K., Tanohata, M. Noda, D. Nakayama: Medically treated steroid-induced epidural lipomatosis. Neuroradiology 30 (1988) 281

Mammone, J. F., M. E. Schweitzer, MRI of occult sacral insufficiency fractures following radiotherapy. Skelet. Radiol. 24 (1995) 101–104

Mascalchi, M., P. Torselli, F. Falaschi, G. D. al Pozzo: MRI of spinal epidural lymphoma. Neuroradiology 37 (1995) 303–307

Mathews, V. P., D. R. Broome, R. R. Smith, J. R. Bognanno, L. H. Einhorn, M. K. Edwards: Neuroimaging of disseminated germ cell neoplasms. Amer. J. Neuroradiol. 11 (1990) 319–324

McKinstry, C. S., R. E. Steiner, A. F. Young, L. Jones, D. Swirsky, V. Aber: Bone marrow in leukemia and aplastic anemia: MR imaging before, during, and after treatment. Radiology 162 (1987) 701–707

Mehta, R. C., M. P. Marks, R. S. Hinks, G. H. Glover, D. R. Enzmann: MR evaluation of vertebral metastases:T1-weighted, short-inversion-time inversion recovery, fast spin-echo, and inversion recovery fast spin-echo sequences. Amer. J. Neuroradiol. 16, (1995) 281–288

Miller, T. J., H. Wang: Case report: radiologic diagnosis of intracranial and intraspinal subarachnoid metastasis from a malignant spinal cord astrocytoma. Med. J. 39 (1990) 471–473

Moore, S. G., C. A. Gooding, R. C. Brasch, R. L. Ehman, H. G. Ringertz, A. R. Ablin et al.: Bone marrow in children with acute lymphocytic leukemia: MR relaxation times. Radiology 160 (1986) 237–240

Morano, J. U., W. F. Russell: Nerve root enlargement in Charcot-Marie-Tooth disease: CT appearance. Radiology 161 (1986) 784

Moulopoulos, L. A., D. G. K. Varma, M. A. Dimopoulos, N. E. Leeds, E. E. Kim, D. A. Johnston et al.: Multiple myeloma: spinal MR imaging in patients with untreated newly diagnosed disease. Radiology 185 (1992) 833–840

Moulopoulos, L. A., M. A. Dimopoulos, R. Alexanian, N. E. Leeds, H. I. Libshitz: Multiple myeloma: MR patterns of response to treatment. Radiology 193 (1994) 441–446

Nakahara, N., M. Uetani, K. Hayashi: Magnetic resonance imaging of sacral insufficiency fractures: characteristic features and differentiation from sacral metastasis. Nippon Igaku Hoshasen Gakkai Zasshi 55 (1995) 281–288

Nittner, K.: Spinal meningiomas, Neurinomas and neurofibromas and hourglass tumors. In Vinken, P. J., G. W.

Bruyn: Tumors of the Spine and Spinal Cord. North Holland, Amsterdam 1976 (pp. 177–322)

Parizel, P. M., D. Baleriaux, G. Rodesch, C. Segebarth, B. Lalmand, C. Christophe et al.: Gd-DTPA-enhanced MR imaging of spinal tumors. Amer. J. Roentgenol. 152 (1989) 1087–1096

Pfluger, T., S. Weil, S. Weis, K. Bise, J. Egger, H. B. Hadorn et al.: MRI of primary meningeal sarcomas in two children: differential diagnostic considerations. Neuroradiology 39 (1997) 225–228

Porter, B. A., A. F. Shields, D. O. Olson: Magnetic resonance imaging of bone marrow disorders. Radiol. Clin. N. Amer. 24 (1986) 269–289

Poser, L. M.: The Relationship Between Syringomyelia and Neoplasm. Thomas, Springfield 1956

Post, M. J. D., R. M. Quencer, B. A. Green, B. M. Montalvo, J. A. Tobias, J. J. Sowers et al.: Intramedullary spinal cord metastasis, mainly of non-neurogenic origin. Amer. J. Roentgenol. 148 (1987) 1015–1022

Pozzi-Mucelli, R., M. Cova, I. Shariat-Razavi, F. Zucconi, M. Ukmar, R. Longo: Comparison of magnetic resonance Spin-Echo sequences and fat-suppressed sequences in bone diseases. Radiol. med. 93 (1997) 504–509

Quint, D. J., R. S. Boulos, W. P. Sanders, B. A. Mehta, S. C. Patel, R. L. Tiel: Epidural lipomatosis. Radiology 169 (1988) 458–490

Ramsey, R. G., C. E. Zacharias: MR imaging of the spine after radiation therapy: Easily recognizable effects. Amer. J. Roentgenol. 144 (1985) 1131–1135

Reiser, M., Th. Kahn, F. Weigert, P. Lukas, F. Büttner: Diagnostik der Spondylitis durch die MR-Tomographie. Fortschr. Röntgenstr. 145 (1986) 320–325

Reiser, M., K. Bohndorf, H.-P. Niendorf, G. Friedmann, R. Erlemann, V. Kunze: Erste Erfahrungen mit Gadolinium-DTPA in der magnetischen Resonanztomographie (MR) von Knochen- und Weichteiltumoren. Radiologe 27 (1987) 467–472

Reiser, M., R. Erlemann, A. Härle, A. Roessner, P. Wuisman, V. Kunze et al.: Radiologische Diagnostik der Knochentumoren – Aussagekraft von konventioneller Röntgendiagnostik, Computertomographie und magnetischer Resonanztomographie. In Heuck/Keck: Fortschritte der Osteologie in Diagnostik und Therapie. Springer, Berlin 1988 (S. 125–136)

Reiser, M., A. Härle, A. Sciuk: Entzündliche Skeletterkrankungen. In Peters, P. E., H. H. Matthias, M. Reiser: Magnetresonanztomographie in der Orthopädie. Enke, Stuttgart 1990 (S. 59–82)

Resnick, D., G. Niwayama: Skeletal metastases. In Resnick, D., G. Niwayama: Diagnosis of Bone and Joint Disorders, 2nd ed. Saunders, Philadelphia 1988 (pp. 3944–4011)

Resnick, D., M. Kyraikos, G. D. Greenway: Tumors and tumor-like lesions of bone: imaging and pathology of specific lesions: In Resnick, D., G. Niwayama: Diagnosis of Bone and Joint Disorders, 2nd ed. Saunders, Philadelphia 1988 (pp. 3616–3888)

Roeder, M. B., J. R. Jinkins, C. Bazan III: Subependymoma of filum terminale: MR appearance. J. Comput. assist. Tomogr. 18 (1994) 129–130

Rosenthal, D. I., J. A. Scott, H. J. Mankin, G. L. Wismer, T. J. Brady: Sacrococcygeal chordoma: magnetic resonance imaging and computed tomography. Amer. J. Roentgenol. 145 (1985) 143–147

Ross, J. S., T. J. Masaryk, M. T. Modic, J. R. Carter, T. Mapstone, F. H. Dengel: Vertebral hemangiomas: MR imaging. Radiology 165 (1987) 165–169

Sardanelli, F., E. Melani, R. Sabattini, R. C. Parodi, A. Castaldi, G. Rescinito et al.: The role of T2*-weighted gradient-echo magnetic resonance sequences in the study of suspected dorsal-lumbosacral vertebral metastases. Radiol. med. 94 (1997) 296–301

Sarrazin, J. L., O. Helie, G. Lefriant, D. Soulie, Y. S. Cordoliani, G. Cosnard: A rare case of chondroid chordoma of the cervical spine. J. Radiol. 77 (1996) 141–144

Sauvage, P. J., P. Thivolle, J. B. Noel, J. Dagognet, V. Quipourt, R. Auberger et al.: MRI in the early diagnosis of spinal metastases of bronchial cancer. J. Radiol. 77 (1996) 185–190

Savader, S. J., R. R. Otero, B. L. Savader: MR imaging of intrathoracic extramedullary hematopoiesis. J. Comput. assist. Tomogr. 12 (1988) 878–880

Schöter, I., J. Wappenschmidt: Die intraspinale Raumforderung im computerassistierten Myelogramm (CAM). Fortschr. Röntgenstr. 133 (1980) 527–530

Schubeus, P., W. Schörner, H. Henkes, G. Hertel, R. Felix: MRT bei primärer und tumorbedingter Syringomyelie. Fortschr. Röntgenstr. 151 (1989) 713–719

Schubeus, P., W. Schörner, N. Hosten, R. Felix: Spinal cord cavities, differentialdiagnostic criteria in magnetic resonance imaging. Europ. J. Radiol. 12 (1991) 219–225

Schulz, E. E., W. L. West, D. B. Hinshaw, D. R. Johnson: Gas in a lumbar extradural juxtraarticular cyst. Sign of synovial origin. Amer. J. Roentgenol. 143 (1984) 875–876

Scotti, G., G. Scialfa, N. Colombo, I. Landoni: Magnetic resonance diagnosis of intramedullary tumors of the spinal cord. Neuroradiology 29 (1987) 130–135

Silbergeld, J., W. A. Cohen, K. R. Maravilla, R. W. Dalley, M. Sumi: Supratentorial and spinal cord hemangioblastomas: Gadolinium enhanced MR appearance with pathologic correlation. J. Comput. assist. Tomogr. 13 (1989) 1048–1051

Silbergleit, R., St. S. Gebarski, J. A. Brunberg, J. McGillicudy, M. Blaiovas: Lumbar synovial cysts: Correlation of myelographic, CT, MR, and pathologic findings. Amer. J. Neuroradiol. 11 (1990) 777–779

Silverstein, A. M., D. J. Quint, P. E. McKeever. Intradural paraganglioma of the thoracic spine. Amer. J. Neuroradiol. 11 (1990) 614–616

Sklar, E., R. M. Quencer, B. A. Green, B. M. Montalvo, M. J. D. Post: Acquired spinal subarachnoid cyst: evaluation with MR, CT, myelography, and intraoperative sonography. Amer. J. Roentgenol. 153 (1989) 1057–1064

Slasky, B. S., G. M. Bydder, H. P. Niendorf, I. R. Young: MR imaging with Gadolinium-DTPA in the differentiation of tumor, syrinx, and cyst of the spinal cord. J. Comput. assist. Tomogr. 11 (1987) 845–850

Smoker, W. R. K., J. C. Godersky, R. K. Knutzon, W. D. Keyes, D. Norman, W. Bergman: The role of MR imaging in evaluation metastatic spinal disease. J. Neuroradiol. 8 (1987) 901–908

Soderlund, V.: Radiological diagnosis of skeletal metastases. Europ. Radiol. 6 (1996) 587–595

Sone, M., S. Ehara, M. Sasaki, T. Nakasato, Y. Tamakawa, H. Shiraishi et al.: Fluid-fluid levels in bone and soft tissue tumors demonstrated by MR imaging. Nippon Igaku Hoshasen Gakkai Zasshi 52 (1992) 1110–1115

Spencer, R. R., W. Jahnke, R. L. Hardy: Dissection of gas into an intraspinal synovial cyst from contiguous vacuum facet. J. Comput. assist. Tomogr. 7 (1983) 886–888

Stäbler, A., R. Beck, R. Bartl, D. Schmidt, M. Reiser: Vacuum phenomena in insufficiency fractures of the sacrum. Skelet. Radiol. 24 (1995) 31–35

Stimac, G. K., B. A. Porter, D. O. Olson, R. Gerlach, M. Genton: Gadolinium-DTPA-enhanced MR imaging of spinal neoplasms: preliminary investigation and comparison with unenhanced spinecho and STIR sequences. Amer. J. Roentgenol. 151 (1988) 1185–1192

Sze, G., G. Krol, R. D. Zimmerman, M. D. F. Deck: Intramedullary disease of the spine: Diagnosis using Gadolinium-DTPA-enhanced MR imaging. Amer. J. Roentgenol. 151 (1988a) 1193–1204

Sze, G., G. Krol, A. Abramson et al.: Gadolinium – DTPA in the evaluation of intradural extramedullary spinal disease. Amer. J. Roentgenol. 150 (1988b) 911–921

Sze, G., G. Krol, R. D. Zimmerman, M. D. F. Deck: Malignant extradural spinal tumors: MR imaging with Gd-DTPA. Radiology 167 (1988c) 217–223

Tabatabai, A., C. A. Jungreis, H. Yonas: Cervical schwannoma masquerading as a glioma: MR findings. J. Comput. assist. Tomogr. 14 (1990) 489–490

Takemoto, K., Y. Matsumura, H. Hashimoto, Y. Inoue, T. Fukuda, M. Shakudo et al.: MR imaging of intraspinal tumors – Capability in histological differentiation and compartmentalization of extramedullary tumors. Neuroradiology 30 (1988) 303–309

Tsuji, H., E. Takazakura, Y. Terada, H. Makino, A. Yasuda, Y. Oiko: CT demonstration of spinal epidural emphysema complicating bronchial asthma and voilent coughing. J. Comput. assist. Tomogr. 13 (1989) 38–39

Uhlenbrock, D., S. Sehlen, H. K. Beyer: Spinechosequenzen und schnelle Bildsequenzen im Vergleich bei Erkrankungen der Wirbelsäule. Fortschr. Röntgenstr. 148 (1988) 79–83

Valk, J.: Gd-DTPA in MR of spinal lesions. Amer. J. Roentgenol. 150 (1988) 1163–1168

Van Heuzen, E. P., M. C. Kaiser, R. G. M. de Slegte: Neurocutaneous melanosis associated with intraspinal lipoma. Neuroradiology 31 (1989) 349–351

Vande Berg, B. C., F. E. Lecouvet, L. Michaux, M. Labaisse, J. Malghem, J. Jamart et al.: Stage I multiple myeloma: value of MR imaging of the bone marrow in the determination of prognosis. Radiology 201 (1996) 243–246

Vande Berg, B. C., L. Michaux, F. E. Lecouvet, M. Labaisse, J. Malghem, J. Jamar et al.: Nonmyelomatous monoclonal gammopathy: Correlation of bone marrow MR images with laboratory findings and spontaneous clinical outcome. Radiology 202 (1997) 247–251

Vanneste, J. A. L.: Subacute bilateral malignant exophthalmos due to orbital medulloblastoma metastases. Arch. Neurol. 40 (1983) 441–443

Wagle, W. A., B. Kaufman, J. E.Mincy: Intradural extramedullary ependymoma: MR-pathologic correlation. J. Comput. assist. Tomogr. 12 (1988) 705–707

Wakamatsu, T., T. Matsuo, S. Kawano, S. Teramoto, H. Matsumura: Extracranial metastasis of intracranial tumor. Acta pathol. jap. 22 (1972) 155–169

Wang, A. M., C. . Gall, J. Shillito, R. Schick, M. L. Brooks, N. Haikal: CT demonstration of extradural thoracic meningioma. J. Comput. assist. Tomogr. 12 (1988) 536–538

Weber, D. M., M. A. Dimopoulos, L. A. Moulopoulos, K. B. Delasalle, T. Smith, R. Alexanian: Prognostic features of asymptomatic multiple myeloma. Brit. J. Haematol. 97 (1997) 810–814

Weigert, F., M. Reiser, K. Pfändner: Die Darstellung neoplastischer Wirbelveränderungen durch die MR-Tomographie. Fortschr. Röntgenstr. 146 (1987) 123–130

Williams, A. L., V. M. Haughton, K. W. Pojunas, D. L. Daniels, D. P. Kilgore: Differentiation of intramedullary neoplasms and cysts by MR. Amer. J. Roentgenol. 149 (1987) 159–164

Wippold, F. J. II, J. G. Smirniotopoulos, C. J. Moran, J. N. Suojanen, D. G. Vollmer: MR imaging of myxopapillary ependymoma: findings and value to determine extent of tumor and its relation to intraspinal structures. Amer. J. Roentgenol. 165 (1995) 1263–1267

Wylie, E. J., B. Kendall: Cranio-vertebral bony changes in a case of congenital lipomatosis. Neuroradiology 31 (1989) 352–353

Yamaguchi, T., K. Tamai, M. Yamato, K. Honma, Y. Ueda, K. Saotome: Intertrabecular pattern of tumors metastatic to bone. Cancer 78 (1996) 1388–1394

Yousem, D. M., P. M. Patrone, R. I. Grossman: Leptomeningeal metastases: MR evaluation. J. Comput. assist. Tomogr. 14 (1990) 255–261

Zanella, F. E., W. Steinbrich, G. Friedmann, A. Koulousakis: Magnetische Resonanztomographie (MR) bei spinalen Raumforderungen. Fortschr. Röntgenstr. 145 (1986) 326–330

Zimmerman, R. A., L. T. Bilaniuk: Imaging of tumors of the spinal canal and cord. Radiol. Clin. N. Amer. 26 (1988) 965–1007

Zülch, K. J.: Brain Tumors. Springer, Berlin 1986

6 Inflammatory Disorders of the Spine and Spinal Canal

D. Uhlenbrock, H. Henkes, W. Weber, S. Felber, and D. Kuehne

Contents

Inflammatory disorders of the vertebral bodies and intervertebral disks are more common than infectious lesions of the base and roof of the skull.

On the other hand, inflammation and infection affect the brain and its meninges far more often than the spinal cord and the spinal meninges.

Inflammatory Disorders of the Spine

D. Uhlenbrock and H. Henkes

MRI diagnostics of inflammatory disorders of the spine and the spinal cord provide verification of location and extent of such lesions and, together with clinical and laboratory findings, allow a differential-diagnostic assessment.

Infectious Spondylodiskitis and Spondylitis

Pathogenesis

Inflammatory disorders of the spine can manifest themselves in the form of a diskitis, spondylitis, or spondylodiskitis. Inflammation may develop in the following ways:

- by the hematogenous route (arterial or venous),
- from direct inoculation with pathogens (e.g. during disk surgery or from a penetrating injury),
- by contiguous spread.

Arterial Spread

By far the most common way is the hematogenous form of development, above all via the arterial vascular system, less often by the venous system. The spread of the inflammation occurs somewhat differently in the adult than in the child because of the differences in arterial vasculature. The intervertebral disk of the child is well vascularized, while the disk of the adult lacks vessels. The blood supply of the vertebral bodies also differs between the child and the adult: the vertebral bodies of the adult has terminal arteries, while in the child there is a marked collateral supply in the region of vertebral body and intervertebral disk. The vascular supply in the adult is via paired segmental arteries which course in the middle of the vertebral body in an anterior to dorsal direction and reach the posterior aspect of the vertebra via the intervertebral foramen. They penetrate the vertebral body via the nutrient foramen. These vessels are accompanied by others coursing from proximal to distal, parallel to the end plates, which are interconnected via collaterals and also communicate all around with the next higher or lower vertebra. These collateral vessels thus span the disk and give off several small nutrient vessels to the vertebral body (Fig. 6.1).

Branches from the paired segmental arteries also supply the dorsal vertebral elements and the paraspinal muscles. In the child there are additional collaterals between the intraosseous vessel

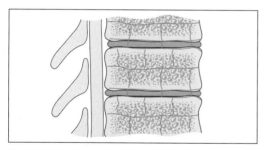

Fig. 6.**1 Arterial supply of a vertebral segment with corresponding intervertebral disk.** The illustration shows the paired segmental arteries, which course in the middle of the vertebral body in an anterior to dorsal direction and reach the posterior aspect of the vertebra via the intervertebral foramen. These vessels are accompanied by others coursing from proximal to distal, parallel to the end plates, which are interconnected via collaterals and also communicate all around with the next higher or lower vertebra. These collateral vessels thus span the disk and give off several small nutrient vessels to the vertebral body.

(nutrient artery) and the paired subchondral extraosseous vessels, which have degenerated by adulthood. There are terminal arteries present in the disk of the neonate that degenerate over the years.

This explains why an isolated diskitis secondary to hematogenous spread is mainly diagnosed in children rather than a spondylitis, even though a concomitant infection of the bone may also be present (Milone *et al.*, 1962; Lascari *et al.*, 1967; Spiegel *et al.*, 1972; Bonfiglio *et al.*, 1973). A diskitis spread by the hematogenous route with secondary invasion of the vertebral bodies also occurs, albeit rarely, in adulthood (Kemp *et al.*, 1973). The mechanism by which an inflammation in the disk and the adjacent vertebral bodies develops is based on the fact that the arterial supply of the disk does not completely degenerate in childhood, but vessels still persist in the disk in a rudimentary form (Smith, 1931; Coventry *et al.*, 1945).

Normally the route of spread in adults is as follows:

- bacterial seeding into the vertebral bodies,
- extension of the inflammatory process on to the adjacent intervertebral disk,
- involvement of the adjacent vertebral body,
- extension on to paravertebral structures, possibly following an epidural to intradural direction.

Over 90 % of infections involve both disk and adjacent vertebral bodies by the time they are diagnosed. Rarely is an isolated spondylitis found.

Bacterial seeding into the vertebral bodies usually occurs from an anterobasal location, i.e. in the region that is regarded as the endpoint of vascular branching. First, a circumscribed infarction develops in the bone secondary to the intraosseous infection. From this focus the inflammation tracks subligamentously and rapidly encroaches on the adjacent structures. Hematogenous spondylodiskitis most commonly affects older patients. There is a predilection for involvement of the lumbar spine.

Venous Spread

A spondylodiskitis can, in rare cases, develop via the venous vascular system (Batson, 1940, 1957; Sherman, 1955; Lame, 1956). The valveless veins emerging from the dorsal aspect of the vertebral body receive their blood from the vertebral periphery and relay it to the epidural venous plexus in the spinal canal, which has connections to the paravertebral venous plexus. Furthermore, the intraosseous veins also have a direct connection with the paravertebral venous plexus via perforating vessels. Since the direction of flow in the valveless paravertebral veins is strongly dependent on intra-abdominal pressure, bacterial spread resulting from reversal of flow is also conceivable. Inflammatory processes in the intestinal tact, the urinary tract collecting system, and the prostrate or gynecological organs can be regarded in this context as potential initial sites for a spondylodiskitis.

Direct inoculation with Pathogens

Direct inoculation with pathogens occurs, for example, iatrogenically or via penetrating injuries. Iatrogenically induced inflammations can develop from:

- puncture of the spinal canal, the vertebral bodies and the paravertebral space,
- surgery of the disk interspace or the spinal canal.

In rare cases a spondylodiskitis can result from penetrating injuries. The most common injuries in this context are gunshot wounds.

Inflammation by Contiguous Spread

The propagation of inflammation by contiguous spread takes its origin from an infectious focus near the spine.

Pathogens

About 80 % of all cases of spondylodiskitis are caused by *Staphylococcus aureus*. Other gram-positive (streptococci, pneumococci) or gram-negative (*Escherichia coli, Salmonella, Pseudomonas*) bacilli are found less commonly. Infections by fungi are an exception. Tuberculous infection has become less common.

Infection from *Staphylococcus aureus* is promoted by the fact that this bacterium has its own proteolytic enzyme, which causes lysis of the structural fibers of the annulus fibrosus and thus contributes in facilitating bacterial spread.

Disease Course

In the case of a bacterial spondylodiskitis, a concomitant involvement of the disk with a corresponding loss of disk-space height typically develops very early (about 1–3 weeks after the onset of the infection) from the spondylitic focus in the bone marrow. During the further course, the infection spreads to the immediately adjacent vertebral body and only later on is there destruction of the cortices of the vertebral body with paravertebral exudation and the development of granulation tissue. Relatively seldom does an epidural abscess develop as a result.

Bacterial Spondylodiskitis

Diagnostics

MRI

Spondylodiskitis is diagnosed at MRI by a pattern of findings that is encountered in more than 90% of all cases and therefore usually allows a secure diagnosis:

- A clear, usually homogeneous reduction in signal intensity of the vertebral body or bodies is displayed on T1-weighted images. The difference in contrast between vertebral body and disk can be lacking, particularly in older patients who regularly display slightly higher bone-marrow signal intensity than disk signal, so that the inflammatory segment reveals a uniformly low signal.
- The contours of the end plates lying within the inflammation are lost or to a large extent disrupted, with the disruption being most pronounced ventrally.
- On T2-weighted images a signal enhancement of the intervertebral disk is seen, displaying higher signal intensity than the healthy disks. The intranuclear cleft is lost. In addition, signal enhancement of those vertebral bodies affected by the inflammation may become apparent.
- After contrast application (depending on the extent of inflammation) a clear contrast enhancement is visible in the inflammatory region, including the disk.

These MRI criteria can be regarded as reliable and hold good for over 90% of all patients. Apart from these there are also less reliable criteria available:

- In about 50% of all patients, additional signal changes of the disk are seen on T1-weighted images in the form of a reduction in signal intensity.
- In less than 50% of cases, the following combined signal changes are found:
  - a reduction in signal intensity of disk and vertebral body on T1-weighted images *and* a signal enhancement of disk and vertebral body on T2-weighted images (Hosten *et al.*, 1995; Dagirmanjian *et al.*, 1996; Wikstroem *et al.*, 1997).

Additional signs are:
- disk space narrowing,
- paravertebral exudate,
- epidural abscess.

Examination technique

STIR sequences have particularly proven themselves for detecting edema. The STIR sequence provides the highest contrast between pathological tissue and adjacent normal bone marrow. The following are recommended for clarifying infectious spondylitis with the aid of MRI:

- T1-weighted images before and after contrast application,
- T2 sequences,
- STIR sequences (Thrush *et al.*, 1990).

Contrast images are particularly helpful for:

- separation of paraspinal abscess from the dural sac,
- differentiation of inflammatory active elements from elements inactive after medicinal treatment.

Post *et al.* (1990) point out that, after application of Gd-DTPA, T1-weighted images are more sensitive in detecting changes relating to diskitis than T2-weighted images. They describe the following pattern of findings for contrast enhancement of inflammatory changes of the disk:

- band-like, broad enhancement of the disk margin,
- thin, contrast-enhancing rim,

- contrast-filling of practically the entire disk space, comparable in its extension to the signal enhancement on T2-weighted representations,
- patchy contrast enhancement in different, non-contiguous, elements of the disk material,
- fine linear contrasting in the periphery of the disk.

The osteomyelitic components are better demonstrated on plain T1-weighted images than after application of Gd-DTPA because the intensity of contrast enhancement seen in inflammatory and normal bone marrow is similar (Post *et al.*, 1990) (Figs. 6.**2**–6.**11**).

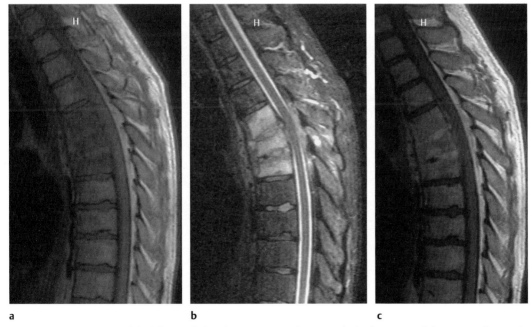

a   b   c

Fig. 6.2 a–c Acute spondylodiskitis of the thoracic vertebrae 4–6:

a T1-weighted sagittal image (TR = 800 ms, TE = 12 ms): Very homogeneous reduction in signal intensity of vertebrae 4–6, with the signal of the vertebrae appearing slightly lower than that of the intervertebral disk. The vertebral end plates are no longer demarcated. The vertebrae have lost somewhat in height, particularly anteriorly. Paravertebral abscess with displacement of the anterior longitudinal ligament.

b T2-weighted sagittal image (STIR sequence): Marked signal enhancement of the affected intervertebral disks, including the disk spaces.

c Sagittal image after contrast application: Clear enhancement of the disks, slight enhancement of the vertebral bodies, and contrast uptake along the paravertebral abscess.

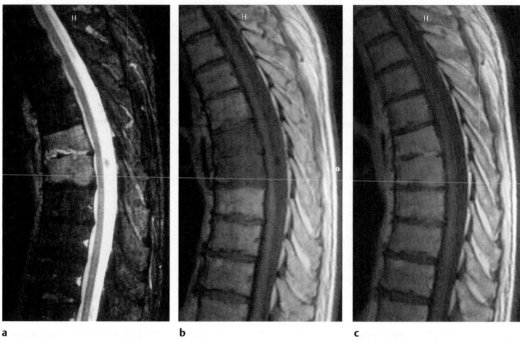

a   b   c

Fig. 6.3 a–c **Spondylodiskitis at the T6/7 level :**

a T2-weighted sagittal image (STIR sequence): Very clear homogeneous signal enhancement in both vertebral bodies and in the disk space.

b T1-weighted plain image (TSE; TR = 800 ms, TE = 12 ms): Clear reduction in signal of both vertebral bodies so that the difference in contrast between disk signal and bone signal appears lost.

c Sagittal image after contrast application: The contrast of the vertebral bodies is brought into line with that of the healthy sections. Band-like contrast enhancement in the disk reflecting the florid inflammatory reaction.

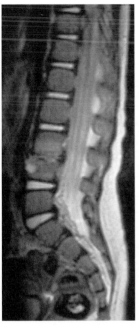
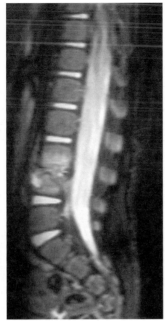
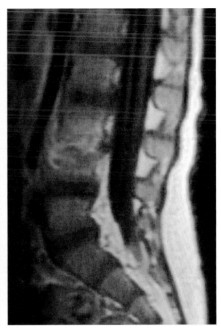

a   b   c

Fig. 6.**4 a−c** **Spondylodiskitis at the level L3/L4. 15-month-old child:**

a T2-weighted sagittal image (TSE; TR = 6000 ms, TE = 120 ms): Slight signal enhancement in the two corresponding vertebral bodies, reduced signal intensity in the disk space. Epidural abscess formation. Circumscribed, hyperintense core in the anterior cortex of L4, to be regarded perhaps as the starting point of the inflammation.

b Sagittal STIR sequence: The destruction of the end plates is better displayed on these images. The signal-intense inflammatory core in L4 demonstrates communication with the disk space.

c Sagittal image after contrast application: Strong, diffuse enhancement of both the disk space and the adjacent vertebral bodies.

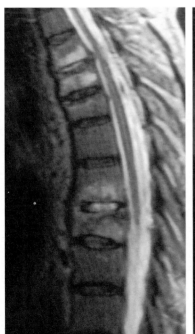
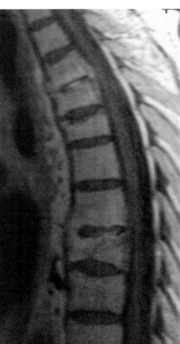

Fig. 6.**5 a, b** **Polysegmental spondylodiskitis T3−T9, sparing the disks T5/6 and T6/7.**

a T2-weighted sagittal image with evidence of clear signal enhancements of the vertebral bodies and corresponding disks in the segmental region T3−T9.

b Sagittal image after contrast application: Somewhat more marked enhancement of the disk T3/4 and disk T7/8. Slight subchondral contrast uptake in the region of the end plates T5 and T9.

b

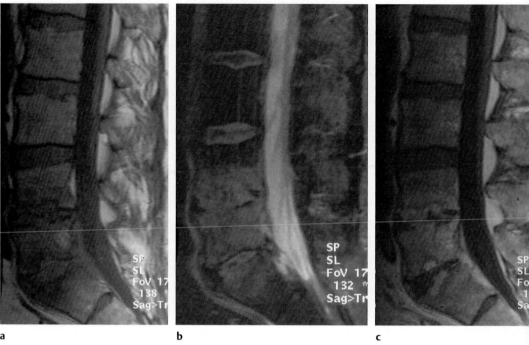

a   b   c

Fig. 6.**6 a–c Spondylodiskitis of the vertebrae L4–S1:**

a T1-weighted sagittal pre-contrast image: Reduced signal intensity of the corresponding vertebral segments L4/L5 and L5/S1 with partial lack of contour delineation of the upper and lower end plates.

b T2-weighted image (STIR): Very clear signal enhancement along the vertebrae L4–S1 with involvement of the disk spaces.

c Sagittal T1-weighted image after contrast application: Patchy enhancement, above all in the disk spaces L4/L5 and L5/S1.

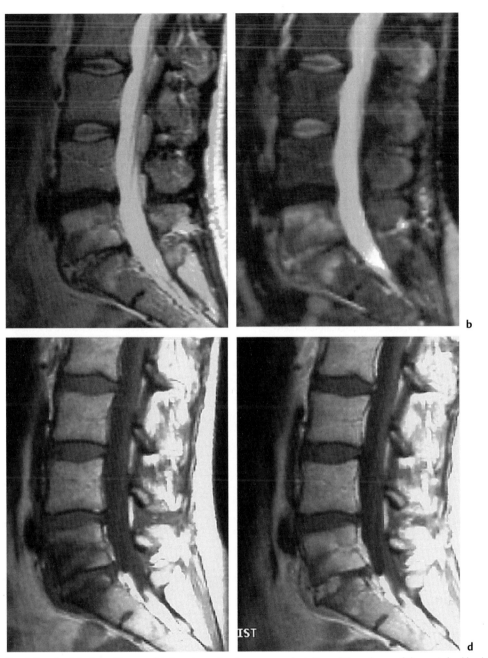

Fig. 6.**7 a–d** **Sciatica.** 38-year-old female patient examined for recurrent sciatica 4.5 months after surgery for disk herniation at the level L5/S1. Greatly elevated ESR:

a T2-weighted sagittal image: Reduced signal intensity of the L4/L5 disk due to degenerative causes, reduced height of the L5/S1 disk with increased signal intensity due to inflammatory causes, and concomitant finding of a hyperintense marrow edema of L5 and S1.

b T2-weighted sagittal image (STIR sequence): Confirmation of the finding with particularly contrast-rich depiction of the edema of the vertebral body and the signal enhancement in the disk space L5/S1.

c T1-weighted sagittal pre-contrast image: Reduced signal intensity of the vertebral bodies L5 and S1.

d Sagittal T1-weighted image after contrast application: Broad, patchy, ventrally accentuated signal enhancement is apparent within the L5/S1 disk, which displays inflammatory changes. Partial hyperemia of the adjacent vertebral bodies, in part with enhanced signal intensity relative to the healthy segments.

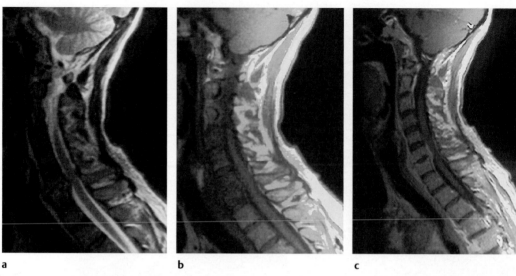

a   b   c

Fig. 6.8 a–c **Spondylodiskitis with epidural abscess.** 58-year-old patient with known diabetes mellitus, cervical pain and slowly progressive tetraparesis:

a Sagittal T2-weighted image: Increased signal intensity of the disk at the level C6/C7. Both vertebral bodies display marrow edema with corresponding signal enhancement.

b Sagittal T1-weighted plain image: The fat signal in the vertebral bodies C4–C7 is reduced.

c Sagittal T1-weighted image after contrast application: This results in an increase of signal intensity, especially in the sixth and seventh cervical vertebra. Dorsal to these two vertebral bodies there is a fringe-like contrast enhancement indicating an epidural abscess formation. The spinal meninges are also thickened at this level, dorsal to the cord. A slight space-occupying effect on the cervical cord takes its origin from this lesion.

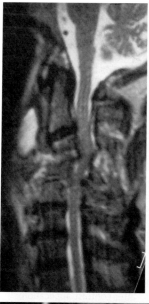

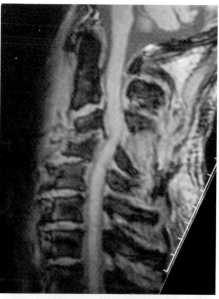

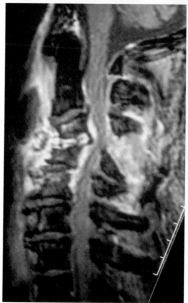

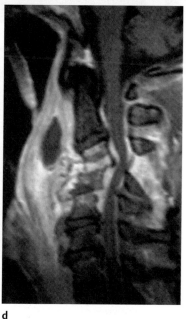

Fig. 6.9 a–d Spondylodiskitis C3–C5 with subluxed position of C3/C4.

a Sagittal T2-weighted image (TSE; TR = 4600 ms, TE = 112 ms): Signal enhancement in the disk space C3/4 and C4/5 with low-grade reactive edema in the adjacent vertebral bodies. Subluxed position of C3/C4. Widening of the interspinal distance between the spinous processes of C3 and C4, here too associated with signal enhancement. Marked paravertebral exudate with retropharyngeal abscess formation. Increased signal intensity along the spinal meninges. Spinal cord compression secondary to frank degenerative changes with posterior osteophytic spurring.

b Sagittal T1-weighted image (FLASH 2D; TR = 403 ms, TE = 11 ms, flip angle α = 90°): Mild reduction in signal intensity in the disk space C3/C4. Subluxed position in the segmental region C3/C4. Widening of the interspinal distance between the spinous processes of C3 and C4. The slight compression of the spinal cord is also recognizable here.

c Sagittal T2-weighted image after contrast application (FLASH 2D; TR = 403 ms, TE = 11 ms, flip angle α = 90°): Very marked contrast enhancement of the disk space C3/C4 and the prevertebral structures with sparing of the retropharyngeal abscess formation reflecting the cavitating process. The epidural structures also demonstrate contrast enhancement as an indication of the epidural abscess formation with involvement of the meninges. Contrast enhancement furthermore in the dorsal appendant structures, especially between the interspinal processes C2/C3, C3/C4, and C4/C5.

d Image after contrast application (SE; TR = 572 ms, TE = 12 ms, with fat saturation): The compression of the spinal cord is more clearly recognizable on this image. There is in addition a better demarcation of the meningeal reaction, both ventrally and dorsally along the spinal canal. The massive retropharyngeal abscess formation with a marked long-segment phlegmonous reaction along the anterior contour of the cervical spine is well delineated.

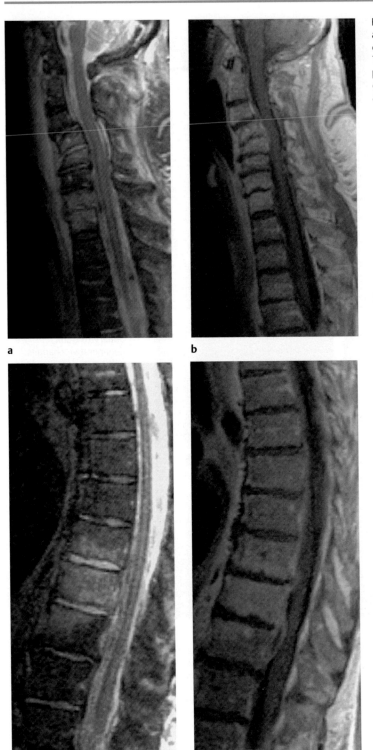

a

b

c

d

Fig. 6.10 a–d Polysegmental acute spondylodiskitis in the cervical and thoracic spine. 79-year-old diabetic. Clinical presentation of a rapidly progressive paraparesis.

a Sagittal T2-weighted image of the cervical spine region: Evidence of spondylodiskitis of the segments C4/C5 and C7/T1. There is a correspondingly clear signal enhancement of both the vertebral bodies and the disks. Clearly recognizable structural instability in this section. Evidence of a prevertebral exudation with elevation of the anterior longitudinal ligament in the C4–C6 section and circumscribed at C7/T1. Mild prevertebral reactive edema.

b Sagittal T1-weighted image after contrast application: Mild enhancement of the vertebral bodies, especially at C4/C5 and to a slight degree in the dorsal area of the disk of this segment.

c Sagittal T2-weighted image: Evidence of spondylodiskitis of the thoracic vertebrae 9–11. A corresponding, relatively homogeneous signal enhancement is visible in T10 and an adjacent, marginal enhancement of the ninth and eleventh thoracic vertebrae. The T9/T10 and T10/T11 disks display signal enhancement.

d Sagittal T1-weighted image after contrast application: The associated epidural abscess at the level of the segments T9/T10 and T10/T11 are well delineated on these images. There is a corresponding enhancement of the abscess membrane. In addition, there is a mild contrast enhancement of the ninth and eleventh vertebrae as well as a strong, homogeneous enhancement of the tenth thoracic vertebra.

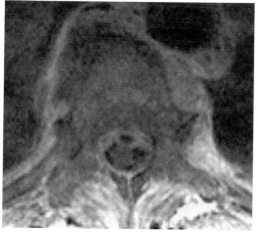

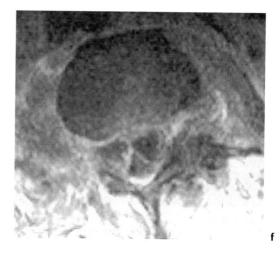

e **f**

Fig. 6.10 e–f
e Corresponding transverse image after contrast application: The epidural abscess formation and the additional paravertebral abscess are well delineated on
this image.

f Transverse image through the level of the abscess
after contrast application: This image shows division
of the ventrally located epidural abscess by the
Trolard membrane (curtain sign).

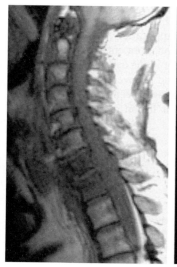

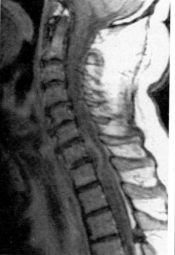

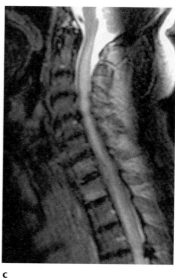

a **b** **c**

Fig. 6.11 a–e **Spondylodiskitis of C7–T1 with extensive epidural abscess.** The 54-year-old patient had
suffered a perforating injury to the esophagus two
weeks previously. Subsequently there was a subacute
development of a progressive paresis of the lower extremities:
a Sagittal T1-weighted plain image: Edema of the
vertebral bodies C7 and T1.

b Image after contrast application: Demarcation of an
extensive compressive epidural abscess.
c Sagittal T2-weighted image: Bone marrow edema at
C7 and T1. The compression of the spinal cord by the
abscess results in a considerable long-segment
edema of the cord, which extends from C2 into the
segments of the thoracic spine.

Fig. 6.11 d and e ▷

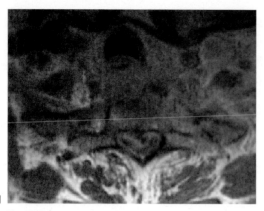

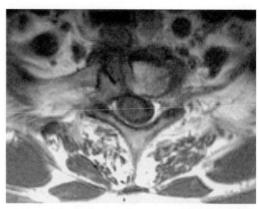

d

Fig. 6.**11 d, e**
d Transverse section after contrast application: The image shows an extensive space-occupying effect by the epidural abscess with corresponding marked compression of the spinal cord.

e After surgical revision of the abscess, the postoperative T1-weighted image after contrast application displays complete regression of the space-occupying effect. The spinal cord edema is still recognizable by the reduction in signal intensity.

Healing

During the healing of spondylodiskitis, a regression of the strong signal reduction on the T1-weighted images, as well as of the signal enhancement on the T2-weighted images, is observed. Instead, patchy and, as the disease progresses, increasingly confluent signal enhancements of the bone marrow are found on T1-weighted plain images, indicating fatty marrow formation. A persistent reduction in signal reflecting sclerosis, as well as a slight signal enhancement due to the formation of fatty marrow, can develop on T2-weighted images. The intervertebral disk displays low signal intensity after a healed spondylodiskitis due to scar formation. After contrast application a reduced, partly mottled, signal enhancement develops, which is totally absent later in the development of the disease. Over a period of several months and years osteophytic bridging is seen and is an indication of the subsequent fusion of the segment (Figs. 6.**12** and 6.**13**).

Fig. 6.**13 a–c Largely healed spondylodiskitis that was followed-up over 1 year:**
a T1-weighted image (SE; TR = 780 ms, TE = 25 ms): Destruction of the inferior and superior end plates of T7 and T8 with loss of disk space height. No larger reduction of signal intensity of the bone marrow. Individual segments of fatty marrow (arrows).
b T2-weighted image (SE; TR = 2100 ms, TE = 80 ms): Uniform reduction in signal intensity. Individual zones of slightly increased signal intensity corresponding to fatty marrow.
c After contrast application (SE; TR = 750 ms, TE = 25 ms): Mottled, stippled signal enhancement of the bone marrow without any larger area of contrast enhancement.

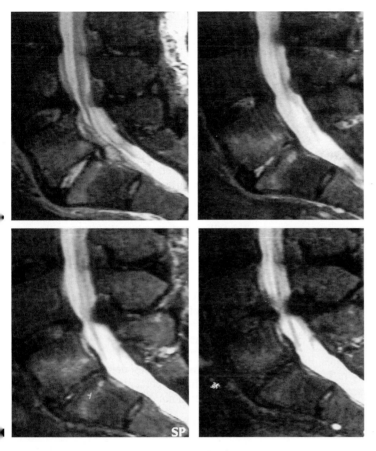

Fig. 6.**12 a–d Clinical course of an L5/S1 spondylodiskitis. Examination series over a period of 1 year. Examinations with a STIR sequence are displayed for comparison:**

a Sagittal image: Evidence of a clear signal enhancement in the disk space L5/S1 and a corresponding reaction in the vertebral segments.

b Examination 1.5 months later: Slightly regressive edema of the intervertebral disk. Strong reactive edema still present in the adjacent vertebral segments.

c Examination 4 months after the initial scan: Further regression of the edema of the intervertebral disk. Strong edema still present in the adjacent vertebral segments.

d Examination 1 year after the initial scan: Complete involution of the disk material, mild marginal signal enhancement still present in the vertebral segments.

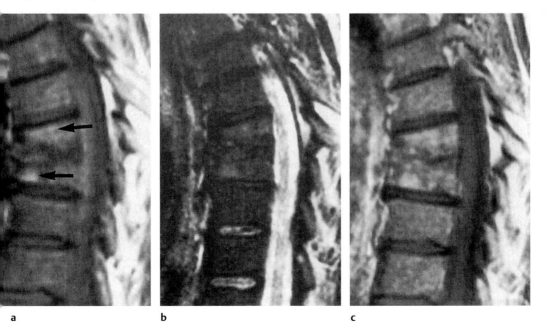

a b c

Fig. 6.**13 a–c**

Tuberculous Spondylodiskitis

Tuberculous spondylodiskitis demonstrates some special features in comparison to nonspecific inflammations, although in individual cases differentiation is only possible by identification of the organism.

Location

In contrast to nonspecific spondylodiskitis, tuberculous spondylodiskitis is most commonly found at a thoracic location, followed by lumbar and cervical ones.

Pathogenesis and Spread

Tuberculous spondylodiskitis typically demonstrates a slow insidious onset and it can take months before changes are detectable on plain radiographs. In about 80 % of all cases, tuberculous spondylodiskitis is not associated with an affection of the lungs, nor even succeeds it, making the diagnosis even more difficult.

The inflammation usually originates in the ventral third of the vertebral body near the end plate. A typical finding is circumscribed areas of subchondral erosion. A mere spondylitis, without involvement of the disk, is more often encountered than with a pyogenic inflammation. This is because, unlike *Staphylococcus aureus*, mycobacteria lack proteolytic enzymes.

Tuberculous spondylodiskitis is rarely limited to the posterior structures of the vertebrae, without involvement of the vertebral body or the disk.

If the posterior longitudinal ligament remains intact, tuberculous spondylodiskitis spreads through several segments, although individual vertebral bodies can be skipped. Polysegmental spread is also possible by the hematogenous route.

Tuberculous spondylodiskitis often results in marked collapse of the vertebral bodies. In many cases this vertebral collapse is associated with a reactive gibbus deformity of the spine. A typical feature is this respect is *telescoping*, where the entire vertebral body, including the disk, collapses into the next higher or next lower vertebra, although the disk can remain more or less intact.

Differential Diagnosis

Due to the often-marked abscess formation associated with tuberculosis, the application of contrast can result in mere marginal enhancement of the inflammatory area instead of a homogeneous distribution. This marginal enhancement is sometimes also encountered within the vertebral body. It defines the region of the intraosseous abscess.

In contrast to bacterial spondylitis, the adjacent disk material is less damaged or is completely spared from the inflammatory changes. Similarly, signal enhancement of the disk on the T2-weighted image is often lacking on the MRI presentation of tuberculous spondylitis.

The following features are helpful in differentiating tuberculous from bacterial spondylitis.

Tuberculous spondylitis:
- expansion into the paraspinal soft tissue is much more strongly developed,
- duration of symptoms is longer (months to years),
- the patient is of a younger age (Smith *et al.*, 1990),
- tuberculous abscesses demonstrate calcifications in a higher percentage of cases, although they are often not detectable on the MR image.

Follow-up studies of tuberculous spondylodiskitis reveal, on the T1-weighted sequences of some of the patients, an increase in signal intensity of those vertebral elements previously damaged by the infection. Smith *et al.* (1990) assume that ischemic or inflammatory effects promote the conversion of hematopoietic bone marrow into fatty marrow.

Differential diagnostic considerations for spondylitis must include erosive osteochondrosis (Staebler *et al.*, 1998) and, particularly in the case of tuberculous spondylitis, metastatic spread to the vertebrae (Thrush *et al.*, 1990) (Figs. 6.**14** and 6.**15**).

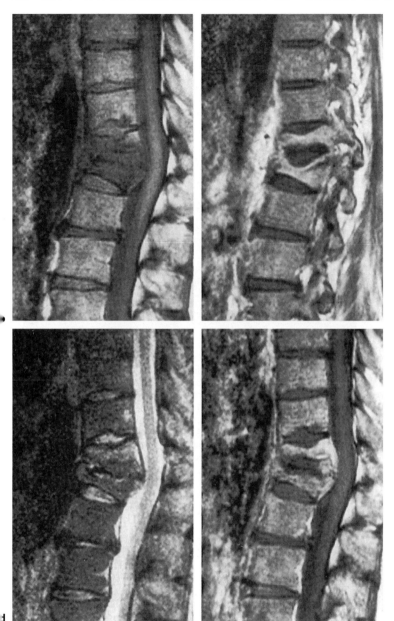

Fig. 6.**14 a–d   Tuberculous spondylodiskitis T11/T12. 46-year-old patient with pulmonary tuberculosis.**

a Sagittal T1-weighted image (SE; TR = 785 ms, TE = 25 ms): Reduced signal intensity of the vertebral bodies T11/T12 with reduction in height and signal loss of the vertebral contours, resulting in lack of demarcation of the disk.

b In the section further laterally, evidence of a prolapse of the largely preserved disk into the adjacent vertebral body.

c T2-weighted image: Slight signal enhancement of the vertebral bodies, especially of T11. No signal enhancement of the disk.

d T1-weighted image after contrast application: Enhancement predominantly in the regions of increased signal intensity. Signal void corresponding to the intervertebral disk.

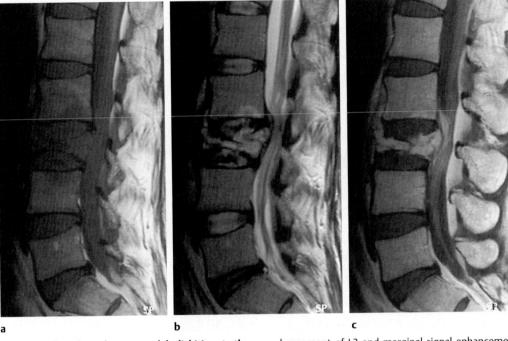

a   b   c

Fig. 6.15 a–d Tuberculous spondylodiskitis at the level L2/3. 38-year-old patient:

a Sagittal T1-weighted image (TSE; TR = 800 ms, TE = 12 ms): More or less complete collapse of L3 with homogeneous reduction in signal intensity. Focal reduction in signal intensity in L2, dorsally, with a hint of interruption in the contour of the inferior end plate.

b Sagittal T2-weighted image (TSE; TR = 4000 ms, TE = 120 ms): Mottled inhomogeneous signal enhancement of L3 and marginal signal enhancement within the focus in L2.

c Sagittal image after contrast application: Marked enhancement both of the bone and paravertebral segments, initial development of an epidural abscess. Slight enhancement of the roots of the cauda equina as a sign of an incipient inflammation of the cauda. Marked elevation of the anterior longitudinal ligament in the region of L2 and L3 secondary to the inflammatory reaction.

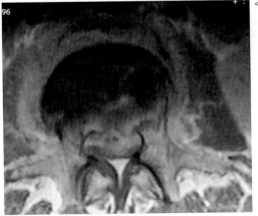

◁ **d** Transverse image after contrast application (SE; TR = 700 ms, TE = 15 ms): Contrast enhancement of the paravertebral structures with involvement of the psoas region on both sides. The epidural abscess formation is clearly recognizable.

Spondylitis

Spondylitis, without involvement of the intervertebral disk, displays the same changes with respect to the bone as does spondylodiskitis. The acute stage reveals a reduction in signal intensity within the bone on the T1-weighted plain image and a more or less marked signal enhancement after contrast application. Nonspecific signal enhancement is seen on the T2-weighted image (Shanley, 1995).

Rheumatoid arthritis

Incidence and etiology

Rheumatoid arthritis (RA; chronic polyarthritis [CP]) is the most common systemic disease of the connective tissue. It primarily affects women, the male to female sex ratio being 3:1. The exact etiology of rheumatoid arthritis is not known. Autoimmune mechanisms could possibly play a role in its pathogenesis since up to 70 % of the patients are HLA-DR4 positive.

Location

In rheumatoid arthritis, the thoracic and lumbar spines are only relatively seldom involved. Destruction of the thoracic and lumbar vertebral bodies by rheumatoid granulomas, however, is seen occasionally. Epidural rheumatoid nodules can result in compression of the spinal cord. The facet joints of the mid to lower spine are also only rarely affected. However, damage to the thoracic and lumbar spine can occur secondary to treatment. Ischemic necrosis of the bone commonly results from the administration of steroids, sometimes affecting thoracic and lumbar vertebrae apart from the typical location within the femoral head. Furthermore, the combination of immobilization due to pain plus corticosteroid therapy can lead to marked osteoporosis with subsequent vertebral collapse (Dihlmann, 1987; Resnick and Niwayama, 1988).

The most important and most common vertebral changes associated with rheumatoid arthritis are seen in the cervical spine, particularly in the region of the craniocervical junction. One of the most common findings in rheumatoid arthritis in the region of the cervical spine is C1/C2 subluxation, of which the following forms are distinguished:

- anterior atlantoaxial subluxation,
- cranial subluxation,
- lateral subluxation,
- rotatory subluxation,
- posterior subluxation.

The *atlantoaxial subluxation* involves a widening of the interval between the anterior atlas arch and the dens axis (anterior atlantodens interval or ADI) by 2.5 mm and more. The *cranial subluxation* results in a basilar impression with a high-riding dens, which can extend far into the foramen. There is concomitant settling of the atlas arch so that it is found in an abnormally low position in relation to C2. The *lateral subluxation* involves a lateralization of the lateral mass of C1 in relation to C2 by more than 2 mm. The *rotatory subluxation* demonstrates a unilateral displacement of the atlas in relation to the joint facets of C2. If the anterior atlas arch is dorsal to the dens then this is referred to as a *posterior subluxation*.

The cause of these changes lies in a laxity or destruction of the atlantoaxial ligamentous structures, especially the transverse ligament, secondary to an inflammatory synovial reaction. In addition, instability of the articular structures develops between the skull base, atlas and axis. An erosion of the dens is also a typical finding and occurs in about 20 % of patients. Synovial proliferation can result in exuberant pannus formation. A distinction is made here between the development of retrodental, predental, supradental and laterodental pannus, with a combination of these types of pannus formation being a common finding. The inflammatory changes can reduce the dens down to a small rudiment. This can result in atlantoaxial subluxation, even in the presence of intact ligamentous structures.

A common result of the pannus reaction and the destruction of the ligamentous and joint structures is compression of the spinal cord at the level of C1 or proximal to it. This compression can be present both in neutral position as well as occurring exclusively during anteflexion of the head. Compression of the spinal cord is particularly common when a combination of atlantoaxial and cranial subluxation is present.

Apart from changes in the region of the atlantoaxial articulation, erosions of the vertebral bodies are observed in rheumatoid arthritis, occurring particularly at the end plates. This results in a reduction in disk space height, which, unlike osteochondrosis, primarily affects the C2–C4 segments and is regarded by some authors as pathognomonic. Erosions of the facet joints is also common and can occur in conjunction with joint space narrowing and articular destruction, even together with ankylosis during late stages.

The erosive changes of the vertebral end plates are often associated with structural instability of the joints so that findings consistent with an anterolisthesis or retrolisthesis are seen, sometimes combined with a marked deformity of the spine. Osteophytes at the vertebral end plates are an uncommon finding, although they can arise in late stages of rheumatoid arthritis and are the result of malposture.

Clinical Presentation

A distinction should be made clinically between local symptoms originating in the affected articular segments and general symptoms. The American Rheumatism Association (ARA) has compiled diagnostic criteria for rheumatoid arthritis (Arnett *et al.*, 1988):

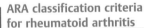

> **ARA classification criteria
> for rheumatoid arthritis**
>
> - Morning stiffness lasting at least one hour.
> - Arthritis of three or more joints.
> - Arthritis involving hand or finger joints.
> - Symmetric arthritis.
> - Rheumatoid nodules.
> - Detection of serum rheumatoid factor.
> - Typical radiographic changes in hand or finger joints.

The first four criteria must have been present for at least six weeks.

General symptoms that may occur include:
- fatigue,
- sweating,
- arteriitis,
- myo- and pericarditis.

The clinical presentation strongly depends on the extent of joint damage. The patients usually present with pain that can be referred to as being in the region of the neck, as well as temporal or retro-orbital in location. Deeper lying lesions can also cause radiation of the symptoms into the shoulder-arm region. Compression of the cervical cord or the medulla oblongata leads to paresthesia and, in marked cases, to paralysis or even tetraplegia. Compromise of cerebral circulation can arise from compression of the vertebral artery, and compromise of spinal cord circulation from impairment of the spinal artery.

Pathogenesis

The pathogenesis is assumed to be an immune complex reaction resulting in the activation of complement secondary to the deposition of immune complexes in the synovial joint structures. This induces the infiltration of lymphocytes, especially T4 helper cells, which maintains the inflammatory process. B lymphocytes and macrophages are also encountered. In the acute inflammatory exudative phase, numerous inflammatory cells are detected in the synovial fluid. Cartilage destruction is seen primarily near the inflammatory changes of the synovia or near the pannus covering the articular cartilage. This tissue consists of proliferative fibroblasts, small blood vessels and mononuclear cells. Proteinases released from here destroy the cartilage.

Histology

Histology reveals proliferation of the synovial lining cells, which demonstrate a palisade-like arrangement and are covered by a fibrin film. Sometimes enlarged lymph follicles and blood vessels with endothelial proliferation are also present. The appearance of rheumatoid granulomas is a rare occurrence. Apart from synovial proliferation, a similar type of granulation tissue also appears in the subchondral medullary cavity. Once the joint space has been bridged, fibrous ankylosis results from fibrotic alterations of the pannus tissue and may be converted further into a bony ankylosis by metaplastic changes.

Diagnostics

MRI

The most impressive findings are encountered at the atlantoaxial junction, especially when extensive pannus formation is present. This pannus displays a moderate signal intensity that corresponds approximately to that of muscle on T1-weighted images and is well delineated from the higher signal of bone.

On the T2-weighted images the pannus can demonstrate either very high signal intensity or a low one. This depends on the water content and extent of fibrosis. If high water content is present then high signal intensity is found, while fibrosed pannus displays a correspondingly low signal. Erosions of the dens are well depicted, although the smallest punctate erosions escape detection by MRI and are better demonstrated by CT. The transverse ligament is often delineated, especially when it is merely displaced by pannus yet otherwise intact.

The application of contrast has proven itself helpful. Pannus tissue usually shows a strong enhancement, which appears less distinctive when the tissue is very edematous and loose. If the other vertebral bodies also exhibit changes, then they are particularly well delineated on contrast-enhanced images. In this case a mild signal enhancement can be found along the vertebral end plates, extending down to the subchondral region and producing a band of diminished signal intensity (Figs. 6.**16**–6.**24**).

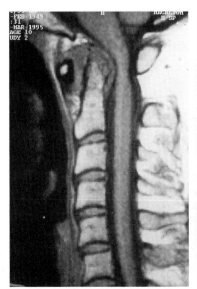 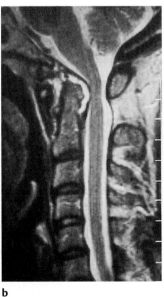 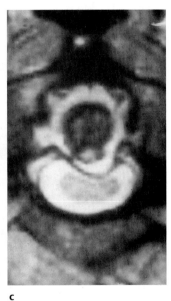

a   b   c

Fig. 6.16 a–c Known long-standing rheumatoid arthritis. 46-year-old female patient:
- **a** Sagittal T1-weighted image (SE): The extensive pre- and retrodental pannus tissue displays a moderate signal intensity. The dens axis is included in the destruction with its point showing structural rarefaction. The atlantoaxial distance is widened.
- **b** Sagittal T2-weighted image (SE): The pannus tissue reveals a clear signal enhancement as an expression of the edematous inflammatory reaction. There is a mild compressive effect in the region of the cervical cord. There is no cord edema.
- **c** Transverse section with T2 weighting: The paradental pannus tissue is well delineated, the retrodental component causes a bulging protrusion of the transverse ligament. Thus the spinal cord is reached and is slightly compromised, especially toward the left.

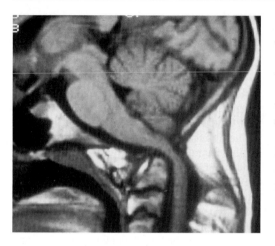

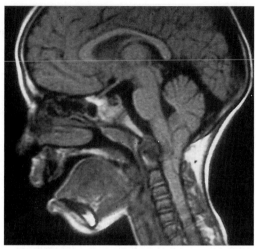

Fig. 6.**17 Rheumatoid arthritis.** 56-year-old female patient with a very long history of chronic rheumatoid arthritis. Sagittal section with T1 weighting (SE technique): Extensive destruction of the apex of the dens with marked widening of the atlantodental interval. Basilar impression with marked compression of the spinal cord. The cervicomedullary angle (the angle formed by lines drawn parallel to the anterior aspects of the medulla and the upper cervical cord; normal value = and >135°) is reduced.

Fig. 6.**18 Rheumatoid arthritis and Arnold–Chiari type I malformation.** 7-year-old girl. The sagittal section with T1 weighting shows marked reactive pannus at the apex of the dens with extensive destruction. A compressive effect occurs at the level of the medulla. Additional narrowing of the spinal canal as a result of the very low position of the tonsils.

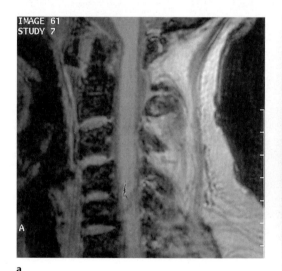

a

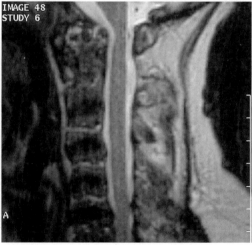

b

Fig. 6.**19 a, b Long-standing rheumatoid arthritis.** 70-year-old female patient:
a Sagittal T1-weighted image (FLASH 2D; TR = 400 ms, TE = 11 ms, flip angle α = 90°): Partial destruction of the apex of the dens and evidence of marked predental pannus with widening of the atlantoaxial distance. Slight pannus reaction also recognizable at the dorsal margin of the tip of the dens. Slight impression of the spinal cord.

b Sagittal T1-weighted image (TSE; TR = 4600 ms, TE = 112 ms): The pannus displays a largely reduced signal intensity as a sign of the remodeling of the fibrous scar tissue. Despite the slight compressive effect at the level of the spinal cord, there is no evidence of edema.

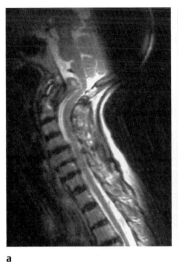
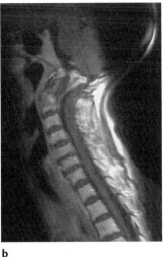

a

b

Fig. 6.**20 a, b Rheumatoid arthritis.** 81-year-old female patient
with marked pannus formation and
progressive high-grade tetraparesis:
a Sagittal T2-weighted image: Presentation of marked pannus
tissue formation dorsal to the
dens producing a considerable
compressive effect along the
course of the medulla oblongata.
The pannus reveals a moderate
and, in parts, slightly increased
signal intensity. Hypointense
tissue situated dorsal to the
eroded dens is distinct from this.
b Sagittal T1-weighted image after
contrast application: An inhomogeneous contrast enhancement
of the inflammatory granulation
tissue has occurred. The sections
of the tissue that are hypointense with T2 weighting dorsal to
the dens show on the whole no
contrast reaction.

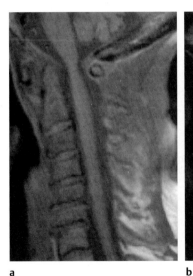
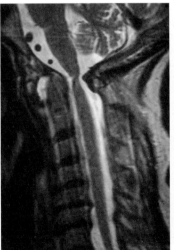
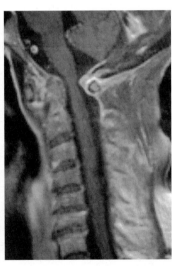

a

b

c

Fig. 6.**21 a–c Long-standing rheumatoid arthritis.**
67-year-old female patient:
a Sagittal T1-weighted image (SE; TR = 572 ms, TE =
12 ms, fat saturation): Widening of the atlantodental
interval secondary to a more extensive predental
pannus. Slight retrodental pannus reaction is recognizable. Inflammatory reaction at the posterior arch
of the atlas with the formation of granulation tissue
extending in a dorsal to intraspinal direction. Structural instability in the segments C4–C7.
b Sagittal T2-weighted image (TSE; TR = 4600 ms,
TE = 112 ms): The pannus tissue displays high signal
intensity. The tissue located along the posterior arch

of the atlas appears hypointense. Pathological signal
enhancements are not detectable within the disks of
the segments C4–C7.
c Sagittal T1-weighted image after contrast application: Clear contrast enhancement of the granulation
tissue along the posterior arch of the atlas, patchy inhomogeneous contrast reaction in the region of the
predental pannus. In addition, there is a subtle linear
contrast enhancement of the disks C5/C6 and C6/C7
with a further contrast reaction in the region of the
posterior longitudinal ligament and the annulus fibrosus at the levels of C3/C4, C4/C5 and C6/C7, reflecting the concomitant inflammatory reaction.

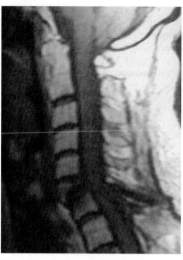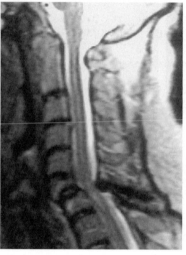

a   b

Fig. 6.**22 a, b** **Long-standing rheumatoid arthritis.**
63-year-old female patient:
a Sagittal T1-weighted image (TSE; TR = 800 ms,
TE = 12 ms): Extensive inflammatory reaction in the
segment C6/C7 with partial destruction of the sixth
cervical vertebra, which displays reduction of the
posterior margin in particular. Decreased signal intensity within the cancellous bone of both vertebral
bodies due to edema. Obvious angulation in the
segmental region C6/C7 with compression of the spinal cord from a ventral and dorsal direction secondary to ligamentous instability.

b Sagittal T2-weighted image (TSE; TR = 5310 ms,
TE = 112 ms): The anterior malalignment of C6 over
C7 is also clearly recognizable on this image. Compression of the spinal cord from a dorsal direction
secondary to the hypertrophy of the ligamenta flava.
Evidence of cord edema in this segment. The slight
signal enhancement of the vertebral bodies C6 and
C7 can also be seen. No destructive changes are delineated in the atlantodental space.

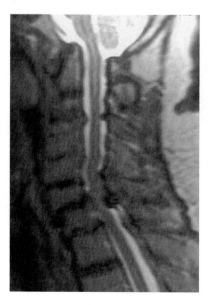

Fig. 6.**23** **Known long-standing rheumatoid arthritis.** 68-year-old female patient. Sagittal T2-weighted
image (TSE; TR = 5310 ms, TE = 112 ms): The image demonstrates a basilar impression in the region of the
atlantodental joint. In addition there are marked structural instabilities of the spine present at C6 and C7 with
partial destruction in the region of the vertebral end
plates. This results in narrowing of the spinal canal with
compression of the spinal cord and mild cord edema.
The vertebrae C4/C5 display partial fusion with extensive collapse of the disk space.

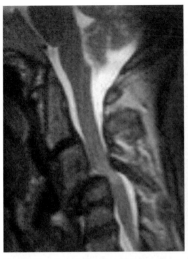
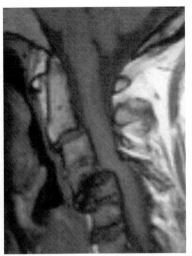

a

b

Fig. 6.**24 a, b** **Extensive destruction of the cervical spine secondary to long-standing rheumatoid arthritis.** 42-year-old female patient:

a Sagittal T2-weighted image (TSE; TR = 5000 ms, TE = 112 ms): Considerable structural instability in the segmental area C4/C5 with frank compression of the spinal cord. Evidence of cord edema. There is partial ossification in segment C3/C4 with disk disintegration and considerable reduction in height of the remaining disk space. Atlantodental joint instability with superior migration of the dens. There is no cord compression here.

b Sagittal T1-weighted image (TSE; TR = 695 ms, TE = 12 ms): The inflammatory tissue in the segmental region C4/C5 extends far ventrally. The vertebral bodies display a normal bone marrow signal; only at C5 is there a slight reduction in signal intensity ventrally. Mild destruction of the end plate at C6 is also recognizable on this image.

It has been shown to be useful to obtain functional images. Placing a cushion beneath the patient's head will suffice to bring it into a stable position of anteflexion. The majority of patients, even those with severe changes of the atlantoaxial junction, are capable of tolerating this position for a limited period of time. T2-weighted sagittal images should be obtained that provide information about possible compression of the spinal cord. It is important here to look out for a possible myelon edema, which can be an indication of damage to the spinal cord. If the patient is capable of sustaining it, the examination in anteflexion can be supplemented by the administration of contrast in order to detect any possible barrier disturbance along the course of the spinal cord. Coronal sections should also be obtained to gain information about a possible compression of the vertebral artery along the course of the C1 loop.

These images are important for the surgeon's preoperative planning with regard to the positional relationship of the bone to the vertebral arteries (Aisen *et al.*, 1987; Beltran *et al.*, 1987; Neuhold *et al.*, 1989; Kroedel *et al.*, 1989; Reiser *et al.*, 1990; Naegele *et al.*, 1992; Roca *et al.*, 1993) (Figs. 6.**25**–6.**30**).

Therapy

Therapy comprises the administration of nonsteroidal antirheumatics, so-called basic therapeutics (chloroquine, gold compounds, D-penicillamine), immunosuppressives and steroids. Chemical synoviorthesis, radiosynoviorthesis and operative or arthroscopic synovectomy can be indicated as local forms of treatment for removing destructive pannus.

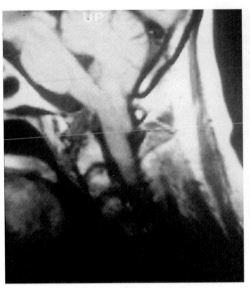

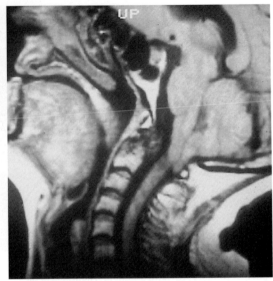

a

b

Fig. 6.25 a, b   Arnold–Chiari type I malformation and long-standing rheumatoid arthritis. Images obtained in anteversion and reclination. The sagittal images display hypointense pannus at the level of the dens with more or less total destruction of its apex. This pannus reaches the medulla oblongata in anteversion. The image obtained in retroflexion reveals a change in the form of the pannus, which now appears spherically delineated and no longer compromises the spinal cord. Frankly low-lying cerebellar tonsils with corresponding additional narrowing of the spinal canal from a dorsal direction.

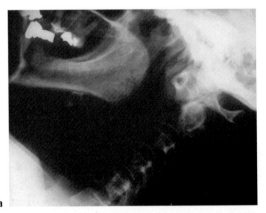

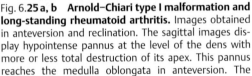

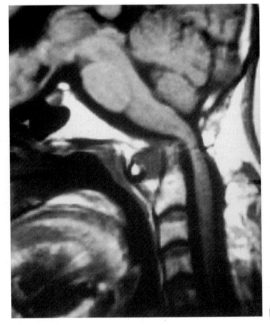

a

b

Fig. 6.26 a, b   Long-standing rheumatoid arthritis. Images of a 64-year-old female patient:

a Conventional functional studies: Demonstration of an obvious widening of the atlantodental interval. The tip of the dens is more or less destroyed and eroded away.

b Sagittal T1-weighted MR image: The widening of the atlantodental interval is also well displayed on this image. The structural atlantodental instability is associated with a mild basilar impression and corresponding superior migration of the dens. Marked compression of the spinal cord.

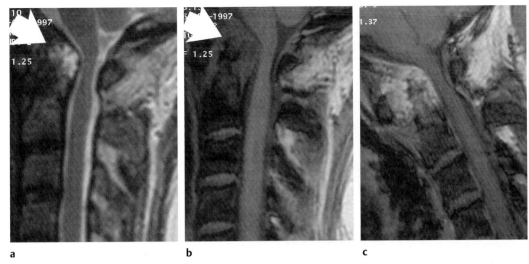

a   b   c

Fig. 6.**27 a–c Long-standing rheumatoid arthritis. 50-year-old female patient:**

a Sagittal T2-weighted image (TSE; TR = 4600 ms, TE = 112 ms): Very signal-intense pannus along the dens, which appears almost completely destroyed (arrow). The spinal canal is narrowed by the pannus tissue. The spinal cord appears compressed.

b Sagittal T1-weighted image (FLASH 2D; TR = 403 ms, TE = 11 ms, flip angle α = 90°): Apart from the pannus

tissue located dorsal to the dens, this image also shows marked granulation tissue ventrally (arrow).

c Functional image in anteflexion with additional contrast application (FLASH 2D; TR = 403 ms, TE = 11 ms, flip angle α = 90°): A very strong contrast enhancement of the whole granulation tissue has developed. The dens also displays signal enhancement, reflecting the hypervascularization. The functional image has resulted in no increase of the compressive effect.

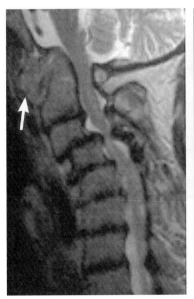
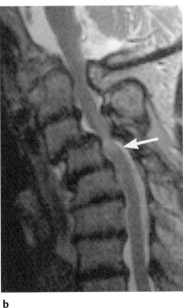

a   b

Fig. 6.**28 a–c Extensive changes secondary to long-standing rheumatoid arthritis.** 70-year-old female patient:

a, b Sagittal T2-weighted images (TSE; TR = 4600 ms, TE = 112 ms): Marked basilar impression with considerable widening of the atlantodental interval due to pannus tissue, which demonstrates moderate signal intensity (arrow). Narrowing of the spinal canal and mild compression of the spinal cord in this segment. There are also massive faults in the segments C3–C6 with a considerable forward translation of C3 over C4, resulting in narrowing of the spinal canal and compression of the spinal cord at the level C3/C4 with cord edema (arrow).

Fig. 6.**28 c** ▷

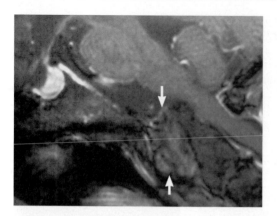

Fig. 6.**28 c** Functional image in anteflexion with additional contrast application (FLASH 2D; TR = 403 ms, TE = 11 ms, flip angle α = 90°): The pannus tissue displays only slight contrast enhancement, which has a patchy inhomogeneous appearance. The compressive effect in the region of the spinal cord does not increase with anteflexion of the head.

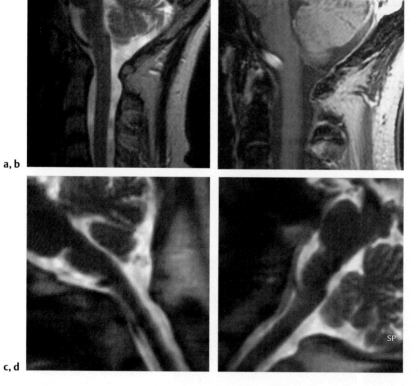

a, b

c, d

Fig. 6.**29 a–d Long-standing rheumatoid arthritis. 58-year-old female patient:**

a Sagittal T2-weighted image of the craniocervical junction (TSE; TR = 4600 ms, TE = 112 ms): Predental patchy inhomogeneous pannus tissue associated with slight widening of the atlantodental interval.

b T1-weighted image after contrast application (FLASH 2D; TR = 403 ms, TE = 11 ms, flip angle α = 90°): Strong contrast enhancement of the predental pannus.

c T2-weighted functional image (HASTE sequence). The image obtained in anteflexion shows mild contact of the dens with the spinal cord. There is no significant compressive effect.

d Image in retroversion: Contact of the dens with the spinal cord has now been counteracted.

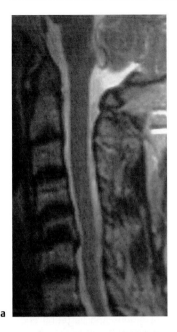

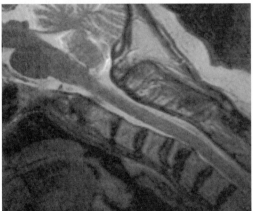

Fig. 6.30 a, b Long-standing rheumatoid arthritis.
60-year-old female patient:
a Sagittal T2-weighted image (TSE; TR = 4600 ms, TE = 112 ms): Structural instability at C5/C6 secondary to a chronic inflammatory reaction with involvement of the inferior end plate C5. Retrolisthesis of C5 on C6. The inflammatory reaction reaches the spinal cord. Mild signal enhancement of an elongated predental pannus, no marked destruction to the dens recognizable.
b Sagittal functional image in anteflexion (TSE; TR = 4600 ms, TE = 112 ms): There is no increase in the compressive effect at the level C5/C6. The predental pannus is also recognizable on this image and displays a somewhat mottled inhomogeneous signal with small nodular signal enhancements.

Spondyloarthropathy

Spondyloarthropathy is clinically characterized most notably by inflammatory spinal pain and by an asymmetric peripheral inflammatory arthritis, predominantly involving joints of the lower limbs. The spinal pain results either from a sacroiliitis or inflammatory changes of the vertebral bodies.

Further typical changes include:
- urogenital and intestinal infections,
- psoriatic skin lesions,
- specific inflammatory bowel disease similar to Crohn's disease,
- enthesopathy,
- dactylitis (sausage digit),
- acute uveitis,
- positive family history,
- presence of HLA-B27 (human leukocyte antigen B27).

The following disorders are subsumed under the term spondyloarthropathy:

- ankylosing spondylitis,
- reactive arthritis,
- psoriatic arthritis,
- arthritis associated with chronic inflammatory bowel disease,
- undifferentiated spondyloarthropathy.

If inflammatory spinal pain is present or the characteristic picture of a peripheral arthritis in combination with an enthesopathy, or if a positive family history is known and the clinical picture is not assignable to any of the above subgroups, then, according to the European Spondyloarthropathy Study Group (ESSG), the diagnosis can be classified as undifferentiated spondyloarthropathy (USpA), the fifth subgroup of spondyloarthropathy. The clinical pictures overlap each other, or sometimes exist side-by-side as subtypes, and also merge. For example, macroscopic and microscopic inflammatory bowel changes have been reported in association with all subtypes of spondyloarthropathy.

The following articular segments are principally involved in the inflammatory process:

- iliosacral joints,
- intervertebral disks including the annulus fibrosus,
- vertebral bodies,

- costovertebral and sternal joints,
- proximal synchondrosis of the symphysis,
- hip joints,
- shoulders,
- tendon attachments in the pelvic region.

The inflammatory changes of the spine can be summarized as follows:

- syndesmophyte formations during the early stage, especially in the T10–L2 region,
- anterior spondylitis (Romanus lesion),
- osteopenia of the spine,
- convex alterations of the vertebral body configuration,
- non-destructive marginal sclerosis of the vertebral body (shiny corner),
- spondylodiskitis (Andersson lesion),
- ossification of the joint capsule and ligaments,
- bamboo spine,
- fractures of the vertebral body,
- pseudarthrosis.

Spondylitis

Spondylitis is usually found after the appearance of sacroiliitis, in some cases even before. The inflammatory changes begin in the region where intervertebral disk, anterior longitudinal ligament and the cortices of the vertebral body converge. Erosive changes of the vertebral bodies, as well as sclerotic alterations, can occur in the further course of the disease.

Posterior spondylitis is less common and is associated with a reactive inflammation and calcification of the posterior longitudinal ligament and the development of posterior syndesmophytes.

Spondylodiskitis (Andersson Lesion)

Incidence

Andersson first described spondylodiskitis in 1937. It is an inflammatory disorder of the diskovertebral region and occurs in about 10–15 % of patients with ankylosing spondylitis (Braun *et al.*, 1998).

In about 30 % of cases the spondylodiskitis is not diagnosed on conventional radiographs and it also often assumes a clinically silent course. Apart from patients with ankylosing spondylitis, it is also not uncommon for spondylodiskitis to be diagnosed in patients with an undifferentiated spondyloarthropathy (USpA), without these patients exhibiting any inflammatory changes of the sacroiliac joints.

This increase in the detection of spondylodiskitis suggests that the diskovertebral segment represents a major target point for the inflammatory disease process.

Pathogenesis

 Classification of the three types of spondylodiskitis, according to Cawley *et al.* (Fig. 6.**31**)

- *Type I:* Diskovertebral lesion in the mid-third of the vertebral body with displacement into the vertebra. These lesions are attributed to osteoporosis, which leads to displacement of diskal components into the vertebral body. A further cause is seen in the reduced mobility of the spine due to ossification of the facet joints, which results in recurrent microtrauma in the region of the disk end plates. These lesions of the cartilaginous and vertebral end plates can promote protrusions of diskal material into the vertebral bodies in the form of Schmorl's nodes. Inflammatory changes of the subchondral bone can lead to destruction of the cartilaginous and vertebral end plates and thus promote the displacement of disk tissue into the bone.
- *Type II:* Type II refers to peripheral diskovertebral lesions, which appear primarily in the anterior and posterior portions of the vertebral body. Inflammation, osteoporosis and enthesopathy with a corresponding reduction of mobility are held responsible for these changes.
- *Type III:* Type III refers to extensive diskovertebral lesions that involve the whole region of a vertebral segment and encompass the inferior and superior end plates as well as the intervertebral disk.

There is some controversy surrounding the pathogenesis of these changes. On the one hand, the cause is believed to lie in an inflammatory reaction, confirmed by the presence of granulation tissue, which destroys the subchondral bone and later contributes to a marked bony sclerosis. On the other hand, repeated trauma is seen as the cause, resulting in what could be regarded as fatigue fractures. They partly result in the

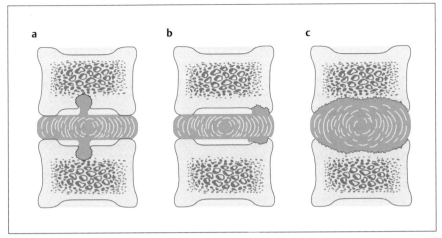

Fig. 6.**31 a–c** **Drawing of spondylodiskitis types I–III** (from Cawley *et al.*):

a Localized central diskovertebral lesion. The defects are associated with herniation of disk material. In these cases marked adjacent edema is detectable on MRI. The contrast series displays enhancement of the corresponding segments of the vertebral bodies.

b Localized peripheral diskovertebral lesion. The defect occurs on either the anterior or posterior aspect of the diskovertebral junction.

c Extensive central and peripheral diskovertebral lesion with destruction of the inferior and superior end plates in the region of the adjacent vertebral bodies. This finding is commonly associated with fractures and pseudarthrosis formation.

development of an inadequate fibrous callus and commonly lead to pseudarthrosis formation. In this respect it is characteristic that mainly the posterior elements of the spine, especially the vertebral arches, are involved in this fracture development.

Uncertainty about its pathogenesis has led to numerous other terms having been introduced for the Andersson lesion:

- spondylodiskitis,
- destructive diskovertebral lesion,
- spinal pseudarthrosis.

It may be assumed that these are all identical findings exhibiting various degrees of expression. The term *spondylodiskopathy* would appear the most suitable to describe these changes.

In cases where a biopsy was taken from the destructive diskovertebral lesion or spondylodiskitis, reactive bone tissue was usually found associated with chronic inflammatory changes, in part with replacement of bone and cartilage by fibrous tissue or associated with the picture of an aseptic chronic osteomyelitis with infiltration by lymphocytes, plasma cells and macrophages. Sometimes the case history of patients with destructive diskovertebral lesions will reveal repeated trauma, but these may also be totally absent.

It may be assumed that Andersson lesions types I–III are in fact different expressions of destructive diskovertebral lesions, possibly graduations, with Andersson lesion type III being regarded as a late form of a long-standing spondylodiskitis or destructive diskovertebral lesion.

Diagnostics

MRI

MRI is in a position to detect a number of cases of spondylodiskitis that would otherwise escape conventional radiography. It should be borne in mind, however, that MRI does not allow a specific diagnosis of spondylitis or spondylodiskitis. Only when an epidural or paraspinal abscess formation or exudation is present, in the case of a bacterial infection, can an unequivocal differentiation be made from a rheumatic disorder. Nevertheless, a reliable diagnosis is possible in the majority of cases when the clinical assessment and observation of the course of the disease over time are taken into account.

MRI of spondylitis or spondylodiskitis displays a variety of findings. The majority of these are consistent with radiographic images as far as location is concerned. In the case of spondylitis, signal changes are often present in the anteroventral and anterocaudal segments of the vertebral bodies. There is a reduction in signal intensity on the T1-weighted images, while the T2-weighted images demonstrate signal enhancement and the contrast-assisted images display a marginal contrast enhancement consistent with the course of the anterior longitudinal ligament as well as with parts of the intervertebral disk. Usually part of the annulus fibrosus of the disk is affected, most notably part of Sharpey's fibers, although a band-like contrast enhancement can appear along the inferior and superior end plates. In addition, there are relatively homogeneous signal changes of the vertebral bodies present, and especially on the T2-weighted images there is a corresponding, almost complete, signal enhancement of the vertebral body or even signal enhancements which follow, in a band-like fashion, the course of the inferior and superior end plates, or fill out one half of the vertebral body.

It is noticeable that, on MRI, changes in the vertebrae are seen in spondyloarthropathy for which there is no radiographic correlation. These are usually changes of the vertebral bodies that correspond to Modic type I, i.e. reductions in signal intensity on the T1-weighted SE image and signal enhancements on the T2-weighted SE image.

There is some discussion in the literature as to whether this is in fact a nonspecific reaction (Remedios, 1998) or whether these findings are more likely early forms of spondylodiskitis (Wienands *et al.*, 1990). Wienands *et al.* (1990) established that marked bone marrow edema found on MRI was associated with a rapid radiological course, the bone marrow edema was less pronounced in older, longer clinical courses of spondylodiskitis, and individual cases revealed a Modic type II signal pattern of the vertebral body. These cases therefore displayed fatty marrow degeneration with a bright signal on T1 weighting and slight signal enhancement on T2 weighting. The bone marrow edema is clearly less well pronounced in

older cases of spondylodiskitis, which emphasizes its importance as an activity parameter. Thus, a rapidly progressive clinical and radiological course is more likely to be expected in the case of a spondylodiskitis with marked bone marrow edema, which would possibly require a more active form of treatment (Figs. 6.**32**–6.**35**).

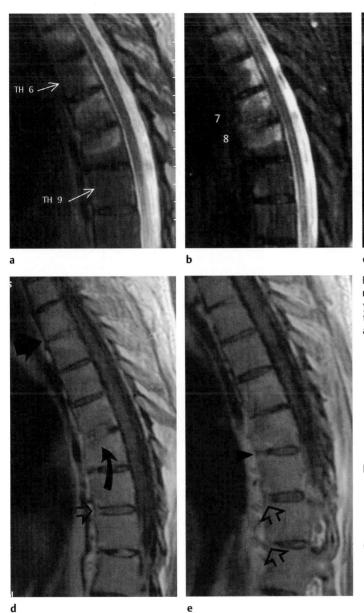

a **b** **c**

d **e**

Fig. 6.**32 a–e** **Extensive inflammatory changes of the spine.** 42-year-old female patient with Bechterew's disease:

a Sagittal T2-weighted image (TSE; TR = 5310 ms, TE = 112 ms): The images show partially inhomogeneous signal enhancement as a sign of edema formation. This involves the depicted vertebrae T4–T8. An Andersson type I lesion is apparent in the segmental region T7 and T8. The image also displays finely speckled signal enhancements in the disk spaces.

b Sagittal T2-weighted image (STIR sequence): Sectional enlargement displaying somewhat more clearly the Andersson lesion in the segmental region T7/T8 in the form of a spondylodiskitis.

c Sagittal T1-weighted image before contrast application (TSE; TR = 800 ms, TE = 12 ms): Marked decrease in signal intensity in the vertebrae T4–T8. There is just a suggestion of the destruction of the inferior end plate of T7 (curved arrow).

d Sagittal image after contrast application: Clear enhancement in the disk space T7/8 (curved arrow). Obvious destruction in the region of the inferior end plate. There are further areas of contrast enhancement, firstly in the vertebral bodies T4 and T5 (straight arrow) and, secondly, ventrally at the level of the vertebral margins and corresponding parts of the annulus fibrosus of T9/T10 (open arrow).

e Parasagittal image after contrast application: Evidence of syndesmophytes (open arrows). Low-grade subchondral contrast enhancement in the region of the corresponding ventral parts of the vertebral bodies in the proximal segment (arrowheads).

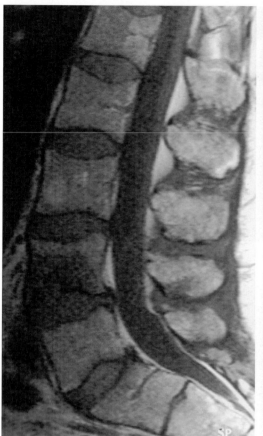
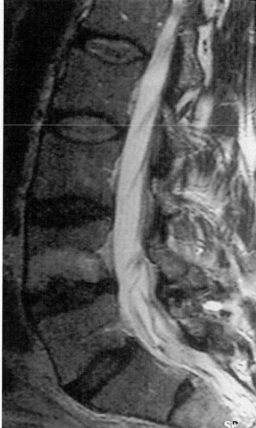

Fig. 6.**33 a, b** **Andersson type I lesion:**

a Sagittal T1-weighted image with signs of a spondylodiskitis in the region L4/L5 (TSE; TR = 800 ms,
TE = 12 ms): The image shows a marked reactive
edema, particularly in the fourth lumbar vertebra.
The inferior end plate is interrupted.

b T2-weighted image (TSE; TR = 5300 ms, TE =
120 ms): Clearly recognizable is the bone marrow
edema of L4. There is interruption of the inferior end
plate of L4 secondary to inflammation with disk
herniation.

Contrast images (not shown) displayed clear enhancement in the fourth lumbar vertebra.

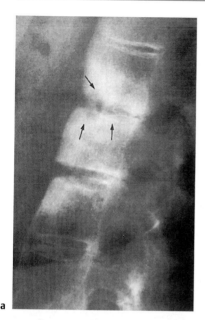

a

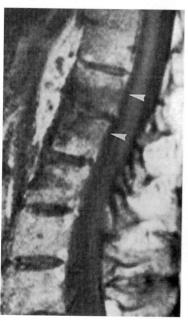

b

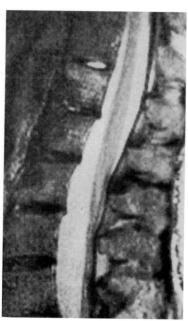

c

Fig. 6.34 a–c Andersson type III lesion:

a Sclerosis near the inferior and superior end plates of T12–L2. The inferior end plate of T12 and the superior end plate of L1 are irregularly contoured, the disk space is narrow (arrows). Osteolysis of the anterior margins. Marked squaring of the 12th thoracic vertebra and the first lumbar vertebra.

b Sagittal T1-weighted image (SE; TR = 726 ms, TE = 20 ms): Circumscribed decrease in signal intensity at T12 and L1 as well as L2 ventrally. The intervertebral disk T12/L1 is reduced in height.

c Sagittal T2-weighted image (SE; TR = 2100 ms, TE = 80 ms): There is a low signal intensity in the affected areas relative to the T1-weighted sequence, reflecting the extensive sclerosis of the bone, as well as a marginal reactive edema which primarily affects the 12th thoracic vertebra. Focal increase in signal intensity in the T11/T12 disk and, in a mottled form, also in the segment T12/L1 as a sign of disk calcifications.

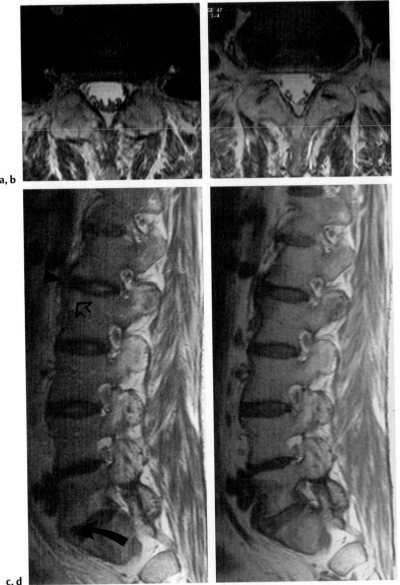

a, b

c, d

Fig. 6.35 a–d **Long-standing Bechterew's disease with extensive bony changes:**

a, b Transverse T2-weighted image (TSE; TR = 4465 ms, TE = 120 ms): Marked ankylosis of the facet joints; the joint space is completely ossified in places, otherwise a residual structure resembling a joint is recognizable.

c Sagittal T2-weighted section (TSE; TR = 5300 ms, TE = 120 ms): The images show syndesmophyte formations at L1/L2 (arrowheads) and L5/S1 (curved arrow). There is also reactive edema of the adjoining parts of the vertebral bodies (open arrow). Frank reactive edema is also recognizable in the region of L5/S1.

d Sagittal T1-weighted section (TSE; TR = 800 ms, TE = 12 ms): The edematous changes in the vertebral segments display a reduction in signal intensity on T1 weighting.

Intervertebral Disk Calcification

Diagnostics

MRI

Intervertebral disk calcification is a common radiographic finding in patients with spondyloarthropathy. Tyrrell *et al.* (1995) performed a correlation analysis between MRI findings and radiographs in patients with disk calcification (Fig. 6.**36**).

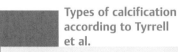

Types of calcification according to Tyrrell et al.

- *Type A:* Calcification of the cartilaginous end plate.
- *Type B:* Calcification within the annulus.
- *Type C:* Calcification within the nucleus pulposus.
- *Type D:* Calcification of the entire intervertebral disk.
- *Type B/D:* Mixed type with calcification of parts of the annulus and at times complete calcification of parts of the disk.

These calcifications demonstrated increased signal intensity on both T1- and T2-weighted images. Disk calcification was usually identified in more than one segment. The majority of patients in which less than 6 disks were affected exhibited a Type A signal pattern. Patients with more than 6 disks involved displayed Type D as the most common pattern. This allows the conclusion that more advanced forms of calcification are seen in cases of progressive disease associated with

corresponding damage to the disks (Figs. 6.**37** and 6.**38**).

Disk calcification did not correlate with changes of the bone marrow signal on the T1- and T2-weighted images.

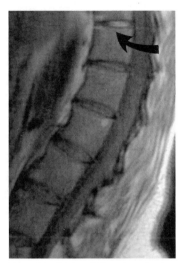

Fig. 6.**37** **Disk calcifications in the uppermost of the depicted segments (T11/T12).** Sagittal T1-weighted image (TSE; TR = 800 ms, TE = 12 ms): Quite homogeneous signal enhancement of the nucleus pulposus of the T11/T12 disk as a sign of calcification.

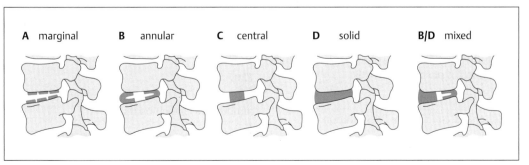

A marginal	B annular	C central	D solid	B/D mixed

Fig. 6.**36** **Typical patterns of disk calcifications.** Patient with long-standing Bechterew's disease (the calcifications are marked red and appear signal intense on MRI).

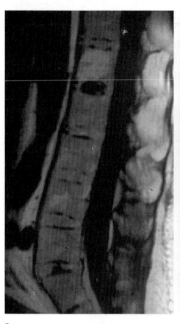
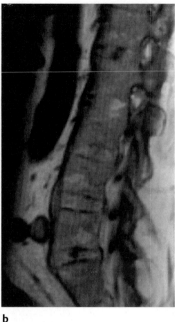

a   b

Fig. 6.38 a, b Long-standing Bechterew's disease. 70-year-old patient:

a Midsagittal section using T1 weighting (TSE; TR = 587 ms, TE = 12 ms): Massive ossification of all depicted spinal segments. Patchy disk changes, in part with signal intense structures, above all of pattern types B and D. In addition there is marked reduction in signal intensity of the nucleus pulposus of L1/L2.

b Parasagittal section using T1 weighting: Here too there are very patchy signal enhancements of the disks together with a segmental reduction in signal intensity. Strong syndesmophyte formations with corresponding elevation of the anterior longitudinal ligament in the regions L1–L3 and L4/L5 and L5/S1.

Subluxations

The changes of the vertebral bodies can manifest themselves in the form of marked subluxations, particularly of the cervical spine, and can result in compression of the spinal cord. In these cases trauma of the cervical spine usually precedes, with the risk of a *trauma-related fracture* being greater in cases of marked ossification and marked ankylosis of the facet joints and ossifications of the ligaments. In individual cases a pre-existing pseudarthrosis may after a trauma lead to frank osteolysis with the formation of substitute fibrous tissue.

Atlantoaxial subluxations are also not infrequently seen and are similar to those found in rheumatoid arthritis. In a study by Ramos-Remus *et al.* (1995), an anterior atlantoaxial subluxation was observed in 21 % of cases and a vertical subluxation in 2 % of cases (Fig. 6.**39**).

Cauda Equina Syndrome

Pathogenesis and Clinical Presentation

A further, infrequently detected complication of ankylosing spondylitis is the cauda equina syndrome. This is a disorder that has not yet been completely clarified. The patients present with marked diverticulum-like herniations of the dura, usually posteriorly into the vertebral arches and spinous processes. The finding is most impressive on myelography because the sac-like diverticula appear well contrasted. The diagnosis presents no difficulties on MRI or CT either.

The clinical picture is commonly associated with a cauda equina syndrome. It is assumed that a chronic inflammation of the spinal meninges, especially the dura, precedes this process.

Diagnostics

Laboratory findings

There are no specific laboratory findings. A mild increase in protein may be present in the CSF, although there is no serious increase in cell count.

EMG

EMG reveals neurological changes in the form of a lumbosacral radiculopathy.

MRI

MRI typically demonstrates characteristic changes and provides a good overview of the entire diverticulum-like meningeal protrusions (Fig. 6.**40**).

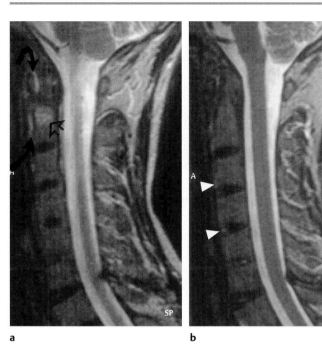

a   b

Fig. 6.**39 a, b** **Long-standing Bechterew's disease. 30-year-old patient.** Sagittal T2-weighted images (TSE; TR = 5300 ms, TE = 112 ms): Low-grade inflammatory reaction with atlantodental pannus tissue (curved arrow) associated with reactive edema of the base of the dens (open arrow). Furthermore the images show small nodular areas of reactive edema in the region of the anterior vertebral margins (arrowheads and straight arrows). In the C4–C6 segment there is a marked syndesmophyte formation in the dorsal and ventral elements with ossification along the annulus fibrosus. The C5/C6 and C7/T1 disks in parts display patchy, in parts relatively homogeneous, signal enhancements, possibly as a sign of calcification.

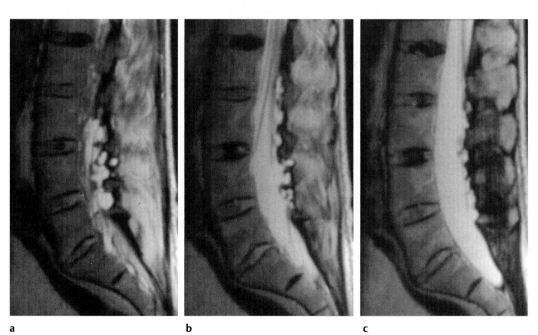

a   b   c

Fig. 6.**40 a–c** **Cauda equina syndrome.** Patient with long-standing Bechterew's disease. (Images courtesy Prof. Kachel, Erfurt Clinical Center, Germany.) Sagittal T2-weighted images with depiction of numerous diverticula extending into the appendant vertebral structures. Syndesmophyte formations and disk calcifications with corresponding signal enhancements.

Fig. 6.**40 d–f** ▷

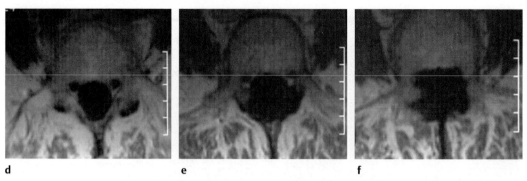

d   e   f

Fig. 6.**40 d–f** **Transverse T1-weighted images.** The dorsal extent of the diverticula is well shown.

Inflammatory Disorders of the Spinal Canal

H. Henkes, W. Weber, S. Felber, and D. Kuehne

Spinal Leptomeningitis

Acute inflammations of the intracranial and spinal meninges do not usually reveal changes of the leptomeningeal structures at MRI. Subacute and chronic courses demonstrate thickening of the leptomeninges, which are particularly well displayed on T1-weighted images after application of Gd-DTPA. Flat or nodular contrast enhancements are demonstrated on the surface of the spinal cord or cauda equina. On the basis of morphological imaging, the finding is not distinguishable from those changes seen in leptomeningeal metastatic dissemination or with primary tumors of the brain (Sugahara *et al.*, 1998; Tamura *et al.*, 1998) (Figs. 6.**41**–6.**47**).

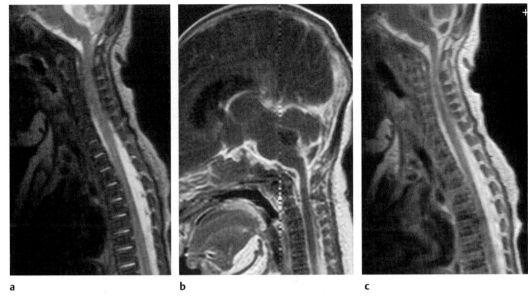

a   b   c

Fig. 6.**41 a–c** **Escherichia coli meningitis.** 4-week-old infant:

a   Sagittal T2-weighted image (TSE; TR = 5300 ms, TE = 120 ms): Image without unequivocal signs of meningitis.

b, c Sagittal images of the craniocervical junction and the cervical and thoracic spine after contrast application: Diffuse, intracranial as well as intraspinal, meningeal enhancement. The inflammation resolved rapidly and completely with the aid of antibiotics.

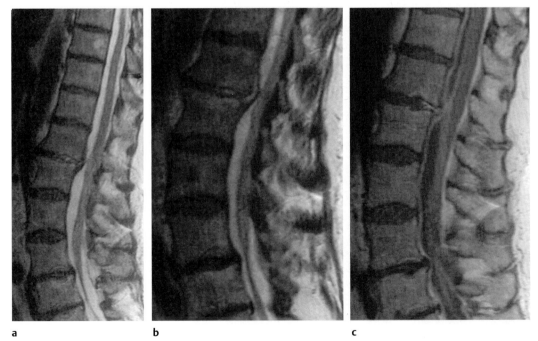

a   b   c

Fig. 6.**42 a–f** **Spondylodiskitis T12/L1 with diffuse pachymeningitis, leptomeningitis, and inflammation of the cauda equina secondary to an epi-subdural abscess in the presence of a staphylococcus infection:**

a, b Sagittal T2-weighted images: Depiction of signal enhancement in the T12/L1 disk space and corresponding mild bone-marrow edema. Small epidural

abscess. Note how the roots of the cauda equina feather out.

c Sagittal image after contrast application: Homogeneous enhancement of the dura, arachnoid membrane, and roots of the cauda equina. Contrast enhancement of the T12/L1 disk.

Fig. 6.**42 d–f** ▷

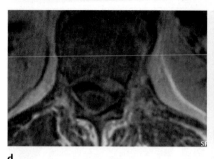
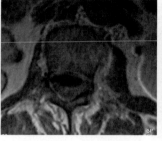
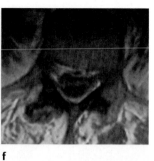

d   e   f

Fig. 6.**42 d–f**

d Transverse image after contrast application at the level of the spondylodiskitis: Enhancement of the abscess, the dura, and the leptomeninges along the spinal cord.

e Image obtained one vertebral level distal to **d**: Enhancement of the roots of the cauda equina and

meninges. Displacement of the cauda equina roots dorsally by subdural effusion.

f Image at the level of L4: Enhancement of the cauda equina roots and meninges. Displacement of the cauda equina roots ventrally by subdural effusion.

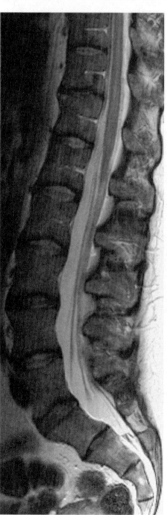
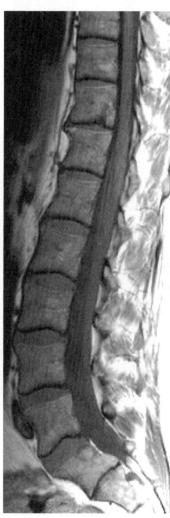

Fig. 6.**43 a–d Arachnoiditis and inflammation of the cauda equina.** 49-year-old female patient with a staphylococcus infection:

a Sagittal T2-weighted images with evidence of thickening of the cauda equina.

b Sagittal T1-weighted images, which also reveal a slight thickening of the cauda equina roots.

a   b

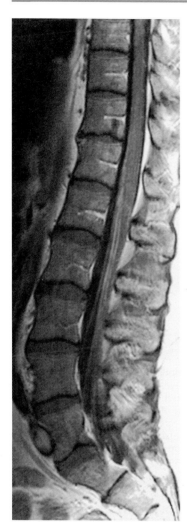

c

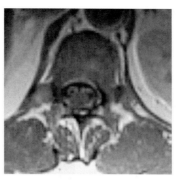

d

Fig. 6.**43 c, d** After contrast application a clear enhancement of the leptomeninges is visible along the conus and the roots of the cauda equina.

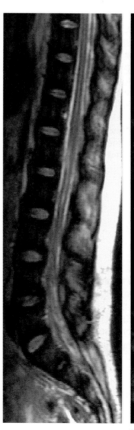

a

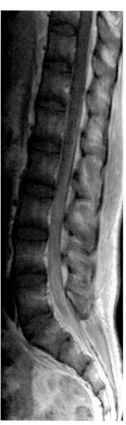

b

Fig. 6.**44 a, b   Arachnoiditis and inflammation of the cauda equina secondary to mucormycosis.** 23-year-old patient with rejection reaction of a transplanted kidney:

a Sagittal T2-weighted image with clear hypointensity of the vertebral bodies indicating the presence of osteoporosis after long-standing steroid therapy. The roots of the cauda equina are shortened and thickened and adherent to one another.

b Diffuse enhancement of the cauda equina roots becomes apparent after contrast application.

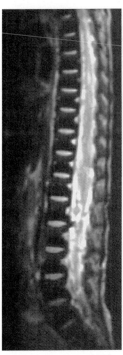
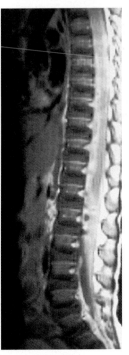
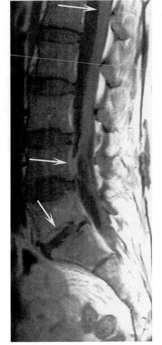

a, b

Fig. 6.**45 a, b** **Arachnoiditis, inflammation of the cauda equina and myelitis.** 13-year-old girl with acute myeloid leukemia and candidiasis. After the fourth cycle of chemotherapy a candida stomatitis developed and subsequently a flaccid paraplegia:

a Sagittal T2-weighted image: Depiction of an irregular margin of the myelon associated with cord edema at the level of T7. There are air inclusions in the lumbar spinal canal.

b Sagittal image after contrast application: There is a diffuse contrast enhancement of the entire subarachnoid space and the roots of the cauda equina.

Fig. 6.**46** **Spondylodiskitis with inflammation of the cauda equina.** 67-year-old patient. In the sagittal T1-weighted image after contrast application there is contrast enhancement of the dural sac and the adjacent roots of the cauda equina at the level of L4 (arrow) in addition to the proximal roots of the cauda equina at the level of the epiconus. Signal enhancement within the L5/S1 disk space (arrow).

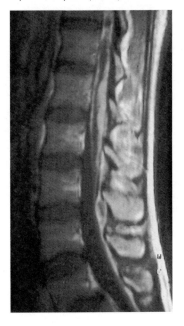

Fig. 6.**47** **Granulomatous, most likely tuberculous, inflammation of the cauda equina and radiculitis.** 28-year-old patient from Mozambique who had suffered from sciatica with radiation to both legs for 4 weeks. At the time of admission to hospital he presented with paraparesis with right-sided predominance and perianal numbness. After contrast application a contrast-enhancing structure is depicted on the sagittal section, surrounding the conus and cauda equina. At laminectomy with opening of the dura at the level of T11–L2, the dorsal nerve roots appeared swollen. Histological examination of the tissue sample revealed epithelioid cell granulomas with central necrosis.

Spinal Epidural Abscess

Epidural abscesses in the spinal canal are less common than inflammatory lesions of the vertebral bodies. Bacterial seeding is more common by the hematogenous route than by direct spread of the pathogen. Abscess formation may be promoted or caused by:

- diabetes mellitus,
- intravenous drug abuse,
- HIV infection,
- other immunocompromising conditions.

Continuous spread only occasionally takes its origin from a spondylitis or a diskitis because the dural sac acts as a barrier to the spread of infection. Potential iatrogenic causes are:

- insertion of an epidural catheter,
- epidural or paravertebral infiltrations,
- chemonucleolysis,
- diskography,
- surgery of the spine or intervertebral disk.

The cervical spinal canal is less commonly affected than the thoracic and lumbar region. Only about one-fifth of spinal epidural abscesses are located ventral to the spinal cord (Lange *et al.*, 1997). Local or radicular pain, paralysis and sensory dysfunction are clinically more indicative than fever and other general signs of inflammation.

The development of an epidural abscess occurs in stages, which are reflected in the MRI findings. During the phlegmonous stage, there is a homogeneous contrast enhancement in the whole of the affected epidural space. This corresponds to an inflammatory thickening of the meninges, which contain microabscesses yet without collections of pus. With increasing abscess formation, there then appears a liquid center of necrotizing tissue that is surrounded by a capsule. The full blown epidural abscess is hypointense to spinal cord tissue on the T1-weighted sequence, is homogeneously hyperintense to spinal cord and isointense with CSF on the T2-weighted sequence, and demonstrates an intensive marginal contrast enhancement, which spares the liquid center of necrotizing tissue, after intravenous administration of Gd-DTPA.

Post *et al.* (1990) describe three patterns of contrast enhancement associated with epidural abscesses:

- diffuse homogeneous,
- diffusely inhomogeneous with circumscribed sparing of contrast,
- thin contrast enhancing rim in the periphery of the abscess.

Epidural abscesses, with or without only little granulation tissue, show only a slight contrast enhancement, even in the presence of larger collections of pus. A definite distinction based on the pattern of contrast enhancement cannot be made between an *acute epidural abscess* and a *chronic epidural inflammation* with proliferation of scarred connective tissue (Post *et al.*, 1990) (Figs. 6.**48**–6.**54**).

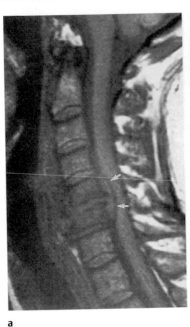

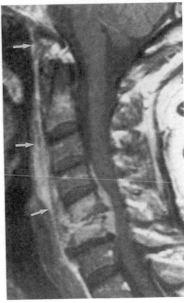

a   b

Fig. 6.48 a, b Spondylodiskitis at C5/C6 with epidural abscess:

a Sagittal T1-weighted plain image (SE; TR = 650 ms, TE = 25 ms): Image with a slight reduction in signal intensity of C5 and C6 and partial loss of the contours of both end plates. A space-occupying structure stands out at an epidural location and appears separated from the spinal cord by the dura in the form of a black fringe-like band (arrows).

b After contrast application: Enhancement within the disk space, the vertebral bodies, and the epidural lesion. At surgery the posterior longitudinal ligament appeared destroyed by the inflammatory epidural lesion. There is also a strong contrast enhancement prevertebrally as an indication of a reactive phlegmonous inflammation with extension as far as the skull base.

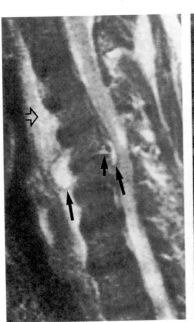

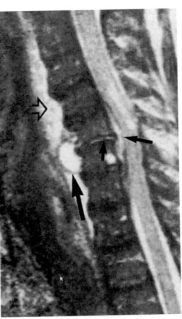

a   b

Fig. 6.49 a, b Diskitis with epidural and prevertebral abscess at C5/C6. There was no apparent involvement of the bone at surgery. Bright signal of the epidural and prevertebral abscess. Signal enhancement in the dorsal part of the disk is particularly distinctive (SE; TR = 2100 ms, TE = 80 ms).

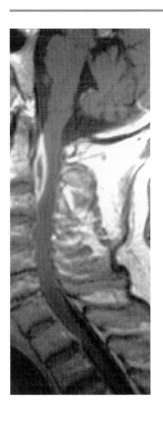

◁ Fig. 6.**50** **Formation of an epidural abscess at the level C2/C3.** 73-year-old patient. This abscess appeared in the course of a staphylococcus sepsis. There were clinical signs of paraplegia. Sagittal section after contrast application: At the level of the atlas there is a ventral epidural abscess formation clearly compromising the spinal cord. There is also contrast enhancement of the spinal meninges. The abscess apparently takes its origin from a diskitis or spondylodiskitis in the segments C5/C6 and C6/C7, revealed by the contrast uptake in both disks of these segments.

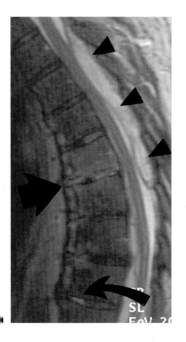

Fig. 6.**51 a–i** **Extensive long-segment epidural abscess formation in the thoracic spinal region of T3–T10 occurring as a result of a spondylodiskitis T6/T7 and concomitant involvement of segments T7/T8 and T8/T9:**

◁ **a** Sagittal T2-weighted image (TSE; TR = 5310 ms, TE = 112 ms): Evidence of spondylodiskitis and corresponding bone-marrow reactions in the region of T6–T9, with T6 displaying a homogeneous signal enhancement and the T6/T7 disk also revealing a clear signal enhancement. In addition there is a subligamentous reaction along the anterior longitudinal ligament with involvement of the thoracic vertebrae 7–9 leading to a ventral signal enhancement within the disk spaces T8/T9 and also, to a small extent, T9/T10 (curved arrow). The anterior longitudinal ligament appears elevated over a long segment in the region of T5 to T10, inclusive, due to the subligamentous exudation (large arrow). A long-segment abscess is recognizable dorsally on the image and is separated in a fringe-like fashion from the subarachnoid space by the dura (arrowheads).

Fig. 6.**51 b–i** ▷

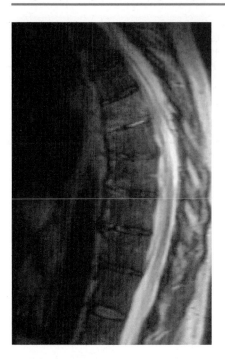

Fig. 6.**51 b Sagittal T2-weighted image (TSE; TR = 5310 ms, TE = 112 ms):** In addition to the dorsal epidural abscess, a ventral abscess formation is also visible on this image extending as far as T10 and taking its origin from the spondylodiskitis 6/7.

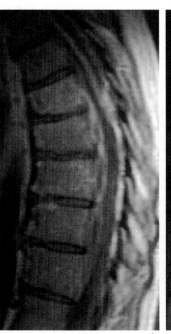

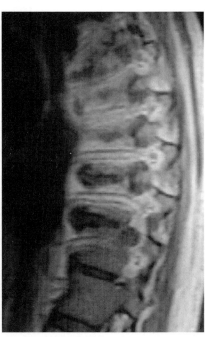

c

d

Fig. 6.**51 c–d**

c Sagittal image after contrast application (TSE; TR = 800 ms, TE = 12 ms): Marginal development of contrast enhancement with signal void of necrotic areas dorsally and ventrally. There is, furthermore, a discrete subligamentous contrast enhancement effect along the anterior longitudinal ligament as well as along the anterior edge of the vertebral bodies and subchondrally.

d Parasagittal image after contrast application with depiction of a marked diffuse contrast enhancement of the adjacent soft-tissue segments as indications of an advanced paravertebral inflammatory co-reaction.

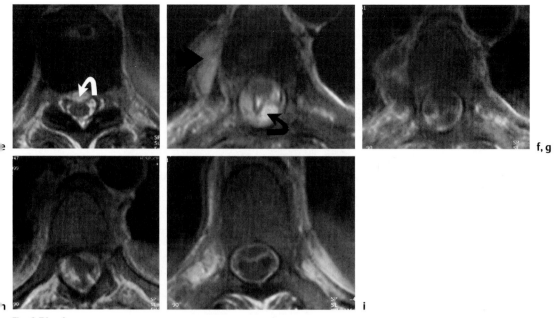

Fig. 6.**51 e–i**

e, f Transverse images using T2 weighting (TSE; TR = 4600 ms, TE = 120 ms): The sections show the signal-intense epidural abscess ventrally and dorsally from which there originates in part a clear compressive effect (curved arrow). In addition, evidence of a more extensive abscess at a right paravertebral location (large arrow).

g–i Transverse images after contrast application: The abscess membrane appears hyperintense on these slices. In part there is a relatively diffuse contrast enhancement of the epidural inflammatory granulation tissue.

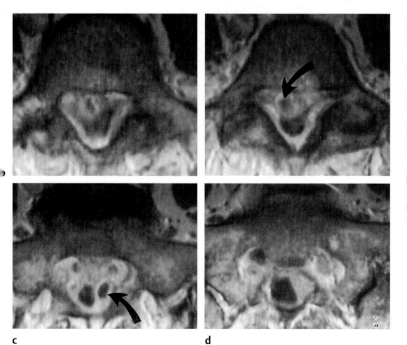

Fig. 6.**52 a–d Lumbosacral epidural abscess formation.** 65-year-old female patient with a long history of diabetes mellitus. Transverse images after contrast application: More extensive epidural abscess formations, in part with clear space-occupying effect, both ventral as well as lateral and dorsal to the dural sac.
b and **c** show larger enclosed liquefactions with reduction of signal intensity (arrows).

c

d

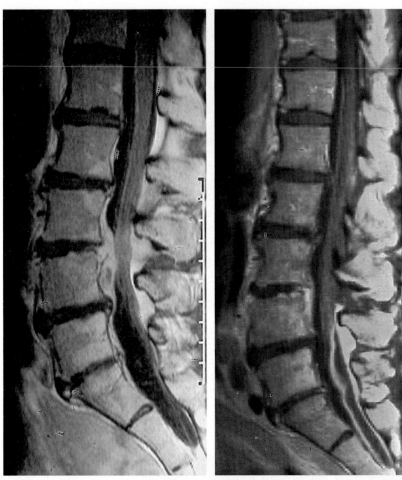

a

b

Fig. 6.**53 a, b Extensive epidural abscess formation after staphylococcal sepsis.** 53-year-old female patient. The probable initial site of entry was a coccygeal furuncle.

a Sagittal T1-weighted image after contrast application: Evidence of dorsally located epidural abscess at the level L3/L4. This abscess was removed via a hemilaminectomy.

b Following persistent attacks of lumbago a further abscess was identified two weeks later, dorsal to the lower roots of the cauda equina at the level of the lumbosacral junction and at a sacral location. Note that the previous abscess located at the level L3/L4 had been completely removed. In addition, this image now showed a long-segment contrast enhancement around the conus and the roots of the cauda in the form of a concomitant inflammation of the cauda equina.

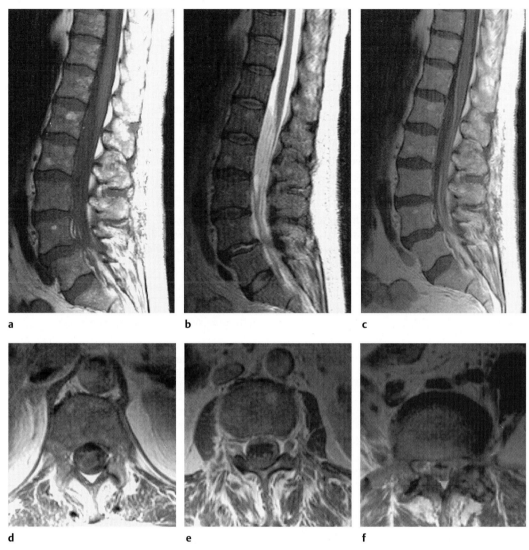

Fig. 6.54 a–f Lumbosacral epi-/subdural abscess. 34-year-old patient with leukemia who developed pneumonia with subsequent sepsis and subacute flaccid paralysis while under chemotherapy:

a Sagittal T1-weighted image: Doubtful portrayal of a space-occupying lesion located ventral to the conus.

b Sagittal T2-weighted image: This doubtful space-occupying lesion shows up as hypointense relative to the CSF.

c After contrast application: Conus and cauda are displaced dorsally.

d Axial T1-weighted image after contrast application: This image now provides evidence of an epidural abscess.

e, f Transverse slice orientation. The subdural abscess is successfully identified here too, together with an inflammation of the cauda equina.

Spinal Cord Abscess

Incidence and Pathogenesis

Unlike abscesses of the brain, abscesses of the spinal cord are extremely rare (Condette-Auliac *et al.*, 1998; Sverzut *et al.*, 1998). They occur preferentially in the second to fourth decades of life, with men being more commonly affected than women. The lesion usually exhibits an expansion in height covering two or three vertebral bodies, with as many as one-third of patients reaching up to five or more vertebral body levels. *Medullary abscesses* are mainly hematogenous in origin, and only in about 20 % do they result from contiguous spread. Predisposing factors are similar to those of the *epidural abscess*. In about one-third of patients the abscess is found in the *thoracic spinal cord*, followed with decreasing frequency by *thoracolumbar* and *cervical abscess* locations. In 10 % of patients *multilocular abscesses* are found (Rachinger *et al.*, 1998).

Clinical Presentation

A distinction is made between the following types of clinical course:

- acute course,
- subacute course,
- chronic course.

The symptoms (cf. also the symptoms of the epidural abscess) can present for a few days, up to six weeks or over the course of more than two months. The most commons pathogens are:

- *Staphylococcus aureus,*
- *Staphylococcus pneumoniae.*

An association has been reported between medullary abscesses and intramedullary ependymomas, as well as with epidermoids and dermal sinuses.

Diagnostics

MRI

The MRI finding is characterized by the fact that the central cavitation, which is filled with pus and necrotic tissue, is surrounded by gliotic and fibrous scar tissue. The spinal cord is enlarged in the region of the abscess and displays increased signal intensity on the T2-weighted sequence. T1-weighted images demonstrate enhancement of the abscess capsule after intravenous administration of Gd-DTPA.

Commonly associated findings include:

- thickening of the meninges, which also enhance with contrast,
- epidural abscess,
- spondylitis.

Therapy

Therapy involves:

- laminectomy,
- myelotomy with drainage of the abscess,
- administration of antibiotics.

Acute Transverse Myelitis

Pathogenesis and Clinical Presentation

Acute transverse myelitis is defined as an acute or subacute spinal dysfunction with paraplegia, sensory level, and bladder and bowel dysfunction. The differential diagnosis must exclude:

- compression of the spinal cord by a tumor,
- epidural hematoma,
- infections,
- vascular malformations,
- trauma,
- local space-occupying manifestation of a malignant disease (Dawson *et al.*, 1991).

Causes of acute transverse myelitis are:
- edema,
- demyelination,
- necrosis of the spinal cord.

Pathogenetically, a distinction is made between:
- infectious diseases (the pathogen directly invades the spinal cord, e.g. borreliosis, infection with herpes simplex virus, syphilis),
- parainfectious diseases (the inflammation is based on an immune reaction of the organism with an antigen e.g. postvaccinal, postinfectious),
- non-infectious diseases (e.g. demyelinating disorders, collagenoses).

Changes involving the white matter are more pronounced that those of the gray matter. The thoracic and lumbar cords are more commonly, and usually more severely, affected than the cervical cord. The prognosis of acute transverse myelitis is not predictable for the individual case. About one-third of the patients experience complete resolution of symptoms, another third makes an incomplete recovery, and a third will lack any improvement at all (Isoda *et al.*, 1998). Rarely during the course of acute transverse myelitis does it recur. As with the spinal manifestations of multiple sclerosis, there is no strict correlation between MRI findings and clinical signs and symptoms during the course of acute transverse myelitis (Choi *et al.*, 1996).

Diagnostics

MRI

As with other inflammatory disorders of the spinal cord, the MRI findings of acute transverse myelitis are nonspecific. The following findings are reported:

- signal-intense lesions of the spinal cord over several vertebral levels on the T2-weighted sequence,
- which are iso- to hypointense on the T1-weighted sequence (hyperintense, hemorrhagic lesions on the T1- and T2-weighted sequences are uncommon in acute transverse myelitis),
- circumscribed expansion of the spinal cord (often with contrast enhancement, Choi *et al.*, 1996),
- contrast enhancements of the spinal cord, reported with varying frequency, which are usually less marked than the contrast-enhanced lesions of medullary tumors and regress during the course, unlike tumorous lesions,
- circumscribed or long-segment atrophies of the spinal cord, reflecting late or secondary stages.

The lesions demonstrated on MRI usually extended for three or more segments cranially above the sensory level (Misra *et al.*, 1996). Long-segmental lesions covering 10 vertebral segments or more are usually associated with an unfavorable neurological outcome (Misra *et al.*, 1996; Imai *et al.*, 1997). It is suggested that, in transverse myelitis, a comparison should be made between spinal cord lesions of patients with and

without multiple sclerosis. In patients with acute transverse myelitis, MRI displays lesions that are associated with a greater extension in length, with enlargement of the spinal cord, and patchy or inhomogeneous contrast enhancement. This differs from multiple sclerosis lesions of the spinal cord, which usually extend over only one to three vertebral body levels. The spinal cord is more frequently not enlarged and contrast enhancement (when present) is more commonly homogeneous (Isoda *et al.*, 1998).

Further criteria for the presence of an acute transverse myelitis without underlying multiple sclerosis are:

- central location and sharp demarcation of the lesions on the T2-weighted sequence,
- expansion of the lesion over more than two-thirds of the cross-sectional area of the spinal cord,
- an area in the center of the lesion appearing signal intense on the T2-weighted sequence and being isointense with spinal cord tissue (central dot sign),
- a fringe-like contrast enhancement in the periphery of the lesion, which appears signal intense on the T2-weighted sequence (Choi *et al.*, 1996). In multiple sclerosis this finding is typically central in location.

Clinical information is of help in individual cases to assist in assessing the MRI findings since the symptoms in patients with acute transverse myelitis are usually symmetric, while in patients with multiple sclerosis they are less marked and asymmetric (Scott *et al.*, 1998).

The following criteria, which are suggestive of the presence of a tumor, can be drawn upon to differentiate between spinal cord tumors and transverse myelitis on the basis of image morphology. With tumors of the spinal cord the following holds true:

- The spinal cord is almost always enlarged.
- The lesion shows as inhomogeneous and hyperintense on the T2-weighted sequence.
- At the level of maximum expansion, the lesion involves the entire cross-sectional area.
- The length of expansion covers four to five vertebral-body levels.
- A secondary syringomyelia is only found in association with tumors. Detection of an intramedullary cavitation therefore militates

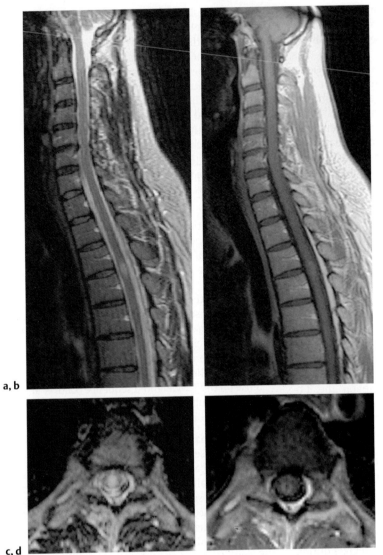

Fig. 6.**55 a–d** **Transverse myeli-tis at the level T2/3.** 48-year-old female patient 2 weeks after a febrile infection:

a Sagittal T2-weighted image: Circumscribed spinal cord lesion at the level T3/4 at a centromedullary location.

b T1-weighted image after contrast application: Enhancement of the lesion.

c Transverse T2-weighted image: Here a circumscribed, sharply delineated signal enhancement can be seen.

d After contrast application: A slight enhancement is apparent with a fringe-like configuration.

a, b

c, d

against the presence of a transverse myelitis, to a great extent.

- Blood degradation products, hyperintense on the T1-weighted sequence, are found more commonly in association with tumors.
- Virtually all tumors of the spinal cord demonstrate marked contrast enhancement, usually affecting the entire cross section of the spinal cord with a pattern of enhancement that is heterogeneous on the whole (Choi *et al.*, 1996) (Figs. 6.**55**–6.**61**).

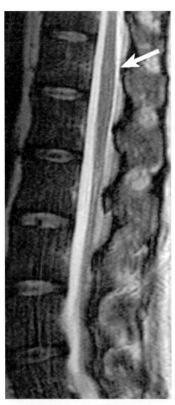

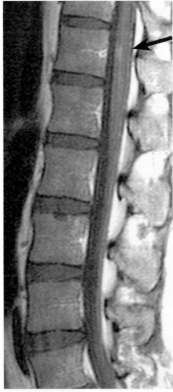

Fig. 6.56 a–e Polysegmental postinfectious transverse myelitis. 40-year-old female patient:

a Sagittal T2-weighted image: A discrete signal enhancement within the spinal cord is apparent at the level T12 (arrow).

b The finding is associated with a mild barrier disturbance after contrast application (arrow).

c Sagittal T2-weighted image: The image of the upper thoracic and cervical spine shows a further, larger lesion at the level C5/C6.

d The lesion at the level C5/C6 enhances strongly with contrast.

e The contrast enhancement applies most notably to the dorsal columns.

b

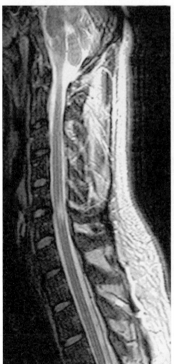

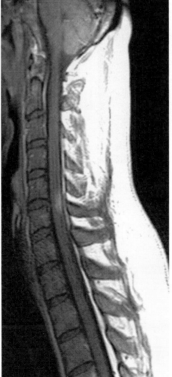

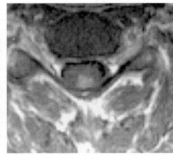

e

d

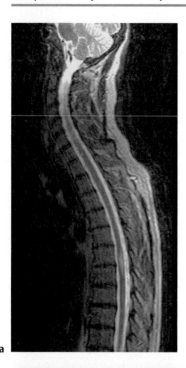

a

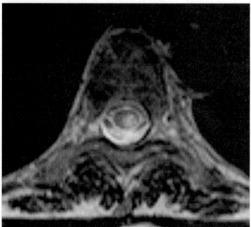

b

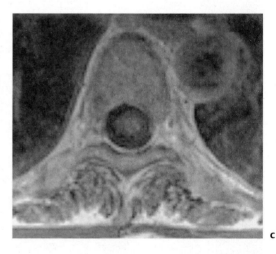

c

Fig. 6.**57 a–c** **Acute transverse myelitis.** 56-year-old patient:

a Sagittal T2-weighted image: The image shows a hyperintense lesion at the level of T6 that has a slight space-occupying effect.

b Axial section: Here the lesion is well circumscribed and involves both the white and gray substances on the left side.

c After contrast application an inhomogeneous contrast enhancement appears on the axial image, indicating transverse myelitis.

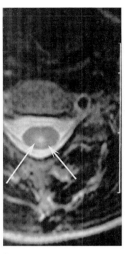
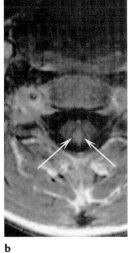

a

b

Fig. 6.**58 a, b** **Transverse myelitis.** 24-year-old female patient:

a Axial T2-weighted image: Evidence of a relatively sharply circumscribed central edema of the spinal cord.

b A faint enhancement appears after contrast application.

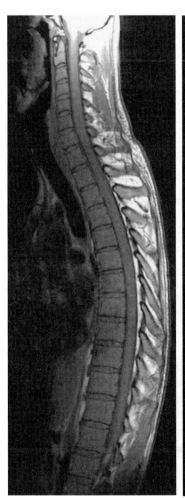
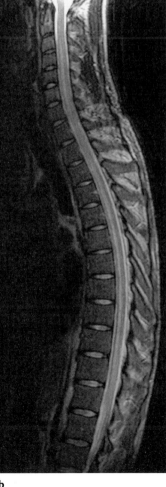
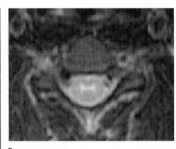

c

a

b

Fig. 6.**59 a–e** **Myelitis.** 18-year-old patient presenting with a flaccid tetraparesis without sensory loss:

a Sagittal T1-weighted image: Depiction of a diffuse swelling of the entire spinal cord.

b Sagittal T2-weighted image: A ventrally accentuated edema of the spinal cord is displayed on this image, extending from C2 down to the conus.

c Axial section: Here there is predominantly involvement of the gray matter of the spinal cord with emphasis of the anterior horns.

Fig. 6.**59 d–e** ▷

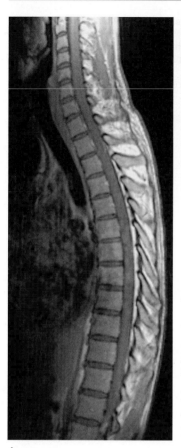

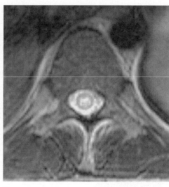

d

e

Fig. 6.59 d, e
d A diffuse enhancement of the cord develops after contrast application.
e Axial section after contrast application: A circumscribed, sharply marginated enhancement of the central cord components and especially of the anterior horns appears.

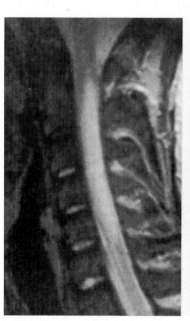

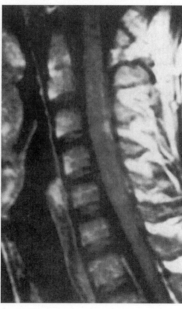

a   b

Fig. 6.60 a, b Transverse myelitis. 20-year-old patient:
a Sagittal section (SE; TR = 1900 ms, TE = 80 ms): Long-segment signal enhancement extending from C2 to the superior edge of C6 with expansion of the spinal cord.
b After contrast application discrete, slightly inhomogeneous enhancement of the dorsal segments of the spinal cord.

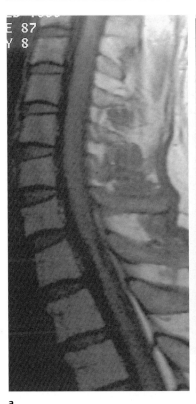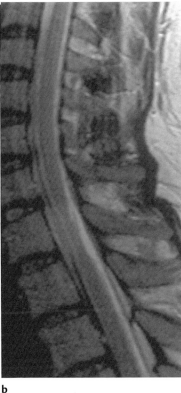

Fig. 6.**61 a, b   Atrophy of the spinal cord secondary to myelitis.** 43-year-old patient:

a Sagittal T1-weighted image: The image shows high-grade atrophy of the spinal cord at the level of T1.

b T2 weighting: Here there is a mild signal enhancement of the spinal cord in the atrophic segment reflecting the gliosis.

a   b

Radiation Myelopathy and Myelitis

Pathogenesis and clinical presentation

Irradiation of the spinal cord can lead to demyelination and necrosis of the cord as a result of direct neuronal damage and secondarily due to vascular reactions to the irradiation (endothelial damage, intima proliferation and fibrosis of the adventitia), i.e. ultimately as a result of thickening of the vascular wall and vascular obliteration (Schultheiss *et al.*, 1997).

Initially sensory symptoms are usually foremost. As the damage to the spinal cord progresses, there is ultimately failure of all functions. There is usually a latency of some months between the irradiation and the onset of symptoms (Abbatucci *et al.*, 1997). Higher radiations doses shorten this free interval.

Diagnostics

MRI

MRI demonstrates thickening of the spinal cord on the T1-weighted sequence with increased signal intensity on the T2-weighted image. Rings of contrast enhancement appear after intravenous application of Gd-DTPA (Yasui *et al.*, 1997). Despite the presence of severe neurological symptoms, radiation myelitis can escape MRI detection during the period of latency. This phenomenon is particularly common after exposition to high radiation doses (Alfonso *et al.*, 1997). The disease leads, at a variable rate, to irreversible damage. There is no known effective treatment (Fig. 6.**62**).

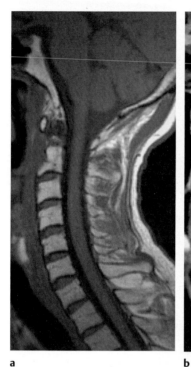

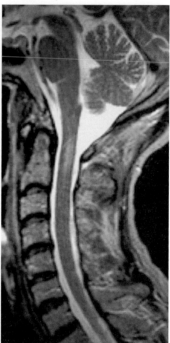

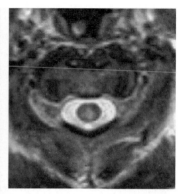

c

a

b

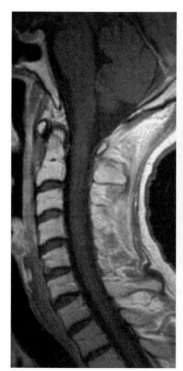

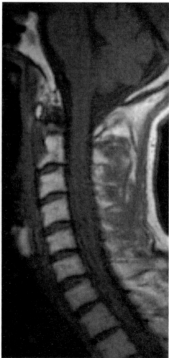

d

e

Fig. 6.62 a–h Radiation myelopathy some months after completion of radiotherapy for posterior tongue carcinoma. The clinical situation deteriorated subsequently: 2 months after radiation myelopathy was noted tetraparesis was superseded by complete tetraplegia. One year after onset of complaints only a minor improvement of the symptoms was detected:

a Sagittal T1-weighted image: The typical signal enhancement of the vertebral bodies after radiotherapy is apparent on this image, reflecting the conversion of hematopoietic bone marrow into fatty marrow.

b T2-weighted image: Here there is a hyperintense intramedullary lesion at the level of C2.

c Axial T2-weighted image: Here the intramedullary lesion at the level of C2 (b) is at a centromedullary location.

d After contrast application there is only a very faint barrier disturbance at the level of C2.

e T1-weighted image: Two months after onset of symptoms a massive swelling of the cervical cord is apparent.

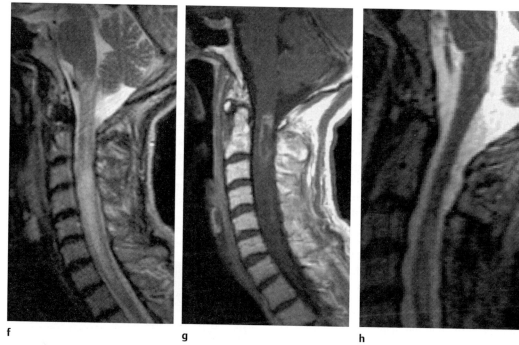

f

g

h

Fig. 6.**62 f–h**

f T2-weighted image: A corresponding extensive intramedullary edema is shown here, extending now as far as the brain stem.

g After contrast application a clear marginal barrier disturbance is visible.

h The follow-up image after 1 year demonstrates atrophy of the cervical cord.

Multiple Sclerosis

Pathogenesis and Clinical Presentation

In multiple sclerosis, lesions develop in the brain or spinal cord that undergo circumscribed demyelination as well as axonal loss.

Diagnostics

The diagnosis rests upon the combination of clinical, electrophysiological, CSF-analytical and imaging findings.

MRI

The MRI findings of spinal manifestations of multiple sclerosis must be considered within this overall context: they should not be evaluated without knowledge of the clinical picture. Large patient populations have revealed a distribution of multiple sclerosis lesions in the brain and spinal cord in a ratio of about 80 % : 20 % (Trop *et al.*, 1998). Multiple sclerosis lesions are more common in the cervical cord than in the thoracic or lumbar region. More than one-half of patients demonstrate more than one lesion. In only 10–15 % of multiple sclerosis patients with spinal involvement is no cerebral lesion detected on MRI.

The following spinal findings are noted at MRI in patients with multiple sclerosis:

- depiction of hyperintense lesions of the spinal cord on the T2-weighted sequence,
- signs of focal barrier disturbance after intravenous administration of Gd-DTPA (nodular, annular or patchy enhancement),
- circumscribed enlargement of the spinal cord in the vicinity of lesions that appear hyperintense on the T2-weighted sequence,

● circumscribed or long-segmental atrophy of the spinal cord.

The hyperintense multiple sclerosis lesions displayed on the T2-weighted sequence are usually two vertebral bodies in length or less, are located in the periphery of the cord and affect less than 50 % of its cross-sectional area (Tartaglino *et al.*, 1995). If the multiple sclerosis plaques acquire a length of more than two vertebral body levels and involve more than 50 % of the cross section of the cord, then the probability increases that enlargement or atrophy of the spinal cord will be present, depending on the stage of the disease.

Cord enlargement has been reported in patients with a relapsing-remitting form of the disease (Tartaglino *et al.*, 1995), but affects less than 10 % of patients who present with multiple sclerosis with spinal involvement.

Cord atrophy occurs with the relapsing-progressive form of multiple sclerosis (Tartaglino *et al.*, 1995) and altogether in about 10 % of all patients with multiple sclerosis and spinal involvement.

Wiebe *et al.* (1992) emphasize that, particularly with multiple sclerosis lesions in the spinal cord, the administration of Gd-DTPA is helpful in assessing disease activity. These authors contest that spinal multiple sclerosis plaques disappear completely. The resolution of GD-DTPA enhancement of spinal multiple sclerosis plaques is often accompanied by clinical improvement (Trop *et al.*, 1998).

Spinal multiple sclerosis lesions very rarely display a reduced signal intensity on the T1-weighted sequence. As regards cerebral multiple sclerosis lesions, van Walderveen *et al.* (1995), among others, were able to show that lesions with reduced signal intensity on the T1-weighted sequence more often cause serious neurological symptoms or disability. It is not clear to what extent this also applies to multiple sclerosis lesions in the spinal cord.

The correlation of clinical symptoms and MRI findings is problematic in multiple sclerosis patients. Patients with relapsing-progressive multiple sclerosis often display no contrast enhancement of the multiple sclerosis lesions or any other MRI correlate, whereas patients with relapsing-remitting forms do not escape detection by MRI. If, however, only a few clinical signs and symptoms of the disease are presented, then

there are hardly any differences between the MRI findings of the different disease courses. Wiebe *et al.* (1992) did find a frequent concordance between clinical and MRI evidence for the presence of disease activity, but the topographic correlation of clinical finding with site of activity at MRI was low. Trop *et al.* (1998) found an agreement between clinical presentation and MRI findings regarding disease activity in only 60 % of patients. Some 40 % of patients demonstrated a new lesion of the spinal cord without any subsequent clinical deterioration, or clinical deterioration occurred without any corresponding correlate on MRI examination (Figs. 6.**63**–6.**67**).

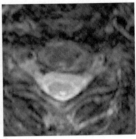

b

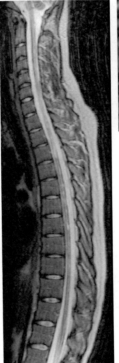

a

Fig. 6.**63 a, b Disseminated encephalomyelitis of 8 years' standing with episodic course.** 24-year-old female patient:
a Sagittal T2-weighted image: The image shows multifocal circumscribed hyperintense lesions. Small-caliber spinal cord with loss of the cervical intumescence.
b Axial T2-weighted image: A left-accentuated lesion in the posterior tracts is apparent on this image through the lower cervical cord.

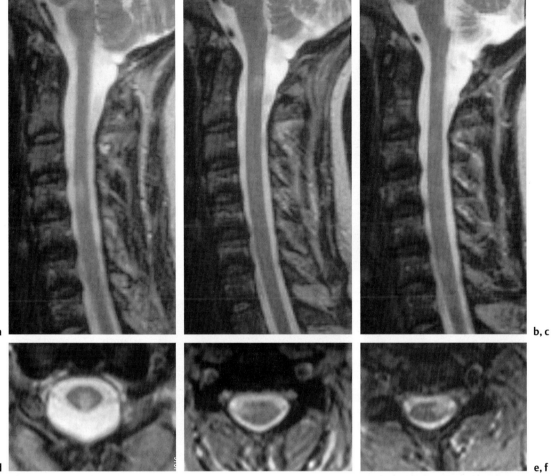

Fig. 6.**64 a–f Long-standing multiple sclerosis.** 33-year-old female patient:

a–c Sagittal T2-weighted images: The images show numerous lesions in the cervical medullary layer.

d–f More or less typical location and size of these lesions.

Spinal manifestations where the lesion is of greater extent both in length and cross section, even to the degree of involving the entire cervical and thoracic cord, have been reported for Devic's syndrome (neuromyelitis optica), a variant of multiple sclerosis. The lesions display inhomogeneous signal intensity on the T2-weighted sequence, and the application of Gd-DTPA results in a patchy, ill-defined contrast enhancement (Tartaglino *et al.*, 1995).

In practice, a combined MRI examination of brain and spinal cord should be obtained for an exact assessment of the disease activity when there is clinical and laboratory evidence of multiple sclerosis with both cerebral and spinal symptomatology. On the other hand, it is usually sufficient to verify the presence of only cerebral lesions to narrow the diagnosis down to multiple sclerosis.

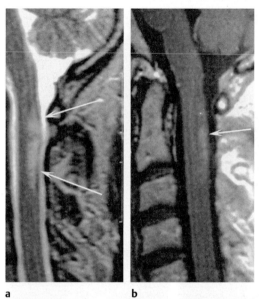

a   b

Fig. 6.**65 a, b   Disseminated encephalomyelitis with focal lesion in the cervical cord.** The patient presented clinically with static and locomotor ataxia and progressive tetraparesis. Six months previously an optic neuritis had developed:
a Sagittal T2-weighted section: The image shows a hyperintense lesion located dorsally in the spinal cord.
b After contrast application a rather strong enhancement becomes apparent.

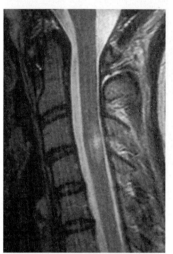

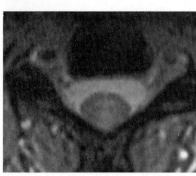

b

a

Fig. 6.**66 a–d   Acute exacerbation of a known long-standing multiple sclerosis.** 32-year-old female patient:
a Sagittal T2-weighted image: Multiple sclerosis lesion in the cervical medullary layer at the level of C3/C4. Slight expansion of the spinal cord due to the edema.
b Transverse T2-weighted image: This image accentuates the dorsal location of the lesion.
c Sagittal T1-weighted image: This image clearly demonstrates the expansion of the spinal cord.
d After contrast application there is a strong enhancement dorsally.

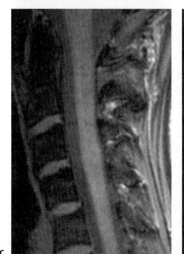

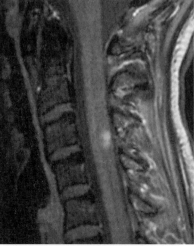

c   d

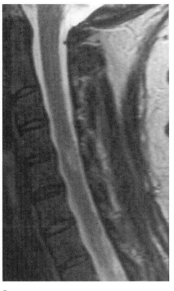
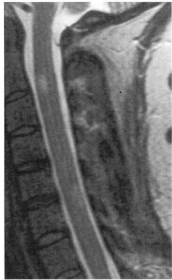
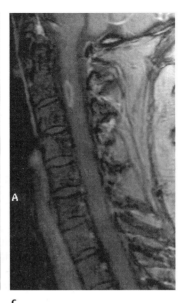

a   b   c

Fig. 6.**67 a–c Acute exacerbation of a known long-standing multiple sclerosis. 27-year-old female patient:**
a, b Sagittal T2-weighted images showing multiple lesions in the cervical cord.

c Sagittal image after contrast application: The lesion situated in the upper cervical cord displays a conspicuous marginal enhancement.

Myelopathy Associated with HIV Infection and AIDS

Lesions of the spinal cord are observed clinically in up to 20 % of all AIDS patients. Autopsy succeeds in detecting such lesions in up to 50 % of cases. With the exception of the rare transverse myelitis during seroconversion, these patients usually present in the advanced stages of the disease. Assessment of MRI findings presents problems because there are no clear-cut differential-diagnostic criteria available. Performing an MRI examination of the skull can be of help because many differential diagnostic considerations for HIV infection of the spinal cord and its meninges can present typical findings of the concomitantly affected brain.

Principally, an HIV infection can manifest itself in the spinal cord in three forms (Quencer *et al.*, 1997):

- lesions with increased signal intensity of the spinal cord:
  - *Vacuolar myelopathy* is the most common medullary manifestation associated with HIV infection (almost 20 %). There is a pre-

dilection for the lateral and dorsal tracts of the thoracic cord. Here vacuolations develop in the white matter that contain lipid-laden macrophages and are surrounded by a thin myelin sheath, but are not associated with demyelination. The foremost clinical symptoms are usually a spastic-atactic paraparesis and incontinence.
  - The *demyelination of the long tracts (tract pallor)* results in demyelination without vacuolization, which is the result of a distal axonal degeneration of the central processes of the dorsal root ganglia. The clinical picture correspondingly consists of a sensory neuropathy.
  - Differential diagnosis: progressive multifocal leukoencephalopathy.
- lesions with focal thickening of the spinal cord and focal thickening of the spinal cord plus meningeal contrast enhancement:
  - HIV myelitis is identified histologically in 5–8 % of AIDS patients. It is characterized by multinuclear giant cells and microglia nodules in the gray mater and often remains clinically asymptomatic.
  - Differential diagnosis: Toxoplasmosis, lymphoma, and, if there is meningeal involve-

ment, tuberculosis and cytomegalic infection (which are commonly associated with AIDS anyway but less often involve the spinal cord). Opportunistic infections of the brain are more common in AIDS patients.

Guillain–Barré Syndrome

Pathogenesis and Clinical Presentation

Guillain-Barré syndrome is an acute inflammatory demyelinating polyradiculoneuropathy. The initial symptoms are typically preceded by a viral or bacterial infection of the respiratory or gastrointestinal tract, resulting in an antibody reaction against peripheral myelin. The patients usually become symptomatic with paresthesias or pain in the lower extremities, normally followed by symmetric ascending flaccid paralysis of the legs. Sensory loss is only slight or is lacking completely. Patients with involvement of the diaphragm muscles are at risk of respiratory failure. The most common cause of death is cardiocirculatory failure with concomitant involvement of the autonomic nervous system. A bilateral facial nerve paralysis occurs in 50% of cases. Central symptoms resulting from concomitant encephalitic involvement are rare (Miller-Fisher syndrome).

Diagnostics

Laboratory findings

Indicative laboratory findings include symmetric ascending paralysis with loss of muscular reflexes in the legs and elevated CSF protein in the absence of pleocytosis.

MRI

Thickening of the cauda equina is demonstrated on MRI and enhances with contrast. The anterior roots are preferentially involved (Fuchigami *et al.*, 1997; Iwata *et al.*, 1997). Spinal cord swelling is also present in rare cases (Delhaas *et al.*, 1998). Concomitant encephalitic involvement manifests itself in the form of hyperintense punctiform lesions of the white matter, which are evident on T2-weighted MR images. On T1 weighting these changes display a barrier breakdown after intravenous contrast application (Borruat *et al.*, 1997). Under treatment, these changes all resolve together with the symptoms (Figs. 6.**68** and 6.**69**).

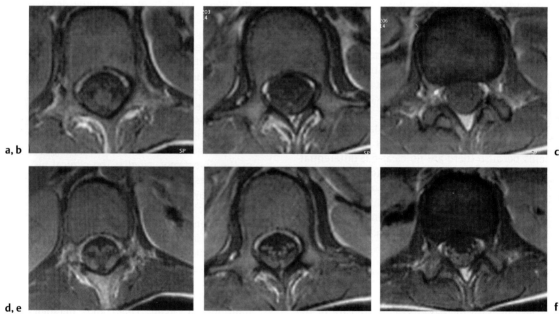

a, b

d, e

c

f

Fig. 6.**68 a–f Guillain-Barré syndrome. 8-year-old girl:**
a–c Pre-contrast images: At the level of the conus (**a**), at the level of the conus-cauda junction (**b**), and at the level of the cauda equina (**c**). A thickening of the roots of the cauda equina is evident on these images.

d–f Images at the same levels after contrast application: A strong enhancement of the ventral and dorsal nerve roots is apparent on these images.

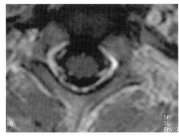 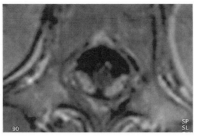

Fig. 6.**69 a, b Guillain–Barré syndrome.** 6-year-old girl. Images after contrast application:
a Transverse image at the level of the upper thoracic spine: Contrast enhancement of the anterior and posterior nerve roots.

b Image at the level of the conus-cauda junction: A strong enhancement of the cauda roots is evident on this image.

Myelitis in Systemic Lupus Erythematosus

Pathogenesis and Clinical Presentation

In up to 60 % of patients with systemic lupus erythematosus (SLE) there is also involvement of the CNS. Transverse myelitis affects 1 % of SLE patients, and, in the majority, it is a late manifestation of the disease, although rarely it can also be the initial syndrome of SLE. The clinical onset often involves belt-like pain, transverse sensory loss, and bladder and rectal disturbances. The further course of the disease involves ascending, initially flaccid (later spastic) para- or tetraparesis. The muscular reflexes are initially absent, CSF shows pleocytosis, CSF glucose concentration is reduced and protein increased. The underlying histological changes are:

- perivascular round cell infiltrates,
- proliferation of connective tissue,
- thrombotic occlusion of small arterioles,
- circumscribed hemorrhage with perivascular gliosis.

The underlying pathogenetic mechanisms currently under discussion are:

- immune complex mediated vasculitis,
- effect of antineural antibodies,
- antiphospholipid- or anticardiolipin antibody-mediated thrombophilia.

The clinical course is most variable and the outcome often does not correlate with the therapeutic regime (Inslicht *et al.*, 1998). Similar cord lesions have also been reported in other autoimmune disorders (mixed connective tissue disease, MCTD). The differential diagnosis includes, among others:

- necrotizing neuromyelitis optica (Devic's syndrome: Mandler *et al.*, 1993),
- Marburg's disease, a malignant variant of multiple sclerosis (Mendez *et al.*, 1988).

Diagnostics

MRI

As in many inflammatory diseases, spinal MRI demonstrates cord enlargement with reduced signal intensity on the T1-weighted sequence and increased signal intensity on the T2-weighted sequence.

Therapy

Treatment involves the use of steroids and cyclophosphamide (Habr *et al.*, 1998).

Intraspinal and Intramedullary Sarcoidosis

Pathogenesis and Clinical Presentation

In sarcoidosis, non-caseating granulomas of unknown origin develop and most commonly affect the lung, eye and skin. Neurological symptoms occur in about 5 % of all patients with sarcoidosis and, if they occur at all, not uncommonly represent the initial manifestation of the disease. Cranial nerve disorders are the most common (> 70 %), while spinal manifestations on the other hand are rare (5–8 %). Apart from involvement of the spinal cord by systemic sarcoidosis, manifestations of the disease limited exclusively to the spine have also been reported (Jaster *et al.*, 1997).

CNS involvement begins with infiltration of the arachnoidea by lymphocytes and non-caseating granulomas. The disease progresses from the surface, down to the brain and spinal cord by centripetal spread via the perivascular spaces. The majority of spinal manifestations of sarcoidosis occur in the fourth decade of life. Men and women are affected with equal frequency. The most common location is the cervical cord (> 50 %), followed by the thoracic cord (< 40 %). Lumbar and sacral manifestations are recorded in less than 10 % of cases.

Diagnostics

MRI

MRI displays the involved cord segment enlarged, with often-circumscribed reductions of signal intensity on the T1-weighted sequence. On the T2-weighted sequence the spinal cord shows circumscribed or diffuse hyperintensity. Intravenous application of Gd-DPTA produces different patterns of enhancement:

- linear leptomeningeal enhancement,
- focal, multifocal or diffuse contrast enhancement of the spinal cord.

The parenchymal lesions commonly demonstrate a broad connection with the surface of the spinal cord and do not usually involve its entire cross section.

Thickenings and contrast enhancement of the cauda equina are found in rare lumbar manifestations (Jallo *et al.*, 1997). Intramedullary calcifications (Waubant *et al.*, 1997) and secondary syringomyelia (Clifton *et al.*, 1997) are very rare.

Junger *et al.* (1993) have proposed a form of classification for spinal sarcoidosis based on MRI findings.

Classification of spinal sarcoidosis according to Junger et al.

- *Phase 1:* Early inflammatory changes: Linear leptomeningeal enhancement along the surface of the spinal cord.
- *Phase 2:* Parenchymal involvement: Spreading within the Virchow-Robin spaces usually associated with contrast-enhancing parenchymal lesions.
- *Phase 3:* Resolution of inflammatory changes: Enlarged spinal cord returns to normal.
- *Phase 4:* Chronic phase: Atrophy of the spinal cord

The MRI findings do not ultimately prove the presence of the disease, so that in cases of doubt the diagnosis must be confirmed by biopsy. However, there have been repeated reports of confusion with gliomas. More than two-thirds of patients with spinal sarcoidosis experience clinical improvement from the long-term administration of corticosteroids (Jaster *et al.*, 1997) (Fig. 6.**70**).

Post-meningitis Syringomyelia

Syringomyelia can develop after meningitis or arachnoiditis with a latency of a few months to many years. Vasculitic changes associated with spinal cord ischemia, traction on the cord secondary to scarring alterations of the meninges, and obstruction of the Virchow-Robin spaces have been postulated as possible pathological correlates of the disorder. Post-meningitis syringomyelia occurs most commonly as a complication of tuberculous meningitis (Fehlings *et al.*, 1997; Kakar *et al.*, 1997). There have also been reports of it affecting neonates following meningitis due to streptococci and other bacteria (Coker *et al.*, 1994; Puvabanditsin *et al.*, 1997).

Spinal Arachnoiditis and Arachnopathy

Pathogenesis and Clinical Presentation

Arachnoiditis can result from the intrathecal administration of steroids, antibiotics, and particularly after the application of oil-based myelo-

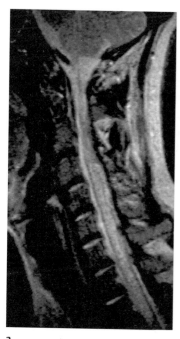

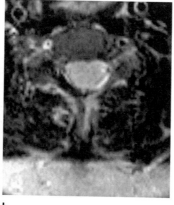

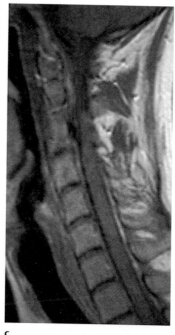

a

b

c

Fig. 6.70 a–g Initial spinal manifestation of sarcoidosis (1987). 48-year-old patient. At first the clinical presentation was that of tetraspasticity, then tetraparesis. Evidence of a pulmonary manifestation in 1991:

a Sagittal T2-weighted image: Image with intramedullary edema and enlargement of the cervical cord.

b Transverse T2-weighted image: The enlargement of the spinal cord is well shown on this image due to the edema.

c Sagittal image after contrast application: A diffuse enhancement of the mid-cervical cord is demonstrated here.

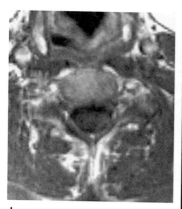

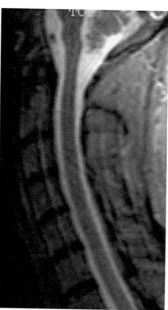

d

e

Fig. 6.**70**

d Axial post-contrast image: The diffuse enhancement of the mid-cervical cord appears accentuated on the left side on this image.

e Follow-up study 8 years later after steroid therapy: The follow-up shows a normal T2-weighted image of the cervical cord.

Fig. 6.**70 f** and **g** ▷

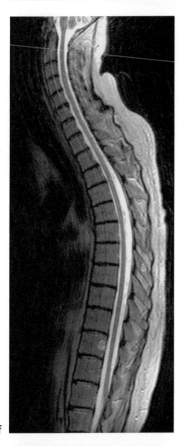

f

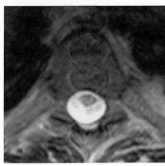

g

Fig. 6.**70f, g** Ten years after the initial manifestation the spinal cord appears somewhat atrophic.

graphic contrast media, which are nowadays no longer in use. Other causes include:

- trauma,
- disk surgery,
- chronic infection,
- intraspinal hemorrhage.

Arachnopathy is the secondary and final stage of spinal arachnoiditis. Arachnoiditis results in a predominantly fibrinous-exudative inflammation with an only slightly developed cellular component secondary to the causes mentioned above. The roots of the cauda equina clump together or adhere to the dura, forming intradural scar and granulation tissue.

Diagnostics

MRI can detect the changes mentioned above, especially when they are more pronounced, although in individual cases they are better demonstrated by myelography and myelo-CT.

MRI

On T1- and, above all, on T2-weighted MR images distinctions can be made among the following diagnostic characteristics (Ross *et al.*, 1987):

- conglomerations of adherent roots of the cauda equina,
- roots adherent to the dural sac,
- obliteration of the lumbar subarachnoid space by inflammatory soft tissue,
- secondary development of arachnoid cysts.

If arachnopathy-like findings of thickening and clumping of the roots of the cauda equina are discovered, yet are also associated with intensive contrast enhancement, then a leptomeningeal metastatic disease must be included in any differential diagnostic considerations (Fig. 6.**71**).

Parasitic Cystic Disorders

Neurocysticercosis. Neurocysticercosis can be associated with the development of intradural, and intra- or extramedullary cysts. Those most commonly found are intradural-extramedullary cysts of the cervical spinal canal. These are particularly well detected by contrast-enhanced T1-weighted images (Schmitz *et al.*, 1993).

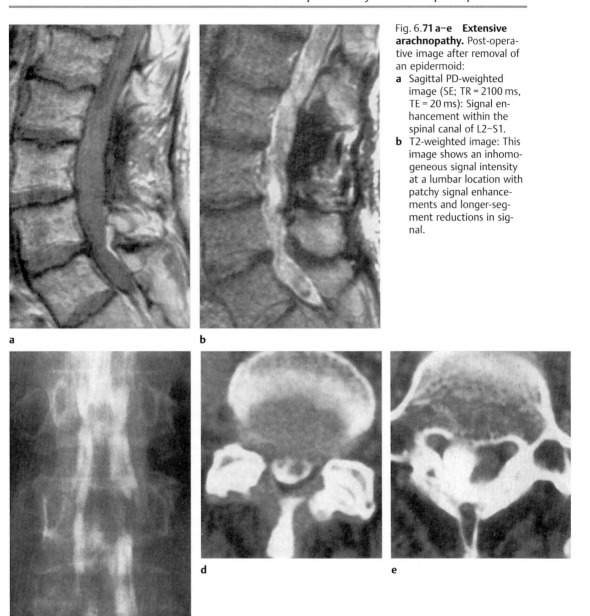

Fig. 6.**71 a–e** **Extensive arachnopathy.** Post-operative image after removal of an epidermoid:

a Sagittal PD-weighted image (SE; TR = 2100 ms, TE = 20 ms): Signal enhancement within the spinal canal of L2–S1.

b T2-weighted image: This image shows an inhomogeneous signal intensity at a lumbar location with patchy signal enhancements and longer-segment reductions in signal.

c Myelography: Here extensive lumbar contrast-free areas are visible.

d, e CT myelography at the level of L4/L5 (**d**) and L5/S1 (**e**): The images show larger contrast-free areas reflecting the proliferative formation of granulation tissue.

Spinal hydatid disease. Spinal hydatid disease can result in the formation of cysts of *Echinococcus alveolaris* in the vertebral bodies, the spinal canal and, very rarely, at an intramedullary location (Jaenisch et al. 1999). The patients are usually adults presenting in the advanced stages of the disease.

Summary

- Inflammatory disorders of the spine can develop by the hematogenous route, from direct inoculation with pathogens, by contiguous spread and in the setting of a rheumatic disease.
- The *hematogenous form of spread* is the most common, particularly by the arterial route.
- The *direct inoculation* with pathogens is due to iatrogenic intervention, such as puncture or surgery, or from penetrating injuries, e.g. gunshot wounds.
- The *propagation of inflammation by contiguous spread* takes its origin from a focus adjacent to the spine.
- Inflammation of the spine occurring in conjunction with a rheumatic disorder is mainly found in *rheumatoid arthritis* and *spondyloarthropathy* where they demonstrate a divergent pattern of distribution.
- A *diskitis* is more commonly seen in children due to the prevailing arterial blood supply to the disk. An arterial blood supply to the disk no longer exists in adults, with the consequence that spread of pathogens is primarily to the vertebral bodies with only secondary involvement of the disk. For this reason a *spondylodiskitis* is usually seen and, less commonly, a *spondylitis*.
- Older patients are preferentially affected by *hematogenous spondylodiskitis*. There is a predilection for the lumbar spine.
- About 80 % of all cases of spondylodiskitis are caused by *Staphylococcus aureus*. The propagation of infection usually begins in the ventral third of the vertebral body from where it proceeds rapidly to the disk, via which it invades the immediately adjacent vertebral body. Only later on does paravertebral exudation develop secondary to destruction of the anterior longitudinal ligament, or the formation of an epidural abscess ensues due to destruction of the structures of the poster longitudinal ligament.
- The following are typically found on MRI examination: a homogeneous reduction in signal intensity of the vertebral bodies on T1-weighted images, with signal loss of the contours of the adjacent vertebral bodies; signal enhancement of the vertebral bodies and intervertebral disk on T2-weighted sequences; enhancement of the disk and adjacent vertebral body segments after contrast application. An additional reduction in signal intensity of the disk is less commonly seen on T1-weighting.
- Further typical changes include:
  - loss of disk height,
  - paravertebral exudate,
  - epidural abscess.
- The MRI examination should be obtained using T1- and T2-weighted sequences. The application of contrast is necessary since it most clearly displays the inflammatory changes of the disk material. Contrast enhancement may be limited here to peripheral segments of the disk as well as filling out the entire disk material. STIR sequences are particularly sensitive for detecting edematous changes of the vertebral body and disk.
- During the healing phase, a regression of the signal reduction on the T1-weighted images is seen and often a partly mottled, partly confluent, signal enhancement secondary to the formation of fatty marrow. After contrast application, enhancement is increasingly lost.
- *Tuberculous spondylodiskitis* can differ in the following respects:
  - less involvement of the disk,
  - marked destruction of the vertebral bodies,
  - vertebral body collapse with development of a gibbus deformity,
  - "telescoping",
  - marginal enhancement,
  - marked paravertebral exudation,
  - calcification,
  - long history,
  - low patient age.
- *Rheumatoid arthritis* is diagnosed by the seven ARA criteria:
  - morning stiffness lasting at least one hour,
  - arthritis of three or more joints,
  - arthritis involving hand or finger joints,
  - symmetric arthritis,
  - rheumatoid nodules,
  - serum rheumatoid factor,
  - typical radiographic changes in hand or finger joints.
- The main changes are found in the upper region of the cervical spine; the thoracic and lumbar spine is affected less often. Epidural rheumatoid nodules can result in compression of the spinal cord.

Summary

- *C1/C2 subluxation* is most commonly seen and can occur in the following forms:
  - anterior atlantoaxial subluxation,
  - cranial subluxation,
  - lateral subluxation,
  - rotatory subluxation,
  - posterior subluxation.
- The cause of these changes is the formation of a proliferative pannus, which can lead to laxity or destruction of the ligamentous structures, especially the transverse ligament, and can also be associated with destruction of the dens axis, in a larger percentage of cases.
- In addition, erosion of the vertebral bodies is observed, especially at the end plates. This results in a reduction in disk space height. Unlike the degenerative forms, these changes notably develop *proximally* in the cervical spine at the level C2–C4. Structural instability of the joints in the form of anterolisthesis or retrolisthesis commonly results from these erosive changes and is sometimes associated with spinal stenoses.
- At MRI the pannus displays moderate signal intensity similar to that of muscle on the T1-weighted plain images, low to moderate signal intensity in the presence of considerable fibrosis, and high signal intensity in the presence of strong vascularization associated with edema. Contrast-assisted images reveal a variably strong enhancement, depending on whether the fibrotic or the edematous-vascularized component is more predominant.
- *Spondyloarthropathy* is characterized clinically by inflammatory spinal pain and by an asymmetric peripheral inflammatory arthritis, predominantly involving joints of the lower limbs. The following disorders are subsumed under the term spondyloarthropathy:
  - ankylosing spondylitis,
  - reactive arthritis,
  - psoriatic arthritis,
  - arthritis associated with chronic inflammatory bowel disease,
  - undifferentiated spondyloarthropathy.
- The following *changes* are seen *in the spine*:
  - formation of syndesmophytes,
  - Romanus lesion,
  - osteopenia,
  - convex alterations of the vertebral bodies,
  - non-destructive marginal sclerosis of the vertebral body,
  - spondylodiskitis (Andersson lesion),
  - ossification of the joint capsule and ligaments,
  - bamboo spine,
  - fractures of the vertebral body,
  - pseudarthrosis.
- *Spondylitis* usually begins in the region where anterior longitudinal ligament, intervertebral disk and the anterior cortices of the vertebral body converge. The occurrence of a posterior spondylitis is less common. About 15% of patients develop a spondylodiskitis, which appears in three forms:
  - in the mid-third of the vertebral body,
  - peripherally,
  - throughout the entire diskovertebral space.
- At MRI, *signal changes* are often found in the anteroventral and anterocaudal segments of the vertebral bodies, in addition to diffuse signal changes. There is a reduction in signal intensity on the T1-weighted images, while the T2-weighted images demonstrate signal enhancement. After contrast application, an enhancement of varying degrees of expression can be found, both in parts of the disk and in parts of the vertebral bodies. The appearance of disk calcification is typical, displaying on MRI high signal intensity on T1 as well as on T2 weighting. Furthermore, marked subluxations of the vertebral bodies can occur, particularly in the cervical spine. A rare complication is the *cauda equina syndrome*.
- Subacute and chronic *inflammations of the leptomeninx* result in reactions that are detectable by MRI, usually in the form of diffuse enhancements along the spinal cord and cauda equina. On the basis of morphological imaging this finding is not distinguishable from those changes seen in metastatic disease.
- *Epidural abscesses* can result from a spondylitis or spondylodiskitis, as well as having iatrogenic causes. Their development can be promoted by diabetes mellitus, drug abuse or immunocompromising diseases such as an HIV infection. The disease begins with a phlegmonous inflammation that is seen at MRI as a homogeneous signal enhancement after contrast application.

Summary

A liquid center of necrotizing tissue then appears, surrounded by a capsule. The full-blown abscess is hypointense on the T1-weighted sequence and hyperintense on the T2-weighted image, and demonstrates after contrast application an intensive marginal contrast enhancement.

- Unlike in the brain, *spinal cord abscesses* are rare. They usually extend over two to three segments and are mainly hematogenous in origin. The spinal cord appears enlarged with a marginal concomitant edema. At MRI there is a reduction in signal intensity on the T1-weighted images with a marked signal enhancement on T2 weighting. After contrast application there is a strong enhancement of the abscess capsule. An inflammatory thickening of the meninges is commonly seen as an associated reaction.

- *Acute transverse myelitis* is a spinal dysfunction associated with edema, necrosis and demyelination. A distinction is made pathogenetically between infectious, parainfectious and non-infectious forms. The changes of the white matter are more pronounced than those of the gray matter. The thoracic cord is predominantly affected. At MRI, long-segmental signal enhancements covering several levels are diagnosed on T2 weighting, which are associated with a slight enlargement of the cord. The signal enhancement is central in location and sharply delineated, occupying more than two-thirds of the cross-sectional area and often displaying a circumscribed central zone of reduced signal enhancement (central dot sign). There is an isointense or slightly hypointense signal on T1 weighting. Contrast application results in a moderate patchy or fringe-like enhancement. Marked cord atrophy can develop in the course of the disease.

- *Irradiation of the spinal cord* can lead to demyelination and necrosis of the cord as a result of neuronal damage and secondarily due to vascular reactions. There is usually a latency of several months between the irradiation and the onset of symptoms. MRI demonstrates enlargement of the spinal cord, signal enhancement on the T2-weighted sequence and an isointense to hypointense signal on the T1-weighted image with a ring-like enhancement after contrast application.

- In *multiple sclerosis* lesions develop in the spinal cord that undergo a circumscribed demyelination as well as axonal loss. The distribution of lesions in the brain and spinal cord is in the ratio of about 80 : 20. Multiple sclerosis lesions are most commonly seen in the cervical cord. More than one-half of patients demonstrate more than one lesion. No cerebral lesion is detected in about 10–15 % of those multiple sclerosis patients with a spinal involvement.

- The multiple sclerosis lesions are usually small at MRI, rarely extending over more than two vertebral body levels and predominantly lying eccentrically in the spinal cord. They occupy less than 50 % of the cross-sectional area of the cord. A circumscribed enlargement of the cord may be present, but is commonly absent. Long segmental lesions will often result in a circumscribed atrophy of the cord on healing. An isointense signal is usually present on T1-weighted images, while the T2-weighted images display a homogeneous signal enhancement. A barrier disturbance is sometimes found after contrast application, displaying a nodular, ring-like or patchy enhancement. Resolution of the barrier disturbance correlates with the clinical course, although in only about 60 % of all patients is a correlation seen between MRI and clinical presentation as regards disease activity.

- Lesions of the spinal cord are observed clinically in up to 20 % of all AIDS patients. The *HIV infection* can manifest itself on MRI in three forms:
  - increased signal intensity (vacuolar myelopathy, demyelination of the long tracts),
  - focal thickening of the cord,
  - focal thickening with meningeal contrast enhancement (HIV myelitis).

- *Guillain–Barré syndrome* is an acute inflammatory demyelinating polyradiculoneuropathy. The patients present clinically with paresthesias or pain in the lower extremities, followed by symmetric ascending flaccid paralysis of the legs. Thickening of the cauda equina is seen on MRI with the anterior roots being particularly involved. Contrast application can lead to a barrier disturbance. Cord enlargement is rarely seen. Punctiform intracerebral signal enhancements of the white matter can also appear.

Summary

- *Systemic lupus erythematosus* is associated with cord involvement, which can manifest itself as transverse myelitis, in only a small percentage of cases. It usually represents a late manifestation of the disease, although, in rare cases, it can also be the initial syndrome of systemic lupus erythematosus. Pathogenetically it is an immune complex mediated vasculitis. Cord enlargement is seen on MRI with reduced signal intensity on the T1-weighted image and an increased signal on the T2-weighted image.

- A *spinal manifestation of sarcoidosis* is rare. The disease begins with infiltration of the arachnoidea by lymphocytes and non-caseating granulomas and progresses by centripetal spread via the perivascular spaces. The most common location is the cervical cord, followed by the thoracic cord. MRI demonstrates thickening of the spinal cord on T1-weighting with decreased signal intensity and a diffuse signal enhancement on the T2-weighted image. Contrast application produces different patterns of enhancement, ranging from linear to diffuse. Thickening of the cauda associated with contrast enhancement is seen in cases of rare lumbar involvement. Disease extension can be classified into four stages, extending from the early leptomeningeal form to the late manifestation with cord atrophy.

- *Spinal arachnoiditis* and *arachnopathy* can be caused by the intrathecal administration of drugs, such as steroids and antibiotics, as well as from trauma, intraspinal hemorrhage, chronic infection and, above all, surgery of the spinal canal. Higher-grade changes are detected well on MRI, while milder forms are better demonstrated by myelography and myelo-CT. Typical findings include:
  - conglomerations of adherent roots of the cauda equina,
  - roots adherent to the dural sac,
  - obliteration of the dural sac by inflammatory soft tissue,
  - secondary development of arachnoid cysts.

- *Neurocysticercosis* can be associated with the development of intradural, intra- or extramedullary cysts. The cervical space is most commonly involved. Detection is best accomplished by contrast-enhanced images where the cyst wall will demonstrate contrast enhancement.

References

Abbatucci, J. S., T. Delozier, R. Quint: Radiation myelopathy in over-irradiated patients. MR imaging findings. Europ. Radiol. 7 (1997) 400–404

Abello, R., M. Rovira, M. P. Sanz, J. Gili, A. Capdevila, J. Escalada et al.: MRI and CT of ankylosing spondylitis with vertebral scalopping. Neuroradiology 30 (1988) 272–275

Adams, C., D. Armstrong: Acute transverse myelopathy in children. Canad. J. neurol. Sci. 17 (1990) 40–45

Aisen, A. M., W. Martel, J. H. Ellis, W. J. McCune: Cervical spine involvement in rheumatoid arthritis: MR imaging. Radiology 165 (1987) 159–163

Alfonso, E. R., M. A. De Gregorio, P. Mateo, R. Esco, N. Bascon, F. Morales et al.: Radiation myelopathy in over-irradiated patients: MR imaging findings. Europ. Radiol. 7 (1997) 400–404

Andrianakos, A. A., J. Duffy, M. Suzuki, J. T. Sharp: Transverse myelopathy in systemic lupus erythematosus. Ann. intern. Med. 83 (1975) 616–624

Angtuaco, E. J. C., J. R. McConnell, W. M. Chadduck, S. Flanigan: MR imaging of spinal epidural sepsis. Amer. J. Neuroradiol. 8 (1987) 879–883

Arnett, F. C., S. M. Edwarthy, D. A. Bloch et al.: The American Rheumatism Association revised criteria for the classification of rheumatoid arthritis. Arthr. and Rheum. 31 (1988) 315–324

Awerbuch, G., W. M. Feinberg, P. Ferry, N. N. Komar, J. Clements: Demonstration of acute post-viral myelitis with magnetic resonance imaging. Pediat. Neurol. 3 (1987) 367–369

Baker, F. J., G. Gossen, J. M. Bertoni: Aseptic meningitis complicating metricamide myelography. Amer. J. Neuroradiol. 3 (1982) 662–663

Barakos, J. A., A. S. Mark, W. P. Dillon, D. Norman: MR imaging of acute transverse myelitis and AIDS myelopathy. J. Comput. assist. Tomogr. 14 (1990) 45–50

Baron, B. A., L. Goldberg, W. E. Rothfus, R. L. Sherman: CT features of sarcoid infiltration of a lumbosacral nerve root. J. Comput. assist. Tomogr. 13 (1989) 364–365

Batson, O. V.: The function of the vertebral veins and their role in the spread of metastases. Ann. Surg. 112 (1940) 138–149

Batson, O. V.: The vertebral vein system. Amer. J Roentgenol. 78 (1957) 195–212

Bell, E. J., S. J. M. Russel: Acute transverse myelopathy and echo-2 virus infection. Lancet II (1963) 1226–1227

Beltran, J., J. L. Caudill, L. A. Herman, S. M. Kantor, P. N. Hudson, A. M. Noto et al.: Rheumatoid arthritis: MR imaging manifestations. Radiology 165 (1987) 153–157

Berman, M., S. Feldman, M. Alter, N. Zilber, E. Kahana: Acute transverse myelitis: Incidence and etiologic considerations. Neurology 31 (1981) 966–971

Bitzan, M.: Rubella myelitis and encephalitis in childhood. A report of two cases with magnetic resonance imaging. Neuropediatrics 18 (1987) 84–87

Bonfiglio, M., T. A. Lange, Y. M. Kim: Pyogenic vertebral osteomyelitis. Disk space infections. Clin. Orthop. 96 (1973) 234–247

Borgstein, B.-J., P. A. Koster, P. Portegies, F. L. M. Peeters: Myelography in patients with acquired immuno deficiency syndrome. Neuroradiology 31 (1989) 326–330

Borruat, F.-X., N. J. Schatz, J. S. Glaser, A. Forteza: Central nervous system involvement in Guillain-Barré syndrome: clinical and magnetic resonance imaging evidence. Europ. Neurol. 38 (1997) 129–131

Brambs, H.-J., K. Weidenhammer, A. Rieber: Spondylodiszitis bei Morbus Bechterew (Andersson-Läsion). Fortschr. Röntgenstr. 151 (1989) 377–378

Braun, J. M. Bollow, J. Sieper: Radiologic diagnosis and pathology of the spondyloarthropathies. Rheum. Dis. Clin. N. Amer. 24 (1998) 697–735

Bundschuh, C., M. T. Modic, F. Kearney, R. Morris, C. Deal: Rheumatoid arthritis of the cervical spine: surface-coil MR imaging. Amer. J. Roentgenol. 151 (1988) 181–187

Castillo, M., R. M. Quencer, M. J. D. Post: MR of intramedullary spinal cysticercosis. Amer. J. Neuroradiol. 9 (1988) 393–395

Cawley, M. I., T. M. Chalmers, J. Ball: Destructive lesions of vertebral bodies in ankylosing spondylitis. Ann. rheum. Dis. 30 (1971) 539–540

Charlesworth, C. H., L. E. Savy, J. Stevens, B. Twomey, R. Mitchell: MRI demonstration of arachnoiditis in cauda equina syndrome of ankylosing spondylitis. Neuroradiology 38 (1996) 462–465

Choi, K. H., K. S. Lee, S. O. Chung, J. M. Park, Y. J. Kim, H. S. Kim et al.: Idiopathic transverse myelitis: MR characteristics. Amer. J. Neuroradiol. 17 (1996) 1151–1160

Claaß, A., U. Piepgras, W. Wussow: Zur Frage der "Kontrastmittelarachnitis" nach lumbosakraler Myelographie mit wasserlöslichem Kontrastmittel. Röntgenpraxis 35 (1982) 174–185

Claudon, M., S. Bracard, F. Plenat, D. Regent, P. Bernadac, L. Picard: Spinal involvement in alveolar echinococcosis: assessment of two cases. Radiology 162 (1987) 571–572

Clifton, A. G., J. M. Stevens, R. Kapoor, P. Rudge: Spinal cord sarcoidosis with intramedullary cyst formation. Brit. J. Radiol. 63 (1990) 805–808

Clifton, A. G., J. M. Stevens, R. Kapoor, P. Rudge: Spinal cord sarcoidosis with intramedullary cyst formation. Neuroradiology 39 (1997) 357–360

Coker, S. B., J. K. Muraskas, C. Thomas.: Myelopathy secondary to neonatal bacterial meningitis. Pediat. Neurol. 10 (1994) 259–261

Condette-Auliac, S., J.-C. Lacour, R. Anxionnat, M. Braun, M. Wagner, C. Moret et al.: Les abcès médullaires, aspects en IRM. J. Neuroradiol. 25 (1998) 189–200

Coventry, M. B., R. K. Ghormley, J. W. Kernohan: The intervertebral disc: Its microscopic anatomy and pathology. J. Bone Jt Surg. 27-A (1945) 105–112

Dagirmanjian, A., J. Schils, M. Mc Henry, M.T. Modic: MR imaging of vertebral osteomyelitis revisited. Am. J Roentgenol. 167 (1996) 1539–1543

Dawson, D. M., F. M. Potts.: Acute nontraumatic myelopathies. In Woolsey, R. M., R. R. Young: Neurologic Clinics, Disorders of Spinal Cord. Philadelphia: Saunders, Philadelphia 1991 (pp. 551–603)

Day, A. L., G. W. Sypert: Spinal cord sarcoidosis. Ann. Neurol. 1 (1977) 79–85

Delhaas, T., D. J. Kamphuis, T. D. Witkamp: Transitory spinal cord swelling in a 6-year-old boy with Guillain-Barré syndrome. Pediat. Radiol. 28 (1998) 544–546

Demirci, M., E. Tan, M. Durguner, T. Zileli, M. Eryilmaz: Spinal brucellosis. A case with "cauliflower" appearance on CT. Neuroradiology 31 (1989) 282–283

Denning, D. W., J. Anderson, P. Rudge, H. Smith: Acute myelopathy associated with primary infection with human immunodeficiency virus. Brit. med. J. 294 (1987) 143–144

Dihlmann, W.: Gelenke, Wirbelverbindungen, 3. Aufl. Thieme, Stuttgart 1987

Dunne, K., I. J. Hopkins, L. K. Shield: Acute transverse myelopathy in childhood. Develop. Med. Child Neurol. 28 (1986) 198–204

Dupuis, M. J. M., S. Atrouni, G. C. Dooms, R. E. Gonsette: MR imaging of schistosomal myelitis. Amer. J. Neuroradiol. 11 (1990) 782–783

Fehlings, M. G., M. Bernstein: Syringomyelia – a complication of meningitis. Spinal Cord 35 (1997) 629–631

Freyschmidt, J.: Knochenerkrankungen im Erwachsenenalter. Röntgenologische Diagnose und Differentialdiagnose. Springer, Berlin 1980

Fuchigami, T., F. Iwata, Y. Noguchi, R. Kohira, H. Yamazaki, O. Okubo, Y. Utsumi, K. Harada: Magnetic resonance imaging of the cauda equina in two patients with Guillain-Barre syndrome. Acta Paediatr Jpn. 1997 Oct; 39(5):607–10

Gelmers, H. J.: Exacerbation of systemic lupus erythematosus, aseptic meningitis and acute mental symptoms, following metrizamide lumbar myelography. Neuroradiology 26 (1984) 65–66

Gero, B., G. Sze, H. Sharif: MR imaging of intradural inflammatory diseases of the spine. Amer. J. Neuroradiol. 12 (1991) 1009–1019

Glew, D., I. Watt, P. A. Dieppe, P. R. Goddard: MRI of the cervical spine: rheumatoid arthritis compared with cervical spondylosis. Clin. Radiol. 44 (1991) 71–76

Goldstick, L., T. I. Mandybur, R. Bode: Spinal cord degeneration in AIDS. Neurology 35 (1985) 103–106

Grose, C., P. M. Feorino: Epstein-Barr virus and transverse myelitis. Lancet I (1973) 892

Habr, F., B. Wu: Acute transverse myelitis in systemic lupus erythematosus: a case of rapid diagnosis and complete recovery. Conn. Med. 62 (1998) 387–390

Henry, A. K., C. M. Brunner: Relapse of lupus transverse myelitis mimicked by vertebral fractures and spinal cord compression. Arthr. and Rheum. 28 (1985) 1307–1311

Hitchon, P. W., A. U. l. Haque, J. J. Olson, S. K. Jacobs, S. P. Olson: Sarcoidosis presenting as an intramedullary spinal cord mass. Neurosurgery 15 (1984) 86–90

Hogan, E. L., M. R. Krigman, C. Hill: Herpes zoster myelitis. Arch. Neurol. 29 (1973) 309–313

Hosten, N., A. J. Lemke, H. M. Mayer, S. W. Dihlmann, E. Pichler, R. Felix: Spondylitis: Grenzbefunde im Magnetresonanztomogramm. Aktuelle Radiologie 5 (1995), 164–168

Imai, T., H. Matsumoto, Y. Ohkubo, H. Shizukawa, S. Chiba, N. Kobayashi: A case of acute transverse Myelitis affecting the entire length of the spinal cord. Europ. Neurol. 37 (1997) 247–248

Inslicht, D. V., A. B. Stein, F. Pomerantz, K. T. Ragnarsson: Three women with lupus transverse myelitis: case reports and differential diagnosis. Arch. phys. Med. 79 (1998) 456–459

Isoda, H., R. G. Ramsey: MR imaging of acute transverse Myelitis (Myelopathy). Radiol. med. 16 (1998) 179–186

Iwata, F., Y. Utsuma: MR imaging in Guillain-Barré syndrome. Pediat. Radiol. 27 (1997) 36–38

Jallo, G. I., D. Zagzag, M. Lee, V. Deletis, N. Morota, F. J. Epstein: Intraspinal sarcoidosis: diagnosis and management. Surg. Neurol. 48 (1997) 514–521

Jänisch, W., H. Henkes, A. de Teyni, W. Weber, D. Kühne: Neuroechinokokkose. In Henkes, H., H. W. Kölmel: Die entzündlichen Erkrankungen des Zentralnervensystems, 5. Erg.-Lief. ecomed, Landsberg 1999

Jaster, J. J., F. C. Dohan, T. E. Bertorini, J. E. Bass, K. E. Mönkemüller, C. R. Handorf et al.: Solitary spinal cord sarcoidosis without other manifestations of systemic sarcoidosis. Clin. Imag. 21 (1997) 17–22

Jensen, M. E., C. W. Hyes, G. G. DeBlois, F. J. Laine: Hemispherical spondylosclerosis: MR appearance. J. Comput. assist. Tomogr. 13 (1989) 540–542

Jevtic, V., B. Rozman, M. Kos-Golja, I. Watt: MR-Bildgebung bei seronegativen Spondyloarthritiden. Radiologe 36 (1996) 624–631

Johnson, C. E., G. Sze, Benign lumbar arachnoiditis: MR imaging with gadopentetate dimeglumine. Amer. J. Neuroradiol. 11 (1990) 763–770

Johnson, D. A., A. W. Eger: Myelitis associated with an echovirus. J. Amer. med. Ass. 201 (1967) 637–638

Jorgensen, J., P. H. Hansen, V. Steenskov, N. Ovesen: A clinical and radiological study of chronic lower spinal arachnoiditis. Neuroradiology 9 (1975) 139–144

Junger, S. S., B. J. Stern, S. R. Levine, E. Sipos, J. F. Marti-Masso: Intramedullary spinal sarcoidosis: clinical and magnetic resonance imaging characteristics. Neurology 43 (1993) 333–337

Kainberger, F., C. Czerny, S. Trattnig, W. Lack, K. Machold, W. Graninger: MRT und Sonographie in der Rheumatologie. Radiologe 36 (1996) 609–616

Kakar, A., V. S. Madan, V. Prakash: Syringomyelia – a complication of meningitis – case report. Spinal Cord 35 (1997) 629–631

Kaplan, P., D. Resnick. M. Murphey, L. Heck, J. Phalen, D. Egan et al.: Destructive noninfectious spondyloarthropathy in hemodialysis patients: A report of four cases. Radiology 162 (1987) 241–244

Karasick, D., M. E. Schweitzer, N. A. Abidi, J. M. Cotler: Fractures of the vertebrae with spinal cord injuries in patients with ankylosing spondylitis: imaging findings. Amer. J. Roentgenol. 165 (1995) 1205–1208

Kelly, R. B., P. D. Mahoney, K. M. Cawley: MR demonstration of spinal cord sarcoidosis: report of a case. Amer. J. Neuroradiol. 9 (1988) 197–199

Kemp, H. B. S., J. W. Jackson, J. D. Jeremiah, A. J. Hall: Pyogenic infections occurring primarily in intervertebral discs. J. Bone Jt Surg. 55-B (1973) 698–714

Kenik, J. G., K. Krohn, R. B. Kelly, M. Bierman, M. D. Hammeke, J. A. Hurley: Transverse myelitis and optic neuritis in systemic lupus erythematosus: a case report with magnetic resonance imaging findings. Arthr. and Rheum. 30 (1987) 947–950

Klastersky, J., R. Cappel, J. M. Snoeck, J. Flament, L. Thiry: Ascending myelitis in association with herpes-simplex virus. New Engl. J. Med. 287 (1972) 182–184

Kramer, J., M. Schratter, N. Pongracz, A. Neuhold, R. Stiglbauer, H. Imhof: Spondylitis: Erscheinungsbild und Verlaufsbeurteilung mittels Magnetresonanztomographie. Fortschr. Röntgenstr. 153 (1990) 131–136

Krödel, A., H. J. Refior, S. Westermann: The importance of functional magnetic resonance imaging (MRI) in the planning of stabilizing operations on the cervical spine in rheumatoid patients. Arch. orthop. traum. Surg. 109 (1989) 30–33

Lame, E. L.: Vertebral osteomyelitis following opreation of the urinary tract or sigmoid. Amer. J. Roentgenol. 75 (1956) 938–952

Lange, M., F. Tiecks, T. Yousry, F. Gückel, R. Oeckler: Spinaler epiduraler Abszeß. In Henkes, H., H. W. Kölmel: Die entzündlichen Erkrankungen des Zentralnervensystems, 3. Erg.-Lief. ecomed, Landsberg 1997

Larsson, E. M., S. Holtas, S. Zygmunt: Pre- and postoperative MR imaging of the craniocervical junction in rheumatoid arthritis. Amer. J. Neuroradiol. 10 (1989) 89–94

Lascari, A. D., M. H. Graham, J. C. Mac Queen: Intervertebral disk infection in children. J. Pediat. 70 (1967) 751–757

Leeb, B. F., K. P. Machold, J. S. Smolen: Diagnose und Therapie der chronischen Polyarthritis. Radiologe 36 (1996) 657–662

Mandler, R. N., L. E. Davis, D. R. Jeffrey, M. Kornfeld: Devic's neuromyelitis optica: a clinicopathological study of 8 patients. Ann. Neurol. 34 (1993) 162–168

Maravilla, K. R., J. C. Weinreb, R. Suss, R. L. Nunnally: Magnetic resonance demonstration of multiple sclerosis plaques in the cervical cord. Amer. J. Neuroradiol. 5 (1984) 685–689

Maritz, N. G. J., J. F. K. de Villiers, O. Q. S. van Castricum: Computed tomography in tuberculosis of the spine. Comput. Radiol. 6 (1982) 1–5

Mendez, M. F., S. Pogacar: Malignant monophasic multiple sclerosis or "Marburg's disease". Neurology 38 (1988) 1153–1155

Merine, D., H. Wang, A. J. Kumar, S. J. Zinreich, A. E. Rosenbaum: CT myelography and MR imaging of acute transverse myelitis. J. Comput. assist. Tomogr. 11 (1987) 606–608

Miller, H. G., J. B. Stanton, J. L. Gibbons: Para-infectious encephalomyelitis and related syndromes. Quart. J. Med. 25 (1956) 427–505

Milone, F. P., A. J. Bianco, J. C. Ivins: Infections of the intervertebral disk in children. J. Amer. med. Ass. 181 (1962) 1029–1033

Misra, U. K., J. Kalita, S. Kumar: A clinical, MRI and neurophysiological study of acute transverse myelitis. J. neurol. Sci. 138 (1996) 150–156

Mitchell, M. J., D. J. Sartoris, D. Moody, D. Resnick: Cauda equina syndrome complication ankylosing spondylitis. Radiology 175 (1990) 521–525

Nägele, M., W. Koch, B. Kaden, B. Wöll, M. Reiser: Dynamische Funktions-MRT der Halswirbelsäule. Fortschr. Röntgenstr. 157 (1992) 222–228

Naidich, J. B., R. T. Mossey, B. McHeffery-Atkinson, M. I. Karmel, P. A. Bluestone, L. U. Mailloux et al.: Spondyloarthropathy from long-term hemodialysis. Radiology 167 (1988) 761–764

Nesbit, G. M., G. M. Miller, H. L. Baker, M. J. Ebersold, B. W. Scheithauer: Spinal cord sarcoidosis: a new finding at MR imaging with Gd-DTPA enhancement. Radiology 173 (1989) 839–843

Neuhold, A., I. Fezoulidis, F. Frühwald, G. Seidl, B. Schwaighofer, K. Wicke et al.: Magnetresonanztomographie des kranio-zervikalen Überganges bei chronischer Polyarthritis. Fortschr. Röntgenstr. 150 (1989) 413–416

Owen, N. L.: Myelitis following type A 2 influenza. J. Amer. med. Ass. 215 (1971) 1986–1987

Paty, D. W., C. M. Poser: Clinical symptoms and signs of multiple sclerosis. In Poser, C. M.: The Diagnosis of Multiple Sclerosis. Thieme & Stratton, New York 1984

Petito, C. K., B. A. Navia, E. S. Cho, B. D. Jordan, D. C. George, B. S. Price et al.: Vacuolar myelopathy pathologically resembling subacute combined degeneration in patients with the acquired immunodeficiency syndrome. New Engl. J. Med. 312 (1985) 874–879

Petito, C. K., E. S. Cho, W. Lemann, B. A. Navia, R. W. Price: Neuropathology of acquired immunodeficiency syndrome (AIDS): An autopsy review. J. Neuropathol. exp. Neurol. 45 (1986) 635–646

Post, M. J. D., R. M. Quencer, B. M. Montalvo, B. H. Katz, F. J. Eismont, B. A. Green: Spinal infection: Evaluation with MR imaging and intraoperative US. Radiology 169 (1988) 765–771

Post, M. J. D., G. Sze, M. Quencer, J. Eismont, A. Green, H. Gahbauer: Gadolinium-enhanced MR in spinal infection. J. Comput. assist. Tomogr. 14 (1990) 721–729

Puvabanditsin, S., E. Wojdylo, E. Garrow, K. Kalavantavanich: Group B streptococcal meningitis: a case of transverse myelitis with spinal cord and posterior fossa cysts. Pediat. Radiol. 27 (1997) 317–318

Quencer, R. M., M. J. Post: Spinal cord lesions in patients with AIDS. Neuroimag. Clin. N. Amer. 7 (1997) 359–373

Rachinger J., J. Trenkler: Zervikaler intramedullärer Abszeß. Fortschr. Röntgenstr. 168 (1998) 631–633

Rafto, S. E., M. K. Dalinka, M. L. Schiebler, D. L. Burk, M. E. Kricun: Spondyloarthropathy of the cervical spine on long-term hemodialysis. Radiology 166 (1988) 201–204

Ragland, R. L., I. F. Abdelwahab, B. Braffman, D. S. Moss: Posterior spinal tuberculosis: A case report. Amer. J. Neuroradiol. 11 (1990) 612–113

Ramus-Remus, C., A. Gomez-Vargas, J. L. Guzman-Guzman et al.: Frequency of atlantoaxial subluxation and neurologic involvement in patients with ankylosing spondylitis. J. Rheumatol. 22 (1995) 2120–2125

Redlund-Johnell, I., E. M. Larsson: Subluxation of the upper thoracic spine in rheumatoid arthritis. Skelet. Radiol. 22 (1993) 105–108

Reiser, M., Th. Kahn, F. Weigert, P. Lukas, F. Büttner: Diagnostik der Spondylitis durch die MR-Tomographie. Fortschr. Röntgenstr. 145 (1986) 320–325

Reiser, M., A. Härle, A. Sciuk: Entzündliche Skeletterkrankungen. In Peters, P. E., H. H. Matthiaß, M. Reiser: Magnetresonanztomographie in der Orthopädie. Enke, Stuttgart 1990a (S. 59–82)

Reiser, M., M. Schneider, H. Sittek, G. Bongartz: Stellenwert der Magnetresonanztomographie (MRT) bei entzündlich-rheumatischen Erkrankungen. Z. Rheumatol. 49 (1990b) 61–69

Remedios, D., C. Natali, A. Saifuddin: Case report: MRI of vertebral osteitis in early ankylosing spondylitis. Clin. Radiol. 53 (1998) 534–536

Resnick, D., G. Niwayama: Ankylosing spondylitis. In Resnick, D., G. Niwayama: Diagnosis of Bone and Joint Disorders, 2nd ed. Saunders, Philadelphia 1988a (pp. 1103–1170)

Resnick, D., G. Niwayama: Rheumatoid arthritis. In Resnick, D., G. Niwayama: Diagnosis of Bone and Joint Disorders, 2nd ed. Saunders, Philadelphia 1988b (pp. 954–1067)

Reynolds, H., S. W. Carter, F. R. Murtagh, G. R. Rechtine: Cervical rheumatoid arthritis: Value of flexion and extension views in imaging. Radiology 164 (1987) 215–218

Rieber, A., H.-J. Brambs, P. Friedl: CT beim Echinokokkus der LWS und den paravertebralen Strukturen. Fortschr. Röntgenstr. 151 (1989) 379–380

Roca, A., W. K. Bernreuter, G. S. Alarcon: Functional magnetic resonance imaging should be included in the evaluation of the cervical spine in patients with rheumatoid arthritis. J. Rheumatol. 20 (1993) 1485–1488

Rodiek, S.-O.: MR-Tomographie der unspezifischen infektiösen Spondylodiszitis. Fortschr. Röntgenstr. 148 (1988) 419–425

Ropper, A. H., D. C. Poskanzer: The prognosis of acute and subacute transverse myelopathy based on early signs and symptoms. Ann. Neurol. 4 (1978) 51–59

Ross, I. S., T. J. Masaryk, M. T. Modic: MR-imaging of lumbar arachnoiditis. Amer. J. Roentgenol. 149 (1987) 885–892

Ross, J. S., T. J. Masaryk, M. T. Modic, R. Delamater, H. Bohlman, G. Wilbur et al.: MR imaging of lumbar arachnoiditis. Amer. J. Roentgenol. 149 (1987) 1025–1032

Rubensein, D. J., O. Alvarez, B. Ghelman, P. Marchisello: Cauda equina syndrome complicating ankylosing spondylitis: MR features. J. Comput. assist. Tomogr. 13 (1989) 511–513

Savoiardo, M., C. Cimino, A. Passerini, L. La Mantia: Mobile myelographic filling defects: spinal cysticercosis. Neuroradiology 28 (1986) 166–169

Schmitz, B., N. Heye, H. Henkes, G. Anuffo-Alonso, C. L. Lancelotti, H. W. Kölmel: Die entzündlichen Erkrankungen des Zentralnervensystems. ecomed, Landsberg 1993 (IV-1, S. 1–30)

Schrader, A., A. Stammler, H. Stickl: Infektiös-entzündliche Erkrankungen des ZNS. Chemie, Weinheim 1988

Schultheiss, T. E., L. C. Stephens: Pathology of radiation myelopathy, widening the circle. Europ. Radiol. 7 (1997) 400–404

Scott, T. F., K. Bhagavatula, P. J. Snyder, C. Chieffe: Transverse myelitis comparison with spinal cord presentations of multiple sclerosis. Amer. Acad. Neurol. 50 (1998) 429–433

Shabas, D., G. Gerard, B. Cunha, V. Malkotra, N. Leeds: MR imaging of AIDS myelitis. Amer. J. Neuroradiol. 10 (1989) 51–52

Shanley, D. J.: Tuberculosis of the spine: imaging features. Amer. J. Roentgenol. 164 (1995) 659–664

Shayamalan, N. C., S. S. Singh, D. B. Bisht: Transverse myelitis after vaccination. Brit. med. J. 1 (1964) 434–435

Sherman, M., G. T. Schneider, Vertebral osteomyelitis complicating postabortal and postpartum infection. Sth. med. J. 48 (1955) 333–338

Smith, A. S., M. A. Weinstein, A. Mizushima, B. Coughlin, S. P. Hayden, M. M. Lakin et al.: MR imaging characteristics of tuberculous spondylitis vs vertebral osteomyelitis. Amer. J. Roentgenol. 153 (1989a) 399–405

Smith, A. S., M. A. Weinstein, A. Mizushima, B. Coughlin, St. P. Hayden, M. M. Lakin et al.: MR imaging characteristics of tuberculous spondylitis vs vertebral osteomyelitis. Amer. J. Neuroradiol. 10 (1989b) 619–625

Smith, N. R.: The intervertebral discs. Brit. J. Surg. 18 (1931) 358–375

Sparenberg, A., B. Hamm, K.-J. Wolf: Ankylosierende Spondylitis: Andersson-Läsion. Fortschr. Röntgenstr. 150 (1989) 744–745

Spiegel, P. G., K. W. Kengla, A. S. Isaacson, J. C. Wilson: Intervertebral discspace inflammation in children. J. Bone Jt Surg. 54-A (1972) 284–296

Stäbler, A., A. Baur, A. Krüger, M. Weiss, T. Helmberger, M. Reiser: Differentialdiagnose der erosiven Osteochondrose und bakteriellen Spondylitis in der Magnetresonanztomographie (MRT). Fortschr. Röntgenstr. 168 (1998) 421–442

Stiskal, M. A., A. Neuhold, D. H. Szolar, M. Saeed, C. Czerny, B. Leeb et al.: Rheumatoid arthritis of the craniocervical region by MR imaging: detection and characterization. Amer. J. Roentgenol. 165 (1995) 585–592

Sugahara, T., Y. Korogi, T. Hirai, Y. Shigematu, Y. Ushio, M. Takahashi: Contrast-enhanced T1-weighted three-dimensional gradient-echo-MR imaging of the whole spine for intradural tumor dissemination. Amer. J. Neuroradiol. 19 (1998) 1773–1779

Sverzut, J. M., C. Laval, P. Smadja, M. Gigaud, A. Sevely, C. Manelfe: Spinal cord abscess in a heroin addict: case report. Neuroradiology 40 (1998) 455–458

Tamura, M., A. Zama, H. Kurihara, H. Fujimaki, H. Imai, T. Kano et al.: Management of recurrent pilocytic astrocytoma with leptomeningeal dissemination in childhood. Child's nerv. Syst. 14 (1998) 617–622

Tartaglino, L. M., D. P. Friedmann, A. E. Flanders, F. D. Lublin, R. L. Knobler, M. Liem: Multiple sclerosis in the spinal cord: MR appearance and correlation with clinical parameters. Radiology 195 (1995) 725–732

Trop, I., P. M. Bourgouin, Y. Lapierre, P. Duquette, C. M. Wolfson, H. D. Duong et al.: Multiple sclerosis of the spinal cord: Diagnosis and follow-up with contrast-enhanced MR an correlation with clinical activity. Amer. J. Neuroradiol. 19 (1998) 1025–1033

Thrush, A., D. Enzmann: MR imaging of infectious spondylitis. Amer. J. Neuroradiol. 11 (1990) 1171–1180

Tyrrell, P. N. M., A. M. Davies, N. Evans, R. W. Jubb: Signal changes in the intervertebral discs on MRI of the thoracolumbar spine in ankylosing spondylitis. Clin. Radiol. 50 (1995) 377–383

Van Loom, K. J., L. E. Kellerhouse, M. N. Pathria, S. I. Moreland, J. J. Brown, M. Zlatkin et al.: Infection versus tumor in the spine: criteria for distinction with CT. Radiology 166 (1988) 851–855

Walderveen, M. A. A., F. Barkhof, O. R. Hommes, C. H. Polman: Correlating MRI and clinical disease activity in multiple sclerosis: Neurology 45 (1995) 1684–1690

Waubant, E., C. Manelfe, A. Bonafé, I. Berry, M. Clanet: MRI of intramedullary sarcoidosis: follow-up of a case. Neuroradiology 39 (1997) 357–360

Wiebe, S., D. H. Lee, S. J. Karlik, M. Hopkins, M. K. Vandervoort, C. J. Wong et al.: Serial cranial and spinal cord magnetic resonance imaging in multiple sclerosis. Amer. Neurol. 32 (1992) 643–650

Wienands, K., P. Lukas, H. J. Albrecht: Klinische Bedeutung der MR-Tomographie von Spondylodiscitiden bei Spondylitis ankylopoetica. Z. Rheumatol. 49 (1990) 356–360

Wikstroem, M., J. Vogel, N. Rilinger, M. Diepers, E. Hartwig, A. Rieber: Die infektiöse Spondylitis. Eine retrospektive Auswertung der MRT-Merkmale. Der Radiologe 37 (1997) 139–144

Wolfe, B. K., D. O'Keeffe, D. M. Mitchell, S. P. K. Tchang: Rheumatoid arthritis of the cervical spine: Early and progressive radiographic features. Radiology 165 (1987) 145–148

Yamamoto, M.: Recurrent transverse myelitis associated with collagen disease. J. Neurol. 233 (1986) 185–187

Yasui, T., H. Yagura, M. Komiyama, Y. Fu, Y. Nagata, K. Tamura et al.: Significance of gadolinium-enhanced magnetic resonance imaging in differentiating spinal cord radiation myelopathy from tumor. J. Neurosurg. 77 (1997) 628–631

Zerbini, C. A. F., T. S. A. Fidelix, G. D. Rabello: Recovery from transverse myelitis of systemic lupus erythematosus with steroid therapy. J. Neurol. 233 (1986) 188–189

Zur Nedden, D., R. Putz: Anatomie und Computertomographie des lumbalen Wirbelkanals. Röntgenpraxis 38 (1985) 153–157

7 Use of MRI in Acute Spinal Trauma

S. E. Mirvis

Contents

MRI is a particularly useful imaging modality for examining the spine, including spinal cord, bony structures and soft tissue, in patients with spinal trauma.

Advantages of MRI

Major advantages of MRI over other techniques include:

- The possibility of obtaining images in all three planes.
- Superior contrast resolution compared with other modalities, providing a higher detection rate for soft-tissue injuries, particularly the spinal ligaments.
- The possibility of generating myelographic-equivalent images to assess the epidural space for evidence of hematoma, bone fragments, herniations and osteophytic changes without the need for administering contrast.
- Contrast-rich imaging of the spinal cord to allow detection of contusion, hematoma or laceration.
- Reliable prognostic information regarding potential for recovery of function based on the MRI appearance of spinal cord injuries.
- The possibility of imaging the paravertebral vessels without the need for contrast application, providing instead various pulse sequences to impart either positive or negative contrast of the vessels.
- MRI is performed without ionizing radiation and is thus free of side effects.

A variety of imaging sequences are required to provide an exact portrayal of both normal anatomy and the various pathological changes. Some new sequences have recently been introduced to improve further the diagnostic reliability of the examinations and reduce scanning time.

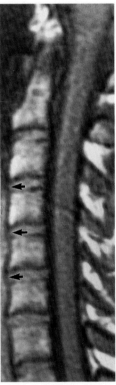

Fig. 7.**1** **Normal sagittal T1-weighted SE image of the cervical spine.** The image displays the spinal cord with moderate signal intensity, surrounded by CSF with less signal intensity. The vertebral bodies show relatively high signal intensity on account of the fatty marrow. The anterior longitudinal ligament and the ventral portion of the annulus fibrosus appear as structures with low signal intensity (arrows) and are therefore well delineated from the higher signal of the disk and prevertebral tissue. The posterior longitudinal ligament and the annulus on the other hand are, together with the ligamentum flavum, somewhat poorly demarcated due to the low contrast relative to CSF.

> **The following scanning regime is generally employed**
>
> - Sagittal T1-weighted SE sequence to highlight basic anatomy (Fig. 7.**1**).
> - Sagittal PD- and T2-weighted SE (or TSE/Fast-Spin-Echo) sequence to identify pathological changes (hemorrhage/edema) or ligament structures (Fig. 7.**2**).
> - Sagittal GRE sequence to optimize identification of hemorrhage and to differentiate between osteophytes and disk material.
> - Axial T1-weighted SE sequence to assess the epidural space, spinal cord and the foramina through areas of interest identified on the sagittal sections (Fig. 7.**3**).
> - Axial GRE sequence to assess spinal cord anatomy, blood vessels (bright signal) and ligaments (Fig. 7.**4**).
> - Optional MR angiography sequence to assess the cervical vessels, depending on the mechanism of injury suffered by the patient (Fig. 7.**5**).

Fig. 7.2 Normal sagittal T2-weighted SE image of ▷ the cervical spine. The image displays CSF with a very high signal in contrast to the moderate signal intensity of the spinal cord. The signal of the vertebral body is lower than on the T1-weighted image, while the intervertebral disks appear brighter because of the high signal of the nucleus. The posterior longitudinal ligament with the annulus (black arrows) and the ligamenta flava (white arrows) are well delineated due to the adjacent structures, which demonstrate higher signal intensity. The dark line in the center of the spinal cord represents an artifact along the phase-encoding direction (Gibbs or truncation artifact) (with permission Mirvis S.E.: Semin. Musculoskelet. Radiol. 1998, 2 27–43).

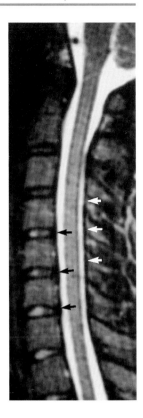

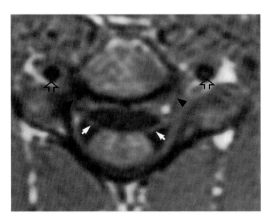

Fig. 7.3 Normal axial T1-weighted SE image through the mid-third of the cervical spine. This image shows the spinal cord surrounded by low-signal CSF. The exiting nerve roots (white arrows) are well delineated as they approach the intervertebral foramina (black arrowheads). Blood flowing in the vertebral arteries appears dark (flow void phenomenon; black open arrows). Cortical bone appears uniformly dark (with permission Mirvis S.E.: Semin. Musculoskelet. Radiol. 1998, 2 27–43).

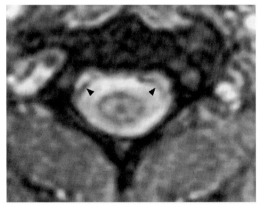

Fig. 7.4 Normal axial T2*-weighted GRE image through the mid-third of the cervical spine. This image shows the internal architecture of the spinal cord (the gray matter appears somewhat brighter than the white matter and displays the typical butterfly- or H-shaped configuration). The myelinated tracts in the periphery of the cord have a lower signal intensity. Bony structures appear relatively dark. The dura (arrowheads) is well delineated from the hyperintense CSF as a dark line.

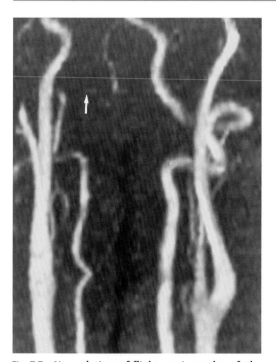

Fig. 7.**5** **Normal time-of-flight angiography of the cervical vessels.** Flowing blood demonstrates a high signal intensity using this two-dimensional GRE time-of-flight technique. The right vertebral artery appears hypoplastic. The horizontal part of the vessel above the loop of the vertebral artery (arrow) shows complete loss of signal due to in-plane signal saturation effects – a typical phenomenon. The suppression of the venous signal is achieved by a saturation pulse applied above the cervical region (with permission Mirvis S.E.: Semin. Musculoskelet. Radiol. 1998, 2 27–43).

Another sequence, the *IR sequence*, is also recommended to identify ligament injuries and to distinguish osteophytes from bulging or herniated disks.

Recently, *three-dimensional volume acquisition of MR data* has been introduced and offers the potential of acquiring the entire cervical region in one scanning procedure and reformatting images through any plane with the resolution of a direct two-dimensional scan. The procedure is particularly useful for exact imaging of the foramina, although with agitated patients image quality is very limited (Ross, 1992; Georgy and Hesselink, 1994).

Echo planar imaging (EPI) or other *fast imaging sequences* can be useful when particularly short acquisition times are required. TSE and fast SE (FSE) sequences are associated with a significant reduction of acquisition time and allow the use of particularly long TR and TE times to achieve more heavily T2-weighted images and improve visualization of the nerve roots within the spinal canal on axial sections (Gundry and Fritts, 1997). TSE sequences also have advantages when imaging patients who have metallic hardware after surgery because metal-induced artifacts appear less pronounced due to decreased magnetic susceptibility effects. However, there is one disadvantage in that these sequences may emphasize CSF motion artifacts (Gundry and Fritts, 1997).

Both GRE and TSE (FSE) sequences are less sensitive in portraying bone-marrow edema than T2-weighted sequences. The combination of TSE (FSE) sequences with fat suppression techniques produces particularly contrast-rich MR myelograms that succeed very well in depicting extradural defects of the nerve roots sleeves. Furthermore, the extent of spinal stenosis can be much better assessed on these images.

Disadvantages of MRI

Disadvantages of MRI include:

- Bone is only poorly demarcated because it contains no hydrogen atoms. Only bone marrow containing fat and blood is depicted as hyperintense. Consequently, only major injuries to the bone are reliably shown on MRI, which should therefore not be considered a sensitive technique for detecting subtle bone injury, particularly injury involving the posterior vertebral elements (Schroeder *et al.*, 1995).
- Currently, an MRI scan of the spine requires somewhat more time than comparable CT studies because of longer data acquisition. However, new imaging acquisition sequences are rendering MRI almost as fast or even faster than CT.
- Hemodynamically unstable patients should not be examined acutely by MRI because cardiopulmonary resuscitation is considerably more difficult to perform in the MR scanning room due to problems associated with the magnetic field.

- Exact monitoring requires MR-compatible supervisory systems that can be used without restriction in the magnet room and without creating radiofrequency noise, which interferes with the image acquisition process (Shellock *et al.*, 1993, 1995).
- The development of non-magnetic neck braces, patient transport systems and remote telemetric monitoring systems now allow MR examination of patients with acute spinal injury, in the majority of cases. However, patients with certain types of ferromagnetic intracranial aneurysm clips, cochlear implants and pacemakers must still be excluded from MR scanning and should be kept away from the magnetic field. Furthermore, patients with metal foreign bodies in the immediate vicinity of vital soft-tissue structures such as the spinal cord, nerve roots, or the orbita are at risk while undergoing MR examination, especially when these metallic foreign bodies show no scar-tissue formation within the tissue (Shellock, 1993). If there is any uncertainty whether the patient has in fact been exposed to metallic foreign bodies, e.g. in the case of welders, then radiographic screening should be performed prior to MR examination.
- It may be assumed that, due to severe claustrophobia, 3 % of patients can only be examined under sedation (Katz *et al.*, 1994).

Indications for the Use of MRI in the Presence of Spinal Trauma

The use of MRI in spinal trauma has clearly increased with improved technology, especially with regard to reduced screening time as well as the introduction of MR-compatible devices for patient positioning and monitoring:

- Today MRI is indicated in the evaluation of all patients with a neurological deficit after spinal injury, especially to the cervical region, when permitted by the patient's overall clinical state and in the absence of any absolute contraindications.
- MRI is particularly indicated in patients with an incomplete or progressive neurological deficit related to spinal trauma.
- Patients with a complete neurological deficit should also undergo MRI assessment if decompression is being considered in an attempt to promote nerve root recovery.
- A further indication for MRI of the spine is given in patients with myelopathy or radiculopathy after spinal trauma in whom previous radiological or CT studies have been negative and in cases where the level of the neurological deficit does not correlate with clinical evidence of location.
- MRI is also useful in deciding the need for internal fixation and the most appropriate surgical approach because MRI best assesses the level or levels of potential mechanical instability secondary to ligament injury, or the presence of spinal-cord compression from epidural processes such as disk herniation or reactive osteophytes.

MRI and Soft-Tissue Injuries

MRI is capable of demonstrating acute injuries to soft tissues secondary to spinal trauma with high contrast resolution and can easily differentiate edema, hemorrhage and direct spinal cord injury. Cord contusions are usually non-hemorrhagic and appear isointense or slightly hypointense relative to the normal cord on T1-weighted SE images, but become brighter in signal intensity than the normal cord on the T2-weighted SE or GRE image sequences (Figs. 7.**6**–7.**9**).

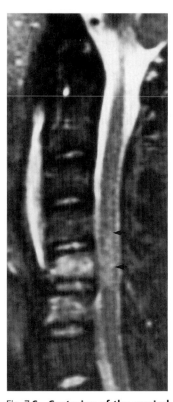

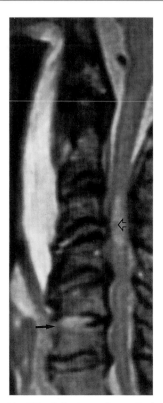

Fig. 7.**6** **Contusion of the cervical cord.** The sagittal T2-weighted image shows a hyperflexion fracture of C5 vertebral body with loss of anterior height. The high signal intensity in the vertebral bodies of C5 and C6 is due to marrow edema and hemorrhage, indicating that both vertebral bodies have been injured. The increased signal within the spinal cord at the levels C4 and C5 (arrows) is an indication of contusion-related edema. In addition, a prevertebral edema is apparent, recognizable by the bright signal anterior to the spine along C2–C6.

Fig. 7.**7** **Spinal cord contusion.** The sagittal T2-weighted SE image shows increased signal intensity within the cord at the level C3/C4 (open arrow). A hyperextension mechanism of injury is indicated by the ventral rupture of the anterior longitudinal ligament at the C5/C6 level (arrow) and the widening and signal enhancement within the disk space C5/C6. There is a disk herniation and hypertrophy of the ligamentum flavum at the C3/C4 level, which have contributed to the contusion of the spinal cord at this level. This image shows a multilevel spinal stenosis at C3-C7. Note, furthermore, the extensive prevertebral edema from C1 to the inferior margin of C4.

When there is significant hemorrhage present within the cord, its appearance on MRI depends on the degree of blood degradation, the field strength of the magnet as well as the imaging sequence used. In the acute to subacute phase after trauma, which ranges approximately from days 1 to 7, blood generally appears dark on the T2-weighted SE images, with this reduction in signal becoming even more intensified on T2*-weighted GRE sequences. Edema, on the other hand, displays a bright signal on T2-weighted images (Figs.7.**10** and 7.**11**).

After about 7 days, when the erythrocyte cell membrane has broken down, extracellular blood develops high signal intensity on both T1- and T2-weighted SE images.

Kulkarni *et al.* (1987) discovered a relationship between the characteristics of signal changes in the spinal cord and the patient's neurological prognosis, suggesting that the signal pattern of the cord on MRI reflects actual cord histopathology.

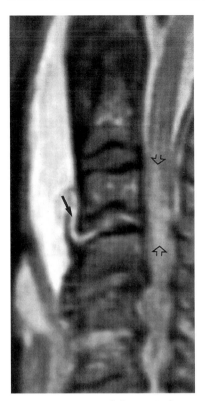

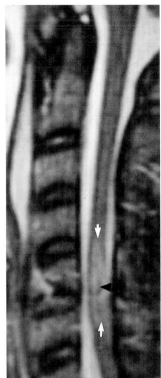

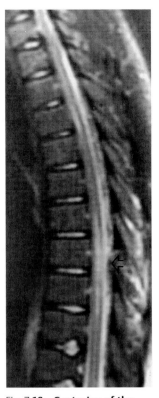

Fig. 7.**8** **Contusion of the cervical cord.** The sagittal T2-weighted SE image in a patient who had sustained cervical spine injury displays increased signal intensity in the cord at C3/C4 level due to cord edema (open arrow). A hyperextension mechanism is assumed to be the cause and is indicated by the signal interruption of the anterior longitudinal ligament and annulus fibrosus at the C3/C4 level (arrow). Note the marked prevertebral edema (with permission Mirvis S.E.: Semin. Musculoskelet. Radiol. 1998, 2 27–43).

Fig. 7.**9** **Contusion of the cervical cord.** T2-weighted TSE sequence in a patient with a teardrop fracture at the C5 level secondary to a hyperflexion trauma. The image demonstrates extensive cord edema in the C4–C6 segment (white arrows). There is also a circumscribed structure with reduced signal intensity recognizable at the C5 level, compatible with intramedullary hemorrhage associated with deoxy- and methemoglobin components (arrowheads). Moderate prevertebral edema.

Fig. 7.**10** **Contusion of the thoracic cord.** Sagittal T2-weighted image in a patient who sustained paraplegia after thoracic hyperflexion injury. The image shows an intramedullary edema at the mid-thoracic level. The ligamentum flavum, which usually displays a low signal intensity, appears disrupted at this level (open arrow). The high signal intensity seen dorsally at several adjacent levels suggests injury of the dorsal soft tissue located in the region of the spinous process (with permission Mirvis S.E.: Semin. Musculoskelet. Radiol. 1998, 2 27–43).

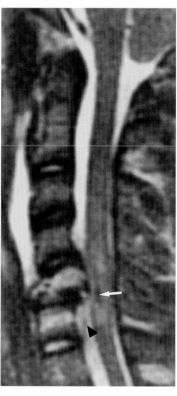

◁ Fig. 7.**11** **Spinal cord injury with development of edema and hemorrhage.** Sagittal T2-weighted image in a patient with a bursting fracture of C5. The image shows a high signal intensity of the cord edema and a low signal in the center of this edematous zone (white arrow) indicating hemorrhage at the C4/C5 level. There is also marrow edema recognizable at C5 and C6 in the region of the vertebral bodies. Extensive prevertebral edema is also present. Retropulsion of C5 has resulted in cord injury. The posterior longitudinal ligament has been separated from the posterior cortex of C6 and is shown as a dark epidural line (arrowhead) (with permission Mirvis S.E.: Semin. Musculoskelet. Radiol. 1998, 2 27–43).

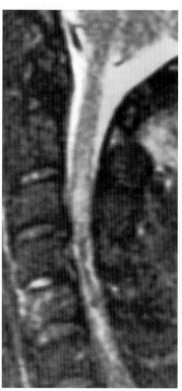

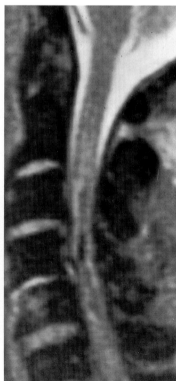

Fig. 7.**12 a, b** **Spinal cord injury with extensive hemorrhage.** 28-year-old patient with tetraplegia secondary to a C5 teardrop fracture. The images show decreased signal intensity in the center of the spinal cord due to intracellular methemoglobin and deoxyhemoglobin with surrounding peripheral edema. The GRE sequence is more sensitive to field inhomogeneity created across the intact erythrocyte membranes and producing larger areas of signal loss. Edema is present in the C4/C5 disk and anterior C5 body:
a Sagittal T2-weighted SE image.
b Sagittal GRE image.

a   b

The significance of these different signal changes within the spinal cord with regard to the patient's prognosis has been verified by several other studies (Mirvis *et al.*, 1988; Schaefer *et al.*, 1992; Silberstein *et al.*, 1992; Mascalchi *et al.*, 1993). Patients with cord lesions containing hematoma generally have a poorer prognosis regarding recovery of neurological function than those with only edema within the cord.

The fact that the MRI finding to a certain extent reflects the histopathology of acute cord injury has been confirmed by direct comparison in experimental studies (Weirich *et al.*, 1990; Quencer *et al.*, 1992).

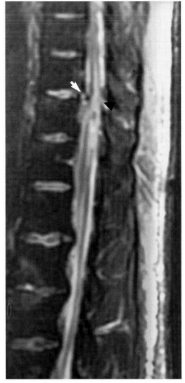

Fig. 7.13   Edema and hemorrhage within the lower thoracic cord. Sagittal T2-weighted TSE image at the dorsolumbar level in a 31-year-old patient with a complete transverse spinal lesion at the lower thoracic level. Edema with central hematoma at the T10/T11 level is recognizable on the image, as well as disruption of the ligamentum flavum (black arrowhead) and the annulus-posterior longitudinal ligament complex (white arrow) (with permission Mirvis S.E.: Semin. Musculoskelet. Radiol. 1998, 2 27–43).

MRI and Ligament Injuries

The mechanism of injury as well as the fracture pattern and alignment of the vertebrae will allow inferences to be drawn on the type of ligament injury sustained from acute spinal trauma. However, even significant ligament injury leading to mechanical instability can go undetected radiographically, particularly in the case of hyperflexion and hyperextension subluxation without concurrent fracture. This is particularly so if concurrent fractures are absent and if the patient is examined radiographically in the supine position, which produces a neutral position or slight extension of the spine. Furthermore, the vertebral alignment shown on plain radiographs may only reveal the main site of mechanical instability, but not demonstrate all segments with ligament injuries and other sites of immediate or potential mechanical instability (Warner *et al.*, 1996).

MRI displays ligaments as structures of low signal intensity due to their lack of mobile hydrogen atoms. Ligament disruption will be seen on MRI as an abrupt interruption of this low signal band, as well as showing thinning or stretching of the ligaments, avulsion of the ligament from its bony attachment, or the combination of a torn ligament with an avulsed bone fragment (an osseous-ligament complex) (Figs. 7.**14**–7.**21**) (Silberstein *et al.*, 1992; Warner *et al.*, 1996; Saifuddin *et al.*, 1996; Benzel *et al.*, 1996; Terk *et al.*, 1997).

The changes to the ligamentous structures of the spine, found at MRI, have a definite bearing on subsequent therapeutic approaches.

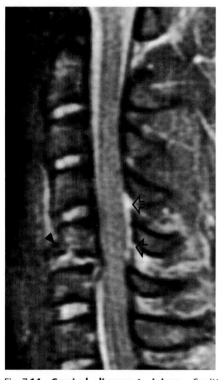

Fig. 7.**14** **Cervical ligament injury.** Sagittal PD-weighted image of a patient who sustained a C5 hyper-flexion teardrop fracture in a motorcycle accident. The interspinous ligaments and the ligamenta flava are disrupted at the C4/C5 and C5/C6 levels (open arrows). The posterior annulus fibrosus of the C5/C6 disk is torn and the posterior longitudinal ligament appears stretched. There is prevertebral edema. The anterior annulus fibrosus at C5/C6 and the anterior longitudinal ligament are probably connected to the bony fracture fragment (arrowhead) (with permission Mirvis S.E.: Semin. Musculoskelet. Radiol. 1998, 2 27–43).

MRI can demonstrate both unsuspected ligamentous injury as well as an extent of injury greater than anticipated based on other available imaging studies (Warner *et al.*, 1996). A study by Warner *et al.* (1996) evaluating MRI examination conducted on 43 trauma patients with cervical spine injury identified a total of 97 ligament injuries. However, a correlation with the intraoperative finding was found in only 11 cases with 14 ligamentous injuries. There were two cases of false positive posterior longitudinal ligament injury diagnosed by MRI. Furthermore, 11 (25 %) of the 43 patients had ligament injuries that were greater than expected (injuries adjacent to the obvious level of osseous pathology or an abnormal alignment). Among these 11 there were also cases in which no ligament injury had been assumed at all, based upon plain radiographs and CT appearance. The study was conducted using PD- and T2*-weighted GRE sequences, with the sagittal image being most sensitive in assessing ligamentous structures.

Benzel *et al.* (1996) reported on MRI examinations in 174 patients with cervical spine trauma who had either minor radiological abnormalities or at least clinical symptoms. They found that 62 patients (36 %) had soft-tissue lesions, including 27 cases of ligament disruption. With one exception, all patients received external stabilization as adequate therapy. In this study, T2-weighted sagittal images proved most useful in assessing the ligament structures, while axial views were of least value.

Terk *et al.* (1997) examined 68 patients with thoracolumbar injury using T1-weighted SE sequences, T2-weighted FSE sequences and fat-suppressed T2-weighted imaging. The posterior ligament complex (PLC) injury was demonstrated in 36 patients (53 %), with flexion-distraction (n = 15) and dislocation fracture being the most common mechanisms of injury. Burst fractures resulted in PLC tears in 10 cases (42 %) and compression fractures in 6 cases (26 %). Thoracolumbar ligament injuries involved the following ligaments in decreasing frequency:

- inter- and supraspinous ligament,
- ligamenta flava,
- posterior longitudinal ligament,
- anterior longitudinal ligament.

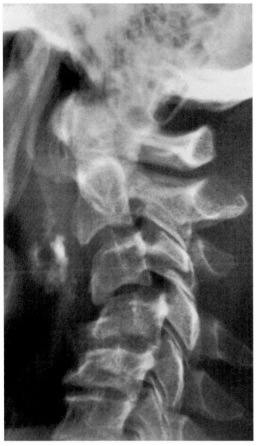

a

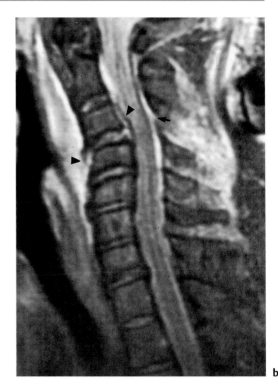

b

Fig. 7.15 a, b   Injury to the ligaments of the thoracic spine:

a Lateral radiograph of the cervical spine: Evidence of a hyperflexion subluxation in the segmental region C3/C4 with focal kyphosis, subluxation of C3 over C4 with anterolisthesis of the C3 body and fanning of the spinous processes C3 and C4.

b PD-weighted SE image of the same patient: Disruption of the anterior and posterior annulus fibers at the C3/C4 level with avulsion of the anterior and posterior longitudinal ligaments from the dorsal cortex of C3 and the anterior cortex of C4 (arrowheads). The ligamentum flava is torn at this level and both prevertebral and posterior soft-tissue structures display extensive edema.

Six patients underwent surgery and in each case the operative finding matched precisely with the MRI result.

Saifuddin *et al.* (1996) discuss the significance of MRI in thoracolumbar injury and refer to the good depiction of ligamentous structures of the spine, emphasizing its value in differentiating between ligament disruption and ligament stretch-

ing, especially with regard to the posterior longitudinal and interspinous ligaments.

The role of MRI in patients sustaining a whiplash injury to the cervical spine without neurological deficits or abnormalities on conventional radiographs is controversial. Pettersson *et al.* (1997) conducted MRI examinations in 39 such patients immediately after the trauma and at a 2-

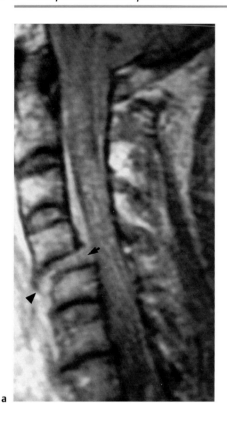

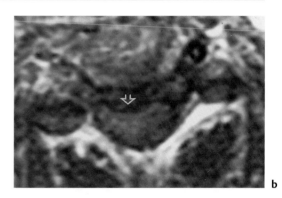

Fig. 7.16 a, b **Injury to the ligaments of the cervical spine at the level C4/C5 in a patient with a unilateral interfacetal dislocation.** Sagittal PD-weighted fast SE image of a patient with a rupture of the posterior longitudinal ligament (arrow) and avulsion of the anterior longitudinal ligament from the anterior cortex of the C5 body (arrowhead). The soft tissues in the C2/C3 and C3/C4 regions demonstrate signal enhancement, probably also indicating an interspinous ligament injury at these levels (open arrow).

year follow-up. They saw no ligament injuries or hematoma formations, so that these authors found no indication for acute MRI after whiplash injury.

Ronnen *et al.* (1996) reach similar conclusions after finding no sequelae of injury at MRI performed on patients with whiplash injuries, yet also no neurological deficits and no radiographic abnormalities. The authors discuss to what extent kyphotic deformities of the cervical spine, as often seen on functional views (flexion/extension views of the spine), in actual fact represent regions of relative hypermobility that compensate for adjacent hypomobile regions resulting from muscle spasm. The authors doubt that kyphotic deformities of the spine are to be regarded as the consequence of injury to soft-tissues.

On the other hand, Davis *et al.* (1991) reported several anterior column injuries in patients with whiplash injury, including MRI findings of separation of the intervertebral disk from the vertebral end plate, anterior longitudinal ligament disrup-

tions, annular tears, and clinically occult vertebral artery injury.

According to the experience gained from our own institution, patients with whiplash injury, on rare occasions, will present with cervical tenderness without apparent radiographic abnormalities or neurological deficit, yet show anterior cervical spine pathology on MRI.

The differences in this experience with MRI examination of whiplash injuries may reflect the different referral patterns at various institutions.

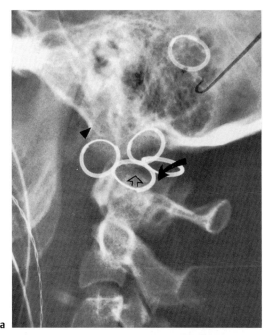

a

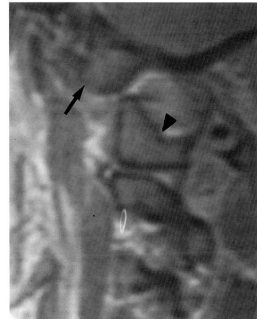

b

Fig. 7.**17 a–c Ligament injury in a tetraplegic patient after a blunt trauma showing an atlanto-occipital dislocation:**

a Lateral radiograph of the cervical spine: Anterior displacement of the occiput relative to the atlas. The distance between the basion (arrowhead) and the tip of the dens (open arrow) is markedly widened (normally less than 12 mm). The condylar fossa of the atlas is uncovered (curved arrow). There is a marked offset between the dorsal contour of the foramen magnum (opisthion) and the spinolaminar line of the atlas.

b Sagittal PD-weighted TSE image: Dislocation between occiput (arrow) and C1 condylar fossa (arrowhead).

c Mid-sagittal T1-weighted SE image after contrast application: Complete disruption of the anterior longitudinal ligament, tectorial membrane, apical dental ligament, and the posterior ligament complex. The spinal cord is markedly narrowed at the C1 level.

c

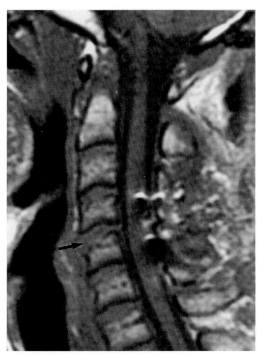

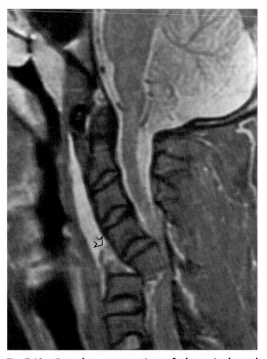

Fig. 7.**18 Injury to the ligaments of the cervical spine at the level C4/C5.** Sagittal T1-weighted image after posterior wire fixation at the C4/C5 level (note artifacts) showing disruption of the anterior longitudinal ligament and the anterior annulus (arrow). The posterior annulus and the posterior longitudinal ligament are not clearly assessable on this sequence, but appeared intact on the T2-weighted images (not shown). C5 shows an anterior compression fracture (with permission Mirvis S.E.: Semin. Musculoskelet. Radiol. 1998, 2 27–43).

Fig. 7.**19 Complete transection of the spinal cord with complete ligament disruption.** Sagittal PD-weighted image of an adolescent after a motorcycle accident, showing a severe hyperflexion dislocation of C5 on C6. The spinal cord is severed. The anterior ligament complex is completely disrupted (open arrow), the posterior ligament complex is torn or markedly stretched. There is marked prevertebral edema. The ligamentum flavum appears thickened above the major injury level (with permission Mirvis S.E.: Semin. Musculoskelet. Radiol. 1998, 2 27–43).

Fig. 7.**21 a–c Posterior complex ligament injury** ▷ **with a flexion teardrop fracture:**

a, b Sagittal PD-weighted (**a**) and T2-weighted fast SE image (**b**): Hyperflexion teardrop fracture of C5 with a correspondingly increased signal in that vertebral body noted on the T2-weighted image. There is widening of the distance between the spinous processes of C5 and C6 with marked signal enhancement along the ligamentum flavum indicating marked attenuation or partial rupture (arrow). The spinal cord appears normal.

c Sagittal image displaying the facet joints. Depiction of widening or distraction of the facet-joint spaces at C5 and C6 with increased signal intensity due to fluid accumulation within the joint space (arrow).

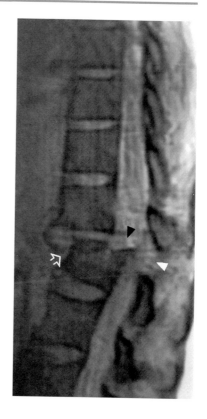

Fig. 7.**20** **Ligament injury at the level of the thora-** ▷
columbar junction. Sagittal PD-weighted image of a
victim of a fall showing a complete ligament disruption
at the level of the thoracolumbar junction secondary to
severe hyperflexion. The anterior parts of the annulus fibrosus and the anterior longitudinal ligament are torn
(open arrow), and the middle column ligaments (black
arrowhead) and the posterior ligament complex (white
arrowhead) are completely disrupted (with permission
Mirvis S.E.: Semin. Musculoskelet. Radiol. 1998, 2 27–
43).

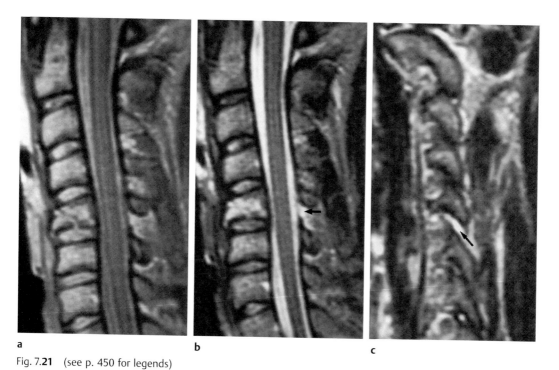

a   b   c

Fig. 7.**21** (see p. 450 for legends)

MRI and Acute Traumatic Epidural Lesions

Intervertebral Disk Herniation

Acute intervertebral disk herniation may accompany fractures or dislocations or even occur as an isolated lesion. If the herniated disk causes compression of the spinal cord or nerve roots, then relevant neurological symptoms may be expected. Evidence of this kind of disk herniation with impingement of neural structures is important for preoperative planning of the surgical management of spinal trauma, with MRI in this case being a most suitable procedure (Figs. 7.**22**–7.**24**).

However, the distinction between disk material and osteophyte poses certain difficulties with SE sequences so that additional GRE sequences should be used for better delineation. Bone displays very low signal intensity on GRE sequences, while disk material, on the other hand, demonstrates a relatively high signal. The advantages of MRI over CT lie in the higher contrast range, which allows a higher detection rate for disk injuries.

Flanders *et al.* (1990) detected 40 % more acute traumatic disk herniations producing neurological deficits by MRI than by CT in patients who had sustained whiplash injuries of the cervical spine.

Rizzolo *et al.* (1991) found a herniated disk in 42 % of 53 patients who were examined using a 1.5-tesla magnetic resonance image scanner within 72 hours of injury. The highest incidence was found in patients with bilateral interfacetal dislocations (80 %) and anterior cord syndromes (100 %).

a

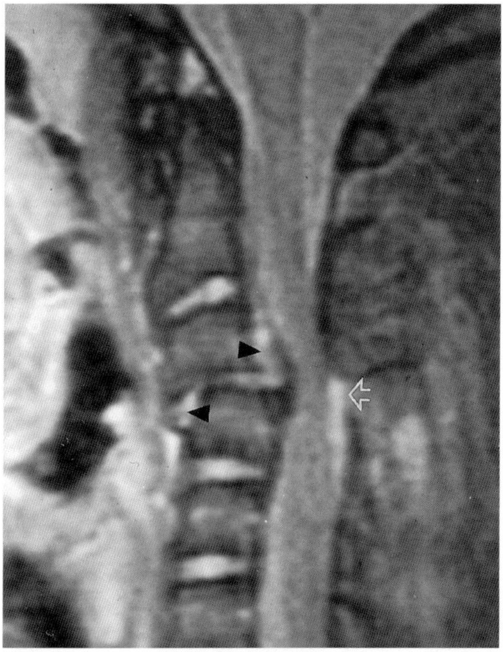

b

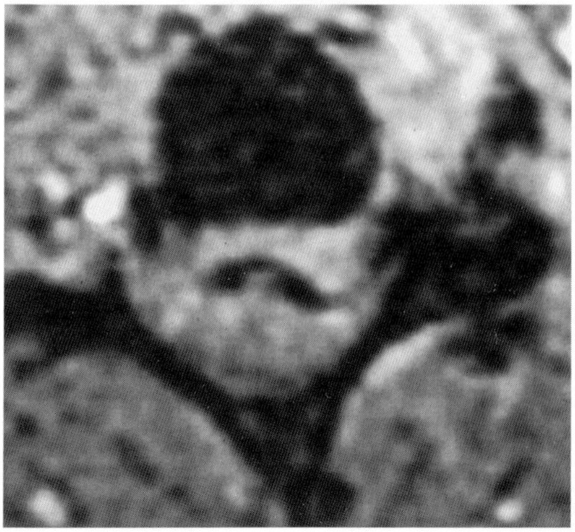

Fig. 7.22 a, b   Disk herniation secondary to bilateral interfacetal dislocation with structural instability between C3/C4:

a Sagittal PD-weighted fast SE sequence: Patient with bilateral interfacetal dislocation. Avulsion of the anterior and posterior longitudinal ligament in the region of C3 and C4 with concomitant complete disruption of the anterior and posterior parts of the annulus fibrosus is shown on this image. The ligamentum flavum is also torn at this level (open arrow). The intervertebral disk appears herniated in an anterior and dorsocranial direction and lies dorsally beneath the posterior longitudinal ligament while the anterior longitudinal ligament bulges anteriorly (black arrowheads).

b Axial GRE sequence through the disk space: Presentation of a marked herniation of disk material and thickened or redundant posterior longitudinal ligament leading to compression of the anterior aspect of the spinal cord.

Doran *et al.* (1993) described a high incidence of traumatic disk herniation in patients with both unilateral and bilateral interfacetal dislocations. Patients with herniated disks secondary to trauma may suffer neurological deterioration from manipulative reduction of the spine because disk material may be displaced into the spinal canal and compromise neural structures (Kathol, 1997). Urgent MRI prior to reduction in patients can avoid this complication with major subluxation or dislocation by identifying herniated disk material that may require anterior diskectomy or intraoperative reduction.

Acute traumatic or chronic posterior disk herniation at the level of the thoracic spine, although relatively uncommon, often tends to produce neurological symptoms due to the relatively narrow spinal canal at this level.

Post-traumatic herniation of disk material is often associated with subligamentous or epidural hematoma (Kathol, 1997).

Epidural Hematoma

Epidural hematomas are an uncommon sequel of spinal trauma and occur in only 1–2 % of cervical spine injuries (Garza-Mercado, 1989). The cervical spine is by far the most common location of epidural hematoma secondary to spinal trauma.

The hematoma typically occurs in the dorsal epidural space due to the close adherence of the ventral dura to the posterior longitudinal ligament (Garza-Mercado, 1989). Bleeding most likely arises from the rich epidural venous plexus due to sudden increases in pressure in these valveless veins (Garza-Mercado, 1989; Olshaker and Barish, 1991). Epidural hematoma may develop acutely after trauma, in a delayed fashion, or after open or closed reduction of the spinal column. Up to 50 % of post-traumatic epidural hematomas develop in patients without overt spinal injuries (Garza-Mercado, 1989). For this reason, the presence of myelopathy without signs of injury to the spine demonstrated by plain radiography or plain CT should suggest an epidural hematoma. It should, however, be kept in mind that an older hematoma is poorly separated from CSF on CT with regard to its density.

Garza-Mercado (1989) reported an increased likelihood of epidural hematoma of the cervical spine in younger patients due to the higher elas-

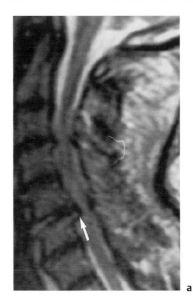
a

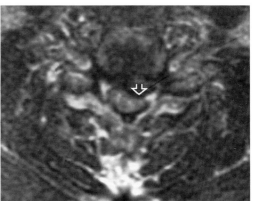
b

Fig. 7.**23 a, b   Probable acute disk herniation:**
a Sagittal T2-weighted image: Presentation of a disk herniation at the level C5/C6 (arrow) compressing the spinal cord. Slight widening of the anterior disk space with increased signal within the disk material and prevertebral edema. Distal to this segment there are additional signs suggesting an acute hyperextension injury.
b T2-weighted image fast SE image: Confirmation of a left mid-lateral disk herniation (open arrow) compressing the spinal cord (with permission Mirvis S.E.: Semin. Musculoskelet. Radiol. 1998, 2 27–43).

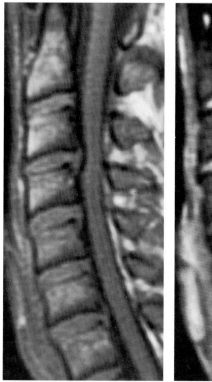
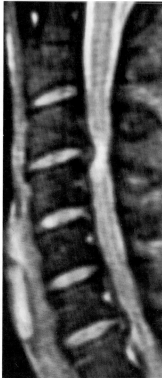

a   b

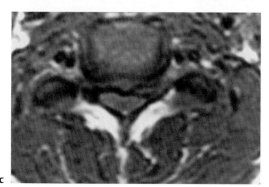

c

Fig. 7.**24 a–c MRI of an acute disk herniation after trauma:**

a, b Sagittal (**a**) and axial (**b**) T1-weighted SE images: 34-year-old male acute trauma victim with clinical evidence of tetraparesis. The images show disk herniation at the C3/C4 level with a corresponding compression of the spinal cord.

c Sagittal T2-weighted SE image: Presentation of cord edema at the C3/C4 level secondary to compression from the herniated disk.

ticity of the spine and in patients with fused cervical spines, including those with ankylosing spondylitis and Forestier disease (diffuse idiopathic skeletal hyperostosis, DISH).

The development of a progressive, unexplained neurological deterioration in patients who have sustained spinal trauma may herald the onset of cord compression from an expanding epidural hematoma.

Epidural hematoma is rarely encountered in the lumbar spine and is poorly distinguishable from a herniated disk if the MR signal characteristics are similar to those of disk material and the hematoma is centered over the disk space (Watanabe *et al.*, 1997).

The signal characteristics of epidural hematoma depend on the following factors:

- age of the blood,
- magnetic field strength,
- imaging sequences used.

In the acute phase 1–3 days after trauma, blood appears isointense with spinal cord on T1-weighted images. At 3–7 days after injury, the central portion of the hematoma, which at this point in time still contains intact red blood cells, displays a low signal on T2-weighted images while the periphery, composed of lysed red blood, shows signal enhancement on both T1- and T2-weighted sequences (Figs. 7.**25**–7.**27**).

In some cases there is a complex mixture of signal intensities, particularly if bleeding has occurred in stages over time (Figs. 7.**26** and 7.**27**).

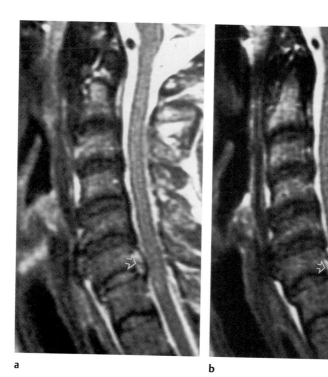

a   b

Fig. 7.**25 a, b** **Subacute epidural hematoma.** Sagittal T2-weighted fast SE images: Trauma patient with an anterior cord syndrome following blunt injury. The images show accumulation of blood with a correspondingly high signal intensity beneath the posterior longitudinal ligament at the C6 level (open arrow). The signal is distinctly different from that of disk material, thus ex-

cluding a disk sequester as a cause of the abnormality. The anterior subarachnoid space is obliterated by the hematoma. The image also suggests disruption of the ligamentum flavum at the C6/C7 level (black arrow). Slightly increased signal along the anterior cord at the C7 level, possibly representing contusion. Mild prevertebral edema.

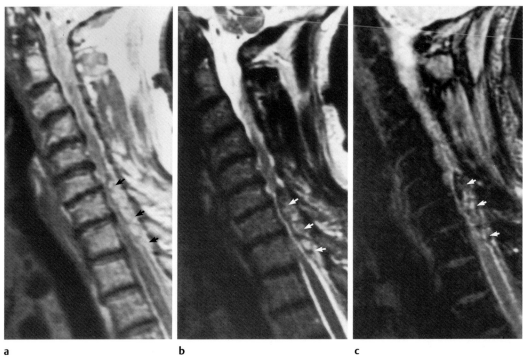

a   b   c

Fig. 7.**26 a–c** **Complex epidural hematoma.** 75-year-old man with tetraplegia and sensory deficits over a 3-day period after lifting a heavy box. The images show an extensive dorsal epidural hematoma (arrows) of complex mixed signal intensity spanning from C6 to T2 and causing marked compression of the spinal cord. The inhomogeneous signal intensity is related to subacute presentation and probable intermittent expansion of the hematoma with episodic bleeding (with permission Mirvis S.E.: Semin. Musculoskelet. Radiol. 1998, 2 27–43).

a Sagittal PD-weighted SE image.
b T2-weighted SE image.
c GRE image.

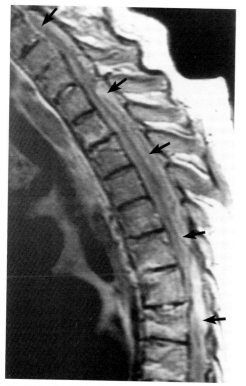

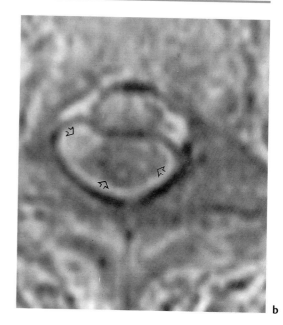

b

a

Fig. 7.**27 a, b** **MRI of a thoracic epidural hematoma:**
a Sagittal PD-weighted fast SE image through the
thoracic and upper lumbar spine: 74-year-old man
with progressive paraplegia after a fall. The image
shows an extensive dorsal epidural hematoma of
mixed signal intensity (arrows). The varied signal intensity of the hematoma is most likely related to
different episodes of hemorrhage. Compression fractures of several thoracic and upper lumbar vertebrae
with corresponding signal enhancements and deformity particularly of the end plates.
b Axial T2-weighted fast SE image: Widespread dorsal
hematoma (arrow) compressing and displacing the
spinal cord.

Degenerative Spondylosis

Spinal cord injury can be caused by impaction of
posterior osteophytes or hypertrophied, calcified
or ossified ligaments, into the anterior cord secondary to a flexion trauma, most commonly in the
cervical region due to the greater mobility of the
cervical spine. Posterior cord injury results not infrequently from hypertrophy or buckling of the
ligamentum flavum secondary to a hyperextension injury. As noted above, prominent posterior
osteophytes in the thoracic spine can also cause
injury to the cord, which overlies the vertebrae in
this region, and because here the spinal canal is
relatively narrow.

In general, patients with congenital or acquired
spinal stenosis from degenerative changes are
more likely to sustain injury from spinal trauma.
If myelopathy is diagnosed in older patients after
trauma, but without radiological evidence of injury, then the cause must be considered to lie in
spinal injury secondary to posterior osteophytes
(Taylor and Blackwood, 1948).

Cervical cord impaction by posterior
osteophytes typically produces a central cord syndrome at the cervical level (Cheng *et al.*, 1992).

MRI performed in the sagittal orientation
clearly demonstrates bony or ligamentous

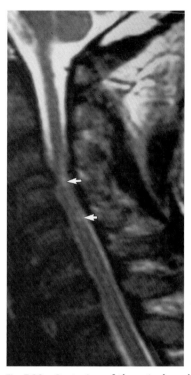

changes of the spinal canal and should be complimented by axial images through levels of spinal stenosis (Fig. 7.**28**).

Comparison of T2-weighted SE and T2*-weighted GRE sequences can be helpful in differentiating acutely herniated disk material from osteophytes surrounding chronic disk herniation. Both sequences give a bright depiction of CSF and thus produce a myelographic appearance, which allows good separation of osteophytes, intervertebral disks and spinal cord. MRI is crucial in planning the extent of posterior surgical decompression by showing underlying bony and ligamentous changes.

Fig. 7.**28 Contusion of the spinal cord after trauma with subsequent spinal stenosis** (arrow). Sagittal T2-weighted GRE image with multifocal areas of canal stenosis in the presence of degenerative disk herniations with posterior osteophyte formation and concomitant hypertrophy of the ligamentum flavum. Increased cord signal at the C3/C4 and C5/C6 levels indicates either chronic myelomalacia or acute contusion. The patient sustained complete motor paralysis after a blunt trauma. The cord atrophy also demonstrated on the image probably contributes to the limited potential for neurological recovery in such cases.

MR Angiography and Injuries to the Cervical Arteries

MR angiography is used as a screening procedure for detecting injury to the cervical vessels, particularly the vertebral arteries. The exact incidence of vertebral artery injury occurring after cervical-spine trauma, especially in association with fracture or dislocation, is unknown, but the injury is being seen and reported with increasing frequency (Gambee, 1986; Louw *et al.*, 1990; Schwartz *et al.*, 1991; Jabre, 1991; Parent *et al.*, 1992; Deen and McGirr, 1992; Friedman *et al.*, 1995; Giacobetti *et al.*, 1997).

Vertebral artery injuries from cervical spine trauma generally involve the second portion of the artery (the V2 segment) coursing intraforaminally from C6 to C2. Fixation of the artery within the confines of the transverse foramina predisposes this vessel to injury from cervical dislocations. Although a variety of cervical spine injuries have been associated with vertebral artery injury, unilateral and bilateral facet dislocations are most commonly implicated. Vertebral artery injury can also occur from fractures extending across the foramen transversarium and has been reported in association with lateral cervical dislocations (Kathol, 1997).

Giacobetti *et al.* (1997) reviewed 61 patients with cervical spine trauma over a period of 7 months after injury. They used MR angiography as a screening procedure to detect lesions to the vertebral arteries. They saw complete occlusion of the vertebral artery in 12 of the 61 patients (19.7%). Ten of these 12 had sustained flexion or flexion-compression mechanisms of injury. The authors found no association between vertebral artery injury and age, sex, degree of neurological impairment, or co-existing injuries.

Friedmann *et al.* (1995) studied 37 patients with non-penetrating acute cervical spine injury and found 9 cases (24%) with uni- or bilateral vertebral artery injury. Only the one patient with bilateral vertebral artery occlusion sustained an extensive, fatal cerebellar infarct, while the others had no neurological deficit related to the vertebral artery injury. The authors therefore reach the conclusion that MR angiography should be a routine part of the diagnostic work-up for cervical spine trauma, even in cases where there is no indication of a vertebral artery injury.

Other studies have shown a prevalence of vertebral artery injury in up to 40% of patients with cervical spine trauma (Giacobetti *et al.*, 1997). The vast majority of these injuries remain clinically silent.

MR angiographic screening of the vertebral arteries is indicated for all patients with blunt trauma of the cervical spine with significant degrees of dislocation or subluxation (more than 1 cm) or fractures crossing the transverse foramina.

Routine examination of the cervical spine should include axial T1-weighted images. These sequences demonstrate flowing blood as a signal void (so-called dark blood). Conversely, GRE sequences show flowing blood as a bright image. Flowing blood can be therefore detected by a combination of these two examination modalities.

However, MR angiography is particularly useful, either in the form of a contrast-assisted examination technique with a three-dimensional FISP sequence or as a three-dimensional time-of-flight sequence (Figs. 7.**29** and 7.**30**).

MR angiography readily displays vascular stenosis or vascular occlusion. Evidence of intimal flaps, intramural dissection or hematoma, pseudoaneurysm formation and vessel thrombosis as causes of vascular stenosis or occlusion are better displayed on axial T1-weighted images. It should be noted that the two vertebral arteries often differ in their degree of development; in about 70% of cases there is hypoplasia of one side with a compensatory hypertrophy of the vessel on the other side. Care must also be taken to distinguish injury from vessel hypoplasia and atherosclerotic disease.

Pathologic findings on MR angiography should be confirmed by DSA, which still offers higher spatial resolution than MR angiography.

Penetrating injury accounts for the majority of cervical vertebral injuries. It should be borne in mind that the presence of retained metal fragments, e.g. from ballistic injury, might constitute a contraindication for MRI examination. The metal fragments also cause signal loss, which in some cases overlaps important areas of the cervical spine, including the vessels, and thus reduces the diagnostic reliability of the examination or even renders reaching a reliable diagnosis impossible. It is sometimes difficult with penetrating ballistic injuries, in particular, to detect subtle intimal injuries by MRI, so that as a rule a DSA examination should be recommended.

Reaney *et al.* (1995) found MR angiography particularly useful in detecting injury to the lumbar spine in association with a Chance-type fracture and abdominal aortic injury.

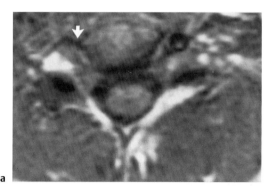

a

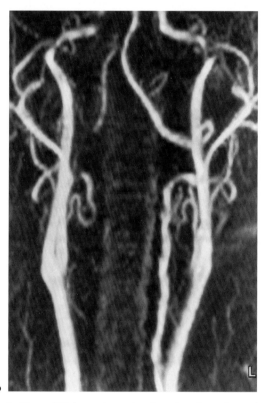

b

Fig. 7.**29 a–c Traumatic injury to the vertebral artery.** 32-year-old woman who sustained a hyperflexion/subluxation injury in the segmental region C5/C6:

a Axial T1-weighted SE image: Evidence of increased signal intensity in the right vertebral artery reflecting loss of blood flow (arrow).

c

b Time-of-flight angiography: Complete loss of signal along the whole course of the right vertebral artery except for a small proximal segment which possibly displays some blood flow from reconstitution of flow by collaterals.

c DSA: Demonstration of complete occlusion of the proximal portion of the right vertebral artery (open arrow). The patient had no neurological symptoms related to this vertebral artery occlusion.

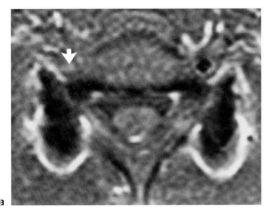

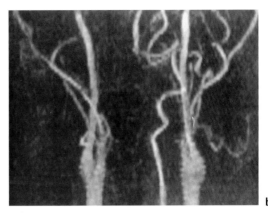

Fig. 7.**30 a, b** **Traumatic occlusion of the right vertebral artery secondary to vertebral artery injury.** 38-
year-old man who sustained a unilateral interfacetal dislocation in the mid-cervical region:

a Axial T1-weighted SE image: After bilateral screw
fixation of the lateral mass, demonstration of signal
enhancement of the right vertebral artery (arrow) reflecting loss of flow-void phenomenon. Normal flow-

void signal in the left vertebral artery as a sign of
flowing blood. The titanium screws are clearly seen
on the right showing artifact formation.

b Time-of-flight angiography: Normal signaling along
the course of the left vertebral artery and complete
loss of right vertebral artery signal. The patient had
no neurological deficit related to the occlusion of the
right vertebral artery.

MRI and Osseous Injuries

MRI has hitherto not been particularly regarded
as being a sensitive examination technique for detecting osseous injury. This is has to do with the
fact that bones do not contain mobile hydrogen
atoms so that the bone signal is only slight or is
missing completely. This lack of sensitivity of MRI
for fracture detection applies particularly to
smaller bony elements, such as:

- lamina,
- pedicles,
- transverse processes (Schaefer *et al.*, 1992;
  Schroeder *et al.*, 1995).

However, osseous damage is associated with
edema and thus with a change in signal, making a
distinction from normal bone easily possible.
Furthermore, the presence of bone damage is
readily separable from inter- and perivertebral
hematoma (Fig. 7.**31**).

With higher spatial resolution, volume acquisition and the use of special sequences (e.g. fat-saturated sequences, STIR sequence), disruption of
cortical bone becomes more apparent by MR imaging. While Schroeder *et al.* (1995) found that
MRI had a sensitivity of only 50 % for C2 fractures,
it detected 89 % of transverse process fractures
and 92 % of lamina fractures in a series of 39
patients.

Salfuddin *et al.* (1996) also refer to the increased accuracy of MRI in demonstrating neural
arch and facet fractures in the thoracic and lumbar region, provided state-of-the-art MR scanners
are used. The use of MRI is recommended, in addition to nuclear bone scintigraphy, for distinguishing between acute and chronic bone damage (e.g.
osteochondrosis) and atypical developmental osseous anomaly.

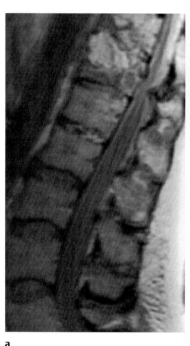 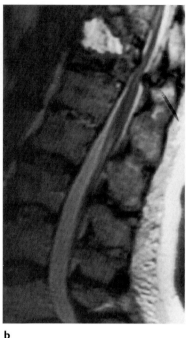

Fig. 7.31 a, b Severe compression fractures of T11 and T12:

a Sagittal PD-weighted lumbar MR image: Evidence of a compression trauma in the region of T11 and T12 with part of the dorsal marginal strip of T12 appearing displaced intraspinally. The conus is contused between the T12 posterior body and the buckled posterior spinal ligaments.

b T2-weighted fast SE image: Depiction of bright hematoma in the region of T11 and T12. Equally well demonstrated on this image is the compression of the conus (with permission Mirvis S.E.: Semin. Musculoskelet. Radiol. 1998, 2 27–43).

a   b

▌MRI and Radicular Symptoms

In the author's experience, MRI is only suitable for detecting nerve root injury to a limited extent.

Volle *et al.* (1992) undertook a comparative study of various imaging modalities for detecting nerve root and brachial plexus injury. They concluded that CT and, in particular CT myelography, were far superior to MRI, with conventional my-elography still the gold standard. MRI detected nerve root injury in only 1 of 18 cases (6 %). These authors therefore recommend the combined use of MRI and CT myelography for diagnosing traumatic meningoceles and myelography with segmental follow-up CT to differentiate pre- and postganglionic nerve root injury.

Summary

- MRI has *advantages* for the examination of patients with spinal trauma:
  - the possibility of obtaining images in all three planes,
  - superior contrast resolution compared with other imaging modalities,
  - the possibility of generating myelographic-equivalent images,
  - contrast-rich imaging of the spinal cord,
  - reliable prognostic information,
  - the possibility of imaging vessels,
  - MRI is performed without ionizing radiation and is thus free of side effects.
- A series of *scanning regimes* is required to obtain an optimal scanning result:
  - sagittal T1-weighted SE sequences for assessing basic anatomy,
  - sagittal T2-weighted TSE sequences to identify pathological changes,
  - sagittal GRE sequence to optimize identification of hemorrhage and osteophytes,
  - axial T1-weighted SE sequence to assess the spinal cord and epidural space,
  - axial images using gradient-echo technique to distinguish ligaments and display spinal cord anatomy and blood vessels.
- The following *disadvantages* of MRI should be noted:
  - since cortical bone produces no signal, fractures of smaller structures, particularly the vertebral appendages, are less well depicted than on CT,
  - screening time is longer than with CT,
  - monitoring patients during screening requires more effort, MR-compatible supervisory systems are required and this means higher costs.
- The development of non-magnetic neck braces, patient transport systems and remote telemetric monitoring systems now allow MR examination of patients with acute spinal injury, in the majority of cases.
- *Indications* for MRI include:
  - the presence of a progressive or incomplete neurological deficit,
  - surgery intended for patients with a complete neurological deficit,
  - when there is discrepancy between clinical presentation and radiological finding with regard to the level of the suspected cord lesion,
  - to detect nerve root damage in the presence of traumatic radiculopathy.
- *MRI readily diagnoses soft-tissue injuries.* A non-hemorrhagic cord contusion appears iso- to hypointense on T1-weighted images and hyperintense on T2-weighted images. When there is significant hemorrhage present within the cord, its signal at MRI depends on age of the blood and thus the degree of hemoglobin degradation. In the acute and subacute phases, hemorrhage appears dark on T2-weighted SE images; after 7 days there is a signal reversal with enhancement both on the T1- and also the T2-weighted sequences. There is nearly always a strong signal reduction on GRE sequences to indicate the hemorrhage.
- There are three different types of spinal-cord contusion:
  - type I: hematoma within the cord,
  - type II: with cord edema,
  - type III: cord edema combined with hemorrhage.

Patients with hematoma generally have a poorer prognosis than those with only edema secondary to contusion.

- The mechanism of injury, the alignment of the vertebrae, as well as the fracture pattern allows inferences to be drawn on the type of *ligament injury* sustained. MRI is capable of depicting ligament injury exactly, with T2-weighted sequences being particularly suitable. Disruption of ligament structures appears as a signal void on these images and is combined with signal enhancement, which can include the adjacent segments. Avulsed bone and stretched ligaments are also readily differentiated.
- Acute traumatic disk *herniations* are well diagnosed by MRI, although the differentiation between osteophyte and disk material can be difficult on SE sequences so that supplementary GRE sequences should be used. Disk herniations are particularly common in patients presenting a traumatic uni- or bilateral interfacetal dislocation.
- An *epidural hematoma* is an uncommon sequel of spinal trauma. It is promoted by the presence of fusion of the vertebral spine or, for example, by a diffuse idiopathic skeletal hyperostosis. The epidural hematoma typically occurs in the dorsal epidural space. It may develop in a delayed

Summary

fashion. MRI readily provides the diagnosis if suitable sequences are used. On SE images the signal depends on the age of the hemorrhage. GRE sequences are more suited for displaying the full extent of the hematoma.

- *Degenerative spondylosis* can promote injury to the spinal cord. Osteophytes can act as a fulcrum and thereby cause anterior cord injury. The same applies to hypertrophy or calcification of the posterior longitudinal ligament. Hypertrophy of the ligamenta flava can cause posterior cord injury during trauma involving retroflexion.
- *MR angiography* is used as a screening procedure for detecting or excluding injury to the cervical vessels, particularly to the vertebral arteries. Injury to the vertebral arteries generally involves the V2 segment, which courses in-

traforaminally from C6 to C2. Fixation of the artery within the confines of the transverse foramina predisposes this vessel to injury. Injuries are particularly common in association with unilateral or bilateral facet dislocations.

- With higher spatial resolution and the use of *fat-saturated sequences* (FS sequences, STIR sequence), depiction of bone by MR imaging becomes more exact. MRI is therefore also well capable of detecting bone damage. Difficulties arise in detecting fractures of the posterior vertebral structures and especially C2 fractures.
- MRI is only suitable to a limited extent for detecting *nerve root injury*. Conventional myelography still serves as the gold standard. Strongly T2-weighted images are used to achieve an effect similar to that of myelography.

References

Benzel, E. C., B. L. Hart, P. A. Ball et al.: Magnetic resonance imaging for the evaluation of patients with occult cervical spine injury. J. Neurosurg. 85 (1996) 824–829

Cheng, C., A. L. Wolf, S. E. Mirvis, W. L. Robinson: Body surfing accidents resulting in cervical spine injury. Spine 17 (1992) 257–260

Davis, S. J., L. M. Terest, W. G. BradleyJr. et al.: Cervical spine hyperextension injuries: MR findings. Radiology 180 (1991) 245

Deen, H. G., S. J. McGirr: Vertebral artery injury associated with cervical spine fractures. Spine 17 (1992) 230–234

Doran, S. E., M. Papadopoulos, T. Ducker, K. O. Lillehei: Magnetic resonance imaging documentation of co-existent traumatic locked facets of the cervical spine and disc herniation. J. Neurosurg. 79 (1993) 341–345

Flanders, A. E., D. M. Schafer, H. T. Doan, M. M. Mishkin, C. F. Gonzales, B. E. Northrup: Acute cervical spine trauma: correlation of MR imaging findings with degree of neurologic deficit. Radiology 177 (1990) 25–33

Friedman, D., A. Flanders, C. Thomas, W. Millar: Vertebral artery injury after cervical spine trauma: rate of occurrence by MR angiography and assessment of clinical consequences. Amer. J. Roentgenol. 164 (1995) 443–447

Gambee, M. J.: Vertebral artery thrombosis after spinal injury: case report. Paraplegia 24 (1986) 350–357

Garza-Mercado, R.: Traumatic extradural hematoma of the cervical spine. Neurosurgery 24 (1989) 410–414

Georgy, B. A., J. R. Hesselink: MR imaging of the spine: recent advances in pulse sequences and special techniques. Amer. J. Roentgenol. 162 (1994) 923–924

Giacobetti, F. B., A. R. Vaccaro, M. A. Bos-Giacobetti et al.: Vertebral artery occlusion associated with cervical

spine trauma. A prospective analysis. Spine 22 (1997) 283–287

Gundry, C. R., H. M. Fritts: Magnetic resonance imaging of the musculoskeletal system. Spine Clin. Orthop. Rel. Res. 138 (1997) 275–287

Jabre, A.: Subintimal dissection of the vertebral artery in subluxation of the cervical spine. Neurosurgery 29 (1991) 912–915

Kathol, M. H.: Cervical spine trauma. What's new? Radiol. Clin. N. Amer. 3 (1997) 507–532

Katz, R. C., L. Wilson, N. Fraser: Anxiety and its determinants in patients undergoing magnetic resonance imaging. J. Behav. Ther. exp. Psychiat. 25 (1994) 131

Kulkarni, M. V., C. B. McArdle, D. Kopanicky, M. Mauer, H. B. Cotler, E. F. Francis et al.: Acute spinal cord injury: MR imaging at 1,5T. Radiology 164 (1987) 837–843

Louw, J. A., N. A. Mafoyane, C. P. Neser: Occlusion of the vertebral artery in cervical spine dislocations. J. Bone Jt Surg. 72-B (1990) 679–681

Mascalchi, M., G. D. Pozzo, C. Dini, V. Zampes, M. D'Andrea, M. Mizzaie, F. Lolli et al.: Acute spinal trauma: prognostic value of MRI appearances at 0,5T. Clin. Radiol. 48 (1993) 100–108

Mirvis, S. E., F. H. Geisler, J. J. Jelinek, J. N. Joslyn, F. E. Gellad: Acute cervical spine trauma evaluation with 1,5T MR imaging. Radiology 166 (1988) 807–816

Olshaker, J. S., R. A. Barish: Acute traumatic cervical epidural hematoma. Ann. Emerg. Med. 20 (1991) 662–664

Parent, A. D., H. L. Harkey, D. A. Touchstone et al.: Lateral cervical spine dislocation and vertebral artery injury. Neurosurgery 31 (1992) 501–509

Pettersson, K., C. Hildingsson, G. Toolanen, M. Fagerland, J. Bjornebrink: Disc pathology after whiplash injury. A prospective magnetic resonance imaging and clinical investigation. Clin. Orthop. 338 (1997) 275–287

Quencer, R. M., R. P. Bunge, M. Egnor et al.: Acute traumatic central cord syndrome: MRI-pathologic correlation. Neuroradiology 34 (1992) 85–94

Reaney, S. M., M. S. Parker, S. E. Mirvis et al.: Abdominal aortic injury associated with transverse lumbar spine fracture – Imaging findings. Clin. Radiol. 50 (1995) 834–838

Rizzolo, S. J., M. R. Piazza, J. M. Cotler et al.: Intervertebral disc herniation complicating cervical spine trauma. Spine 16 (1991) 187–189

Ronnen, H. R., P. J. de Korte, P. R. Brink, H. J. van der Bijl, A. J. Tonino, C. L. Franke: Acute whiplash injury: Is there a role for MR imaging? A prospective study of 100 patients. Radiology 210 (1996) 93–96

Ross, J. S.: MR imaging of the cervical spine. Techniques for two- and three-dimensional imaging. Amer. J. Roentgenol. 159 (1992) 779–786

Saifuddin, A., H. Noordeen, B. A. Taylor, I. Bayley: The role of imaging in the diagnosis and management of thoracolumbar burst fractures: current concepts and a review of the literature. Skelet. Radiol. 25 (1996) 603–613

Schaefer, D. M., A. E. Flanders, J. L. Osterholm, B. E. Northrup: Prognostic influence of magnetic resonance imaging in the acute phase of cervical spine injury. J. Neurosurg. 173 (1992) 219–224

Schröder, R. J., T. Vogt, N. Hidajat et al.: Comparison of the diagnostic value of CT and MRI in injuries of the cervical vertebrae. Akt. Radiol. 5 (1995) 197–202

Schwartz, N., W. Buchinger, T. Gaudernak et al.: Injuries to the cervical spine causing vertebral artery trauma: case reports. J. Trauma. 31 (1991) 127–133

Shellock, F. G., S. Morisoli, E. Kanal: MR procedures and biomedical implants, materials, and devices: 1993 update. Radiology 189 (1993) 587–599

Shellock, F. G., H. Lipczak, E. Kanal: Monitoring patients during MR-procedures. Appl. Radiol. 24 (1995) 11–17

Silberstein, M., B. M. Tress, O. Hennessey: Prediction of neurologic outcome in acute spinal cord injury. The role of CT and MR. Amer. J. Neuroradiol. 13 (1992a) 1597–1608

Silberstein, M., B. M. Tress, O. Hennessey: Prevertebral swelling in cervical spine injury: Identification of ligament injury with magnetic resonance imaging. Clin. Radiol. 46 (1992b) 318–323

Taylor, A. R., W. Blackwood: Paraplegia in hyperextension cervical injuries with normal radiographic appearance. J. Bone Jt Surg. 30-B (1948) 245–248

Terk, M. R., M. Hume-Neal, M. Fraipont et al.: Injury of the posterior ligament complex in patients with acute trauma: evaluation by MR imaging. Amer. J. Roentgenol. 168 (1997) 1481–1486

Volle, E., J. Assheuer, J. P. Hedde, R. Gustorf-Aeckerle: Radicular avulsion resulting from spinal injury: assessment of diagnostic modalities. Neuroradiology 34 (1992) 235–240

Warner, J., K. Shanmuganathan, S. E. Mirvis, D. Cerva: Magnetic resonance imaging of ligamentous injury of the cervical spine. Emerg. Radiol. 3 (1996) 9–15

Watanabe, N., T. Ogura, K. Kimori, H. Hase, Y. Hirawasa: Epidural hematoma of the lumbar spine simulating extruded disk herniation: clinical, discographic, and enhanced magnetic resonance imaging features. A case report. Spine 22 (1997) 105–107

Weirich, S. D., H. B. Cotler, P. A. Narayana et al.: Histopathologic correlation of magnetic resonance image signal patterns in a spinal cord model. Spine 15 (1990) 630–638

8 Vascular Disorders of the Spinal Canal

A. Felber, S. Felber, H. Henkes, and D. Kuehne

Contents

▍Vascular Anatomy of the Spinal Cord

Knowledge of the normal vascular anatomy of the spinal cord is essential for understanding vascular disorders of the spinal canal.

Arterial Blood Supply

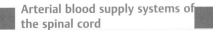

Arterial blood supply systems of the spinal cord

- Longitudinal system
- Horizontal system

The *longitudinal system* comprises the singular anterior spinal artery and the paired posterior spinal arteries. The spinal arteries arise from the vertebral arteries and the posterior inferior cerebellar arteries at the craniocervical junction. The anterior spinal artery is reinforced along the spinal canal by the anterior radicular arteries, and the posterior spinal arteries are reinforced by the posterior radicular arteries (*horizontal system*). On average there are 6 anterior and 11–16 posterior radicular arteries that are formed by the nervomedullary arteries. The nervomedullary arteries are supplied from arterial branches coming off the vertebral arteries and also, in the cervical region, from arterial branches coming off the deep cervical, the ascending cervical and the deep intercostal arteries, in the thoracolumbar region from branches derived from the intercostal and lumbar arteries, and in the sacral region from branches of the internal iliac artery. These radicular arteries are less prominent in the mid-thoracic cord. The anterior radicular artery in the thoracolumbar region is the artery with the largest caliber and is known as the *great radicular artery* or *artery of Adamkiewicz* (Adamkiewicz, 1882; Lazorthes *et al.*, 1973).

The *anterior spinal artery* courses in the anterior median fissure from the craniocervical junction to the filum terminale. Together with the anterior radicular arteries, the anterior spinal artery forms the anterior pial arterial plexus and, via segmental penetrating branches (sulcal arteries), supplies about 70 % of the spinal cord, including the corticospinal tracts and the gray matter but excluding the posterior horns (Friedman and Flanders, 1992). The sulcal arteries are arranged

in a centrifugal fashion and demonstrate no anastomoses with one another within the spinal cord (terminal arteries; Friedman and Flanders, 1992).

Together with the posterior radicular arteries, the paired *posterior spinal arteries* form a pial arterial plexus around the dorsal part of the spinal cord. This pial arterial plexus is divided by the denticulate ligament into a dorsal and lateral (vasa corona) pial plexus. Via deep penetrating branches from the dorsal and lateral pial plexus, the posterior spinal arteries supply about 30 % of the spinal cord, including the posterior horns and the dorsal columns (Fig. 8.**2**) (Friedman and Flanders, 1992). Here the penetrating branches are arranged in a centripetal fashion and demonstrate numerous anastomoses with each other.

In the region of the conus medullaris the anterior spinal artery anastomoses with the paired posterior spinal arteries to form an *arterial "basket"* (Lazorthes *et al.*, 1958, 1966, 1973; Manelfe, 1973; Lasjaunas and Berenstein, 1990). The blood supply to the filum terminale proceeds around the conus via this "basket" (Djindjian *et al.*, 1988).

The so-called *watershed zone* of the spinal cord is situated along the gray mater, between the centrifugal (anterior spinal artery) and the centripetal (posterior spinal arteries) penetrating branches (Friedman and Flanders, 1992).

Spinal Cord Veins

Drainage of the spinal cord into the epidural venous plexus is via an intrinsic and an extrinsic venous system.

Intrinsic venous system. Sulcal and horizontal veins are formed from a network of venous capillaries, which exhibit numerous interconnecting horizontal anastomoses and together form sulcal and horizontal veins. Together with transmedullary veins, they form a longitudinal venous plexus that follows the tracts of the gray and white matter.

Extrinsic venous system. The extrinsic system consists of the pial venous plexus, the longitudinal veins (anterior and posterior spinal veins) and the radicular veins. The pial venous plexus, which forms a network of numerous anastomoses on the surface of the spinal cord, connects the intrinsic perforating veins to a system of longitudinal venous anastomoses on the surface of the spinal cord (anterior and posterior spinal veins). The anterior and posterior spinal veins are interconnected by numerous anastomoses and have contact with the radicular veins. Usually (in 60 % of cases) the radicular veins penetrate the dura together with the nerve roots. The radicular veins can also penetrate the dura separately (Lasjaunias and Berenstein, 1990). Although the radicular veins have no valves, they usually display a narrowing at the point of penetration through the dura that assumes the function of an *antireflux valve* (Tadie *et al.*, 1979). Blood reaches the epidu-

ral venous plexus via the anterior and posterior radicular veins.

Epidural venous plexus. There is an extensive network of intercommunicating veins extending from the skull base to the sacrum, which forms the epidural venous plexus. The radicular veins flow either directly into the epidural venous plexus in the region of the neuroforamina or into the anterior epidural venous plexus via a dural pool. The anterior epidural venous plexus is primarily located in the upper cervical and lumbar segments (Rodesch *et al.*, 1992; Gelber *et al.*, 1992). The epidural venous plexus drains into the basivertebral venous plexus located in the vertebral bodies via the radicular veins in the region of the exit points of the foramina intervertebralia.

Spinal Hemorrhage

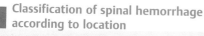

Classification of spinal hemorrhage according to location

- Spinal epidural hematoma.
- Spinal subdural hematoma.
- Spinal subarachnoid hemorrhage.
- Hematomyelia.

Spinal Epidural Hematoma

Etiology and Pathogenesis

Spinal epidural hematomas arise from hemorrhages of the epidural venous plexus. The hemorrhage is situated between the periosteum of the vertebral bodies and the dura mater. The hemorrhage usually extends over several segmental levels and has a predominantly dorsal location. The hemorrhage rapidly leads to compression of the dural sac and subsequently to symptoms of a transverse spinal lesion. It is an urgent indication for MRI (Cowie, 1992; Johnston, 1993).

The most common causes of a spinal epidural hematoma (Gingrich, 1965; Langmayr *et al.*, 1995) are:

- treatment with anticoagulants,
- trauma.

Hemorrhages from vascular malformations are rare.

Incidence, Age and Sex

Spinal epidural hematomas are rare. The age peak lies in the fifth decade of life (Langmayr *et al.*, 1995). Men are more commonly affected than women (Gingrich, 1965).

Clinical Presentation

Spinal epidural hematoma begins with intense, often radiating radicular pain at the level of the hemorrhage. Symptoms of a transverse spinal lesion appear within a few hours.

Diagnostics

MRI

An intraspinal, extramedullary, unenhancing space-occupying lesion appears on MRI, displaying a signal pattern which varies according to the age of the hematoma (Fig. 8.**1**). GRE sequences are most sensitive for detecting acute hemorrhages, being particularly sensitive to the susceptibility artifacts caused by deoxyhemoglobin. The hematoma itself usually demonstrates a biconvex configuration on sagittal and axial images (Bernsen *et al.*, 1988; Avrahami *et al.*, 1989; Di Lorenzo *et al.*, 1990) and, when located in the anterior part of the epidural space, shows the typical *curtain sign*, which, because of the Trolard membrane, does not transgress the midline (Fig. 8.**2**). Hematomas

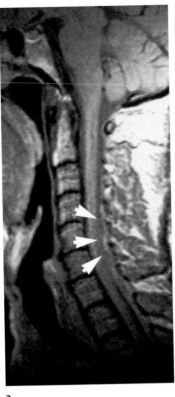

a

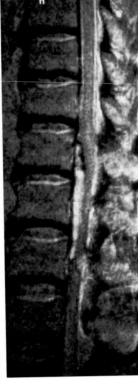

b

Fig. 8.1 a, b   Acute epidural hematoma:

a Acute epidural hematomas can be isointense with the spinal cord on the T1-weighted image (arrowheads).

b This patient was in a peracute stage. In this stage the hematoma can have such high water content that it appears predominantly hyperintense on the T2-weighted image, even at 1.5 tesla.

located in the posterior epidural space are not distinguishable by MRI from a subdural hematoma (Fig. 8.3). The surrounding meningeal structures exhibit increased contrast enhancement and may render differentiation from an abscess difficult, depending on the age of the hemorrhage.

Spinal Subdural Hematoma

Etiology and Clinical Presentation

The etiology of spinal subdural hemorrhage and its clinical presentation are similar to those of an epidural hematoma (Edelson, 1976; Russel and Benoit, 1983). Subdural hematomas are also an urgent indication for MRI (Mattle *et al.*, 1987). The hemorrhage is situated between the layers of the dura mater. Since major blood vessels are lacking below the foramen magnum, a spinal subdural hematoma is very rare. It mainly affects women (Cowie, 1992).

Diagnostics

MRI

Like the epidural hematoma, an unenhancing, intraspinal, extramedullary, space-occupying lesion appears on MRI (Fig. 8.4). Subdural hematomas have a concave configuration on the sagittal image and demonstrate an irregular shape on the axial image (Langmayr *et al.*, 1995).

MRI can only distinguish a subdural hematoma from an epidural hematoma when it is situated in the anterior subdural space and crosses the midline. As already pointed out, the surrounding meninges exhibit increased contrast enhancement and can render differentiation from an abscess difficult, depending on the age of the hemorrhage.

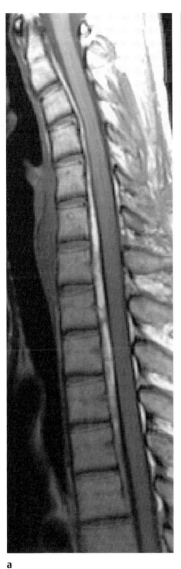

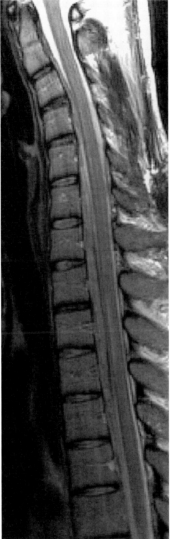

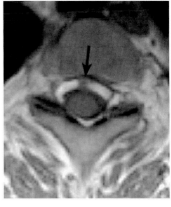

c

Fig. 8.**2 a–c** **Epidural hematoma in a 29-year-old female patient with known systemic lupus erythematosus.** Incomplete transverse spinal lesion of 10 days' duration:
a Sagittal T1-weighted image: Depiction of an intraspinal extramedullary space-occupying lesion extending anteriorly to the spinal cord from C1–T4 and appearing hyperintense. This corresponds to a subacute stage of hemorrhage.
b Sagittal T2-weighted image: The hemorrhage also appears slightly hyperintense on this image. Compression of the spinal cord secondary to edema at the level T1–T3.
c Transverse T1-weighted image: Typical curtain sign indicating that the hematoma is divided into two parts by the Trolard membrane (arrow). This finding is proof of the epidural location.

a   b

Spinal Subarachnoid Hemorrhage

Etiology and pathogenesis

The spinal subarachnoid hemorrhage is by far less common than the intracranial subarachnoid hemorrhage. The hemorrhage is located between the spinal cord (pia mater) and the arachnoid membrane.

The most common causes of a spinal subarachnoid hemorrhage are:

- intradural vascular malformations,
- tumors of the spinal cord.

A traumatic spinal subarachnoid hemorrhage is rare. Bleeding from a spinal aneurysm is also a rarity.

Clinical Presentation

Sudden back pain located at the level of the lesion, followed by bilateral sciatica and meningism, is characteristic for a spinal subarachnoid hemorrhage. Intense headache, nausea and vomiting usually ensue within minutes.

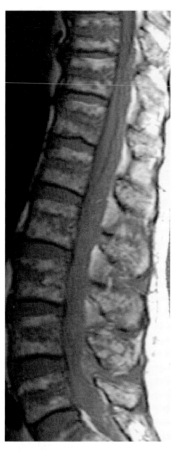

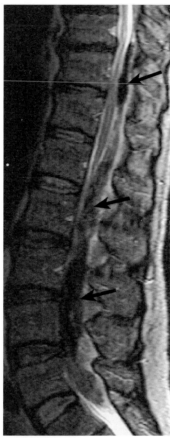

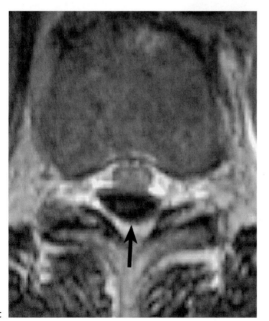

a

b

c

Fig. 8.**3 a–c** **Dorsal intraspinal hemorrhage in a 68-year-old patient under anticoagulant therapy.** Acute denervation at the L4 level on the left side with bilateral loss of quadriceps reflex and neurogenic bladder:

a Sagittal T1-weighted image: Presentation of an intraspinal space-occupying lesion, which appears isointense, corresponding to a hemorrhage in the acute stage.

b T2-weighted image: The hemorrhage appears hypointense and is associated with a massive intraspinal extramedullary space-occupying effect (arrow).

c Transverse T2-weighted image: Here the hemorrhage appears dorsal in the spinal canal, which makes any reliable differentiation between epi- and subdural location impossible.

Diagnostics

MRI

Like the acute intracranial subarachnoid hemorrhage, the acute spinal subarachnoid hemorrhage is difficult to diagnose by MRI. Distribution and, consequently, dilution of the blood in the CSF renders difficult the detection of susceptibility-type changes caused by deoxyhemoglobin and lead to loss of signal on the T2-weighted images. Detection is easier in the subacute phase due to the paramagnetic effect. The subarachnoid space appears hyperintense on the T1-weighted images. The picture of a spinal CNS siderosis appears during the chronic phase (Fig. 8.**5**).

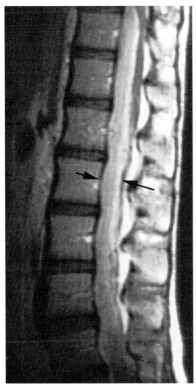

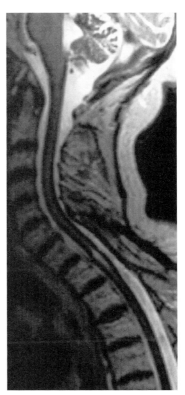

Fig. 8.**4 Rare case of a spinal subdural hematoma (arrows) without previous trauma.** Signal-intense presentation on the T1-weighted image due to methemoglobin in the subacute stage. Conus and cauda have been displaced dorsally. Sagittal T1-weighted image.

Fig. 8.**5 Idiopathic siderosis of the CNS.** Sagittal T2-weighted MRI of a 77-year-old female patient. The cervical cord displays the typical superficial reduction in signal due to the susceptibility artifact of the incorporated iron degradation products.

Hematomyelia

Hemorrhage into the spinal cord produces a severe clinical picture and usually extends over several segments.

Etiology and Pathogenesis

Possible causes of hematomyelia are:

- treatment with anticoagulants,
- trauma.

More commonly a tumor of the spinal cord, or a vascular malformation, is the root cause of an intramedullary hemorrhage.

Clinical Presentation

The neurological symptoms with an acute incomplete cord transection syndrome, often in the form of dissociated sensation, are clinically difficult to distinguish from an anterior spinal artery syndrome. Hematomyelia and spinal cord infarction are often clinically inseparable and in these cases MRI is of decisive importance.

Diagnostics

MRI

MRI reveals an intramedullary space-occupying lesion. The signal pattern is related to the age of the hemorrhage. A fresh hemorrhage appears hypointense on T2-weighted images (Fig. 8.**6**), being displayed most sensitively on GRE sequences due to the higher susceptibility for deoxyhemoglobin.

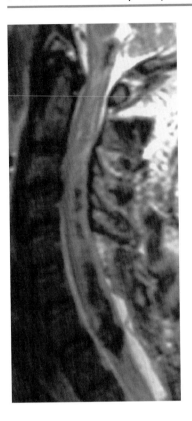

During the acute stage, the hemorrhage appears hyperintense on all weightings due to the paramagnetic effect of methemoglobin. In the chronic stage, hemosiderin causes signal loss, showing up primarily on the T2-weighted images.

◁ Fig. 8.**6 Acute intramedullary hematoma after a traffic accident.** A laminectomy to provide relief of symptoms has been performed at the cervicothoracic junction. The acute hemorrhage appears hypointense on the T2-weighted image due to deoxyhemoglobin.

Aneurysms

Spinal aneurysms are rare and usually appear in association with spinal arteriovenous malformations.

Etiology and Pathogenesis

Spinal aneurysms are circumscribed, saccular dilations of the spinal cord arteries or the feeding branches of the spinal cord arteries. Spinal aneurysms are usually associated with arteriovenous malformations (Biondi *et al.*, 1992).

Incidence, Age and Sex

Isolated spinal aneurysms are rare (Rengachary *et al.* 1993). The incidence is 20 % in patients with intramedullary arteriovenous malformations. The age peak lies between 10 and 40 years. There is no sex predilection (Biondi *et al.*, 1992).

Location

Spinal aneurysms with intramedullary arteriovenous malformations are located on the major feeding branches, which demonstrate, increased blood flow. The majority (70 %) is located on the anterior spinal artery (Biondi *et al.*, 1992). Unlike intracranial aneurysms, spinal aneurysms rarely appear at bifurcations (Rengachary *et al.*, 1993).

Clinical Presentation

In 85 % of cases spinal aneurysms become symptomatic secondary to a subarachnoid hemorrhage. In 15 % of cases they manifest themselves with symptoms of a progressive neurological deficit. Untreated spinal aneurysms usually lead to recurrent hemorrhage (Biondi *et al.*, 1992).

Diagnostics

MRI

To date it has not been possible to demonstrate spinal aneurysms by MRI. MRI is primarily intended to detect a subarachnoid hemorrhage or an intramedullary arteriovenous malformation or to exclude another cause for spinal symptoms. MRI therefore aids in reaching an indication for *spinal catheter angiography*. The diagnostic reliability of this new method of contrast-enhanced three-dimensional *MR angiography* is promising, but still requires evaluation.

Spinal Vascular Malformations

Vascular malformations of the spine and spinal cord are rare.

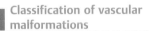
Classification of vascular malformations

- Vascular malformations of the spinal canal:
  - intramedullary arteriovenous malformations,
  - intramedullary cavernous hemangiomas (cavernomas),
  - perimedullary arteriovenous fistulae,
  - dural arteriovenous fistulae with medullary venous drainage.
- Vertebral body hemangiomas.
- Paravertebral arteriovenous malformations (located paraspinally or in the intervertebral foramen).

Arteriovenous Malformations

Etiology and Pathogenesis

Arteriovenous malformations are classified according to their location, their feeding arteries and their nidus (Manelfe, 1988; Anson and Spetzler, 1992):

Direct arteriovenous fistula. A direct arteriovenous fistula is an intradural, extramedullary arteriovenous shunt. The vascular malformation is situated outside the spinal cord and the pia mater. The arterial inflow is provided by the anterior spinal artery, draining directly into a dilated, elongated venous plexus of varying size. The fistula site demonstrates a high flow rate. The majority of direct arteriovenous fistulae are located anterior to the spinal cord at the level of the conus medullaris.

Arteriovenous malformations with nidus. Arteriovenous malformations with nidus display a perior intramedullary, compact vascular convolute (nidus) which is supplied by numerous arterial feeding vessels originating from the anterior spinal artery and the posterior spinal artery. Arteriovenous malformations drain into a dilated, arterialized perimedullary venous plexus and are usually located dorsally in the cervical cord.

Microarteriovenous malformations. A microarteriovenous malformation comprises a small nidus, which exhibits feeding and draining vessels, each of small caliber.

Metameric arteriovenous malformation. The metameric arteriovenous malformation is composed of complex vascular masses of intraspinal (intra- and extramedullary) and usually also extraspinal location. Metameric arteriovenous malformations are generally fed by multiple transdural arteries originating from several vertebral segments. The involvement of skin, vertebral body and spinal cord, with the constant exception of the dura, in the same segmental dermatome is known as *Cobb's syndrome* (metameric angiomatosis) (Cobb 1915).

Spinal dural arteriovenous fistula. The spinal dural arteriovenous fistula is an acquired lesion, as opposed to the congenital malformations mentioned above. The arteriovenous shunt is located in the spinal canal, most commonly in the lateral surface of the dura of the lower thoracic and upper lumbar spine. The feeding vessel is a radiculomeningeal artery and drainage is via dilated radicular veins. These draining veins often extend over many segments, are considerably dilated and display a tortuous course (Nichols *et al.*, 1992).

Incidence, Age and Sex

With an incidence of more than 60%, spinal dural arteriovenous fistulae are the most common. Arteriovenous malformations with nidus are more common than direct arteriovenous fistulae. Metameric arteriovenous malformations are rare.

Sometimes direct arteriovenous fistulae already become symptomatic in childhood.

The spinal arteriovenous malformation with nidus usually manifests itself in younger patients by a progressive neurological symptomatology or an intramedullary hemorrhage (Anson and Spetzler, 1992).

The spinal dural arteriovenous fistula primarily occurs in men between the fifth and eighth decade of life (Anson and Spetzler, 1992). Nearly 60% of all spinal dural arteriovenous fistulae occur spontaneously, while a history of trauma is noted in about 40% (Beaujeux *et al.*, 1992).

Location

The location varies with the type of arteriovenous malformation. More than one half of arteriovenous malformations are located in the thoracolumbar segment; 40% of arteriovenous malformations occur in the region of the cervical cord (Rodesch *et al.*, 1992).

Clinical Presentation

The symptoms and clinical course of arteriovenous malformations depend upon their angioarchitecture and location.

The most common symptoms are:
- paresis,
- sensory loss,
- bladder and bowel dysfunction,
- impotence.

Hemorrhage occurs in about 50% of cases (Rodesch *et al.*, 1992). Venous hypertension is decisive for the course of spinal symptoms. The arteriovenous malformation with nidus usually becomes manifest by symptoms of a transverse spinal lesion with an acute onset secondary to an intramedullary hemorrhage, while the direct arteriovenous fistula typically leads to a progressive neurological symptomatology (Anson and Spetzler, 1992).

Acquired spinal dural arteriovenous fistulae do not lead to hemorrhage, unlike intracranial dural arteriovenous fistulae. The symptoms (paresis, bladder dysfunction, bowel dysfunction, impotence, lumbago, or sciatica) are caused by the disturbed drainage of the spinal cord as a result of the arterialized epidural veins.

Diagnostics

MRI

The MRI diagnosis of a spinal arteriovenous malformation rests upon the detection of pathologic changes of the spinal cord and the depiction of dilated vessels in the spinal canal (Figs. 8.**7** and 8.**8**). The spinal cord changes can include congestive edema, which in the further course usually leads to a glial scar within the medulla and to local spinal cord atrophy, or intramedullary hemorrhage. Intramedullary contrast enhancement depends upon the age of the presenting lesion, given that congestive edema can enhance with contrast during the acute phase, as can the marginal areas of a fresh hemorrhage.

The dilated vessels in the spinal canal appear as punctiform hypointense areas on sagittal and transverse images, corresponding to the signal loss of fast-flowing blood. These findings should be distinguished from CSF pulsations. Depending on the flow rate, contrast medium may be detected within the vessel lumina. The new method of contrast-enhanced three-dimensional *MR angiography* can provide helpful details about the location of the arteriovenous shunt. Definite diagnosis and classification of a spinal arteriovenous malformation requires *catheter angiography* of the spinal vessels, which will also clarify the therapeutic options. The function of MRI and MR angiography is the targeted selection of patients requiring such a catheter angiography.

Cavernous Hemangiomas (Cavernomas)

Etiology and Pathogenesis

Spinal cavernomas are usually soft circumscribed formations consisting of small cavernous, dilated, blood-filled cavities strung together. These cavities are lined by endothelium and contain neither elastic fibers nor smooth muscle cells (Ogilvy *et al.*, 1992). Blood tends to develop a thrombosis in these

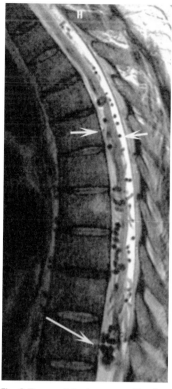

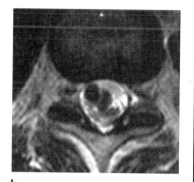

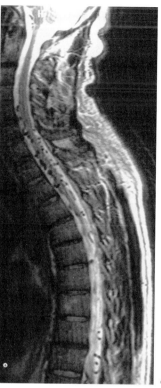

Fig. 8.**7a–c Arteriovenous fistula:**
a Perimedullary arteriovenous fistula ventral to the conus medullaris (long arrow).
b There is a convolute of massively dilated veins at the fistula site.

c The engorged veins (small arrows in **a**) are traceable up to the level of the foramen occipitale magnum.

sinusoids. Calcifications can appear in the cavernous matrix (Anson and Spetzler, 1993). Cavernomas are congenital vascular malformations; rare cases demonstrate a familial disposition.

Incidence, Age and Sex

Spinal cavernomas are rare. Purely exophytic cavernomas along the roots of the cauda equina are extremely rare. Most cavernomas become symptomatic between the third and sixth decade of life. There is a female predominance of 2:1 (Anson and Spetzler, 1993).

Location

Cavernomas can be located in the spinal cord. *Cavernomas of the vertebral body* can affect any vertebral body, occurring singularly or multilocularly.

The majority of *cavernomas of the spinal cord* are of purely intramedullary location. *Intramedullary cavernomas* can demonstrate an exophytic component. A purely exophytic location in the subarachnoid space or along the roots of the cauda equina is rare. Intramedullary cavernomas are located in the thoracic cord in slightly more than one half of cases (Ogilvy *et al.*, 1992). *Multilocular intramedullary cavernomas* are rare (Anson and Spetzler, 1993).

Clinical Presentation

Cavernomas of the vertebral body usually remain asymptomatic. However, extensive cavernomas of the vertebral body can lead to local pain or elicit radicular symptoms that are topographically related to the intervertebral foramen. Compression of the spinal cord can result from expansive cavernomas of the vertebral body.

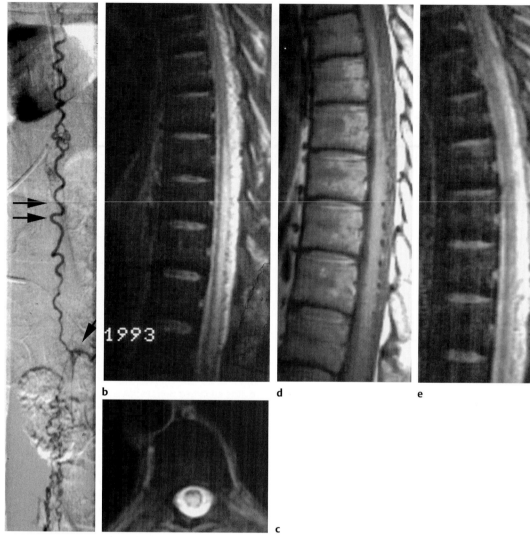

Fig. 8.8 a–e Arteriovenous fistula:

a Spinal catheter angiography using a sagittal beam projection with injection of the T10 segmental artery. The arteriovenous fistula appears in the foramen intervertebrale and is fed by the radiculomeningeal artery (arrow). The dilated and very tortuous pial drainage vein is recognizable dorsal to the spinal cord (double arrows).

b The typical triad of medullary edema, swelling of the spinal cord and dilated dorsal veins is apparent on the T2-weighted image.

c Characteristically, the edema is of a dorsal location on the axial T2-weighted image. Circumferential reduction of signal of the spinal cord periphery, regarded by some authors as a typical sign.

d The dilated vessels are also found on the sagittal T1-weighted image on the dorsal aspect of the spinal cord.

e Spinal cord swelling and edema are diminished on the T2-weighted image after endovascular obliteration of the fistula.

Intramedullary cavernomas usually produce sensorimotor symptoms with a progressive painful paraparesis. The clinical symptoms vary from slowly progressive neurological deficits to acute tetraplegia secondary to intramedullary cavernous hemorrhage (Bourgouin *et al.*, 1992).

Diagnostics

MRI

Cavernomas of the vertebral body are circumscribed lesions appearing hyperintense on all weightings and demonstrating an intense contrast enhancement. A fat-saturated T1-weighted sequence is helpful in discriminating from lipomas of the vertebral body.

Intramedullary cavernomas characteristically present in the form of so-called *popcorn lesions* (Fig. 8.**9**). This refers to circumscribed regions demonstrating a central mixed signal pattern resulting from blood degradation products at various stages and slow-flowing blood. The lesion is surrounded by a hypointense margin on T2-weighted images and on GRE sequences, corresponding to an impregnation with hemosiderin. Contrast enhancement varies, depending on the rate of blood flow and the degradation stage of the thrombosis in the cavernous cavities. If the MRI finding is not characteristic, then a catheter angiography is required to verify or rule out a spinal arteriovenous malformation. On detection of a spinal cavernoma, an MRI examination of the brain should be conducted to exclude further associated cavernomas (Bourgouin *et al.*, 1992).

Capillary Telangiectasia and Venous Malformations

Capillary telangiectasia of the spinal cord is often an incidental finding. At MRI they appear in the form of discrete punctate or linear hypointensities on T2-weighted sequences and do not demonstrate contrast enhancement. Venous malformations, like transparenchymal veins, are often seen as incidental findings in the cerebrum and, if detected at all, are rare in the spinal cord.

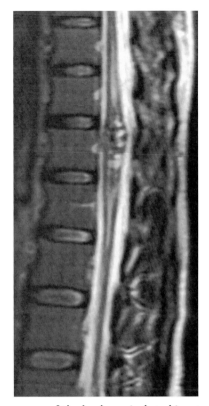

Fig. 8.**9** **Cavernoma of the lumbar spinal cord in an 18-year-old female patient with acute symptoms of a transverse spinal lesion.** The cavernoma appears on the sagittal T2-weighted image as a space-occupying lesion with hypo- and hyperintense components. Because of recent hemorrhage, the cranial and caudal parts of the adjacent spinal cord demonstrate central edema.

Both entities are an indication for spinal catheter angiography to rule out an underlying small spinal arteriovenous malformation.

Hemangioblastoma

Etiology and Pathogenesis

Hemangioblastomas of the spinal cord are densely vascular, nodular, circumscribed tumors, which may contain an intramedullary cyst. Hemangioblastomas are vascular tumors comprising thin-walled, tightly packed blood vessels (Silbergeld *et al.*, 1989). Multiple occurrences are suggestive of von Hippel–Lindau disease. This disorder is often combined with a retinal angiomatosis. Other associated tumors are also encountered and can be decisive for the life expectancy of the patients:

- pancreatic tumors,
- renal cell carcinomas,
- pheochromocytomas.

The von Hippel–Lindau disease is inherited by autosomal dominant transmission. The diagnosis may be regarded as certain if involvement of the eyes, CNS or visceral organs is found in one patient and at the same time a first-degree relative is also affected.

Incidence, Age and Sex

Hemangioblastomas are rare and account for 1–5 % of all spinal cord tumors. In over 80 % of patients the initial symptoms appear before the age of 40 years (Murota and Symon, 1989).

Location

Some 75 % of hemangioblastomas are of intramedullary location, and 10–15 % exhibit in-

tramedullary and extramedullary-intradural components. Extradural hemangioblastomas are rare (Avila *et al.*, 1993).

One-half of all hemangioblastomas are located in the thoracic cord, while 40 % are located in the cervical cord. A solitary occurrence is found in 80 % of hemangioblastomas.

Classification

Lindau tumors demonstrate a low tendency for growth and can recur after incomplete removal. The WHO classifies them as grade 1 tumors.

Clinical Presentation

The initial symptoms usually include sensory dysfunction, typically in the form of reduced depth perception (Murota and Symon, 1989). One-third of patients with a hemangioblastoma have von Hippel–Lindau disease. Hemangioblastomas have a slow growth and if untreated lead to para- or quadriplegia (Avila *et al.*, 1993).

Diagnostics

MRI

The majority of cases demonstrate a diffuse enlargement of the spinal cord, which appears hyperintense on T2-weighted, and isointense with the spinal cord on T1-weighted images. In addition, punctate hypointensities are revealed on all weightings, corresponding to the signal loss of fast-flowing blood in the elongated and dilated arterial feeding branches and draining pial veins. From 50–70 % of cases are associated with intramedullary cysts or a syrinx (Murota and Symon, 1989). The signal intensity of the cysts depends on the cystic contents. If it contains fluid similar to CSF, then there will be a corresponding signal intensity. If, however, the protein content of the fluid is higher, there will be T1 shortening, and thus signal enhancement, on the T1-weighted sequences. A high signal is virtually always found on the T2-weighted sequences. The signal on the T1-weighted sequences can be so strongly increased that the cyst becomes only poorly delineated from the spinal cord. The tumor nodule enhances intensely with contrast (Figs. 8.**10**–8.**14**). Contrast-enhanced three-dimensional *MR angiography* demonstrates a distinct tumor blush and can reveal arteriovenous shunt-

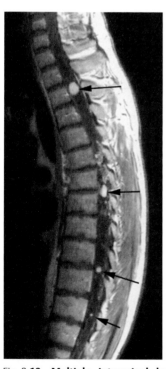

Fig. 8.**10 Multiple intraspinal hemangioblastomas in a 23-year-old patient with von Hippel–Lindau disease.** Multiple contrast-enhancing tumors (arrows) are apparent on the T1-weighted image after intravenous application of Gd-DTPA.

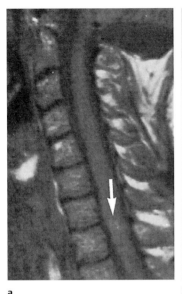
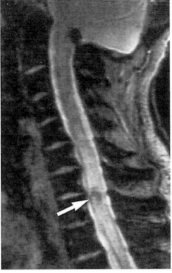
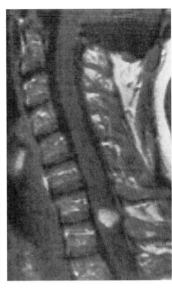

a   b   c

Fig. 8.**11 a–c Hemangioblastoma.** 50-year-old woman:

a T1-weighted plain image (SE; TR = 550 ms, TE = 25 ms): Slight enlargement of the cervical cord and a circumscribed, nodular signal enhancement at T1 (arrow). Postoperative image after surgery for a hemangioblastoma of the cerebellum.

b T2-weighted image (FFE; TR = 600 ms, TE = 20 ms, flip angle α = 10°): Cervicothoracic signal enhancement of C6–T3 representing edema or myelomalacia. Circumscribed nodular reduction in signal at T1, corresponding to the lesion on the T1-weighted image (arrow).

c After contrast application: Strong enhancement of the hemangioblastoma at T1.

ing. A spinal catheter angiography is required for exact presentation of the arterial feeding branches and the draining veins.

MRI can also be used for screening patients with von Hippel–Lindau tumors if they present without symptoms associated with CNS involvement. The lesions are often very small and demonstrate multiple distribution throughout the CNS. In individual cases they may only be detected by contrast application (Filling-Katz *et al.*, 1989; Silbergeld *et al.*; 1989).

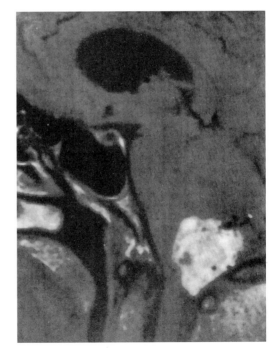

Fig. 8.**12 Hemangioblastoma in the region of the craniocervical junction.** Sagittal section after contrast application showing a patchy, yet on the whole strong, contrast enhancement of the tumor.

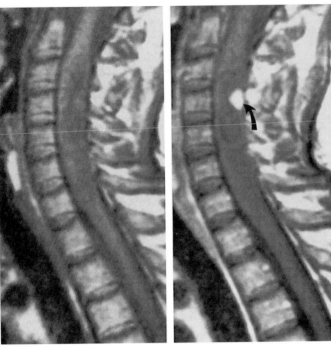
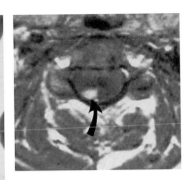

Fig. 8.**13 a–c** **Hemangioblastoma.** 49-year-old woman:

a Sagittal T1-weighted image (SE; TR = 680 ms, TE = 28 ms): Enlargement of the cervical cord between C2 and C7. Slight reduction in signal in this segment.

b After contrast application: Evidence of the tumor nodule displaying a strong homogeneous enhance-

ment (arrow). A cystic structure is also demarcated within the enlarged spinal cord and demonstrates signal intensity that is higher than that of CSF.

c Transverse section: The hemangioblastoma is situated eccentrically in the cyst wall (arrow).

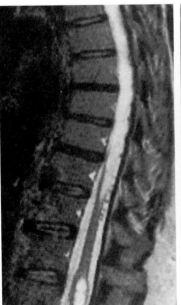
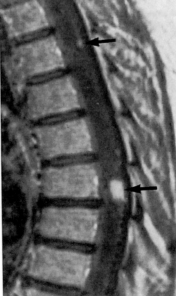

Fig. 8.**14 a–d** **Von Hippel-Lindau disease.** Apart from involvement of the CNS, retinal angiomatosis and renal carcinoma were also present. 59-year-old female patient:

a Sagittal T2-weighted section (SE; TR = 2100 ms, TE = 80 ms): Diffuse signal enhancement in the thoracic cord extending to include T10. Cyst at the level of L1.

b After contrast application: Enhancement in two hemangioblastomas at the levels T4 and T7. Diffuse enlargement of the spinal cord secondary to an extensive edema (arrows).

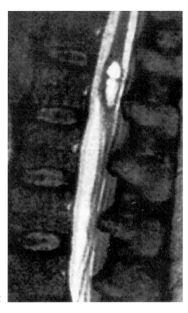

c

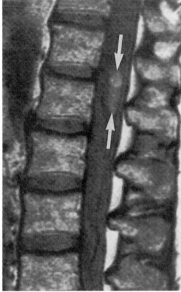

d

Fig. 8.**14 c–d**
c Sagittal T2-weighted section distal to Fig. **a** (SE; TR = 2100 ms, TE = 80 ms): The large cyst at the level of L1 displays marked signal enhancement and results in enlargement of the conus medullaris.
d T1-weighted image (SE; TR = 660 ms, TE = 25 ms): There is signal enhancement present (arrows), most likely due to methemoglobin secondary to previous hemorrhages into the hemangioblastoma cyst.

Spinal Cord Ischemia

A distinction is made between the following types of infarction secondary to spinal cord ischemia:

- arterial spinal cord infarction,
- venous spinal cord infarction.

Arterial Spinal Cord Infarction

Etiology and Pathogenesis

The arterial blood supply of the spinal cord is primarily based upon three longitudinal arteries:

- a singular anterior spinal artery,
- paired posterior spinal arteries (Yuh *et al.*, 1992).

The penetrating intramedullary branches of the anterior spinal artery are terminal arteries, whereas the intramedullary branches of the posterior spinal arteries demonstrate numerous anastomoses between each other. Therefore, an arterial spinal cord infarction is, in the majority of cases, an ischemia in the distribution of the anterior spinal artery. Ischemia in the distribution of the posterior spinal arteries is rare.

Spontaneous infarctions in the distribution of the anterior spinal artery are seen in patients with marked arteriosclerosis or an aneurysm or dissection of the aorta.

Rare causes of arterial spinal cord infarctions include (Friedman and Flanders, 1992; Mikulis *et al.*, 1992):

- syphilis,
- vasculitis,
- fibrocartilaginous emboli in the presence of disk herniation,
- cervical subluxation,
- hypotension,
- hematological disorders,
- pregnancy,
- diabetes,
- thrombophlebitis,
- trauma,
- tuberculosis.

Incidence, Age and Sex

Arterial spinal cord infarction is very rare. The reported age of the patients lies between 15 and 75 years (Friedman and Flanders, 1992).

Location

The most common locations are the lower thoracic cord and the conus medullaris, which are very vulnerable to impaired perfusion. The extent of the infarction can be limited to one segment or spread across several segments (Yuh *et al.*, 1992).

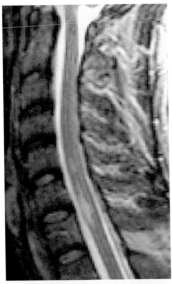

a

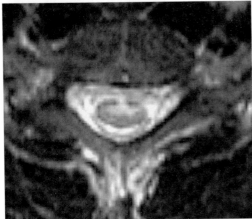

b

Fig. 8.15 a, b   Acute infarction in the territory of the anterior spinal artery. 36-year-old patient with apoplectiform pain in the cervical region and a bilateral triceps paralysis of 2 days' duration:

a Sagittal T2-weighted image: Presentation of an intramedullary lesion in the cervical cord at the level C5–C7.

b T2-weighted transverse section: Note that the lesion is located in the anterior part of the gray matter and corresponds to the distribution of the anterior spinal artery.

Clinical Presentation

The clinical symptoms are not uniform. The classic anterior spinal artery infarction presents with an acute or flaccid paraparesis or tetraparesis with or without burning or sharp pain. Characteristic is a dissociated sensation with loss of depth perception (Takahashi *et al.*, 1992).

Diagnostics

MRI

Swelling of the spinal cord is sometimes detectable in the acute phase. Signal enhancement is recognizable on the T2-weighted images centrally or in the anterior part of the spinal cord (Fig. 8.**15**). Contrast enhancement depends on the age of the spinal cord infarction. It usually occurs a few days after the acute episode and is still detectable for several weeks (Fig. 8.**16**) (Mikulis *et al.*, 1992; Takahashi *et al.*, 1992; Hirono *et al.*, 1992). Follow-up examinations usually reveal a circumscribed atrophy of the spinal cord, which appears hyperintense on the T2-weighted images (Fig. 8.**17**).

The most important differential diagnoses are:
- transverse myelitis,
- demyelinating disorders.

Venous Spinal Cord Infarction

Etiology and Pathogenesis

Little is known about venous ischemia and venous spinal cord infarction. The so-called *Foix–Alajouanine syndrome*, also referred to as subacute necrotizing myelitis, is supposed to correspond to an infarction secondary to venous stagnation and thrombosis (Rodesch *et al.*, 1992). Pathological studies in such cases reveal elongated, dilated veins, which are usually thrombosed. The result is characteristically a coagulation necrosis involving the gray and white matter (Enzmann, 1990).

Diagnostics

MRI

A spinal cord edema is observed on MRI, appearing hyperintense on the T2-weighted images and being located diffusely over the cross-section of

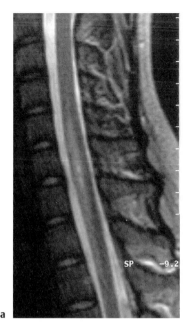

a

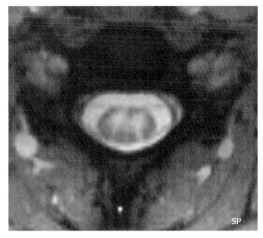

b

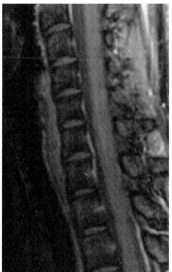

c

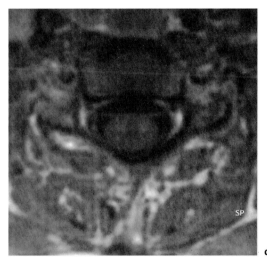

d

Fig. 8.16 a–d Acute anterior spinal artery infarction in a 20-year-old female patient. Rapidly developing tetraparesis, evidence of dissociated sensation and a more or less complete loss of depth perception. Possible inflammatory causes were excluded by lumbar puncture for CSF and by the disease course:

a Sagittal T2-weighted image: Signal enhancement in the anterior and middle section of the spinal cord at the level C4–T2. Slight enlargement of the spinal cord.

b Transverse section: Note the predominant involvement of the gray matter.

c Sagittal section after contrast application: Subtle linear barrier disruption in the C4–C7 segment.

d Transverse section after contrast application: Note the contrast enhancement in the gray matter, in particular at the level of the anterior horns.

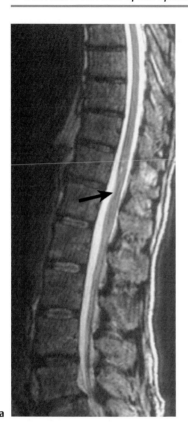

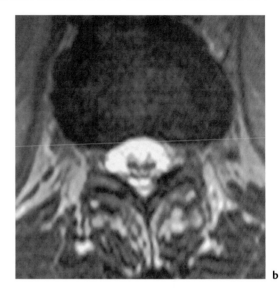

Fig. 8.**17 a, b Image following an anterior spinal artery infarction in a 75-year-old patient which occurred after surgery for a dissecting aortic aneurysm:**
a Circumscribed atrophy of the spinal cord with slight anterior retraction at T11/T12 (arrow).
b T2-weighted transverse section: The atrophy primarily involves anterior sections and includes the gray matter in particular.

the spinal cord. Dilated thrombosed vessels are also recognizable, coursing garland-like in the subarachnoid space, and which are diagnostically inseparable from a spinal vascular malformation.

On the other hand, it is a widely known fact that pathological spinal cord changes secondary to an arteriovenous malformation or a spinal dural arteriovenous fistula are usually attributable to venous congestive edema. The congestive edema is the result of venous hypertension or, less commonly, thrombosis in the draining veins.

Summary

■ The arterial blood supply of the spinal cord is based upon two systems:
  - longitudinal system,
  - horizontal system.

The *longitudinal* system comprises the singular anterior spinal artery and the paired posterior spinal arteries. The *horizontal* system comprises the anterior and posterior radicular arteries. Both systems are interconnected. The artery with the largest caliber is the artery of Adamkiewicz, which courses in the thoracolumbar region.

■ Together with the anterior radicular arteries, the *anterior spinal artery* forms the anterior pial arterial plexus and supplies via segmental penetrating branches about 70 % of the spinal cord, including the pyramidal tracts and the gray matter, but excluding the posterior horns. The arteries are arranged in a centrifugal fashion. Together with the posterior radicular arteries, the paired *posterior spinal arteries* form a pial arterial plexus around the dorsal part of the spinal cord from which the remaining 30 % of the spinal cord, including the dorsal columns and the posterior horns, are supplied. The vessels are arranged in an intramedullary centripetal fashion.

■ The *watershed zone* of the spinal cord is situated along the gray matter, between the centrifugal branches of the anterior spinal artery and the centripetal penetrating branches of the posterior spinal arteries.

■ *Venous drainage* into the epidural venous plexus is via an intrinsic and an extrinsic system. The *intrinsic system* consists of a network of venous capillaries that exhibit numerous interconnecting horizontal anastomoses and together form sulcal and horizontal veins. Together with transmedullary veins, these veins form a longitudinal venous plexus. The *extrinsic system* consists of the pial venous plexus, the longitudinal veins (anterior and posterior spinal veins) and the radicular veins. Blood reaches the epidural venous plexus via the anterior and posterior radicular veins.

■ The *epidural venous plexus* is an extensive network extending from the skull base to the sacrum. It is drained via the radicular veins in the region of the exit points of the foramina in tervertebralia into the basivertebral venous plexus located in the vertebral bodies.

■ *Spinal hemorrhage* can occur in the form of an epidural or subdural hematoma, a subarachnoid hemorrhage or a hematomyelia.

■ *Spinal epidural hematomas* arise from hemorrhages from the epidural venous plexus. They usually develop dorsally and extend over several segmental levels. The peak age is in the fifth decade of life. An intraspinal, extramedullary, space-occupying lesion is seen at MRI and demonstrates a biconvex configuration on axial and sagittal slice orientations. When located anteriorly, the hematoma does not transgress the midline, but rather is limited by the Trolard membrane. Hematomas located posteriorly are not distinguishable from a subdural hematoma. The signal intensity depends on the age of the hemorrhage.

■ *Subdural hematomas* develop between the layers of the dura mater. Since major blood vessels are lacking below the foramen magnum, a subdural hematoma is very rare. It mainly affects women. Subdural hematomas have a concave configuration on the sagittal image and demonstrate an irregular shape on the axial section. MRI can only distinguish a subdural hematoma from an epidural hematoma when it is situated anteriorly and crosses the midline.

■ The *spinal subarachnoid hemorrhage* is far less common than its intracranial counterpart. The most common causes are:
  - intradural vascular malformations,
  - tumors of the spinal cord.

Spinal subarachnoid hemorrhages are difficult to diagnose by MRI. Detection is easier in the subacute phase due to the paramagnetic effect of hemoglobin degradation products. The subarachnoid space appears hyperintense on the T1-weighted image. The clinical picture of a spinal CNS siderosis appears during the chronic phase.

■ *Hemorrhage into the spinal cord* is rare. It occurs secondary to treatment with anticoagulants or trauma. MRI reveals an intramedullary space-occupying lesion. The signal pattern is related to the age of the hemorrhage.

■ *Spinal aneurysms* are rare and usually appear in association with spinal arteriovenous malformations. They are circumscribed, saccular dilations of the spinal cord arteries and are located on the major feeding branches, which demonstrate in-

Summary

creased blood flow. The majority of aneurysms become symptomatic secondary to a subarachnoid hemorrhage. It is virtually impossible to demonstrate spinal aneurysms on account of their small size.

- Spinal vascular malformations are classified into:
  - intramedullary arteriovenous malformations,
  - intramedullary cavernous hemangiomas (cavernomas),
  - perimedullary arteriovenous fistulae,
  - dural arteriovenous fistulae with medullary venous drainage.
- *Arteriovenous malformations* are classified according to their location, their feeding arteries and their nidus. A *direct arteriovenous fistula* is an intradural, extramedullary arteriovenous shunt. The vascular malformation is located outside the spinal cord and the pia mater. The majority of direct arteriovenous fistulae are located anterior to the spinal cord at the level of the conus medullaris.
- *Arteriovenous malformations with nidus* display a peri- and/or intramedullary, compact vascular convolute which is supplied by numerous arterial feeding vessels originating from the anterior spinal artery and the posterior spinal artery.
- *Microarteriovenous malformations* comprise a small nidus that exhibits feeding and draining vessels, each of small caliber.
- The *metameric arteriovenous malformation* is composed of complex vascular masses of intraspinal and usually also extraspinal location. The involvement of skin, vertebral body and spinal cord in the same segmental dermatome is known as Cobb's syndrome.
- The *spinal dural arteriovenous fistula* is an acquired lesion. It is most commonly located in the lateral surface of the dura of the lower thoracic and upper lumbar spine. The feeding vessel is a radiculomedullary artery and drainage is via dilated radicular veins.
- With an incidence of more than 60%, spinal dural arteriovenous fistulae are the most common. They primarily occur in men between the 5th and 8th decade of life, more than one half of fistulae are located in the thoracolumbar segment. The MRI diagnosis of a spinal arteriovenous malformation rests upon the detection of pathologic changes of the spinal cord and

the depiction of dilated vessels in the spinal canal. The spinal cord displays a congestive edema with a corresponding bright signal on T2-weighted images. Individual cases may exhibit a slight enlargement. The congestive edema can enhance with contrast. The dilated vessels in the spinal canal appear as punctiform hypointense areas on the sagittal and transverse images.

- *Spinal cavernomas* are usually circumscribed formations consisting of small cavernous, dilated, blood-filled cavities strung together. Cavernomas tends to form thromboses and calcifications. *Intramedullary cavernomas* can demonstrate an exophytic component. Intramedullary cavernomas demonstrate a mixed signal pattern. The lesion is surrounded by a hypointense margin on T2-weighted images, corresponding to hemosiderin deposits. Depending on the extent of thrombosis, signal enhancement can be found on T1-weighted images. Cavernomas vary considerably in their degree of contrast enhancement.
- *Capillary telangiectasia of the spinal cord* is often an incidental finding. At MRI it appears in the form of punctate or linear hypointensities on T2-weighted images. They do not demonstrate contrast enhancement.
- *Hemangioblastomas of the spinal cord* are strongly vascularized, nodular, circumscribed tumors, which may contain an intramedullary cyst. Multiple occurrences are suggestive of von Hippel–Lindau disease. This disorder is often combined with a retinal angiomatosis. Furthermore, associated tumors are also encountered, including pheochromocytomas, renal cell carcinomas, and pancreatic tumors. At MRI an enlargement of the spinal cord is seen which appears hyperintense on T2-weighted, and isointense on T1-weighted images. In addition, punctate hypointensities are revealed on all weightings, corresponding to the signal loss of fast-flowing blood in the elongated and dilated arterial feeding branches and draining pial veins. The nodules enhance intensely, with small nodules only becoming recognizable after contrast application. Such pinhead-sized nodules are primarily associated with von Hippel–Lindau disease.

Summary

- An *arterial spinal cord infarction* is usually an ischemia in the distribution of the anterior spinal artery. The reported age of the patients lies between 15 and 75 years. The most common locations are the lower thoracic cord and the conus medullaris. The infarction can be spread across several segments. Swelling of the spinal cord is seen in the acute phase. Signal enhancement is recognizable on the T2-weighted images centrally or in the anterior part of the spinal cord. Subacute infarctions can enhance with contrast. Follow-up examinations usually reveal atrophy of the spinal cord.

- The *Foix–Alajouanine syndrome* corresponds to an infarction secondary to venous stagnation and thrombosis. Histology reveals elongated, dilated veins, which are usually thrombosed. A spinal cord edema is seen at MRI with a corresponding signal enhancement on the T2-weighted image, which extends diffusely over the entire cross-section of the spinal cord. Also recognizable on MRI are elongated and dilated vessels in the subarachnoid space rendering the disorder diagnostically inseparable from a spinal vascular malformation.

References

Adamkiewicz, A.: Die Blutgefäße der menschlichen Rückenmarksoberfläche. Sitzungsblatt D. K. Akad. D. Wissensch: in Wien Math. Natural Klasse 82 (1882) 101

Anson, J. A., R. F. Spetzler: Classification of spinal arteriovenous malformations and implications for treatment. BNI Quarterly 8 (1992) 2–8

Anson, J. A., R. F. Spetzler: Surgical resection of intramedullary spinal cord cavernous malformations. Neurosurg. 781 (1993) 446–51

Avila, N. A., T. H. Shaweker, P. L. Choyke, E. H. Oldfield: Cerebellar and spinal hemangioblastomas: evaluation with intraoperative gray-scale and color Doppler flow US. Radiology 188 (1993) 43–147

Avrahami, E., R. Tadmor, Z. Ram, M. Feibl, Y. Itzhak: MR demonstration of acute epidural hematoma of the thoracic spine. Neuroradiology 89 (1989) 89–92

Beaujeux, R. L., D. C. Reinzine, A. Casasco et al.: Endovascular treatment of vertebral arteriovenous fistulas. Radiology 183 (1992) 361–367

Bernsen, P. L. J. A., J. Haan, G. J. Vielvoje, K. M. J. Peerlinck: Spinal epidural hematoma visualized by magnetic resonance imaging. Neuroradiology 30 (1988) 280

Biondi, A., J. J. Merland, J. E. Hodes et al.: Aneurysms of spinal arteries associated with intramedullary arteriovenous malformations. I. Angiographic and clinical aspects. Amer. J. Neuroradiol. 13 (1992) 913–922

Bourgouin, P. M., D. Tampieri, W. Johnston et al.: Multiple occult vascular malformations of the brain and spinal cord: MRI diagnosis. Neuroradiology 34 (1992) 110–111

Cobb, S.: Hemangiomas of the spinal cord, associated with skin nevi of the same metamere. Ann. Surg. 62 (1915) 641–649

Cowie, R. A.: Acute spinal hematoma. In Findlay, G., R. Owen: Surgery of the Spine. Blackwell, Oxford 1992 (pp. 823–827)

Di Lorenzo, N., A. Rizzo, A. Fortuna: Spontaneous spinal epidural hematoma: preoperative diagnosis by MRI. Clin. Neurol. Neurosurg. 92 (1990) 357–359

Djindjian, M., A. Ribeiro, E. Ortega, A. Gaston, J. Poirier: The normal vascularization of the intradural filum terminale in man. Surg. radiol. Anat. 10 (1988) 201–209

Edelson, R. N.: Spinal subdural hematoma. In Vinken, P. J., G. W. Bruyn: Handbook of Clinical Neurology, Vol 26. Injuries of the Spine and Spinal Cord, Pt II. Elsevier, Amsterdam 1976 (pp. 31–38)

Enzmann, D. R.: Vascular diseases. In Enzmann, D. R., R. DeLaPaz, J. Rubin: Magnetic Resonance Imaging of the Spine. Mosby, St. Louis 1990 (pp. 510–537)

Filling-Katz, M. R., P. L. Choyke, N. J. Patronas et al.: Radiologic screening for von Hippel-Lindau disease: the role of GD-DTPA enhanced MR imaging of the CNS. J. Comput. assist. Tomogr. 13 (1989) 743–755

Friedman, D. P., A. E. Flanders: Enhancement of gray matter in anterior spinal infarction. Amer. J. Neuroradiol. 13 (1992) 983–985

Gelber, N. D., R. L. Ragland, J. L. Knorr: Gd-DTPA enhanced MRI of cervical anterior epidural venous plexus. J. Comput. assist. Tomogr. 16 (1992) 760–763

Gingrich, T. F.: Spinal epidural hematoma following continuing epidural anesthesia. Anesthesiology 29 (1968) 162–163

Hirono, H., A. Yamadori, M. Komiyama et al.: MRI of spontaneous spinal cord infarction: serial changes in gadolinium-DTPA enhancement. Neuroradiology 34 (1992) 94–97

Hurst, R. W., R. I. Grossman: Peripheral spinal cord hypertensity on T2-weighted MR images: a reliable imaging sign of venous hypertensive myelopathy. Amer. J. Neuroradiol. 21 (2000) 781–787

Johnston, R. A.: The management of acute spinal cord compression. J. Neurol. Neurosurg. Psychiat. 56 (1993) 1046–1054

Langmayr, J. J., M. Ortler, A. Dessl, K. Twerdy, F. Aichner, S. Felber: Management of spontaneous extramedullary hematomas: results in eight patients after MRI diagnosis and surgical decompression. J. Neurol. Neurosurg. Psychiat. 59 (1995) 442–447

Lasjaunias, P., A. Berenstein: A Surgical Neuroangiography, Vol. 3. Functional Vascular Anatomy of Brain, Spinal Cord and Spine. Springer, Berlin 1990 (pp. 15–87)

Lazorthes, G., H. Poulhès, G. Bastide, J. Roulleau, A. R. Chancholle: La vascularisation artérielle de la moelle. Neurochirurgie 4 (1958) 3–19

Lazorthes, G., A. Gouazè, G. Bastide, J. H. Soutoul, O. Zadeh, J. J. Santini: La vascularisation artérielle du renflement lombaire. Etude des variations et supléances. Rev. neurol. 114 (1966) 109–122

Lazorthes, G., A. Gouazè, R. Djindjian: Vascularisation et circulation de la moelle épinière. Masson, Paris 1973

Manelfe, C.: Vascular anatomy of the spinal cord: angiographic study: 338 Int. Congress. Radiol. Except. Med. 1 (1973) 377–383

Manelfe, C.: Imaging of the Spine and Spinal Cord. Raven, New York 1989 (pp. 565–597)

Mattle, H., J. P. Sieb, M. Rohner, M. Mumenthaler: Nontraumatic spinal epidural and subdural hematomas. Neurology 37 (1987) 1351–1356

Mikulis, D. J., C. S. Ogilvy, A. McKee et al.: Spinal cord infarction and fibrocartilagenous emboli. Amer. J. Neuroradiol. 13 (1992) 155–160

Murota, T., L. Symon: Surgical management of hemangioblastomas of the spinal cord: a report of 18 cases. Neurosurgery 25 (1989) 699–708

Naidich, T. P., D. G. McLone, D. C. Harwood-Nash: Vascular malformations. In Newton, T. H., D. G. Potts: Modern Neuroradiology, Vol 1: Computed Tomography of the Spine and Spinal Cord. 1983; 397–400

Nichols, D. A., D. A. Rufenacht, C. R. Jack Jr., G.Forbes: Embolization of spinal dural arteriovenous fistulas with polyvinyl alcohol particles: experience in 14 patients. Amer. J. Neuroradiol. 13 (1992) 933–940

Ogilvy, C. S., D. N. Louis, R. G. Ojeman: Intramedullary cavernous angiomas of the spinal cord: clinical presentation, pathological features, and surgical management. Neurosurgery 31 (1992) 219–230

Rengachary, S. S., D. A. Duke, F. Y. Tsai, P. J. Kragel: Spinal artery aneurysm: case report. Neurosurgery 33 (1993) 125–130

Rodesch, G., P. Lasjaunias, A. Berenstein: Embolization of spinal cord arteriovenous malformations. Riv. Neuroradiol. 5 (1992a) 67–92

Rodesch, G., P. Lasjaunias, A. Berenstein: Functional vascular anatomy of the spine and cord. Riv. Neuroradiol. 2 (1992b) 63–66

Russel, N. A., B. G. Benoit: Spinal subdural hematoma. A review. Surg. Neurol. 20 (1983) 133–137

Silbergeld, J., W. A. Cohen, K. R. Maravilla et al.: Supratentorial and spinal cord hemangioblastomas: gadolinium-enhanced MR appearance with pathologic correlation. J. Comput. assist. Tomogr. 13 (1989) 1048–1051

Tadie, M., J. Hemet, C. Aaron, C. Bianco: Le dispositif protecteur anti-reflux des veines de la molle. Neurochirurgie 25 (1979) 28–30

Takahashi, S., T. Yamada, K. Ishii et al.: MRI of anterior spinal artery syndrome of the cervical spinal cord. Neuroradiology 35 (1992) 25–29

Yuh, W. T. C., E. E. March, A. K. Wang et al.: MR imaging of spinal cord and vertebral body infarction. Amer. J. Neurroradiol. 13 (1992) 145–154

9 Functional Analysis and Surgery of the Spine in an Open MR System

P. Hilfiker and J. F. Debatin

Contents

Excellent soft tissue contrast and high spatial resolution combined with multiplanar three-dimensional imaging are the characteristic features of MRI. By using different weightings, inherent signal intensities allow CSF to be distinguished from the spinal cord and nerve roots from intervertebral disks without the application of a contrast medium. The most complex of morphological relationships are comprehensively displayed with the aid of three-dimensional acquisitions. Because there is no radiation load, examinations can also be repeated any number of times. It is therefore not surprising that MRI has been able to establish very quickly such a significant position in spinal diagnostics.

Soft- and hardware innovations over recent years now allow images to be obtained in real time (Debatin *et al.*, 1998). In combination with the increasing availability of open-configuration scanners, the high temporal resolution of the image acquisition allows, on the one hand, functional examinations to be carried out for the entire musculoskeletal system (Schenck *et al.*, 1995), as well as real-time guidance of minimally invasive interventions (Jolesz and Kikinis, 1995; Lufkin, 1995). As this chapter will show, both aspects are of direct relevance to the spinal column.

Open Configured MR Systems

Two goals are pursued with the open construction of MR systems:

- improved access to the patient during image acquisition (Lenz and Dewey, 1995),
- the patient should be allowed more freedom of movement during the examination.

Furthermore, sufficient room must be available for instruments (surgery) or for positioning aids (functional examinations).

Open-configuration scanners are primarily judged by the strength of the "main magnet," which generates the static magnetic field and is the deciding factor for the type of system. In this respect, it should be borne in mind that the signal-to-noise ratio is proportional to the field strength. The signal in a 1.5 tesla environment is therefore three times higher than at 0.5 tesla. The gradient coils used determine the degree of spatial resolution and the rate of data acquisition. High-performance gradients have so far only been used in high-field systems. Furthermore, the systems also differ with respect to their radio-frequency coils (RF coils) for transmission and reception of the MR signal. As regards the "gap," systems are available with a vertical patient access and others with a horizontal access. The currently commercially available open MR systems can be divided into three categories.

> **Categories of open MR systems**
>
> - Closed high-field system with a wide short-bore magnet (Example: 1.5 tesla Gyroscan ACS-NT).
> - Open mid-field system with a vertical access (Example: 0.5 tesla Signa SP).
> - Open low-field system with a horizontal access (Example 0.2 tesla Magnetom Open).

Furthermore, there are numerous other systems whose description would be beyond the scope of this chapter. The open MR systems can also be combined with other systems, such as a fluoroscopy unit or an ultrasound apparatus, to form what are known as "hybrid units."

The different systems have their various advantages and disadvantages. High-field systems, for example, allow better image quality at a higher acquisition rate. On the other hand, access to the patient is markedly poorer with high-field systems than with the open mid- and low-field systems. This makes interactive operations difficult in the high-field system. Low-field systems allow better access and more freedom of movement, yet at the price of a markedly reduced image quality and, above all, a clearly restricted temporal resolution. The horizontal gap usually associated with the majority of low-field systems is clearly inferior to the vertical access as far as freedom of movement for the patient and the interventionalist is concerned.

The mid-field system cited above was designed as a dedicated interventional MR system (Fig. 9.**1**).

The system is provided with a vertical, 58-cm-wide gap between the coils of the main magnetic field and there is enough room for direct access to the patient as well as for freedom of movement for functional examinations. There are two liquid crystal monitors mounted in the gap on to which the acquired MR images are projected (Fig. 9.**2**).

It is not possible to use volume coils due to the open construction of the MR system. Signal transmission and reception are accomplished by flexible transmitter and receiver coils of various sizes (Fig. 9.**3**).

To depict the spine, a homogenous high-frequency field is generated using a butterfly coil with two opposing elements (attached anteriorly and posteriorly onto the patient). Care should be taken that the high-frequency field is not parallel to the B_0 field when the patient is seated. The image quality achieved in this way lies between that of high- and low-field systems. Spatial resolution is sufficient for a comprehensive diagnostic work-up of the spinal column.

An open mid-field system (Signa SP, GE Medical Systems) was installed in the MR Center of the University Hospital of Zurich in autumn 1995. The practical knowledge reported in this chapter is based primarily on our experience gained with this system.

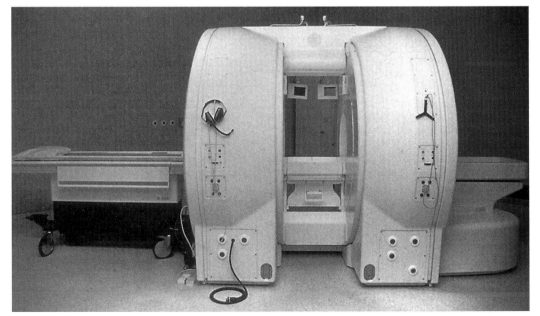

Fig. 9.**1 Open superconducting interventional 0.5 tesla MR system** (Signa SP, General Electrics). Between the two magnets that induce the main magnetic field is a gap 58 cm wide offering room for additional installations or free access to the patient during interventions.

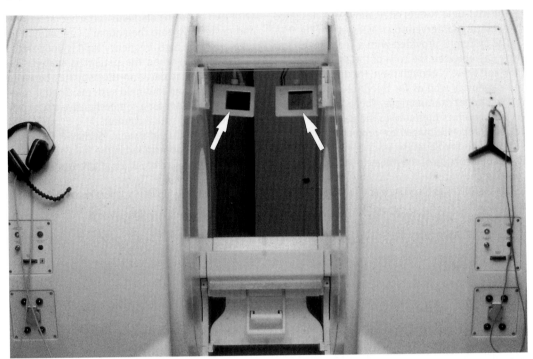

Fig. 9.2 Detail picture of the open MRI scanner. The latest image data are conveyed to the examiner via two LCD monitors (arrows), e.g. for the intervention guidance. The examiner can communicate with the patient directly from the control desk via headphones or, during interventions, the radiologist with assistants outside the scanning room.

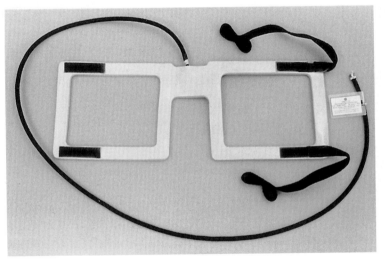

Fig. 9.3 Butterfly coil required for transmission and reception. The coil is attached to the patient over the site to be examined and connected to the magnet via a cable.

Functional Analysis of the Spine

Functional studies of the spine are performed for a large number of disorders, including degenerative diseases. Compression of the spinal cord can develop secondarily to degenerative diseases, resulting in their final stage in cord atrophy and producing the clinical picture of cervical myelopathy (Kunze and Arlt, 1991). Functional examinations, however, have also proven themselves in inflammatory diseases of the spine, as in for example rheumatoid arthritis (Roca *et al.*, 1993) and trauma-related disorders (Mirvis *et al.*, 1988; Rothhaupt and Liebig, 1994).

All available imaging techniques, including myelography, CT and MRI, have already been studied with regard to their suitability for the assessment of spinal function (Muhle *et al.*, 1995). MR examinations were usually performed in closed systems, simulating motion sequences or changes in posture with mechanical aid appliances (such as non-metallic, MR-compatible positioning devices) (Naegele *et al.*, 1992). However, all of these studies were of a static nature, i.e. spinal morphology was compared in at least two or several static conditions. Only fluoroscopy has hitherto allowed demonstration of the actual dynamic sequence of motion and the pathological aspects arising from this. Limited contrast and problems of overlapping, however, considerably restrict the use of fluoroscopy for the functional assessment of the spinal column, even if myelographic contrast media is applied (Wildermuth *et al.*, 1997).

Given the use of fast data acquisition strategies, examinations using the open MRI, on the other hand, allow the presentation of dynamic motion sequences with the aid of tomographic data, in any slice orientation and with an inherently high soft-tissue contrast. In addition, the vertical type of gap allows the examination of the patient in both the seated and standing positions.

Examination of the Spine in the Seated Position

There are a few precautions to be taken in the interests of optimum image quality when examining the spine by MRI in the seated position. GRE sequences should be used because of their shorter acquisition time and low sensitivity to field inhomogeneities. In order to minimize arbitrary patient movements and to prevent coil movements relative to the spine, the patient should be secured as well as possible in a rigid corset or on a special chair (Fig. 9.**4**).

Only those movements relevant to the functional examination should be allowed. The examination parameters, such as phase encoding in the craniocaudal direction, field of view and image matrix, must be adjusted to individual needs. By taking these aspects into consideration, the lumbar spine can be comprehensively displayed in the seated position in high image quality (Schoenenberger *et al.*, 1996).

Intervertebral Disk Height in Relation to the Time of Day and Examination Position

Assessment of intervertebral disks is often based on their height, which is subject to change during the course of the day, however, and is above all dependent upon position. Since the majority of patients have hitherto only been examined lying down, these aspects were only of minor consequence. In order to quantify these interrelations, which may well be of some significance in the assessment of functional MR images, the height as well as the proton density (as an indication of the water content) of lumbar intervertebral disks were assessed over the course of the day in 10 healthy volunteers in the sitting and lying positions (Schoenenberger *et al.*, 1996; Duwell *et al.*, 1996).

There was a marked reduction in disk height throughout the day, especially in the seated position. The most conspicuous difference in height was detected in the L4/L5 segment (0–2 mm). Interestingly, the proton density of the interverte-

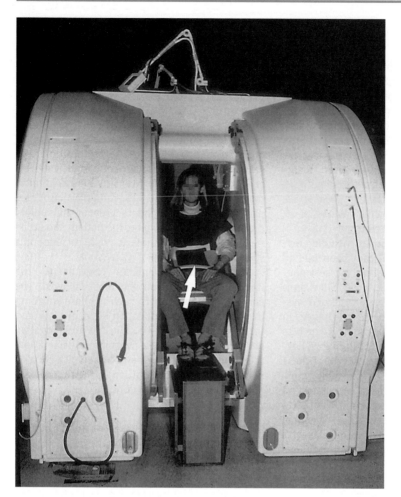

Fig. 9.**4** **Examination of the lumbar spine in the seated position.** The vertical part of the butterfly coil is well visible (arrow).

bral disks did not demonstrate any significant differences at the various times of day. Yet, on the other hand, the transition from the lying to the seated position was characterized by a considerable reduction in proton density (Fig. 9.**5**).

Considering these results, two aspects appear to influence disk elasticity:

- slow morphological changes within the disk during the course of the day,
- fast changes resulting from fluid content displacements when position is altered (Duwell *et al.*, 1996).

The second aspect deserves particular attention when assessing examinations of the spine in the seated position.

Functional MR Myelography of the Lumbar Spine

Stenosis of the spinal canal, the lateral recesses and the neuroforamina are usually indications of degenerative changes of the spinal column, which generally get worse in the course of ageing (Andersson and McNeill, 1992; Hasegawa *et al.*, 1995). These stenoses can appear at several segmental levels. Their exact location and characterization are of great importance prior to initiating therapy, especially before performing decompressive surgery (Bell and Ross, 1992).

Even though it is possible to demonstrate the spinal canal comprehensively using a conventional closed MR system, many surgeons still prefer conventional myelography for preoperative

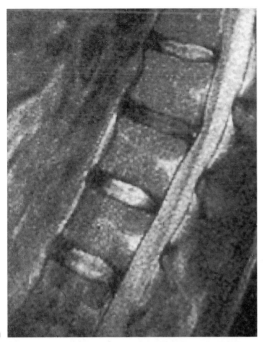

a

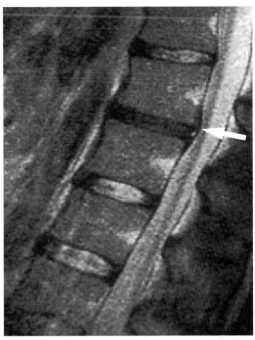

b

Fig. 9.**5 a, b** **T2-weighted sagittal images of the lumbar spine:** Image on the left (**a**) acquired at 9 a.m. and the image on the right (**b**) at 6 p.m. The L2/L3 intervertebral disk is dehydrated, the inferior plate of L2 displays a small posterior spondylophyte (arrow). The L3/L4 and L4/L5 disks have lost 2 mm in height during the course of the day.

planning, especially for patients with severe scoliosis, implants, or if an important functional component is expected (Jeanneret and Forster, 1993). For this purpose, conventional myelograms are obtained in different functional positions. The fact that the diameters of the spinal canal and neuroforamina are dependent upon position is given consideration by performing measurements in different positions (Schumacher, 1986; Mayoux-Benhamon *et al.*, 1989). Although indispensable for conventional myelography, the intradural application of contrast medium is considered unpleasant by the majority of patients and subsequently leads to a considerable headache in up to 75 % of those examined (Peterman, 1996). Functional MR myelography in the open MR system is just as capable of obtaining the same diagnostic information for the surgeon, yet in a completely non-invasive manner. This has been documented in a recently concluded study (Fig. 9.**6**) (Wildermuth *et al.*, 1997).

The lumbar spines of 30 patients were subject to functional studies before surgery, both by using conservative myelography and in the open MR system (Wildermuth *et al.*, 1997). Sagittal T2-weighted SE sequences were acquired for functional MRI examinations in the lying and seated positions (flexion and extension views) using the following parameters:

- TR = 3000 ms, TE = 85 ms,
- echo train length 8,
- bandwidth 16 kHz,
- slice thickness 5 mm with a slice increment of 1.5 mm,
- field size 20 cm,
- 256 × 256 matrix.

Three excitations were averaged. Using the MRI images, the largest sagittal diameter of the spinal canal, on the one hand, and the size of the neuroforamina using electronic measuring points, on the other, were measured from the imaged disk levels of the lumbar spine.

Comparison with data obtained from conventional myelographs produced a good correlation for the sagittal spinal canal diameters (correlation

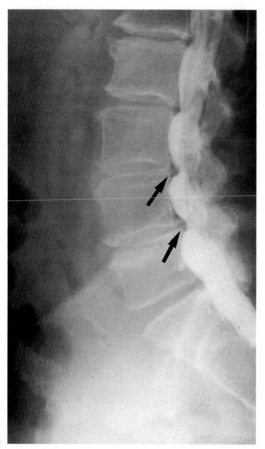

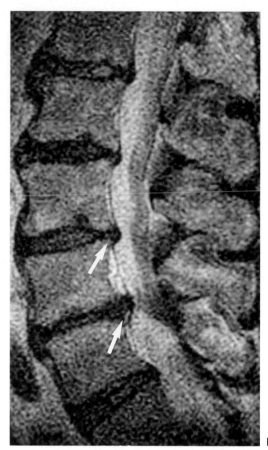

Fig. 9.**6 a, b** **Examination of the lumbar spine in the lying position.** The multisegmental protrusions with narrowing of the dural sac (arrows) are visible both on conventional myelography and on the median sagittal T2-weighted image:

a Conventional myelography.
b Sagittal T2-weighted image.

quotient r = 0.94). It was demonstrated that the diameter of the spinal canal varies only little during different types of movement, at least in a symptomatic orthopedic patient population. This result is all the more surprising since in a preceding study on healthy volunteers considerable differences in spinal canal width were shown to be related to movement (Schmid *et al.*, 1997) (Fig. 9.**7**).

Increase in volume of the ligamentum flavum during extension resulted in a significant reduction in the cross-sectional area of the spinal canal, especially at the level of the intervertebral disk. The discrepant results between healthy volunteers and orthopedic patients are most probably

due to the limited mobility and immobile herniations without segmental instability of the patients.

The qualitative measurements of the size of the neuroforamina on MR images during different functional states produced results that were examiner-dependent ($x = 0.62$). Here too, there were considerable discrepancies between patients and volunteers with regard to the degree of dependency of the measurements on function. While the values of the patients remained unchanged, the volunteers demonstrated marked reductions in neuroforamen cross-section in the extension position. This was due to bulging of the intervertebral disk, increase in volume of the liga-

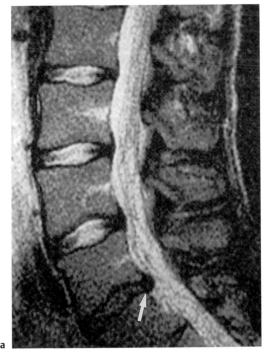

a

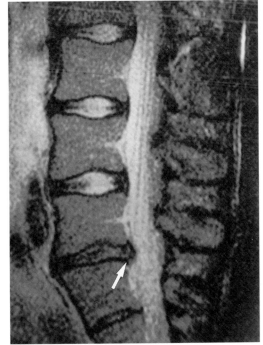

b

Fig. 9.**7 a, b** **Median sagittal plane through the lumbar spine.** T2-weighted images. Healthy volunteer. In comparison with the upright flexed position, protrusion of the intervertebral disk occurs at the L5/S1 level (arrows) in the upright extended position:

a Upright extended position.
b Upright flexed position.

mentum flavum and reduction of the craniocaudal diameter of the bony neuroforamen (Fig. 9.**8**).

In comparison with conventional myelography, functional MR images were regarded to be of particular advantage for demonstrating the course of the nerve root through the neuroforamina.

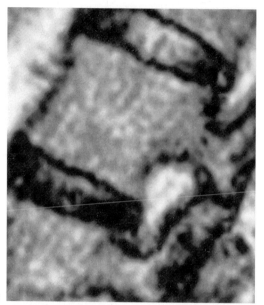
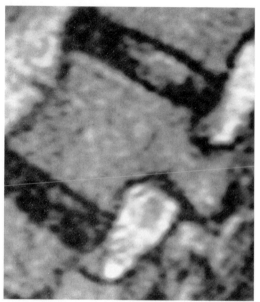

a

b

Fig. 9.**8 a, b** **Parasagittal plane through the neu-roforamen of the lumbar spine.** Healthy volunteer. Marked reduction in the neuroforamen cross-section in the extension position as compared with the neutral position. Bulging of the intervertebral disk, an increase in volume of the ligamentum flavum and a reduction of the craniocaudal diameter of the osseous neuroforamen cause this:

a Extension position.
b Neutral position.

MR-Guided Spinal Surgery

The availability of open MR systems allows the use of MR imaging for the guidance and monitoring of minimally invasive operations. The majority of these procedures are performed on outpatients under local anesthesia. The possibilities of MR-supported guidance and monitoring not only improve safety and accuracy of current interventions, but also provide a basis for the implementation of new minimally invasive techniques. Multiplanar imaging capabilities and temperature sensitivity of the MR imaging experiment have turned out to be particularly helpful aspects of MRI, in addition to its excellent soft-tissue contrast. The former allows the optimization of the percutaneous approach, while with the latter the energy propagation of thermosensitive applicators can be monitored and regulated.

With the introduction of fluoroscopy and CT, a large number of open surgical operations soon found themselves replaced by minimally invasive techniques. This was an important contribution to cost saving, on the one hand, and reducing risks, on the other. With the introduction of open MR systems it was merely the next logical step that the advantages of MR imaging should be exploited for the guidance and monitoring of minimally invasive interventions.

All-round visualization of the instruments within the body relative to the surrounding tissues is a prerequisite for the safe and successful implementation of MR-guided operations. The instruments must be easy to identify on the image and, in particular, remain trackable throughout the whole duration of the operation. An ideal method should clearly contrast the instrument against the tissue (contrast difference) and at the same time enable high spatial resolution to allow an exact placement of the instruments even in the smallest of target areas.

Passive visualization. Passive visualization refers to any technique that makes an instrument visible with the aid of normal image processing (Ladd, 1998). Today, the utilization of susceptibility artifacts is the most common passive visualization method in use (Fig. 9.**9**) (Frahm *et al.*, 1996).

This technique was primarily used for MR-guided biopsies (van Sonnenberg *et al.*, 1988), although it also finds use in vascular interventions for visualizing guide wires and catheters (Koechli *et al.*, 1994).

Combining it with an optical tracking system can considerably extend the possibilities of passive visualization. The Signa SP MR system has an integrated stereotactic puncture system with spatial orientation for simplifying percutaneous interventions (Flashpoint 5000; Image Guided Technologies, Boulder, USA) (Fig. 9.**10**).

This system consists of two main components:
- three infrared cameras with a viewing angle of 70° mounted on the connecting element between the two magnets 83 cm above the isocenter,
- a "needle handle" on which two or three infrared emitting diodes (LEDs) are located.

With the aid of the signals received by the infrared sensors, the position and orientation of the instrument, which is contained within the needle handle and inserted percutaneously, are calculated relative to the surrounding tissue depicted on the MR images. Once the position has been calculated, the acquisition of the subsequent MR slices can be interactively controlled. The prerequisite for the correct functioning of this procedure is the straight course of the percutaneously introduced instrument. Even small deflections of the needle can lead to considerable errors in calculating the position of the needle tip. For this reason, the computer calculation should always be verified by visualizing the signal loss caused by the instrument (Fig. 9.**11**) (Steiner *et al.*, 1996).

Active visualization. Active visualization refers to the positioning of the instrument using a signal reception from a radio-frequency receiver coil incorporated directly into an instrument (Ackermann *et al.*, 1986; Dumoulin *et al.*, 1993). This methodology is referred to in the literature as MR tracking (Leung *et al.*, 1995a, b). The coils can also be integrated in a miniaturized form into the

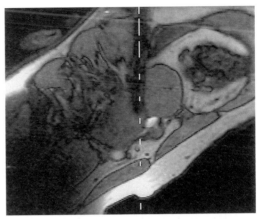

Fig. 9.**9** **Puncture of a disk space of the lumbar spine of a pig.** The puncture needle is visible as a black line due to the susceptibility artifact. The stereotactic "Flashpoint" system was used for puncturing. The dashed white line indicates the direction of the puncture needle as calculated by the computer, assuming it would follow a straight line.

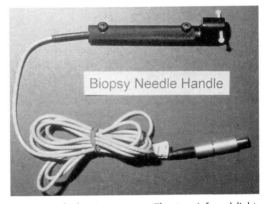

Fig. 9.**10** **Flashpoint system.** The two infrared light-emitting diodes (LED) are visible on the handle. The system is connected to the main magnet. The puncture needle is inserted into the handle and secured by two arresting screws. The handle is measured in space by three cameras in the main magnet so that its actual position is always known.

finest of instruments, such as catheters, guide wires or even biopsy needles (Fig. 9.**12**) (Wildermuth *et al.*, 1997).

The spatial coordinates of the receiver coils are calculated within a three-dimensional space with only four MR imaging experiments. It is therefore possible to depict the position of the coils simultaneously in various planes in a multiplanar fash-

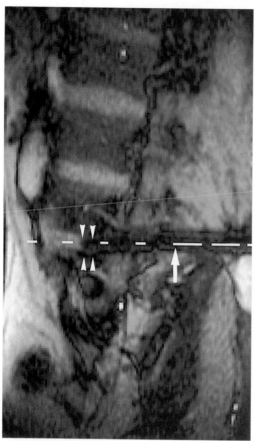

ion up to 20 times per minute on previously obtained road-map images (Leung *et al.*, 1995b). Up to four coils can be displayed simultaneously without delay. This allows the spatial relationship of various instruments to be monitored in real time. This active means of determining position also permits the recording of the next MR slices in various planes to be actively controlled.

The development of the so-called MR profiling method should be regarded as an extension of the active visualization of instruments in the MR environment (McKinnon *et al.*, 1996; Ladd *et al.*, 1997). Here, a wire up to 10 cm in length is incorporated into the instrument and used as an active receiver coil (Fig. 9.**13**).

With a temporal resolution of 1 image/sec, the whole tip of a flexible instrument, such as a guide wire or catheter, can be depicted in three dimensions.

◁ Fig. 9.**11 Parasagittal plane during puncture of a facet joint.** The position of the needle point (arrow) as calculated by the computer does not comply with the actual position of the needle point due to the susceptibility artifact (arrowheads). The computer system received false information concerning the length of the puncture needle.

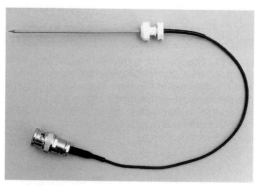

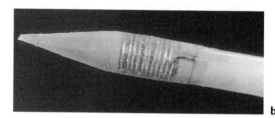

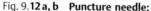

Fig. 9.**12 a, b Puncture needle:**
a MR-compatible puncture needle for linkage to the main magnet via a connecting cable.

b The small receiving coil is located on the tip of the mandrin (the "soul of the needle") and after puncturing is removed to take biopsy material.

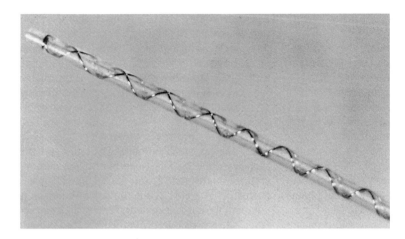

Fig. 9.**13 Flexible catheter.** The catheter tip is wrapped in wire for a length of 10 cm. In this way a larger part of the instrument is visualized on the MR image (so-called profiling).

MR-Guided Bone Biopsy

MR-guided bone biopsies have already been conducted as part of everyday clinical routine in several centers for some time now (Neuerburg *et al.*, 1996). Here MRI plays a complementary role to CT. The use of MRI is practically inevitable if the target lesion cannot be made visible by any other procedure. This may be the case with intramedullary lesions in particular. The use of MRI is also beneficial for lesions with difficult access routes, such as in the region of the spine or skull base (Fig. 9.**14**) (Kacl *et al.*, unpublished data).

Otherwise, the indication for an MR-guided puncture is not essentially different from that of a CT-guided biopsy (Laredo *et al.*, 1994; White *et al.*, 1995).

The requirements placed on the instruments differ according to the lesion to be punctured (osteolytic or osteosclerotic). Generally speaking, the needle design is the same as that for a biopsy under CT control. A non-ferromagnetic material such as titanium, tantalum or aluminum alloys, however, must replace the ferromagnetic material. A large number of MR-compatible needles of various sizes and designs are commercially available today for the recovery of cytological as well as histological tissue samples from osteolytic and soft-tissue lesions. When taking biopsies of osteosclerotic lesions, such as osteoid osteomas or osteoplastic metastases, or when the bone cortex is intact, the recovery of tissue is considerably more difficult. MR-compatible tracer systems have already been developed and some are already commercially available. Even a drill system

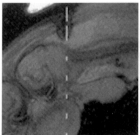
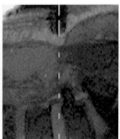
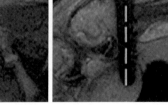
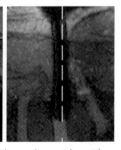

Fig. 9.**14 Puncture of a disk space with the Flashpoint system:**
Left image: Axial slice orientation. The needle tip is located in the paravertebral soft tissues. The further direction of the puncture as simulated by the computer is displayed as an interrupted white line.

Mid-left image: Parasagittal oblique plane with an identical location of the needle tip.
Mid-right image: Axial slice orientation. The needle tip is now in the intervertebral disk.
Right image: Confirmation of the needle position in the parasagittal oblique plane.

with an MR-compatible motor drive has already been assessed (Neuerburg *et al.*, 1996).

The technique of aspiration and the actual biopsy are in fact complementary procedures (Fig. 9.**15**) (Schweitzer *et al.*, 1996).

Fine-needle puncture is preferably recommended for small osteolytic lesions, whereas a biopsy is of more advantage in cases of larger osteolysis and osteosclerotic lesions. If need be, very hard lesions will require the use of a pneumatic drill.

Bone biopsies of the spine can generally be performed under local anesthesia on an outpatient basis. This also has the advantage that communication with the patient is possible during the intervention. The position of the needle can be corrected immediately should the nerve root be touched and corresponding radicular symptoms are elicited during the intervention.

The use of the "Flashpoint" system is a considerable simplification of the puncture technique. Multiplanar imaging allows optimization of the percutaneous puncture site with regard to safety and distance to the target lesion. This allows simulation of the entire intervention without the needle even being introduced into the subcutaneous tissue.

A generous amount of local anesthetic is always recommended for bone biopsy because penetration of the periosteum, in particular, can be very painful. After a small skin incision, the trocar system or the biopsy needle is advanced as far as the periosteum. Here, the use of the interactive optical control system allows immediate corrections to be made under real-time conditions. The computer-animated position of the needle can be compared at any time with the actual needle artifact. Depending on the lesion, the biopsy needle is introduced directly into the lesion, or the bone cortex has to be drilled or penetrated. Bone biopsy specimens are fixed in 10 % formalin, while cytological samples are spread out directly on to a slide for fixation to be done by the pathologist. Of course, bacteriological cultures are also taken where infection is suspected.

The, as yet, small number of MR-guided bone biopsies done so far (Neuerburg,1998) demonstrate similarly good results to CT-guided biopsies (Laredo *et al.*,1994). While the risk of infection is comparable, damage to neural and vascular structures is less probable, given the improved visualization under MR guidance. There is a general consensus that MR-guided biopsy can be regarded as at least an equivalent alternative to CT-guided puncture.

Minimally Invasive Spinal Surgery

Under fluoroscopic or CT control, many percutaneous forms of therapy are already in use today for the treatment of chronic back pain. These procedures are mainly performed under local anesthesia. MRI has already been used for some time in some centers as an alternative technique for guiding these interventions. Considerable advances have been made in this field, almost at a weekly rate.

The most prevalent MR-guided therapeutic interventions are described below:

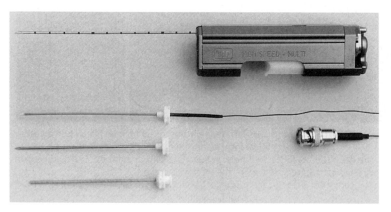

Fig. 9.**15** **MR-compatible holding device for cutting biopsies.** MR needle with active visualization via a receiver coil on its tip (MR tracking). The cable connects the radio-frequency coil with the MR system.

■ Percutaneous Pain Therapy

Low lumbar back pain often arises from degenerative changes of the facet joints, most commonly (in 80% of cases) at the segmental levels L4/L5 and L5/S1 (Bell and Ross, 1992). Percutaneous pain therapy involves the MR-guided application of a mixture of corticosteroid and local anesthetic into the facet joint. Alternatively, denervation can be achieved by applying ethanol and using the same technique (Seibel *et al.*, 1990). Monitoring the intervention and the distribution of the ethanol can be readily performed using CT as well as MRI (Fig. 9.**16**).

■ Periradicular Therapy

Periradicular therapy involves the repeated application of a mixture of corticosteroid and local anesthetic into the neuroforamen. Guidance of the puncture needle can again be done either by CT or MRI (Seibel *et al.*, 1990). The authors report good results with this method for failed back surgery syndrome and for cases of foraminal stenosis.

■ Percutaneous Laser Diskectomy

Percutaneous laser diskectomy (PLDD, percutaneous laser disk decompression) was initially undertaken by Ascher *et al.* (1989). The use of lasers in open surgery of disk hernias has meanwhile become quite widespread. Destruction of the nucleus pulposus relieves the affected nerve roots and so alleviates the symptoms. Monitoring laser application was hitherto only possible by using technically demanding endoscopic procedures, and even then, monitoring the extent of the depth of the thermoenergy was still not possible. Such monitoring is, however, possible with high temporal resolution, given the temperature sensitivity of the MR imaging equipment. The energy spread can be demonstrated after MR-guided percutaneous introduction of the laser probe. In this way, the energy can be directed towards the target lesion, while at the same time avoiding damage to contiguous neural structures. These are the reasons why our working group has already been engaged for some time in the possibilities of MR guidance of PLDD (Steiner *et al.*, 1996; Schoenenberger *et al.*, 1997).

The patient is placed in the prone position for the intervention. After prior application of a local anesthetic, an 18-gauge titanium needle is advanced with the aid of the stereotactic MR guid-

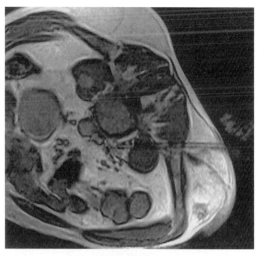

Fig. 9.**16** **Axial T1-weighted image.** The needle was introduced percutaneously under MR control and lies with its tip at a right-paravertebral location. This position is suitable for a MR-guided lumbar sympathectomy with ethanol (permission of Prof. R. Seibel, Institute for Diagnostics and Interventional Radiology, Witten/Herdecke University, Germany).

ing system into the intervertebral disk via a dorsolateral approach. Using this access method, the laser fiber is inserted into the disk and positioned under MR (real time) control (Steiner *et al.*, 1996). The disk is subsequently heated up with a Nd-YAG laser (Nd-YAG = neodymium yttrium aluminum garnet). Temperature monitoring is done with the aid of a modified T1-weighted sequence. This makes real-time control of the heat-spread possible (Fig. 9.**17**) (Schoenenberger *et al.*, 1997).

Experience to date with this therapeutic option is quite encouraging, despite the small number of patients treated. Follow-up examinations of the 15 patients treated so far have shown good results. MR-guided and -monitored PLDD is, however, still in its early stages. Further optimization of the laser fibers appears essential, as does improvement of the temperature-sensitive MR imaging. The compensation of motion artifacts in particular deserves more attention.

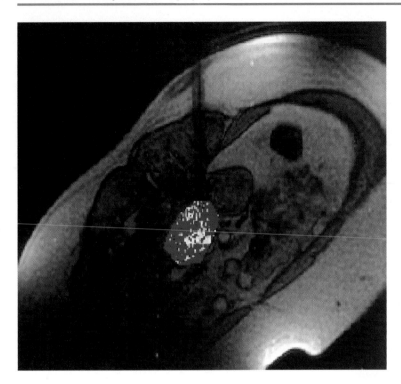

Fig. 9.**17** **Percutaneous laser diskectomy (PLDD, percutaneous laser disk decompression).** The paravertebral approach is easily visible from the susceptibility artifact. The temperature changes in the intervertebral disk are displayed color-coded.

Assessment

There are still some obstacles in the way of widespread use of MR imaging for functional diagnostics and guidance of minimally invasive therapeutic interventions of the spine. Even today, the availability of open MR systems is still limited. The generally poorer image quality as compared with closed high-field systems limits the diagnostic options of these systems.

Despite the need for critical evaluation, it is nevertheless important to point out that MR imaging in open systems is still at the very outset of its development. The potential advantages of MR imaging in the functional analysis of the spine and the guidance of minimally invasive forms of therapy will in the future doubtlessly lead to a rapidly progressive improvement of both hardware and software. With such optimization, it is indeed conceivable that all functional examinations and interventions of the spine will be conducted in open MR systems, in the not too distant future.

Summary

- The aim of *open configured systems* is improved access to the patient. The patient should also be allowed more freedom of movement during the examination. Open systems are particularly well suited for interventional surgery, including for example surgery of the spine.
- As with closed systems, the *signal-to-noise ratio* is proportional to the field strength, bearing in mind that this is a linear relation. The signal in a 1.5 tesla system is therefore three times higher than at 0.5 tesla.
- A distinction is made in *open systems* between those with a vertical and those with a horizontal patient access. In this respect, systems with a horizontal gap for patient access are far inferior to systems with a vertical opening.
- The *midfield system of the General Electric Company* is exemplary as far as patient access is concerned, having been designed as a dedicated interventional MR system. It is not possible to use volume coils because of the open construction of the MR system. Flexible transmitter and receiver coils of various sizes transmit and receive signals.
- To depict the spine, a homogeneous high-frequency field is generated using a *butterfly coil* with two opposing elements (attached anteriorly and posteriorly on to the patient). The image quality achieved in this way lies between that of high- and low-field systems. Spatial resolution is sufficient for a comprehensive diagnostic work-up of the spinal column.
- An examination using open MRI with a vertical access allows *presentation of a dynamic motion sequence* with the aid of tomographic data, in any slice orientation and with an inherently high soft-tissue contrast. In addition, the patient can be examined both in the seated and standing positions.
- When using MRI to examine the spine in the *seated position,* the patient should be secured as well as possible in a *rigid corset* or on a *special chair* to prevent any unwanted movements. Only those movements relevant for the functional analysis should be allowed.
- A *marked reduction in disk height* can occur *throughout the day* in the seated position, with changes of 2 mm in the segment L4/L5 being the most conspicuous. The proton density of the intervertebral disks, however, does not change during the day, except in connection with a change from the lying into the seated position when a reduction in proton density resulted when sitting.
- Using the open MR system with a *vertical access,* the examination of the spine can be undertaken according to the same principles as those of functional myelography. During a comparative study between *functional myelography* and *MR myelography* in an open system, a good correlation was detected for measurements of the sagittal diameter of the spinal canal. It was demonstrated that the diameter of the spinal canal varies only little during different types of movement in a symptomatic orthopedic patient population. Measurements taken from a healthy population, however, revealed considerable differences in the values, depending on the position of the spine. These differences are most likely due to the limited motion and immobile herniations without segmental instability shown by the patients as compared with the normal population.
- The qualitative *measurements of the size of the neuroforamina* on MR images during different functional states produced *results that were examiner-dependent.* Here too, there were considerable discrepancies between patients and volunteers with regard to the degree of dependency of the measurements on function. The volunteers demonstrated marked reductions in neuroforamen cross-section in the extension position. This was not detected in the patients. These changes were due to:
  - bulging of the intervertebral disk,
  - increase in volume of the ligamentum flavum,
  - reduction of the craniocaudal diameter of the bony neuroforamen.

  MR myelographic images offer particular advantages in comparison with conventional myelography in demonstrating the course of the nerve roots through the neuroforamina.
- MRI is particularly well suited for conducting *minimally invasive interventional operations* with the use of open systems. The advantages of MRI lie in the high soft-tissue contrast, muliplanar imaging capabilities and temperature sensitivity of the procedure. Controlling the operations requires visualization of the instruments. Here, a

Summary

distinction is made between *passive* and *active visualization*. Passive visualization primarily uses susceptibility artifacts, while with active visualization the positioning of the instruments is accomplished by signal reception using a mini receiver coil incorporated into the tip of the instrument. This method is referred to as *MR tracking*. An extension of active visualization is the development of the so-called *MR profiling method* in which a wire up to 10 cm in length is incorporated into the instrument and used as an active receiver coil.

■ Indications for an *MR-guided bone biopsy* are no different from those for a CT-guided biopsy. The procedure begs an alternative, however, when it comes to taking puncture samples of alterations that cannot be made visible by CT, such as bone marrow infiltrates. For this purpose, an instrument is required that contains non-ferromagnetic alloys such as titanium, tantalum or aluminum. A large number of sets are available for the puncture of osteolytic lesions, while puncturing osteosclerotic lesions requires materials such as a drill or trocar systems, which hitherto are not so readily obtainable. It is possible to perform MR-guided operations with less risk because vascular and neural structures can be demonstrated with more precision by producing images in three planes.

■ *Percutaneous interventions of the spine* are commonly undertaken for therapeutic purposes. CT has so far played an almost exclusive role as the guiding tool. In the future, open MR systems will be more significant for needle placement. Percutaneous laser diskectomy can also exploit the possibility of MRI-guided temperature sensitization, thus allowing the dose of laser energy to be delivered more exactly.

References

Ackermann, J. L., M. C. Offutt, R. B. Buxton et al.: Rapid 3D tracking of small RF coils., Proceedings of the 5th Annual Meeting of the Society of Magnetic Resonance in Medicine. Montreal 1986

Andersson, G. B. J., T. W. McNeill: Definition and classification of lumbar spinal stenosis. In Andersson, G. B. J., T. W. McNeill: Lumbar Spinal Stenosis. Mosby Year Book, St. Louis 1992 (pp. 9–15)

Ascher, P. W., D. S. J. Choy, H. Yuri: Percutaneous nucleus pulposis denaturation and vaporization of protruded discs. Amer. Soc. Laser Med. Surg. Abstr. Suppl 1 (1989) 202

Bell, G. R., J. S. Ross: Diagnosis of nerve root compression. Myelography, computed tomography and MRI. Orthop. Clin. N. Amer. 23 (1992) 405–419

Debatin, J. F., G. C. Mc Kinnon: Ultrafast MRI: techniques and applications. Springer, Berlin 1998

Dumoulin, C. L., R. D. Darrow, J. F. Schenck et al.: Tracking system to follow the position and orientation of a device with radiofrequency field gradients. US patent 5,211,165. US Patent and Trademark Office. Department of Commerce, Arlington 1993

Duwell, S., A. W. Schönenberger, S. C. Göhde, P. Steiner, J. F. Debatin, J. Hodler: MR Imaging of the loaded lumbar spine: quantitative assessment of the intervertebral disk with patient in a sitting position. RSNA, Chicago 1996

Frahm, C., H. B. Gehl, H. D. Weiss, W. A. Rossberg: Technik der MR-gesteuerten Stanzbiopsie im Abdomen an einem offenen Niederfeldgerät: Dürchführbarkeit und erste klinische Ergebnisse. Fortschr Röntgenstr 164 (1996) 62–67

Hasegawa, T., H. S. An, V. M. Haugthon, B. H. Nowicki: Critical heights of the intervertebral discs and foramina. J. Bone Jt Surg. 77-A (1995) 32–38

Jeanneret, B., T. Forster: Anamnesis and myelography in the preoperative assessment of the lumbar spinal stenosis. Results of a postoperativ follow-up study. Orthopäde 22 (1993) 217–231

Jolesz, F. A., R. Kikinis:. Intraoperative imaging revolutionizes therapy. Diagn. Imag. 9 (1995) 62–68

Köchli, V. D., G. C. McKinnon, E. Hofmann, G. K. von Schulthess: Vascular interventions guided by ultrafast MR-imaging: evaluation of different materials. Magn. Reson. Med. 31 (1994) 309–314

Kunze, K., A. Arlt: Klinik und Differentialdiagnose der zervikalen Myelopathie. Die Wirbelsäule in Forschung und Praxis. Hippokrates, Stuttgart 1991

Ladd, M. E.: Principles of passive visualization. In Debatin, J. F., G. Adams: Interventional Magnetic Resonance Imaging. Springer, Berlin 1998

Ladd, M. E., P. Erhart, J. F. Debatin et al.: Guidewire antennas for MR fluoroscopy. Magn. Reson. Med. 37 (1997) 891–897

Laredo, J. D., L. Bellaiche, B. Hamze, J. F. Naouri, J. M. Bondeville, J. M. Tubiana: Current status of musculoskeletal interventional radiology. Radiol. Clin. N. Amer. 32 (1994) 377–398

Lenz, G. W., C. Dewey: An open MRI system used for interventional procedures: current research and initial clinical results. In Lemke, H. U., K. Inamura, C. C. Jaffe, M. W. Vannier: Computer Assisted Radiology. Springer, Berlin 1995 (pp. 1180–1187)

Leung, D. A., J. F. Debatin, S. Wildermuth et al.: Intravascular MR tracking catheter: preliminary experimental evaluation. Amer. J. Roentgenol. 164 (1995) 1265–1270

Leung, D. A., J. F. Debatin, S. Wildermuth et al.: Real-time biplanar needle tracking for interventional MR imaging procedures. Radiology 197 (1995) 485–488

Lufkin, R. B.: Interventional MR Imaging. Radiology 197 (1995) 16–18

Mayoux-Benhamou, M. A., M. Revel, C. Aaron, G. Chomette, B. Amor: A morphometric study of the lumbar foramen. Influence of flexion-extension movements and of isolated disc collapse. Surg. radiol. Anat. 11 (1989) 97–102

McKinnon, G. C., J. F. Debatin, D. A. Leung, S. Wildermuth, D. J. Holtz, G. K. von Schulthess: Towards active guidewire visualization in interventional magnetic resonance imaging. MAGMA 4 (1996) 13–18.

Mirvis, S. E., J. H. Geisler, J. J. Jelinek, J. N. Joslyn, F. Gellad: Acute cervical spinal trauma: evaluation with 1,5 T imaging. Radiology 166 (1988) 807–816

Muhle, C., J. Wiskirchen, G. Brinkmann et al.: Kinematische MRT bei degenerativen Halswirbelsäulenveränderungen. Fortschr. Röntgenstr. 163 (1995) 148–154

Nägele, M., W. Koch, B. Kaden, B. Wöll, M. Reiser: Dynamische Funktions-MRT der Halswirbelsäule. Forschr. Röntgenstr. 157 (1992) 222–228

Neuerburg, J. J.: MR-guided biopsy of the bone. In Debatin, J. F., G. Adams: Interventional Magnetic Resonance Imaging. Springer, Berlin 1998

Neuerburg, J., G. Adam, T. Schmitz-Rode et al.: Neues MR-kompatibles Knochenbiopsiesystem. Fortschr. Röntgenstr. 165 (1996) 316

Peterman, S. B.: Postmyelography headache: a review. Radiology 200 (1996) 765–770

Roca, A., K. Bernreuter, G. S. Alarcon: Functional magnetic resonance imaging should be included in the evaluation of the cervical spine in patients with rheumatoid arthritis. J. Rheumatol. 20 (1993) 1485–1488

Rothhaupt, D., K. Liebig: Diagnostik, Analyse und Bewertung von Funktionsstörungen der oberen HWS im Rahmen von Beschleunigungsverletzungen unter Einsatz der Kernspintomographie. Orthopäde 23 (1994) 278–281

Schenk, J. F., F. A. Jolesz, P. B. Roemer: Superconducting open-configurated MR imaging system for image-guided therapy. Radiology 195 (1995) 804–814

Schönenberger, A. W., S. C. Göhde, P. Steiner, J. Hodler, J. F. Debatin, S. Duwell: Untersuchung der Lumbalwirbelsäule in sitzender Position am interventionellen MR-Gerät (0,5 T), SGMR 83. Jahresversammlung, Lausanne 1996

Schönenberger, A. W., P. Steiner, J. F. Debatin et al.: Real time monitoring of laser diskectomies with a superconducting, open configuration mr system. Amer. J. Roentgenol. 169 (1997) 863–867

Schmid, M. R., G. Stucki, J. F. Debatin, B. Romanowski, S. Duwell: Influence of inclined and reclined position to cross sectional area of the spinal canal: experience with functional imaging of the lumbar spine in the upright position on an open MR system, ISMRM, 5th Scientific Meeting and Exhibition (Vol. 428). Vancouver 1997

Schumacher, M.: Die Belastungsmyelographie. Fortschr. Röntgenstr. 245 (1986) 642–648

Schweitzer, M. E., F. H. Gannon, D. M. Deely, B. J. O'Hara, V. Juneja: Percutaneous skeletal aspiration and core biopsy: complementary techniques. Amer. J. Roentgenol. 166 (1996)

Seibel, R. M. M., D. H. W. Grönemeyer, T. H. Grumme: New treatments of the spinal column diseases using interventional radiological techiques. In Seibel, R. M. M., D. H. W. Grönemeyer: Interventional Computed Tomography. Blackwell, Oxford 1990 (pp. 95–97)

van Sonnenberg, E., P. Hajek, V. Gylys-Morin et al.: A wire sheath system fpr MR-guided biopsy and drainage: laboratory studies and experience in 10 patients. Amer. J. Roentgenol. 151 (1988) 815–817

Steiner, P., A. W. Schönenberger, E. A. Penner et al.: Interaktive, stereotaktische interventionen im supraleitenden, offenen 0,5 T MR-Tomographen. Fortschr. Röntgenstr. 165 (1996) 276–280

White, L. M., M. E. Schweitzer, D. M. Deely, F. Gannon: Study of osteomyelitis: utility of combined histologic and microbiologic evaluation of percutaneous biopsy samples. Radiology 197 (1995) 840–842

Wildermuth, S., J. F. Debatin, D. A. Leung et al.: MR Imaging-guided intravascular procedures: initial demonstration in a pig model. Radiology 202 (1997) 578–583

Wildermuth, S., M. Zanetti, S. Duwell et al.: Functional (upright flexion and extension) MR imaging and myelography of the lumbar spine: Quantitative and qualitative assessment in 30 patients, RSNA, 83rd annual meeting, Chicago 1997

Index